# Human Health Engineering

# Human Health Engineering

Special Issue Editor
**Jean-Marie Aerts**

MDPI • Basel • Beijing • Wuhan • Barcelona • Belgrade • Manchester • Tokyo • Cluj • Tianjin

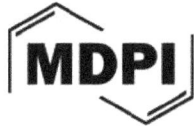

*Special Issue Editor*
Jean-Marie Aerts
Katholieke Universiteit Leuven
Belgium

*Editorial Office*
MDPI
St. Alban-Anlage 66
4052 Basel, Switzerland

This is a reprint of articles from the Special Issue published online in the open access journal *Applied Sciences* (ISSN 2076-3417) (available at: https://www.mdpi.com/journal/applsci/special_issues/Human_Health_Engineering).

For citation purposes, cite each article independently as indicated on the article page online and as indicated below:

LastName, A.A.; LastName, B.B.; LastName, C.C. Article Title. *Journal Name* **Year**, *Article Number*, Page Range.

**ISBN 978-3-03928-408-5 (Pbk)**
**ISBN 978-3-03928-409-2 (PDF)**

© 2020 by the authors. Articles in this book are Open Access and distributed under the Creative Commons Attribution (CC BY) license, which allows users to download, copy and build upon published articles, as long as the author and publisher are properly credited, which ensures maximum dissemination and a wider impact of our publications.

The book as a whole is distributed by MDPI under the terms and conditions of the Creative Commons license CC BY-NC-ND.

# Contents

**About the Special Issue Editor** . . . . . . . . . . . . . . . . . . . . . . . . . . . . . . . . . . . . . . . . . . . . . . . . . . ix

**Jean-Marie Aerts**
Special Issue on "Human Health Engineering"
Reprinted from: *Applied Sciences* **2020**, *10*, 564, doi:10.3390/app10020564 . . . . . . . . . . . . . . . 1

**Muhammad E. H. Chowdhury, Amith Khandakar, Belayat Hossain and Khawla Alzoubi**
Effects of the Phantom Shape on the Gradient Artefact of Electroencephalography (EEG) Data in Simultaneous EEG–fMRI
Reprinted from: *Applied Sciences* **2018**, *8*, 1969, doi:10.3390/app8101969 . . . . . . . . . . . . . . . . 9

**Yu-Min Fang, Lin Chun and Bo-Cheng Chu**
Older Adults' Usability and Emotional Reactions toward Text, Diagram, Image, and Animation Interfaces for Displaying Health Information
Reprinted from: *Applied Sciences* **2019**, *9*, 1058, doi:10.3390/app9061058 . . . . . . . . . . . . . . . . 23

**Rolandas Gircys, Agnius Liutkevicius, Egidijus Kazanavicius, Vita Lesauskaite, Gyte Damuleviciene and Audrone Janaviciute**
Photoplethysmography-Based Continuous Systolic Blood Pressure Estimation Method for Low Processing Power Wearable Devices
Reprinted from: *Applied Sciences* **2019**, *9*, 2236, doi:10.3390/app9112236 . . . . . . . . . . . . . . . . 43

**Shriram Mukunthan, Jochen Vleugels, Toon Huysmans, Kalev Kuklane, Tiago Sotto Mayor and Guido De Bruyne**
Thermal-Performance Evaluation of Bicycle Helmets for Convective and Evaporative Heat Loss at Low and Moderate Cycling Speeds
Reprinted from: *Applied Sciences* **2019**, *9*, 3672, doi:10.3390/app9183672 . . . . . . . . . . . . . . . . 59

**Arthur van der Have, Sam Van Rossom and Ilse Jonkers**
Squat Lifting Imposes Higher Peak Joint and Muscle Loading Compared to Stoop Lifting
Reprinted from: *Applied Sciences* **2019**, *9*, 3794, doi:10.3390/app9183794 . . . . . . . . . . . . . . . . 77

**Dwi Basuki Wibowo, Achmad Widodo, Gunawan Dwi Haryadi, Wahyu Caesarendra and Rudiansyah Harahap**
Effect of In-Shoe Foot Orthosis Contours on Heel Pain Due to Calcaneal Spurs
Reprinted from: *Applied Sciences* **2019**, *9*, 495, doi:10.3390/app9030495 . . . . . . . . . . . . . . . . . 97

**Saranda Bekteshi, Marco Konings, Ioana Gabriela Nica, Sotirios Gakopoulos, Inti Vanmechelen, Jean-Marie Aerts, Hans Hallez and Elegast Monbaliu**
Development of the Dyskinesia Impairment Mobility Scale to Measure Presence and Severity of Dystonia and Choreoathetosis during Powered Mobility in Dyskinetic Cerebral Palsy
Reprinted from: *Applied Sciences* **2019**, *9*, 3481, doi:10.3390/app9173481 . . . . . . . . . . . . . . . . 109

**Jimmy Aurelio Rosales-Huamani, Rita Rocio Guzman-Lopez, Eder Eliseo Aroni-Vilca, Carmen Rosalia Matos-Avalos and Jose Luis Castillo-Sequera**
Determining Symptomatic Factors of Nomophobia in Peruvian Students from the National University of Engineering
Reprinted from: *Applied Sciences* **2019**, *9*, 1814, doi:10.3390/app9091814 . . . . . . . . . . . . . . . . 123

**Nilakash Das, Kenneth Verstraete, Marko Topalovic, Jean-Marie Aerts and Wim Janssens**
Estimating Airway Resistance from Forced Expiration in Spirometry
Reprinted from: *Applied Sciences* **2019**, *9*, 2842, doi:10.3390/app9142842 . . . . . . . . . . . . . . . . 139

**Yanming Fu, Xin Wang and Tianbiao Yu**
Simulation Analysis of Knee Ligaments in the Landing Phase of Freestyle Skiing Aerial
Reprinted from: *Applied Sciences* **2019**, *9*, 3713, doi:10.3390/app9183713 . . . . . . . . . . . . . . . 153

**Gian Carlo Cardarilli, Luca Di Nunzio, Rocco Fazzolari, Francesca Silvestri and Marco Re**
Improvement of the Cardiac Oscillator Based Model for the Simulation of Bundle Branch Blocks
Reprinted from: *Applied Sciences* **2019**, *9*, 3653, doi:10.3390/app9183653 . . . . . . . . . . . . . . . 165

**Hervé Mukenya Mwamba, Pieter Rousseau Fourie and Dawie van den Heever**
PANDAS: Paediatric Attention-Deficit/Hyperactivity Disorder Application Software
Reprinted from: *Applied Sciences* **2019**, *9*, 1645, doi:10.3390/app9081645 . . . . . . . . . . . . . . . 179

**Joren Buekers, Jan Theunis, Alberto Peña Fernández, Emiel F. M. Wouters, Martijn A. Spruit, Patrick De Boever and Jean-Marie Aerts**
Box-Jenkins Transfer Function Modelling for Reliable Determination of VO$_2$ Kinetics in Patients with COPD
Reprinted from: *Applied Sciences* **2019**, *9*, 1822, doi:10.3390/app9091822 . . . . . . . . . . . . . . . 193

**Ali Youssef, Anne Verachtert, Guido De Bruyne and Jean-Marie Aerts**
Reverse Engineering of Thermoregulatory Cold-Induced Vasoconstriction/Vasodilation during Localized Cooling
Reprinted from: *Applied Sciences* **2019**, *9*, 3372, doi:10.3390/app9163372 . . . . . . . . . . . . . . . 207

**Hema Sekhar Reddy Rajula, Veronika Odintsova, Mirko Manchia and Vassilios Fanos**
Overview of Federated Facility to Harmonize, Analyze and Management of Missing Data in Cohorts
Reprinted from: *Applied Sciences* **2019**, *9*, 4103, doi:10.3390/app9194103 . . . . . . . . . . . . . . . 227

**Ali Youssef, Jeroen Colon, Konstantinos Mantzios, Paraskevi Gkiata, Tiago S. Mayor, Andreas D. Flouris, Guido De Bruyne and Jean-Marie Aerts**
Towards Model-Based Online Monitoring of Cyclist's Head Thermal Comfort: Smart Helmet Concept and Prototype
Reprinted from: *Applied Sciences* **2019**, *9*, 3170, doi:10.3390/app9153170 . . . . . . . . . . . . . . . 239

**Ali Youssef, Ahmed Youssef Ali Amer, Nicolás Caballero and Jean-Marie Aerts**
Towards Online Personalized-Monitoring of Human Thermal Sensation Using Machine Learning Approach
Reprinted from: *Applied Sciences* **2019**, *9*, 3303, doi:10.3390/app9163303 . . . . . . . . . . . . . . . 259

**Jasper Gielen and Jean-Marie Aerts**
Feature Extraction and Evaluation for Driver Drowsiness Detection Based on Thermoregulation
Reprinted from: *Applied Sciences* **2019**, *9*, 3555, doi:10.3390/app9173555 . . . . . . . . . . . . . . . 279

**Ahmed Y. A. Amer, Julie Vranken, Femke Wouters, Dieter Mesotten, Pieter Vandervoort, Valerie Storms, Stijn Luca, Bart Vanrumste and Jean-Marie Aerts**
Feature Engineering for ICU Mortality Prediction Based on Hourly to Bi-Hourly Measurements
Reprinted from: *Applied Sciences* **2019**, *9*, 3525, doi:10.3390/app9173525 . . . . . . . . . . . . . . . 293

**Alberto Peña Fernández, Ali Youssef, Charlotte Heeren, Christophe Matthys and Jean-Marie Aerts**
Real-Time Model Predictive Control of Human Bodyweight Based on Energy Intake
Reprinted from: *,,,* doi: . . . . . . . . . . . . . . . 311

**Xin Zhang, Jiehao Li, Zhenhuan Hu, Wen Qi, Longbin Zhang, Yingbai Hu, Hang Su, Giancarlo Ferrigno, Elena De Momi**
Novel Design and Lateral Stability Tracking Control of a Four-Wheeled Rollator
Reprinted from: , , , doi: . . . . . . . . . . . . . . . . . . . . . . . . . . . . . . . . . . . 335

**Shanhai Jin, Xiaogang Xiong, Dejin Zhao, Changfu Jin and Motoji Yamamoto**
Long-Term Effects of a Soft Robotic Suit on Gait Characteristics in Healthy Elderly Persons
Reprinted from: *Applied Sciences* **2019**, *9*, 1957, doi:10.3390/app9091957 . . . . . . . . . . . . . . . 355

**Dimas Adiputra, Mohd Azizi Abdul Rahman, Ubaidillah, Saiful Amri Mazlan, Nurhazimah Nazmi, Muhammad Kashfi Shabdin, Jun Kobayashi and Mohd Hatta Mohammed Ariff**
Control Reference Parameter for Stance Assistance Using a Passive Controlled Ankle Foot Orthosis—A Preliminary Study
Reprinted from: *Applied Sciences* **2019**, *9*, 4416, doi:10.3390/app9204416 . . . . . . . . . . . . . . . 369

**Iñigo Aramendia, Ekaitz Zulueta, Daniel Teso-Fz-Betoño, Aitor Saenz-Aguirre and Unai Fernandez-Gamiz**
Modeling of Motorized Orthosis Control
Reprinted from: *Applied Sciences* **2019**, *9*, 2453, doi:10.3390/app9122453 . . . . . . . . . . . . . . . 383

**Quy-Thinh Dao, Manh-Linh Nguyen and Shin-ichiroh Yamamoto**
Discrete-Time Fractional Order Integral Sliding Mode Control of an Antagonistic Actuator Driven by Pneumatic Artificial Muscles
Reprinted from: *Applied Sciences* **2019**, *9*, 2503, doi:10.3390/app9122503 . . . . . . . . . . . . . . . 399

# About the Special Issue Editor

**Jean-Marie Aerts** holds a M.S. and a Ph.D. in bio-engineering from KU Leuven (former Catholic University of Leuven) in Belgium. Currently, he is heading the Measure, Model & Manage Bioresponses (M3-BIORES) Group of the Division Animal and Human Health Engineering (A2H) at the Department of Biosystems (BIOSYST) of the KU Leuven. He is a full professor and chair of Leuven Health Technology Centre (L-HTC). His research focuses on data-based mechanistic modelling of biological systems as a basis for developing human health engineering technology. Jean-Marie Aerts is an IEEE member and has been a visiting researcher at the Engineering Department of Lancaster University and at the Institute of Biomedical Engineering of the University of Oxford.

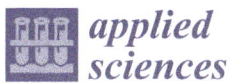 

*Editorial*

# Special Issue on "Human Health Engineering"

### Jean-Marie Aerts

KU Leuven, Department of Biosystems, Division Animal and Human Health Engineering, Measure, Model & Manage Bioresponses Group, Kasteelpark Arenberg 30, 3000 Leuven, Belgium; jean-marie.aerts@kuleuven.be

Received: 6 January 2020; Accepted: 7 January 2020; Published: 13 January 2020

## 1. Referees for the Special Issue

A total of 52 manuscripts were received for our Special Issue (SI), of which eight manuscripts were directly rejected without peer review. The remaining 44 articles were all strictly reviewed by no less than two reviewers in related fields. Finally, 25 of the manuscripts were recommended for acceptance and published in Applied Sciences-Basel. Referees from 10 different countries provided valuable suggestions for the manuscripts in our SI, the top five being the USA, Italy, Japan, Australia, and Spain. The names of these distinguished reviewers are listed in Table A1. We would like to thank all of these reviewers for their time and effort in reviewing the papers in our SI.

## 2. Main Content of the Special Issue

In the 1930s Walter Cannon introduced the term 'homeostasis', reflecting the idea that complex organisms, such as humans, are able to maintain their internal environment quasi-constantly in the face of (external) perturbations [1]. Although homeostasis was originally not discussed in terms of regulatory mechanisms, this changed in the 1950s and 1960s with the work of pioneers such as Norbert Wiener and Ludwig von Bertalanffy who envisioned complex organisms as complex systems that can be studied from an engineering system and/or control perspective [2–4]. This has been the start of the fast growing field of health engineering that uses concepts from control theory and fault-detection and diagnosis to study, monitor, and/or control health processes [2,5,6].

According to modern model-based monitoring and control theory there at least two conditions necessary to study and develop monitoring and control systems, namely continuous information of the relevant process variables (inputs and outputs) and a (mathematical) model describing the relationships between the process inputs and outputs [6,7]. The first condition stresses the need for sensors and sensing systems that allow capturing the necessary information on the considered biosystem, and the latter assumes access to advanced mathematical modelling approaches.

The field of sensor development and sensing systems for biological signals has evolved tremendously the last couple of decades and has resulted in advanced sensing elements that can, among others, harvest their own energy from the human body [8], measure real-time physiological information in biofluids, such as sweat, tears, saliva, and interstitial fluid [9,10], or continuously measure physiological variables (e.g., activity, heart rate, respiratory rate, and body temperature) using wearable technology [11]. In addition to this, the Internet of Things has also made it possible to interconnect many of these sensing systems with the internet, allowing the capture and exchange of information between connected devices, data storage systems, and relevant stakeholders [12].

The field of signal analysis and modelling has also evolved during recent decades. Although the more classic approaches of mechanistic modelling and data-based (or empirical) modelling are still very relevant and offer yet unexploited added value for health engineering (e.g., [13–15]), it can be expected that recent trends in artificial intelligence (e.g., big data approaches and deep learning algorithms [16,17]) will change the health engineering landscape (and life in general) in a radical way.

The fusion of sensing systems with powerful (real-time) modelling algorithms creates opportunities to, among others, monitor chronic patients at home [18], connect patients within a smart city environment with relevant caregivers [19], or even actively control physiological variables using smart actuators, such as wheelchairs [20] or electric bikes [21], to enhance physical condition of thermal comfort [22]. Last, but not least, also human-robot, interactions can be considered as means for actively controlling human health conditions, e.g., by supporting human gait using exoskeletons or exosuits [23].

In this special issue on "Human Health Engineering", we invited submissions exploring recent contributions to the field of human health engineering, i.e., technology for monitoring the physical or mental health status of individuals in a variety of applications. Contributions can focus on sensors, wearable hardware, algorithms, or integrated monitoring systems. We organized the different papers according to their contributions to the main parts of the monitoring and control engineering scheme applied to human health applications, namely papers focusing on measuring/sensing of physiological variables [24–31], contributions describing research on the modelling of biological signals [32–38], papers highlighting health monitoring applications [39–42], and finally examples of control applications for human health [43–48]. In comparison to biomedical engineering, we envision that the field of human health engineering also covers applications on healthy humans (e.g., sports, sleep, and stress) and thus not only contributes to develop technology for curing patients or supporting chronically ill people, but also for disease prevention and optimizing human well-being more generally.

The first series of articles in this SI describes methods for (improved) measuring, sensing, or communication of physiological signals. The work of Chowdhury et al. [24] contributes to solving the problem of gradient artefacts (GA) in electroencephalography (EEG) signals when measured in combination with functional magnetic resonance imaging (fMRI) in MR scanners. They demonstrated that the use of realistically human head-shaped phantoms outperformed the standard used spherical phantoms for the characterization of GA in EEG data and thus improves the GA removal in the signal post-processing step. Fang et al. [25] investigated the usability of four different types of interfaces (text, diagram, image, and animation) for wearable devices with health management applications (app) for elderly people. Their research demonstrated that most (older as well as younger) users preferred animation interfaces for communicating health information, but that older adults, in contrast to younger users, were also open to text interfaces. Such research can contribute significantly to the development of useful health management apps for the growing elderly population.

Gircys et al. [26] developed a method for continuously measuring systolic blood pressure (SBP) using photoplethysmography (PPG) sensing elements. Since their method is based on cheap PPG sensing elements that can be integrated in wearables, this approach can significantly contribute to (preventive) health monitoring as, compared to classical (expensive) cuff-based methods, as it allows 24/7 measurements. The work of Mukunthan et al. [27] describes the use of a nine-zone thermal manikin head for measuring convective and evaporative heat losses from a human head wearing a bicycle helmet. They demonstrated that the design of the helmet, mainly characterized by the number and position of vent openings and the presence of internal air channels, has a significant effect on the heat losses of a human head when covered by a bicycle helmet. The results of this work demonstrate the use of thermal manikins for improving comfort and safety of cycling activities.

In their work, van der Have et al. [28] studied the effect of squat lifting versus stoop lifting in terms of joint and muscle loading when handling heavy materials. Their study demonstrates that squat lifting imposes higher peak full body musculoskeletal loading compared to stoop lifting, but similar lower back loading, which is an important factor in work-related musculoskeletal disorders (WMSDs). These results show the usefulness of 3D movement trajectory and force analysis in combination with electromyography for optimizing ergonomic guidelines. Wibowo et al. [29] studied the effects of in-shoe foot orthosis contours on heel pain due to calcaneal spurs. The applied method made use of force sensors for measuring 2D pressure information on the foot in combination with an algometer for quantifying pain. By combining these measurements the authors were able to optimize insole geometry resulting in improved comfort by significantly reducing pain.

In their work, Bekteshi et al. [30] developed a dyskinesia impairment mobility scale (DIMS) for measuring the presence and severity of dystonia and choreoathetosis during powered mobility (electric wheelchair) in dyskinetic cerebral palsy. Such a scale could be a promising tool in clinical practice for assisting in accelerating the learning process of using a powered mobility wheelchair and for tailoring individualized mobility training programs. Rosales-Huamani et al. [31] studied the possible adverse effects of indiscriminate mobile phone use in Peruvian students, more specifically focusing on mental complaints when having no access to a mobile phone, also known as 'nomophobia' (no mobile phone phobia). Using a self-designed questionnaire, they identified three symptomatic factors of nomophobia. Their work was additionally relevant for this SI in demonstrating also the possible adverse health effects of wearable technology on users in daily life.

The second series of articles focuses on research related to modelling of biological signals in the framework of human health. Das et al. [32] used a mechanistic model to describe forced expiration in patients suffering from chronic obstructive pulmonary disease (COPD). In their work, they demonstrated that data of forced expiration maneuvers in combination with a physical knowledge-based model allowed to estimate airway resistance in the lungs. Such a model-based approach has especially clinical relevance for screening patients for COPD using classical spirometry in primary care. In their work, Fu et al. [33] developed a mechanistic finite element model to simulate forces and stresses inside knee joints during the landing phase in freestyle skiing aerial. These simulations helped quantifying which types of landings are most challenging in terms of ligament damage. Such results have high relevance for training design and nicely demonstrate how models can help preventing injuries in sports.

In their study, Cardarilli et al. [34] improved an existing mechanistic cardiac model based on four modified Van der Pol oscillators, each representing one of the main natural pacemakers. Their model allowed to reproduce healthy dynamic heart dynamics, as well as pathological rhythms in case of right bundle branch block (RBBB) and left bundle branch block (LBBB). The clinical relevance of such a model is that it allows simulation and evaluation of heart activity and dynamics under different types of pacemaker couplings. The study of Mwamba et al. [35] contributed to the diagnosis and management of attention-deficit/hyperactivity disorder (ADHD) by developing a tablet-based application (app) software using support vector machine (SVM) approaches from machine learning. Their approach demonstrated that (serious) games in combination with modelling approaches from the field of artificial intelligence can offer a useful tool for first line screening of children for ADHD by their parents and/or teachers.

Buekers et al. [36] applied a dynamic Box-Jenkins transfer function modelling approach for quantifying the $VO_2$ kinetics in patients with COPD performing a constant working rate test (CWRT). The added value of this work is that it contributes in optimizing clinical tests for objectively quantifying the physical capacity of patients. As such, measuring and modelling the kinetics of metabolic variables in COPD patients can contribute in managing their disease and in preventing hospital admissions due to exacerbations. Youssef et al. [37] applied a combination of a data-based transfer function modelling approach with a mechanistic model to develop a so called data-based mechanistic (or grey box) model to describe the thermoregulatory mechanisms of vasoconstriction and vasodilation to control body temperature during localized cooling. In their research, they demonstrated that dynamic data-based models are not only useful for monitoring or controlling complex biological systems, but can also be used to generate new insights (i.e., reverse engineering) in the working of biological control systems.

In their review article, Rajula et al. [38] describe methodological aspects related to the construction of a federated facility to optimize the analyses of multiple datasets, the impact of missing data and methods for handling missing data in cohort studies. The described database management systems permits the increase of the statistical power of medical multi-center studies, allowing for more advanced statistical analyses and answering research questions that might not be addressed by a single study.

The third series of articles describes applications of human health monitoring. Youssef et al. [39] showed in their work the possibilities and added value of integrating wearable sensors (heart rate, air temperature, and air humidity) in bicyclists' helmets. They developed a prototype of a smart helmet for monitoring thermal comfort based on adaptive personalized models. Such technology could be used in a next step to actively control thermal comfort of cyclists' head. Another thermal comfort application was studied in the work of Youssef et al. [40]. Here, the authors focused on developing a system for online personalized monitoring of thermal sensation. They used measurements of heart rate, metabolic rate, skin temperature, heat flux between skin and ambient air, and aural temperature in combination with least-squares support vector machine algorithms to estimate an individual's thermal sensation. The combination of these algorithms with wearable sensors allow, in a next step, to develop personalized indoor climate control systems by integrating online information from the occupants.

Gielen and Aerts [41] used physiological variables linked to thermoregulation to develop a drowsiness monitor for drivers. Since the process of falling asleep is accompanied by a shift/decrease in body temperature, online estimations of heat loss and heat production of drivers' can be used to monitor drowsiness. In their work, they measured heart rate, as indirect estimate of heat production, and nose tip and wrist temperature, as an indirect estimate of heat loss, to monitor changes in driver's thermoregulation. This proof-of-principle shows that wearable technology in combination with algorithms from machine learning can contribute to traffic safety.

In a another health monitoring study, Youssef et al. [42] demonstrated that a set of five vital signs (heart rate, respiration rate, oxygen saturation, arterial blood pressure, and body temperature) measured bi-hourly on patients in an intensive care unit (ICU) could be used to predict mortality. They combined a linear hard margin support vector machine (SVM) with a feature engineering approach to classify survivors and non-survivors during their stay at the ICU, demonstrating the added value of combining vital signs monitoring with machine learning for monitoring critically ill patients.

Finally, the fourth series of articles in this SI discusses examples of control applications for human health management. The study of Peña Fernández et al. [43] describes a model predictive controller (MPC) approach for managing human bodyweight using energy intake as the control input. Based on the data of the Minnesota starvation experiment, they show that the combination of weekly bodyweight and energy intake measurements with model predictive control theory allows to calculate future energy intake for following a predefined bodyweight trajectory. This nicely demonstrates how control theory could have a significant contribution in solving one of the major health challenges of today, namely obesity. However, the same technology could also be used to help elderly people suffering from underweight conditions.

Another application of MPC is described by Zhang et al. [44]. In their work, they demonstrate that MPC can also be successfully used to design smart four-wheeled rollators for elderly and/or disabled people. Their work focused on developing a lateral stability control for four-wheeled rollators allowing users to move in more smooth trajectories. Such smart rollators can improve the mobility of elderly and disabled people significantly and contribute to their overall physical and mental health. Also Jin et al. [45] describe the development of walking assistive devices for elderly people. However, in their case the assistive device is a soft robotic suit. They demonstrate that such robotic suits have positive long-term effects by helping improving gait characteristics of elderly people when using these suits. Furthermore, such robot-assisted tools could also help elderly people during gait rehabilitation when recovering from bone and/or joint surgery.

Adiputra et al. [46] described the results of a preliminary study focusing on a passive controlled ankle foot orthosis. The device they developed, aimed at assisting walking during the gait stance phase of people suffering from abnormal gaits, such as weak ankle, spasticity or foot drop, conditions that typically result after stroke. Whereas the previous three studies focused on control applications for assisting/improving walking behaviour, the work of Aramendia et al. [47] studied a robotic arm orthosis to assist arm movements. The authors developed a numerical model of a muscle, arm, and orthosis and used this model for simulating different scenarios. They demonstrated that by optimizing the controller algorithm, the needed force of the biceps muscle to overcome a load added to the orthosis control system could be reduced to nearly half of the force needed without optimized orthosis control algorithm.

Finally, Dao et al. [48] investigated pneumatic artificial muscles (PAM) as a basis for antagonistic actuators in assistive rehabilitation robots. They developed a discrete-time second order model describing the dynamic characteristics of PAMs and a fractional order integral sliding mode controller to improve the trajectory tracking performance. They demonstrated that the system could be used a basis for a robotic gait training system, contributing in this way to enhancing human health and quality of life for people suffering from gait disabilities.

## 3. Conclusions

This SI clusters recent contributions in the field of human health engineering. The contributions demonstrate that research is focusing on different aspects of the monitoring and control engineering scheme (sensors, sensing systems, data analysis, modelling approaches, and control algorithms) as applied to human health. Health monitoring and control applications on both healthy as well as (chronically) ill people are covered and this is in relation to physical as well as mental processes.

Thanks to the (r)evolution in sensors and (wearable) sensing technology in combination with the ever growing possibilities in artificial intelligence, it can be expected that human health engineering applications will become more and more ubiquitous in our society and will increasingly assist people of all ages in living healthy, high quality, and productive lives.

**Funding:** This research was funded by the European Union's Horizon 2020 research and innovation programme under the Marie Skłodowska-Curie grant number 645770.

**Acknowledgments:** Furthermore, we would like to sincerely thank our Section Managing Editor, Marin Ma (marin.ma@mdpi.com), for all the efforts she has made for this special issue in the past year.

**Conflicts of Interest:** The author declares no conflict of interest.

## Appendix A

Table A1. Special Issue (SI) reviewer list.

| | | | |
|---|---|---|---|
| Dean Picone | Shiang-Feng Tang | Mariana Domnica Stanciu | Modar Hassan |
| Warwick Butt | Angelos Karatsidis | Arcady Putilov | Mikito Ogino |
| Kurt Ammer | E. Mark Williams | Xinqin Liao | Ghulam Hussain |
| Johannes C. Ayena | Seungyeon Lee | U Rajendra Acharya | Joo-Young Lee |
| Raphael Vallat | Munish Chauhan | Roger Ho CM | Paweł Mazurek |
| Claudia Flexeder | Xiaoliang Zhu | Miguel Damas Hermoso | Cátia Tavares |
| Chrysovalantou Ziogou | Helen J. Huang | David Bienvenido-Huertas | Venkatraman Balasubramanian |
| Christina Zong-Hao Ma | Changhong Wang | Ana Belen Ortega Avila | Shahab Tayeb |
| Walter Franco | Huanyu (Larry) Cheng | Wen-Yu Su | Balaraman Rajan |
| Caterina Ledda | Derya Akleman | Cheng-Hung Chuang | Elisa Passini |
| Andrea Viggiano | Aiping Liu | Takao Sato | Ehsan Rashedi |
| Vincenzo Minutolo | Ibrahim Faruqi | Quy-Thinh Dao | Maryam Panahiazar |
| Baojun Chen | Mojtaba Yazdani | Roland K. Chen | In Cheol Jeong |

## References

1. Cannon, W.B. *The Wisdom of the Body*; Norton & Company Inc.: New York, NY, USA, 1932.
2. Modell, H.; Cliff, W.; Michael, J.; Mcfarland, J.; Wenderoth, M.P.; Wright, A. A physiologist's view of homeostasis. *Adv. Physiol. Educ.* **2015**, *39*, 259–266. [CrossRef] [PubMed]
3. Wiener, N. *Cybernetics or Control and Communication in the Animal and the Machine*; MIT Press: Cambridge, MA, USA, 1948.
4. Von Bertalanffy, L. *General System Theory—Foundations, Development, Applications*; George Braziller Inc.: New York, NY, USA, 1968.

5. Fossion, R.; Rivera, A.L.; Estañol, B. A physicist's view of homeostasis: How time series of continuous monitoring reflect the function of physiological variables in regulatory systems. *Physiol. Meas.* **2018**, *39*, 084007. [CrossRef] [PubMed]
6. Isermann, R. Model-based fault-detection and diagnosis—Status and applications. *Annu. Rev. Control* **2005**, *29*, 71–85. [CrossRef]
7. Camacho, E.F.; Bordons, E. *Model-Predictive Control*; Springer-Verlag: Berlin, Germany, 1999.
8. Madhusoodanan, J. Self-powered biomedical devices tap into the body's movements. *Proc. Natl. Acad. Sci. USA* **2019**, *116*, 17605–17607. [CrossRef] [PubMed]
9. Kim, J.; Campbell, A.S.; Esteban-Fernández de Ávila, B.; Wang, J. Wearable biosensors for healthcare monitoring. *Nat. Biotechnol.* **2019**, *37*, 389–406. [CrossRef]
10. Heikenfeld, J.; Jajack, A.; Feldman, B.; Granger, S.; Gaitonde, S.; Bergtrup, G.; Katchman, A. Assessing analytes in biofluids for peripheral biochemical monitoring. *Nat. Biotechnol.* **2019**, *37*, 407–419. [CrossRef]
11. Peake, J.M.; Kerr, G.; Sullivan, J.P. A critical review of consumer wearables, mobile applications, and equipment for providing biofeedback, monitoring stress, and sleep in physically active populations. *Front. Physiol.* **2018**, *9*, 743. [CrossRef]
12. Ornes, S. The internet of things and the explosion of interconnectivity. *Proc. Natl. Acad. Sci. USA* **2016**, *113*, 11059–11060. [CrossRef]
13. El-Samahy, E.; Mahfouf, M.; Linkens, D.A. A closed-loop hybrid physiological model relating to subjects under physical stress. *Artif. Intell. Med.* **2006**, *38*, 257–274. [CrossRef]
14. Tambuyzer, T.; Ahmed, T.; Taylor, C.J.; Berckmans, D.; Balschun, D.; Aerts, J.-M. System identification of mGluR-dependent long-term depression. *Neural Comput.* **2013**, *25*, 650–670. [CrossRef]
15. Aerts, J.-M.; Haddad, W.H.; An, G.; Vodovotz, Y. From data patterns to mechanistic models in acute illness. *J. Crit. Care* **2014**, *29*, 604–610. [CrossRef] [PubMed]
16. Prosperi, M.; Min, J.S.; Bian, J.; Modave, F. Big data hurdles in precision medicine and precision public health. *BMC Med. Inform. Decis. Mak.* **2018**, *18*. [CrossRef] [PubMed]
17. Tobore, I.; Li, J.; Yuhang, L.; Al-Handarish, Y.; Kandwal, A.; Nie, Z.; Wang, L. Deep learning intervention for health care challenges: Some biomedical domain considerations. *JMIR mHealth uHealth* **2019**, *7*, e11966. [CrossRef] [PubMed]
18. Buekers, J.; Theunis, J.; De Boever, P.; Vaes, A.W.; Koopman, M.; Janssen, E.; Wouters, E.F.M.; Spruit, M.; Aerts, J.-M. Wearable finger pulse oximetry for continuous oxygen saturation measurements during daily home routines of patients with COPD during a 1-week observational study. *JMIR mHealth uHealth* **2019**, *7*, e12866. [CrossRef] [PubMed]
19. Venkatesh, J.; Aksalani, B.; Chan, C.S.; Akyurek, A.S.; Rosing, T.S. Modular and personalized smart health application design in a smart city environment. *IEEE Internet Things J.* **2018**, *5*, 614–623. [CrossRef]
20. Cooper, R.A.; Fletcher-Shaw, T.L.; Robertson, R.N. Model reference adaptive control of heart rate during wheelchair ergometry. *IEEE Trans. Control Syst. Technol.* **1998**, *6*, 507–514. [CrossRef]
21. De La Iglesia, D.H.; De Paz, J.F.; Villarubia González Barriuso, A.L.; Bajo, J.; Corchado, J.M. Increasing the intensity over time of an electric-assist bike based on the user and route: The bike becomes the gym. *Sensors* **2018**, *18*, 220. [CrossRef]
22. Hong, S.; Gu, Y.; Seo, J.K.; Wang, J.; Liu, P.; Meng, S.; Xu, S.; Chen, R. Wearable thermoelectrics for personalized thermoregulation. *Sci. Adv.* **2019**, *5*, eaaw0536. [CrossRef]
23. Kim, J.; Lee, G.; Heimgartner, R.; Revi, D.A.; Karavas, N.; Nathanson, D.; Galiana, I.; Eckert-Erdheim, A.; Murphy, P.; Perry, D.; et al. Reducing the metabolic rate of walking and running with a versatile, portable exosuit. *Science* **2019**, *365*, 668–672. [CrossRef]
24. Chowdhury, M.; Khandakar, A.; Hossain, B.; Alzoubi, K. Effects of the Phantom Shape on the Gradient Artefact of Electroencephalography (EEG) Data in Simultaneous EEG–fMRI. *Appl. Sci.* **2018**, *8*, 1969. [CrossRef]
25. Fang, Y.; Chun, L.; Chu, B. Older Adults' Usability and Emotional Reactions toward Text, Diagram, Image, and Animation Interfaces for Displaying Health Information. *Appl. Sci.* **2019**, *9*, 1058. [CrossRef]
26. Gircys, R.; Liutkevicius, A.; Kazanavicius, E.; Lesauskaite, V.; Damuleviciene, G.; Janaviciute, A. Photoplethysmography-Based Continuous Systolic Blood Pressure Estimation Method for Low Processing Power Wearable Devices. *Appl. Sci.* **2019**, *9*, 2236. [CrossRef]

27. Mukunthan, S.; Vleugels, J.; Huysmans, T.; Kuklane, K.; Mayor, T.; De Bruyne, G. Thermal-Performance Evaluation of Bicycle Helmets for Convective and Evaporative Heat Loss at Low and Moderate Cycling Speeds. *Appl. Sci.* **2019**, *9*, 3672. [CrossRef]
28. van der Have, A.; Van Rossom, S.; Jonkers, I. Squat Lifting Imposes Higher Peak Joint and Muscle Loading Compared to Stoop Lifting. *Appl. Sci.* **2019**, *9*, 3794. [CrossRef]
29. Wibowo, D.; Widodo, A.; Haryadi, G.; Caesarendra, W.; Harahap, R. Effect of In-Shoe Foot Orthosis Contours on Heel Pain Due to Calcaneal Spurs. *Appl. Sci.* **2019**, *9*, 495. [CrossRef]
30. Bekteshi, S.; Konings, M.; Nica, I.; Gakopoulos, S.; Vanmechelen, I.; Aerts, J.; Hallez, H.; Monbaliu, E. Development of the Dyskinesia Impairment Mobility Scale to Measure Presence and Severity of Dystonia and Choreoathetosis during Powered Mobility in Dyskinetic Cerebral Palsy. *Appl. Sci.* **2019**, *9*, 3481. [CrossRef]
31. Rosales-Huamani, J.; Guzman-Lopez, R.; Aroni-Vilca, E.; Matos-Avalos, C.; Castillo-Sequera, J. Determining Symptomatic Factors of Nomophobia in Peruvian Students from the National University of Engineering. *Appl. Sci.* **2019**, *9*, 1814. [CrossRef]
32. Das, N.; Verstraete, K.; Topalovic, M.; Aerts, J.; Janssens, W. Estimating Airway Resistance from Forced Expiration in Spirometry. *Appl. Sci.* **2019**, *9*, 2842. [CrossRef]
33. Fu, Y.; Wang, X.; Yu, T. Simulation Analysis of Knee Ligaments in the Landing Phase of Freestyle Skiing Aerial. *Appl. Sci.* **2019**, *9*, 3713. [CrossRef]
34. Cardarilli, G.; Di Nunzio, L.; Fazzolari, R.; Re, M.; Silvestri, F. Improvement of the Cardiac Oscillator Based Model for the Simulation of Bundle Branch Blocks. *Appl. Sci.* **2019**, *9*, 3653. [CrossRef]
35. Mwamba, H.; Fourie, P.; van den Heever, D. PANDAS: Paediatric Attention-Deficit/Hyperactivity Disorder Application Software. *Appl. Sci.* **2019**, *9*, 1645. [CrossRef]
36. Buekers, J.; Theunis, J.; Peña Fernández, A.; Wouters, E.; Spruit, M.; De Boever, P.; Aerts, J. Box-Jenkins Transfer Function Modelling for Reliable Determination of VO2 Kinetics in Patients with COPD. *Appl. Sci.* **2019**, *9*, 1822. [CrossRef]
37. Youssef, A.; Verachtert, A.; De Bruyne, G.; Aerts, J. Reverse Engineering of Thermoregulatory Cold-Induced Vasoconstriction/Vasodilation during Localized Cooling. *Appl. Sci.* **2019**, *9*, 3372. [CrossRef]
38. Rajula, H.S.R.; Odintsova, V.; Manchia, M.; Fanos, V. Overview of Federated Facility to Harmonize, Analyze and Management of Missing Data in Cohorts. *Appl. Sci.* **2019**, *9*, 4103. [CrossRef]
39. Youssef, A.; Colon, J.; Mantzios, K.; Gkiata, P.; Mayor, T.; Flouris, A.; De Bruyne, G.; Aerts, J. Towards Model-Based Online Monitoring of Cyclist's Head Thermal Comfort: Smart Helmet Concept and Prototype. *Appl. Sci.* **2019**, *9*, 3170. [CrossRef]
40. Youssef, A.; Youssef Ali Amer, A.; Caballero, N.; Aerts, J. Towards Online Personalized-Monitoring of Human Thermal Sensation Using Machine Learning Approach. *Appl. Sci.* **2019**, *9*, 3303. [CrossRef]
41. Gielen, J.; Aerts, J. Feature Extraction and Evaluation for Driver Drowsiness Detection Based on Thermoregulation. *Appl. Sci.* **2019**, *9*, 3555. [CrossRef]
42. Youssef, A.; Amer, A.; Vranken, J.; Wouters, F.; Mesotten, D.; Vandervoort, P.; Storms, V.; Luca, S.; Vanrumste, B.; Aerts, J. Feature Engineering for ICU Mortality Prediction Based on Hourly to Bi-Hourly Measurements. *Appl. Sci.* **2019**, *9*, 3525. [CrossRef]
43. Peña Fernández, A.; Youssef, A.; Heeren, C.; Matthys, C.; Aerts, J. Real-Time Model Predictive Control of Human Bodyweight Based on Energy Intake. *Appl. Sci.* **2019**, *9*, 2609. [CrossRef]
44. Zhang, X.; Li, J.; Hu, Z.; Qi, W.; Zhang, L.; Hu, Y.; Su, H.; Ferrigno, G.; Momi, E. Novel Design and Lateral Stability Tracking Control of a Four-Wheeled Rollator. *Appl. Sci.* **2019**, *9*, 2327. [CrossRef]
45. Jin, S.; Xiong, X.; Zhao, D.; Jin, C.; Yamamoto, M. Long-Term Effects of a Soft Robotic Suit on Gait Characteristics in Healthy Elderly Persons. *Appl. Sci.* **2019**, *9*, 1957. [CrossRef]
46. Adiputra, D.; Rahman, A.; Ubaidillah; Mazlan, S.; Nazmi, N.; Shabdin, M.; Kobayashi, J.; Mohammed Ariff, M. Control Reference Parameter for Stance Assistance Using a Passive Controlled Ankle Foot Orthosis—A Preliminary Study. *Appl. Sci.* **2019**, *9*, 4416. [CrossRef]

47. Aramendia, I.; Zulueta, E.; Teso-Fz-Betoño, D.; Saenz-Aguirre, A.; Fernandez-Gamiz, U. Modeling of Motorized Orthosis Control. *Appl. Sci.* **2019**, *9*, 2453. [CrossRef]
48. Dao, Q.; Nguyen, M.; Yamamoto, S. Discrete-Time Fractional Order Integral Sliding Mode Control of an Antagonistic Actuator Driven by Pneumatic Artificial Muscles. *Appl. Sci.* **2019**, *9*, 2503. [CrossRef]

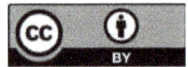

© 2020 by the author. Licensee MDPI, Basel, Switzerland. This article is an open access article distributed under the terms and conditions of the Creative Commons Attribution (CC BY) license (http://creativecommons.org/licenses/by/4.0/).

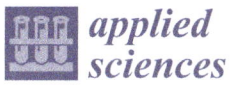 

Article

# Effects of the Phantom Shape on the Gradient Artefact of Electroencephalography (EEG) Data in Simultaneous EEG–fMRI

Muhammad E. H. Chowdhury [1,*], Amith Khandakar [1], Belayat Hossain [2] and Khawla Alzoubi [1]

[1] Department of Electrical Engineering, College of Engineering, Qatar University, Doha 2713, Qatar; amitk@qu.edu.qa (A.K.); kalzoubi@qu.edu.qa (K.A.)
[2] Department of EECS, Graduate School of Engineering, University of Hyogo, Kobe 650-0047, Japan; belayat@ieee.org
* Correspondence: mchowdhury@qu.edu.qa; Tel.: +974-3101-0775

Received: 11 September 2018; Accepted: 16 October 2018; Published: 18 October 2018

**Abstract:** Electroencephalography (EEG) signals greatly suffer from gradient artefacts (GAs) due to the time-varying field gradients in the magnetic resonance (MR) scanner during the simultaneous acquisition of EEG and functional magnetic resonance imaging (fMRI) data. The GAs are the principal contributors of artefacts while recording EEG inside an MR scanner, and most of them come from the interaction of the EEG cap and the subject's head. Many researchers have been using a spherical phantom to characterize the GA in EEG data in combined EEG–fMRI studies. In this study, we investigated how the phantom shape could affect the characterization of the GA. EEG data were recorded with a spherical phantom, a head-shaped phantom, and six human subjects, individually, during the execution of customized and standard echo-planar imaging (EPI) sequences. The spatial potential maps of the root-mean-square (RMS) voltage of the GA over EEG channels for the trials with a head-shaped phantom closely mimicked those related to the human head rather than those obtained for the spherical phantom. This was confirmed by measuring the average similarity index (0.85/0.68). Moreover, a paired $t$-test showed that the head-shaped phantom's and the spherical phantom's data were significantly different ($p < 0.005$) from the subjects' data, whereas the difference between the head-shaped phantom's and the spherical phantom's data was not significant ($p = 0.07$). The results of this study strongly suggest that a head-shaped phantom should be used for GA characterization studies in concurrent EEG–fMRI.

**Keywords:** artefact correction; head-shaped phantom; spherical phantom; gradient artefact; simultaneous EEG–fMRI

## 1. Introduction

The simultaneous recording of electroencephalography (EEG) and functional magnetic resonance imaging (fMRI) has enabled many researchers to investigate and study new possibilities in functional neuroimaging to understand the human brain and help in diagnosing and treating brain-related diseases and disabilities [1]. Because of the fusion of the excellent spatial resolution of fMRI [1,2] and the high temporal resolution of EEG in combined EEG–fMRI studies, this technique has enabled us to better understand the relationship between spontaneous or evoked electrical activity and hemodynamic response in the human brain [3–5].

In concurrent EEG–fMRI recordings, the magnetic fields of the MRI scanner generate artefacts in the EEG data [6,7]. These artefacts are larger than the neuronal activity of interest by an order of magnitude or more [8]. The major induced artefact voltage, known as gradient artefact (GA), in EEG data is produced by magnetic field gradients [6,7]. The GA ranges between 10 and 100 mv, which is far greater than the typical EEG signal (less than 200 µV). Mullinger et al. [8] suggested that the position of the head and EEG cap with respect to the applied magnetic field gradients could affect the induced GA. The GA could be reproduced provided that the position of the head or the EEG cap remains steady during data recording [9]. This, in turn, helps to remove the GA using a post-processing method called Average Artefact Subtraction (AAS) [6].

There are two other kinds of artefact: pulse artefact (PA) and motion artefact (MA) [10,11]. The magnitude of the PA is in the order of a few hundred microvolts in a 3T static magnetic field [12]. In contrast, head rotation is responsible for the MA, which could be in the order of 10 mV [13]. The induced MA due to head rotation could be temporally correlated with the task response in fMRI experiments, which could lead to cofounding effects in simultaneously acquired EEG–fMRI data [14]. Since the GA forms the largest artefact in EEG data recorded during simultaneous EEG–fMRI experiments, it is very essential to minimize this kind of artefact to avoid amplifier saturation [15]. Furthermore, GA amplitude reduction could also help in easing the constraints on the dynamic range and the bandwidth of the EEG amplifier and, thus, it could be beneficial in the future for many EEG–fMRI studies.

In EEG–fMRI studies testing new configurations or settings with the aim to reduce or eliminate the GA from the EEG data, it is not always safe to use human subjects, because there is a risk of heating the subject's tissues following the emission of radiofrequency (RF) energy during the slice excitation procedure [16], which couples into the loops of the electrodes' cable and leads to dissipating energy in the human tissues or in the loop materials themselves in the form of heat [17,18]. Thus, there is a common practice among EEG–fMRI researchers to use a phantom in the initial setup of any EEG artefact correction technique in simultaneous EEG–fMRI recording [8,9,15,19,20]. This is a primary step when testing and preparing any hardware-based methods and configurations or software-based EEG artefact reduction (more specifically, GA correction) techniques, before acquiring EEG data from a human subject. Furthermore, the use of a phantom helps the researchers to avoid PA and MA that are due to blood circulation and head movement, as it is not possible to prevent a human subject from moving their head. Thus, the use of a phantom could facilitate the study, allowing to focus only on the reduction of the GAs as they are the largest artefacts in EEG data. Moreover, it is not easy to conduct experimental tests on human subjects because ethical approval is required for EEG–fMRI analyses. Therefore, it could be more convenient and safe to conduct experiments on a phantom rather than on a human subject.

While some studies suggested a different hardware configuration, such as an EEG cap lead reconfiguration, a specific cap-cable configuration, etc., [8,15,19] for GA reduction, according to the recent literature, no study has investigated the effect of a phantom shape when characterizing the GA in EEG data, which is done in this work. In this study, EEG data were acquired three times using the same experimental setup with a spherical phantom, a head-shaped phantom, and six healthy volunteers. The primary contribution of this work is the investigation of how the shape of the phantom affects the magnitude of the GA generated by each of the three orthogonal gradients (anterior–posterior (AP), right–left (RL), and foot–head (FH)). Secondly, we discuss our findings obtained from the different experimental setups. Finally, we use the quantitative measurement of the EEG data recorded using a standard echo-planar imaging (EPI) sequence to confirm the findings of this study.

This paper is organized into five sections. A discussion about phantom production is given in Section 2; a detailed discussion of the experimental setup, hardware configuration, study design, and data acquisition is given in Section 3; Section 4 presents the details of the analysis applied for data processing; experimental findings, performance measures, experimental evaluations, and possible impacts are discussed in Section 5; finally, the paper's conclusions are presented in Section 6.

## 2. Method of Phantom Production

To produce a phantom, it is essential to make a mold in the desired phantom's shape. In this study, two different molds were custom-made to obtain a spherical and a head-shaped phantom. The spherical and head-shaped molds were built in an engineering workshop at the University of Nottingham. The spherical mold (Figure 1) was made from plastic, using two hollow hemispheres finely polished at the inner and outer surface, with inner and external diameters of 15 cm and 15.5 cm, respectively. The head-shaped mold was made using a Styrofoam male head model and plastic, which could be unscrewed into two cross-sectional pieces (Figure 2). The spherical and head-shaped molds were kept upright using a clamp to pour liquid agar into them, and the phantoms were made, as shown in Figure 3.

*Agar Preparation*

In order to calculate the amount of agar and salt necessary for making the phantoms, the following Equations (1) and (2) were used:

$$\frac{a}{a+s+w} = 4.0\% \tag{1}$$

$$\frac{s}{a+s+w} = 0.5\% \tag{2}$$

where $a$, $s$, and $w$ are the agar, salt, and water weights, respectively (1 mL of water is equivalent to 1 g of water). Typically, the percentages of agar and salt were 4% and 0.5%, respectively. Solving this pair of simultaneous Equations (3) and (4) yields:

$$a = \frac{100}{2487}w \tag{3}$$

$$s = \frac{13}{2487}w \tag{4}$$

The volume of the spherical mold was equal to 4000 mL approximately and, therefore, 4300 mL of agar was prepared.

Firstly, water was heated with the required amount of salt and few drops of sterilizing fluid (Milton) to prevent bacterial growth, then agar was added, and finally the temperature was decreased. Attention was paid while adding agar, as very hot water would produce a viscous solution with the first addition of agar powder, causing the agar added subsequently to become encapsulated and thus preventing its full dissolution. This would produce a speckled phantom, impossible to correct even with appropriate stirring.

Constant stirring of the solution was required to avoid burning the agar. It was necessary to boil the agar solution without burning it, as this would lead to a speckled phantom. Strong stirring ensured a uniform distribution of the heat. It was necessary to proceed by trial and error to distinguish between properly boiled agar and burnt agar.

When the vortex at the top, created by the magnetic stirrer, became visible, it was assumed that the agar had reached the right consistency. The ideal phantom can be made when the sticky mix becomes viscous. The mold was initially filled by pouring the liquid agar through the hole on the top of it but, as the agar cooled and contracted, it became partially empty (~75 mL) at the top. To preserve the spherical shape of the phantom, about 300 mL of agar was kept aside (mildly heated) to be added to the mold whenever necessary. A similar approach was used for the head-shaped phantom. Figure 3 shows the spherical and head-shaped phantoms, which were prepared following the method described above.

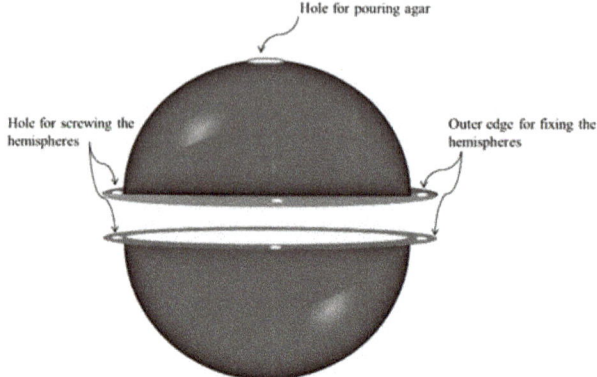

**Figure 1.** Mold for making the spherical phantom.

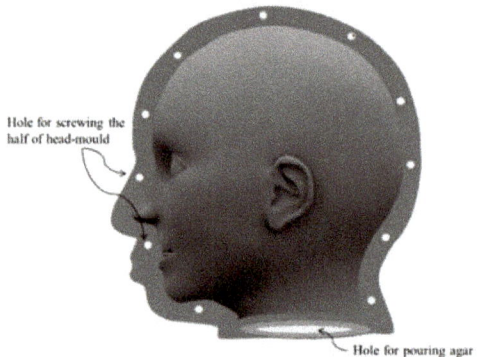

**Figure 2.** Mold for making the head-shaped phantom.

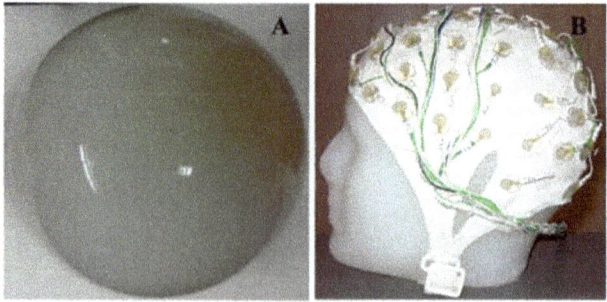

**Figure 3.** Spherical agar phantom (**A**), and human head-shaped agar phantom (**B**).

## 3. Methodology and Experiments

In this study, an EEG cap of 32 standard Ag/AgCl electrodes from BrainProduct (Munich, Germany) was utilized to record EEG data at 5 kHz sampling rate, and the electrodes were positioned according to the extended international 10–20 system with FCz as a reference electrode. Additionally, an electrode was attached beneath the left eye of the subject for electrooculography (EOG) recording. A BrainAmp MR-plus EEG Amplifier (BrainProducts, Munich, Germany) was placed behind a Philips Achieva 3T MR scanner (Best, The Netherlands) at the Sir Peter Mansfield Magnetic Imaging Centre (SPMIC), University of Nottingham, for acquiring the EEG data while the MR scanner was running, and the data were finally recorded into a personal computer by Vision Recorder (Version 1.10) software (Figure 4).

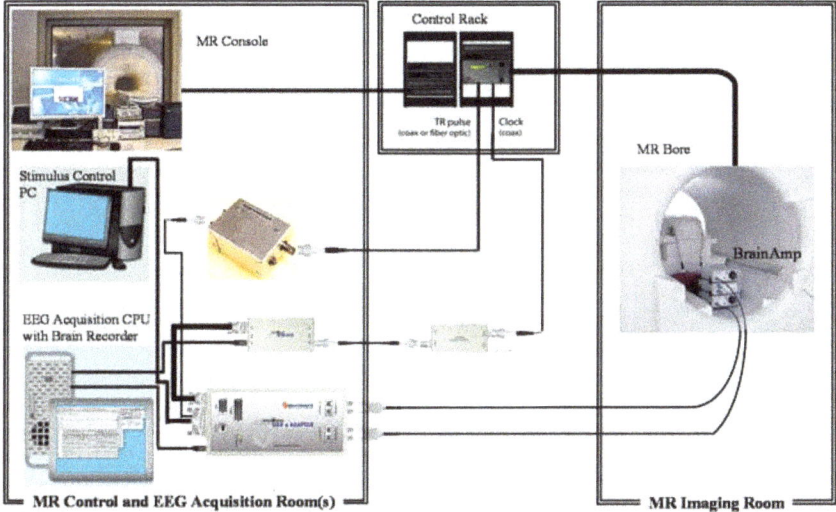

Figure 4. Schematic diagram of the experimental setup of the study.

The EEG and MR scanner clocks were synchronized throughout the experiments to guarantee a reliable sampling of the waveforms [7,21]. An 8-channel radio frequency (RF) head coil was used to acquire the fMRI data. As shown in Figure 5A, the amplifier was placed outside the MR bore to isolate it from the vibrations of the MR scanner. Similarly, the cables were run along the cantilever beam and then were coupled to the EEG cap (Figure 5B). Suspending the cable above the mounting of the scanner bed also minimized the scanner's vibrations [8].

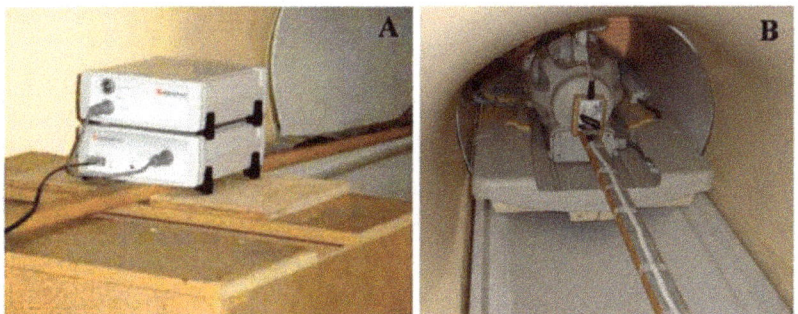

Figure 5. Arrangement of the amplifier (**A**) and cables attachment to a cantilever beam (**B**), utilized to separate it from the scanner's vibrations.

### 3.1. Study 1: Orthogonal Gradients

EEG recordings were carried out individually from the spherical phantom, the head-shaped phantom, and six human subjects during the execution of a modified echo-planar imaging (EPI) sequence. The purpose of this work was to investigate how the shape of the phantom affects the magnitude of the GA generated by each of the three orthogonal gradients (AP, RL, and FH). Prior to each slice acquisition, three additional gradient pulses, shown in Figure 6, were applied sequentially along the AP, RL, and FH directions. This study was approved by the local Ethics Committee of the University of Nottingham, and each subject provided written informed consent.

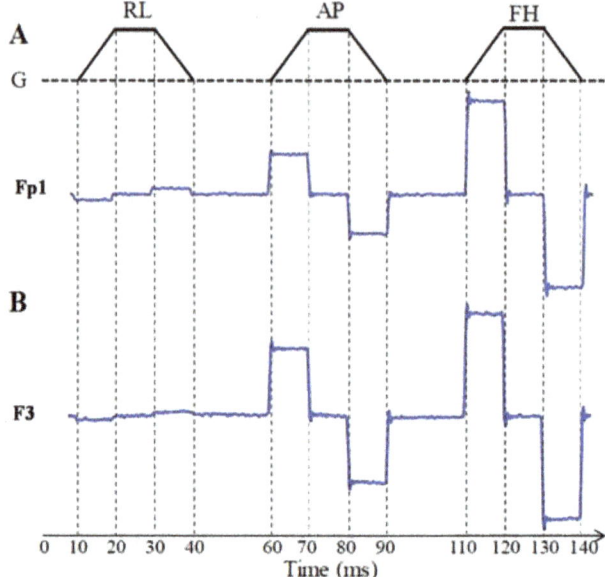

**Figure 6.** Representation of the three gradient pulses which were applied along the three orthogonal directions (right–left, RL, anterior–posterior, AP, and foot–head, FH) (**A**) and the corresponding induced artefact voltages (in µV) in two example leads (Fp1 and F3) for the head-shaped phantom (**B**).

The trapezoidal gradient pulse for 30 ms duration consisted of two 10 ms ramps, during which the gradient was changed at a rate of 2 Tm$^{-1}$s$^{-1}$ and was kept constant between the consecutive ramps (Figure 6). Successive gradient pulses had a gap of 20 ms. The modified pulse sequence provided clearly defined intervals during which just a single gradient varied in time, allowing the easy separation of the effects of the three different gradients. In a standard gradient echo (GE) EPI acquisition, time-varying gradients are simultaneously applied along multiple axes at high frequencies, and the typical EEG system's low-pass filtering significantly attenuates and affects the induced voltages, which in turn makes it difficult to differentiate the voltages produced by individual gradient pulses. This introduces a challenge to compute the outcome of the applied time-varying gradient pulse along one specific direction. Therefore, the EEG data were recorded with a frequency range of 0.016–1000 Hz, which ensured the reliability of the acquisition of the EEG data (assuring a higher bandwidth) during the usage of gradient pulses.

*3.2. Study 2: EPI Sequence*

In the second study, a standard axial, multi-slice GE EPI sequence (repetition time (TR) = 2 s, echo time (TE) = 40 ms, 84 × 84 matrix, 3 × 3 mm$^2$ in-plane resolution, 4 mm slice thickness, flip angle = 85°, fold-over direction = AP, SENSE factor = 2, i.e., a two-fold reduction in the number of lines of k-space acquired) was executed while EEG data were recorded. Twenty equidistant slices were acquired within a 2 s TR period, with a resulting slice acquisition frequency of 10 Hz. This standard GE EPI sequence is popular among researchers for characterizing the GA in combined EEG–fMRI data acquisition. Seventy volumes of EEG data were recorded on the phantoms, and 150 volumes were acquired on the human subjects. In this study, the EEG data were recorded with a typical bandwidth

(0.016–250 Hz) conventionally used in combined EEG–fMRI studies to keep the EEG signal amplitude in the dynamic range of the EEG amplifier.

EEG data were recorded using the spherical and head-shaped phantoms for six trials in a single recording session and six human subjects in different sessions. Table 1 shows the main characteristics of the human test subjects. The subjects were asked to stay as stable as possible to avoid any motion artefacts in the EEG data. Subjects' EEG data were visually inspected during the EEG recording, and any particular dataset was discarded and re-recorded if any noticeable motion artefacts were observed. In each session, the subjects were placed in the same axial position (+4 cm axial [8]) inside the MRI scanner to avoid any variation due to subject positioning. However, there was some obvious variation due to the head shape and orientation. In the case of the phantoms, in each trial, the phantom was taken out of the scanner and then replaced inside it to mimic the possible variation experienced with the subjects in different recording sessions.

**Table 1.** Characteristics of the six human subjects tested in the study.

| Subjects | Age | Sex | Height (cm) | Weight (lb) |
|---|---|---|---|---|
| Sub1 | 29 | M | 177 | 160 |
| Sub2 | 24 | F | 160 | 140 |
| Sub3 | 31 | M | 180 | 150 |
| Sub4 | 35 | M | 165 | 154 |
| Sub5 | 22 | F | 180 | 135 |
| Sub6 | 25 | F | 158 | 120 |

## 4. Analysis

Brain Vision Analyzer 2 (Version 2.0.1.3417) from BrainProducts and MATLAB (The MathWorks, Natick, MA, USA) were used to analyze the EEG data. Each gradient pulse in the customized EPI sequence commenced with a 10ms period during which the gradient ramped up linearly to a value of 20 mT m$^{-1}$ giving a rate of change of gradient, dG/dt, of 2 Tm$^{-1}$s$^{-1}$. This was followed 10 ms later by a 10 ms period during which the gradient ramped down to zero with dG/dt = $-2$ Tm$^{-1}$s$^{-1}$ (Figure 6). Thus, equal and opposite artefact voltages (in µV) were induced during both periods. The induced GAs were averaged over 30 pulses (Figure 6) to measure the artefact voltage of each electrode, and then we evaluated the average voltage over the central 5 ms of each ramp period, before taking the difference between the positive and negative values. In this way, the effect of any baseline offset and high-frequency fluctuations were eliminated. The severity of the GA depending on the phantom shape was characterized by calculating the root-mean-square (RMS) amplitude of the artefact voltage for each orthogonal gradients across the 31 electrodes (excluding the EOG electrode) located on the phantoms' or subjects' head and, finally, by averaging these measures over the phantom trials and human subjects. To graphically depict the difference between the effects of the phantom shape on the GA, spatial voltage maps of average RMS artefact voltages, for each gradient (RL, AP, and FH), were produced using Brain Vision Analyzer 2 for the different phantoms and human subjects. Additionally, the structural similarity (SSIM) was also calculated for the head-shaped phantom and the spherical phantom spatial maps in comparison to the subjects' spatial maps for each gradient. The SSIM index is a standard method to evaluate the similarity between two images (test and reference images). SSIM assesses [22] the visual impact of three characteristics of an image: luminance l(x,y), contrast c(x,y), and structure s(x,y) with respect to a reference image. The overall index is a multiplicative combination of the three terms:

$$SSIM(x,y) = [l(x,y)]^{\alpha} \cdot [c(x,y)]^{\delta} \cdot [s(x,y)]^{\gamma} \qquad (5)$$

where $\alpha$, $\delta$, and $\gamma$ are exponents with the value of 1. $l(x,y)$, $c(x,y)$, and $s(x,y)$ are calculated from the local means, standard deviations, and cross-covariance for images $x$, $y$. In this work, the SSIM index was computed to quantify how close or different the spatial maps are.

The EEG artefact waveform of each channel in the study 2 was acquired for a 100 ms (slice) duration. Each waveform was baseline-corrected by subtracting the average channel artefact voltage in the corresponding slice duration. The baseline-corrected voltages were averaged over the slices while excluding the periods of the EEG signal with unacceptable head movements for the subject data. To assess the effect of the phantom shape on the induced GA, the RMS over the slice acquisition period was then calculated for the average artefact on each lead. The average and standard deviation of the EEG data over phantom trials and subjects were also calculated. A paired $t$-test was applied to the phantoms' and subjects' data to assess if there were significant differences between the GAs, which were induced by the EPI sequence due to the variation of the geometric shapes.

The MR data were realigned by using SPM8 [23] to check the head movement, so to keep them stable during the repeated MRI acquisitions. The RMS of the mean corrected realignment parameters (pitch, yaw, and roll, and $x$, $y$, and $z$ translation) were calculated for each dataset, and then the average and standard deviation of the phantom and subject trails were computed.

## 5. Results and Discussion

To demonstrate how the phantom shape in concurrent EEG–fMRI recording affected the induced GA that confounded the EEG data inside the MR scanner, the average contribution of the RMS voltage for each orthogonal gradients was mapped to a 2D spatial voltage representation, as shown in Figure 7. The potential map of the RL gradient of the spherical phantom showed that the frontal, fronto-central, and temporal lobe electrodes contributed to the largest negative voltages, whereas the occipital and parietal lobe electrodes contributed to the largest positive voltages, respectively. However, the potential maps of the RL gradient of the head-shaped phantom and subjects were significantly different from the spherical phantom's fronto-parietal and parietal lobe electrodes data. In the case of the AP gradient, which is one of the largest artefact-contributing gradient, as shown in previous work by one of this study's authors [15], the largest positive and negative voltages were recorded in the right and left side of the head-shaped phantom and human subjects. However, the left temporal and parietal lobes of the spherical phantom showed the largest negative voltage contribution. In the FH gradient, there were significant variations reported in previous works [15,19,24] due to the variation of the subjects' head positions and shapes in the MR scanner bore. In addition, the patterns of the potential maps (induced voltage distribution) of the FH gradient for the head-shaped phantom and human subjects were similar, whereas the map for the spherical phantom was significantly different (Figure 7).

Although it was observed that the head-shaped phantom's spatial map was very similar to that of the subjects for each orthogonal gradient, it was necessary to quantify this similarity using a mathematical method. The SSIM variation is shown in Figure 8 for each gradient to the compare head-shaped phantom with the spherical phantom in reference to the human subjects. The SSIM was significantly higher (average value, 0.85) for the head-shaped phantom in comparison to the spherical phantom (average value, 0.68) (Figure 8). Interestingly, it was observed that the difference of potential map between the head-shaped phantom and the spherical phantom for the FH gradient was significantly high (Figure 7), but the SSIM value did not reflect this difference. This was due to the variations in the range of the potential for the spherical phantom (i.e., there were several electrodes that contributed to high positive and negative potentials); however, this did not occur for most of the electrodes. It is also important to note that the observed variations of the SSIM values reflected by the error bar in Figure 8, show that the SSIM values varied more significantly for the spherical phantom than for the head-shaped phantom.

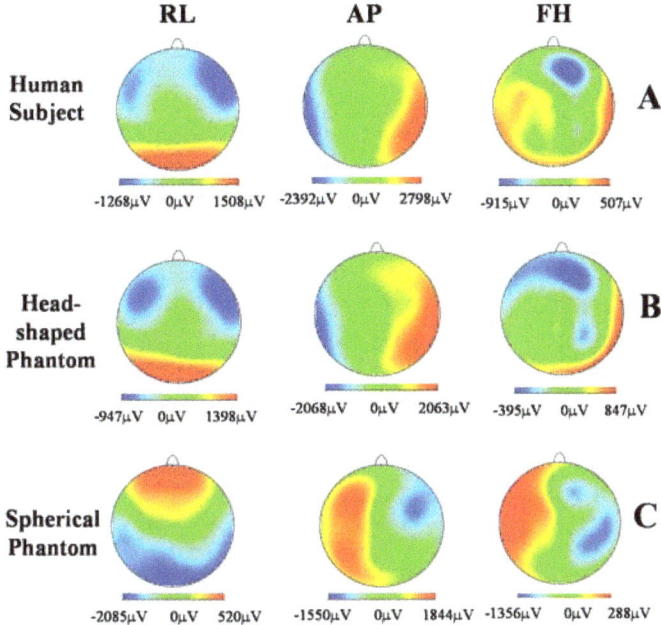

**Figure 7.** Spatial maps of the average root-mean-square (RMS) voltage of the induced gradient artefact (GA) in the electroencephalography (EEG) data for each orthogonal gradient (RL, AP, and FH) related to the subjects' head (**A**), the head-shaped phantom (**B**), and the spherical phantom (**C**).

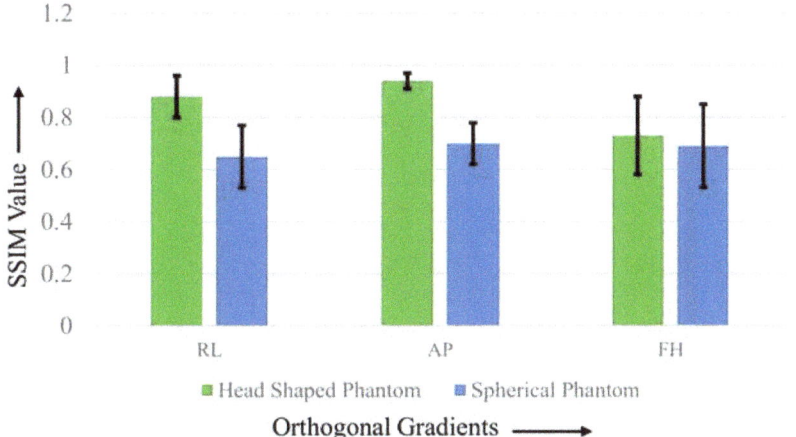

**Figure 8.** The structural similarity (SSIM) variation between the subjects' map and the head-shaped phantom map (green) and between the subjects' map and the spherical phantom map (blue). The error bar shows the standard deviation of the SSIM variation over the trials. Note: SSIM is a unitless quantity, in the range 0–1.

To clarify the observed differences in AP and RL in the subjects' data (as shown in Figure 7), we considered the average RMS voltage for each channel, for the AP gradient (the most contributing gradient), for the subject, the head-shaped phantom, and the spherical phantom (Figure 9). In Figure 9, the means RMS of the induced voltage for the subject data appear highly correlated to the head-shaped phantom data, although the standard deviations for subjects' data re significantly higher than those of the head-shaped phantom data. This could be explained easily by considering the pulse artefacts and small involuntary movements of subjects' head during data acquisition, in addition to the brain signal.

Moreover, in the different sessions, even though the subjects were set in the +4 cm axial position inside the scanner, the shape and orientation of the heads did not match completely, which, we believe, greatly contributed to the variation of the standard deviations. To mimic the variation of the orientations of human's head in different sessions, we took the head-shaped phantom out of the scanner bore and returned it to its position (+4 cm axial position) in different trials, thus slightly altering its orientation. Even though the shape of the phantom remained the same, and no PA and MA occurred in the head-shaped phantom, the observed standard deviation in the head-shaped phantom was due to the altered orientation in different trials. However, Figure 9 shows that the patterns of the potential distribution across different channels for the AP gradients were significantly different for the spherical phantom in comparison to the human head. This clearly revealed that any characterization study of GA to reduce these artefacts in EEG data in concurrent EEG–fMRI experiments might not be accurate when the spherical phantom is used.

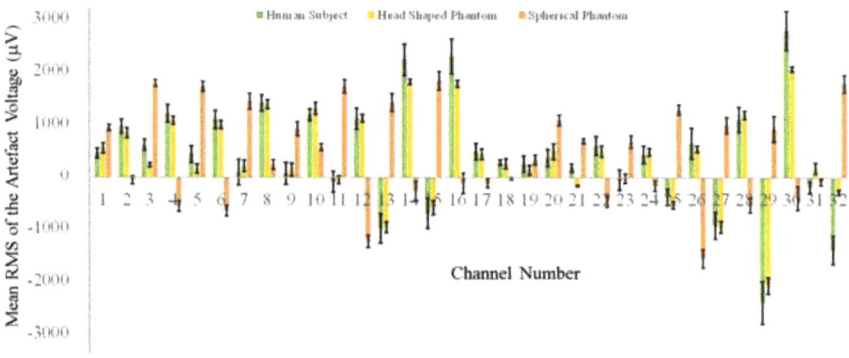

**Figure 9.** The average RMS of the induced GA recording for repeats of the AP orthogonal gradient for each channel on the subjects' head, head-shaped phantom, and spherical phantom. Error bars show the corresponding standard deviation of the mean RMS over trials.

In the study 2, the induced voltages for different trials (subjects and phantoms) were not significantly different. Moreover, the average RMS of the EEG data over time over the channels were 455 ± 21 µV, 368 ± 13 µV, and 383 ± 16 µV for subjects, head-shaped phantom, and spherical phantom trials, respectively. It is clear from Figure 10 that the highest gradient peaks occurred for the same gradients in the human subjects' and head-shaped phantoms' data, whereas some variations were observed in the beginning of the R period (fat suppression and slice select). However, the mean RMS value and standard deviation for the human subjects were much higher than those of the phantoms, which also agrees with the findings, as shown in Figures 7 and 9. It can be noted that a higher variation of the standard deviation for the human subjects can be expected, due to the variations of the size and shape of the human head. Moreover, it is evident from the average potential map of the FH gradient for the human subjects (Figure 7) that it is quite different from that of the phantoms, possibly in relation to the shape of the human subjects and of their head. The paired $t$-test to compare the different trials with the phantoms with the sessions with the subjects showed that the head-shaped phantom and spherical phantom data were significantly different ($p < 0.005$) from the subjects' data, whereas the difference between the head-shaped phantom's and spherical phantom's data was not significant ($p = 0.07$).

Furthermore, the movement parameters were identified in the different experimental sessions for all subjects, and no significant deviation among the parameters was observed. The maximum average displacements were smaller than a 0.5 mm translation (z-translation) and a 0.005 rotation (pitch) for all subjects. These movements were small, which implies that the related MA could not be the reason of the similarity of the subjects' data with the head-shaped phantom's data. Moreover, the consistency of the RMS amplitude of the induced voltage in time over the channels (small standard deviation) also indicates that this might not be due to MA but, rather, could be the result of the induced voltage.

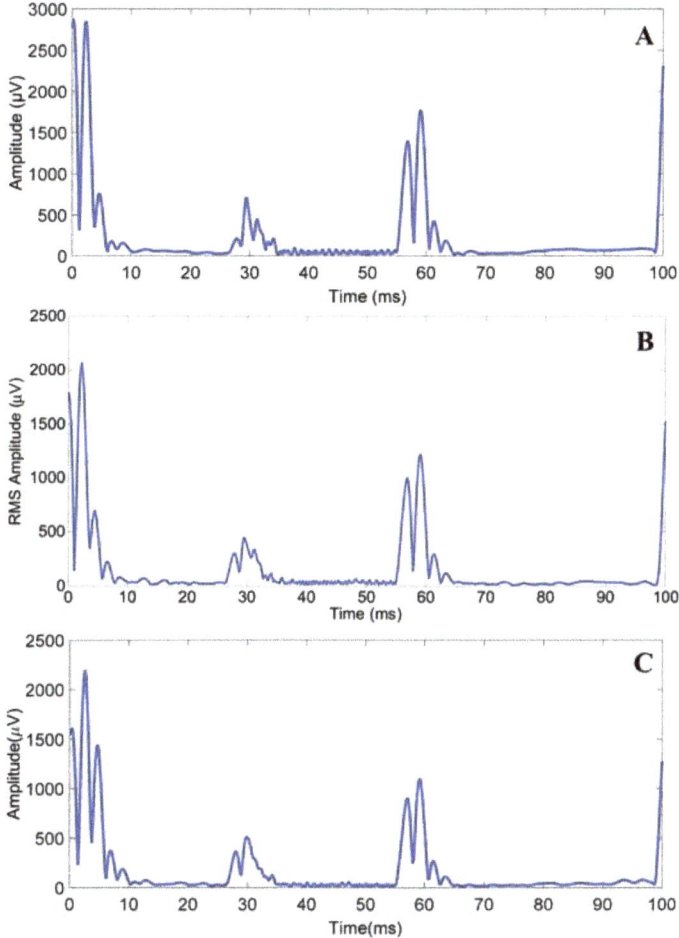

**Figure 10.** Variation of the average RMS amplitude of the GA over the channels with respect to time in the TR period for the human subjects (**A**), the head-shaped phantom (**B**), and the spherical phantom (**C**).

## 6. Conclusions

In this study, we investigated experimental EEG data obtained from the simultaneous EEG–fMRI recording of six human subjects and six trials using ahead-shaped phantom, and a spherical phantom in order to study the effects of the phantom shape on the induced GA voltages in the EEG data inside the MR scanner. All the conducted experiments had the same settings and configurations in terms of EEG cap, wiring, and MR scanner. The only uncontrolled difference among the different experiments were caused by the marginal placement shifts of the phantoms in different trials or of the subjects in different sessions inside the MR scanner along with the variations of the orientations. It was found that the head-shaped phantom well mimicked the effects of the GA induced in EEG data by the human head in comparison to the spherical phantom. The SSIM values also supported similar findings. The mean RMS amplitudes of GA in time over the channels for the head-shaped phantom and the spherical phantom were significantly different from that of the subjects, but the difference between the phantoms was not significant. This implies that, even though both phantom shapes mimicked the human head for the overall GA characteristics, the head-shaped phantom reliably mimicked the spatial characteristics of the GA induced by the human head. Therefore, this study recommends the use of a head-shaped phantom instead of a spherical phantom in the future to investigate new cap and wiring configuration designs in order to reduce the induced GA in EEG data derived from the MR scanner.

**Author Contributions:** Experiments were designed by M.E.H.C. and B.H.; Experiments were performed by M.E.H.C.; Results were analyzed by M.E.H.C., B.H. and A.K. All authors were involved in interpretation of data and paper writing.

**Funding:** The publication of this article was funded by the Qatar National Library, Engineering, and Physical Sciences Research Council (EPSRC) with the grant (EP/J006823/1).

**Acknowledgments:** The authors would like to thank the Engineering and Physical Sciences Research Council (EPSRC) for the grant (EP/J006823/1) which made this work possible. The authors would like to thank Richard Bowtell and Karen Mullinger from the Sir Peter Mansfield Imaging Center, University of Nottingham, UK, for their help during data acquisition and analysis and for useful discussions.

**Conflicts of Interest:** The authors declare no conflict of interest.

### References

1. Laufs, H. A personalized history of EEG–fMRI integration. *Neuroimage* **2012**, *62*, 1056–1067. [CrossRef] [PubMed]
2. Mullinger, K.J.; Cherukara, M.T.; Buxton, R.B.; Francis, S.T.; Mayhew, S.D. Post-stimulus fMRI and EEG responses: Evidence for a neuronal origin hypothesised to be inhibitory. *Neuroimage* **2017**, *157*, 388–399. [CrossRef] [PubMed]
3. Andreou, C.; Frielinghaus, H.; Rauh, J.; Mußmann, M.; Vauth, S.; Braun, P.; Leicht, G.; Mulert, C. Theta and high-beta networks for feedback processing: A simultaneous EEG–fMRI study in healthy male subjects. *Transl. Psychiatry* **2017**, *7*, e1016. [CrossRef] [PubMed]
4. Brueggen, K.; Fiala, C.; Berger, C.; Ochmann, S.; Babiloni, C.; Teipel, S.J. Early Changes in Alpha Band Power and DMN BOLD Activity in Alzheimer's Disease: A Simultaneous Resting State EEG-fMRI Study. *Front. Aging Neurosci.* **2017**, *9*, 319. [CrossRef] [PubMed]
5. Fouragnan, E.; Queirazza, F.; Retzler, C.; Mullinger, K.J.; Philiastides, M.G. Spatiotemporal neural characterization of prediction error valence and surprise during reward learning in humans. *Sci. Rep.* **2017**, *7*, 4762. [CrossRef] [PubMed]
6. Allen, P.J.; Josephs, O.; Turner, R. A method for removing imaging artifact from continuous EEG recorded during functional MRI. *Neuroimage* **2000**, *12*, 230–239. [CrossRef] [PubMed]
7. Mullinger, K.J.; Morgan, P.S.; Bowtell, R.W. Improved artifact correction for combined electroencephalography/functional MRI by means of synchronization and use of vectorcardiogram recordings. *J. Magn. Reson. Imaging* **2008**, *27*, 607–616. [CrossRef] [PubMed]
8. Mullinger, K.J.; Yan, W.X.; Bowtell, R. Reducing the gradient artefact in simultaneous EEG-fMRI by adjusting the subject's axial position. *Neuroimage* **2011**, *54*, 1942–1950. [CrossRef] [PubMed]
9. Yan, W.X.; Mullinger, K.J.; Brookes, M.J.; Bowtell, R. Understanding gradient artefacts in simultaneous EEG/fMRI. *Neuroimage* **2009**, *46*, 459–471. [CrossRef] [PubMed]
10. Debener, S.; Mullinger, K.J.; Niazy, R.K.; Bowtell, R.W. Properties of the ballistocardiogram artefact as revealed by EEG recordings at 1.5, 3 and 7 T static magnetic field strength. *Int. J. Psychophysiol.* **2008**, *67*, 189–199. [CrossRef] [PubMed]
11. Allen, P.J.; Polizzi, G.; Krakow, K.; Fish, D.R.; Lemieux, L. Identification of EEG events in the MR scanner: The problem of pulse artifact and a method for its subtraction. *Neuroimage* **1998**, *8*, 229–239. [CrossRef] [PubMed]
12. Mullinger, K.J.; Havenhand, J.; Bowtell, R. Identifying the sources of the pulse artefact in EEG recordings made inside an MR scanner. *Neuroimage* **2013**, *71*, 75–83. [CrossRef] [PubMed]
13. LeVan, P.; Zhang, S.; Knowles, B.; Zaitsev, M.; Hennig, J. EEG-fMRI gradient artifact correction by multiple motion-related templates. *IEEE Trans. Biomed. Eng.* **2016**, *63*, 2647–2653. [CrossRef] [PubMed]

14. Jansen, M.; Whitea, T.P.; Mullinger, K.J.; Liddle, E.B.; Gowland, P.A.; Francis, S.T.; Bowtell, R.; Liddle, P.F. Motion-related artefacts in EEG predict neuronally plausible patterns of activation in fMRI data. *Neuroimage* **2012**, *59*, 261–270. [CrossRef] [PubMed]
15. Chowdhury, M.E.; Mullinger, K.J.; Bowtell, R. Simultaneous EEG–fMRI: Evaluating the effect of the cabling configuration on the gradient artefact. *Phys. Med. Biol.* **2015**, *60*, N241. [CrossRef] [PubMed]
16. Steyrl, D.; Krausz, G.; Koschutnig, K.; Edlinger, G.; Müller-Putz, G.R. Reference layer adaptive filtering (RLAF) for EEG artifact reduction in simultaneous EEG-fMRI. *J. Neural Eng.* **2017**, *14*, 026003. [CrossRef] [PubMed]
17. Hoffmann, A.; Jäger, L.; Werhahn, K.J.; Jaschke, M.; Noachtar, S.; Reiser, M. Electroencephalography during functional echo-planar imaging: Detection of epileptic spikes using post-processing methods. *Magn. Reson. Med.* **2000**, *44*, 791–798. [CrossRef]
18. Gutberlet, I. Recording EEG signals inside the MRI. *Simul. EEG fMRI Rec. Anal. Appl.* **2010**, *2*, 69–83.
19. Mullinger, K.J.; Chowdhury, M.E.; Bowtell, R. Investigating the effect of modifying the EEG cap lead configuration on the gradient artifact in simultaneous EEG-fMRI. *Front. Neurosci.* **2014**, *8*, 226. [CrossRef] [PubMed]
20. Bonmassar, G.; Hadjikhani, N.; Ives, J.R.; Hinton, D.; Belliveau, J.W. Influence of EEG electrodes on the BOLD fMRI signal. *Hum. Brain Mapp.* **2001**, *14*, 108–115. [CrossRef] [PubMed]
21. Mandelkow, H.; Halder, P.; Boesiger, P.; Brandeis, D. Synchronization facilitates removal of MRI artefacts from concurrent EEG recordings and increases usable bandwidth. *Neuroimage* **2006**, *32*, 1120–1126. [CrossRef] [PubMed]
22. Zhou, W.; Bovik, A.C.; Sheikh, H.R.; Simoncelli, E.P. Image Qualifty Assessment: From Error Visibility to Structural Similarity. *IEEE Trans. Image Process.* **2004**, *13*, 600–612.
23. Ashburner, J.; Barnes, G.; Chen, C.; Daunizeau, J.; Flandin, G.; Friston, K.; Gitelman, D.; Kiebel, S.; Kilner, J.; Litvak, V. SPM8, 2012. Functional Imaging Laboratory, Institute of Neurology. Available online: https://www.fil.ion.ucl.ac.uk/spm (accessed on 10 September 2018).
24. Chowdhury, M.E.; Mullinger, K.J.; Bowtell, R. Simultaneous EEG-fMRI: Evaluating the effect of the EEG cap cabling configuration on the gradient artefact. Presented at the International Society for Magnetic Resonance in Medicine (ISMRM), Miami Beach, FL, USA, 7–13 May 2005.

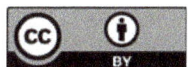

© 2018 by the authors. Licensee MDPI, Basel, Switzerland. This article is an open access article distributed under the terms and conditions of the Creative Commons Attribution (CC BY) license (http://creativecommons.org/licenses/by/4.0/).

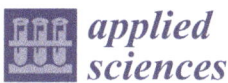 

*Article*

# Older Adults' Usability and Emotional Reactions toward Text, Diagram, Image, and Animation Interfaces for Displaying Health Information

Yu-Min Fang *[ID], Lin Chun and Bo-Cheng Chu

Department of Industrial Design, National United University, Miaoli 36003, Taiwan;
wildchaser07@gmail.com (L.C.); lkp53412@yahoo.com.tw (B.-C.C.)
* Correspondence: FanGeo@nuu.edu.tw; Tel.: +886-37-38-1664

Received: 1 February 2019; Accepted: 11 March 2019; Published: 13 March 2019

**Featured Application: Wearable devices design and personal health management.**

**Abstract:** Technology can facilitate the provision of healthcare to older adults. Wearable devices are thus increasingly prevalent amidst perpetual component miniaturization and cost reduction. This study aimed to determine whether existing application (app) interfaces are suitable for older adults by comparing the perceived usability and emotional reactions of younger users and older users to the health information display formats of wearable interfaces. Based on the outcomes of a literature review and expert recommendations, four health display interfaces—text, diagram, image, and animation—were developed and revised. Thirty respondents in Miaoli, Taiwan, were invited to participate in a questionnaire and interviews. The collected data were analyzed and discussed to develop design recommendations. The findings of this study were as follows: (1) the diagram interface had the lowest performance; (2) the respondents preferred the animation interface, which produced strong affective valence, thereby suggesting that animation generated positive emotions, yielding a result consistent with expert views and existing design principles; and (3) older users were more accepting of the text interface than the younger users, who exhibited negative emotions toward the text interface, highlighting a significant generation gap.

**Keywords:** health information; interface formats; older adults; wearable devices; usability; emotional reaction

## 1. Introduction

In an aged society, technology can facilitate the provision of healthcare to older adults [1–3]. The role of artificial intelligence (AI) and machine learning technologies is growing and is expected to be used across the entire healthcare ecosystem [4–7]. A majority of consumers are willing to consider AI technologies for managing their health, including monitoring heart condition (e.g., pulse, blood pressure, electrocardiography, etc.), providing customized advice for health based on their personal preferences and health records [7,8]. Furthermore, people are becoming more and more involved in managing their personal health using the internet of things (IoT) and wearable devices [9,10].

Wearable devices are becoming increasingly prevalent amidst perpetual component miniaturization and cost reduction. According to consumer data research, the healthcare wearables market is expected to reach $14.4 billion by 2022 [11,12]. These devices have enabled older users to track and manage their health information anytime, anywhere. In addition, as the voice user interfaces, such as Apple's Siri and Amazon's Alexa, becomes standard on wearables devices, these interactions increase ease of use for healthcare management [13,14]. In today's market, developers are constantly launching new health management applications (apps), providing more opportunities for older adults to use health information interfaces.

Wearable devices serve as both accessories and trackers of personal information. This information can be simultaneously transferred to the wearer and relevant parties. Wearable devices must be compatible with the user and their environment. Therefore, they are complex microdevices that facilitate human–computer interaction. With the evolution and innovation of new technology for this interaction, the design of visual display for older adults' health information was concerned in this study. Considering how older adults' physical and mental functions deteriorate with age, questions have arisen as to whether existing app interface designs are suitable for older adults and whether the perceived usability of these app interfaces differs for younger users and older adults. Many scholars asserted that products become more acceptable to users when they are able to incite positive emotions [15–17]. Therefore, it is important to elucidate how visual health information interfaces incite affective valence and arouse older adults. This study analyzed the display formats of health information on wearable interfaces to determine perceived usability and emotional reactions, with the goal of improving healthcare for older adults.

A literature review and a sample analysis were performed to identify four different interface formats, namely text, diagram, image, and animation, and a questionnaire was conducted to test them. This study examined the differences in how the four interfaces are used by younger users and older adults, and highlighted the advantages and disadvantages of the interfaces. Several design suggestions are presented based on the research findings.

The objectives of this study were as follows:

1. To analyze the display formats for visualizing health information and test the usability of these formats.
2. To investigate users' acceptance and comprehension of the display formats and determine the affective valence and arousal elicited by these formats.
3. To compare the responses of younger users and older users to the different formats.

This research, however, is subject to several limitations. Providing sound feedback can enhance the user interface design. Furthermore, applying the technology of voice user interfaces to assist communication is growing as the rapid development of AI [18,19]. This research only focuses on different types of visual interfaces and regards sound/voice as a controlled variable. Therefore, as with the majority of studies, the findings of this study have to be seen in light of some limitations.

## 2. Literature Review

### 2.1. Wearable Devices and Aging

Wearable devices are defined as apparel or accessories embedded with electronic components or computers. These devices adhere comfortably to the human body and provide a variety of functions. The purpose of wearable devices is to satisfy the demand for stable, convenient, comprehensive, and hands-free electronics. Wearable devices focus on user communication, providing information in real-time. In certain situations, these devices are superior to handheld devices, such as when tracking vital signs [20,21].

A United Nations report predicted that the global elderly population in the twenty-first century will exceed the total world population in the previous century [22]. Monitoring the health conditions of older adults through wearable devices helps delay the aging process, improves quality of life, promotes independent lifestyles, minimizes hospitalization and mortality rates, and reduces healthcare cost [1,23]. To achieve these objectives, wearable devices can be coupled with wireless technologies to track vital signs and health conditions on-the-go, achieving effective information management [24].

Older adults' physical and mental functions gradually deteriorate with age. Therefore, a specific set of design principles should be followed when designing products for older users [25–28].

Understanding the characteristics of older adults' physical and mental functions enables designers to create products suitable for these users. In the future, wearable device designs will focus more on fashion trends, practicality, and functionality. The findings of a previous study on older adults' perceptions of wearable computers showed that they preferred wearable devices that were concealed [3].

## 2.2. Information Visualization: Definition and Classification

Information visualization refers to the conversion of information into different visual formats that can be easily viewed on small interfaces. Information visualization effectively reduces the effort required to process information, helping users quickly understand large amounts of information [29,30]. One example is the Health App on Apple Watch, a wearable device launched in 2015, which uses circles and numbers to represent health information (Figure 1). Apple also introduced a new interactive mode for this device, comprising images, audio messages, haptic touch, and information sharing. Another example is the TrackMeo app for Android (Figure 2). The app, designed largely for patients with cardiovascular diseases, provides cardiovascular and health information on smart devices.

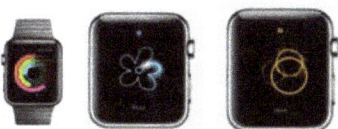

**Figure 1.** Health App by Apple.

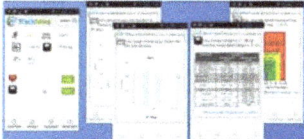

**Figure 2.** TrackMeo by Google.

According to past conversion accuracy analyses (from concrete to abstract) [31,32], information display models can be classified into three dimensions (Table 1): information indices, images, and symbols. Each dimension contains several interface formats. Information indices comprise measuring instruments, maps, and photographs. Images can be drawings, doodles, caricatures, or metaphors. Symbols can be linguistic (text and numeric) or abstract.

**Table 1.** Information display dimensions and formats.

| Accuracy | Information Display Model | Example | Interface Format |
|---|---|---|---|
| Concrete to abstract | Information indices | | Measuring instruments, maps, photographs |
| | Images | | Drawings, doodles, caricatures |
| | | | Metaphors |
| | Symbols | | Linguistic (letters and numbers) |
| | | | Abstract |

## 2.3. Health Information Interface Formats

In this study, 60 health information display interfaces on hardware equipment (traditional and digital sphygmomanometers), digital hardware equipment, mobile devices (smartphones and tablets), and wearable devices were selected to analyze the formats of different health information interfaces. Previous studies have highlighted that information presentation and content are crucial aspects of display design and that text, graphics, images, and color serve to express informational content [33,34]. However, people's demand for human–computer interaction has increased due to technological advancement. Animation has become a key element for enhancing design attractiveness and usability [32]. In this study, the aforementioned classifications were consolidated, and a classification comprising four formats (text, diagrams, images, and animation) was developed for subsequent analysis.

Text is a basic, easy-to-understand information display format [35,36]. Therefore, it has been used in numerous devices, including traditional hardware and wearable devices (Figure 3). Diagrams typically present statistics, allowing users to easily interpret statistical significance and variance. The diagram format is widely applied in mobile and wearable devices (Figure 4). For example, bar charts are often used to show repeated test results, allowing users to quickly track their long-term health information. Line charts can also help users interpret changes at various points in time. Images refer to small metaphoric depictions of real-world objects. These images facilitate learning and memorization (Figure 5) [33]. Animation has become a favored design element among designers. When effectively applied, it can help first-time users of an app quickly adapt to the design. Meaningful animation enhances the attractiveness of the design and guides users in operating the interface [37]. Animating health information not only improves storytelling but also makes the information interesting and affective (Figure 6).

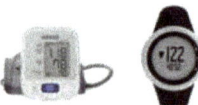

**Figure 3.** Omron upper-arm sphygmomanometer HEM-7121 and Suunto M1 heart rate monitor.

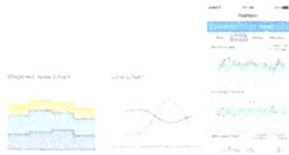

**Figure 4.** Charts for Google developers and iHealth Gluco-Smart.

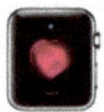

**Figure 5.** Images: Apple Watch.

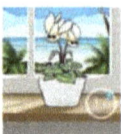

**Figure 6.** Animation: Plant Nanny.

*2.4. SAM, SUS, and QUIS Scales*

The Self-Assessment Manikin (SAM) was adopted in this study to measure emotion. The SAM is a pictorial assessment developed by Mehrabian and Russell to measure affective responses [38]. This semantic scale describes three emotional aspects: emotional valence, arousal, and dominance. These aspects are measured with emotional images to rate 18 different emotional states. The scope of the application of this tool is the emotional measurement used in the computer interaction procedure [38,39]. Two emotional aspects, valence and arousal, were measured and rated on a nine-point scale. Antonymous semantic adjectives were added to the left and right to help respondents interpret the pictures.

The System Usability Scale (SUS) and the Questionnaires for User Interaction Satisfaction (QUIS) were adopted in this study to measure usability. The SUS is a widely applied measuring tool proposed by John Brooke in 1986. The scale can be used to measure subjective perceptions concerning the use of product interfaces, desktop applications, and website interfaces [40,41]. These perceptions are scored on a scale of 1 to 100.

The QUIS was proposed by Chin and Norman in 1987. This scale can be used to measure users' subjective satisfaction with specific aspects of human–computer interaction [42–44]. The QUIS is executed on a seven-point scale and divided into five categories: overall reaction, screen, terminology/system information, learning, and system capabilities [45]. It was modified in this study for health information display interfaces; "overall reaction" and "screen" were the only categories used.

**3. Materials and Methods**

A survey was conducted to determine the perceived usability of different interface formats based on the emotional reactions of younger and older respondents. Different visualization formats for health information were developed as the sample designs in the survey. A preliminary questionnaire regarding the four types of health information display interfaces was developed for the pretest. Experts were invited to test the questionnaire and provide suggestions. These suggestions were adopted to revise the samples and the questionnaire.

A total of 30 respondents were invited to participate in the formal survey, which was divided into three stages. First, the respondents provided personal information and completed a health knowledge test. Then, a portable computer was used to present the four interface samples. Each interface was presented to the respondents for 5 s, in which time they were required to interpret the health information. Thereafter, they completed the interface interpretation questionnaire. Finally, the respondents were instructed to complete the main questionnaire to measure their level of comprehension, information adequacy, preferences, affective valence and arousal (SAM), and perceived usability (SUS, QUIS) concerning the four interfaces. After the formal survey, all respondents participated in a semistructured interview.

A one-way analysis of variance (ANOVA) was performed on the data collected from the questionnaire survey and interviews to validate the relationships between the variables. A least significant difference (LSD) test and Scheffé test were adopted for post-hoc validation.

*3.1. Subjects*

The pretest participants were four graduate students from National United University, Taiwan (two men and two women) and older male expert. All had prior experience using smart devices, and four had prior experience using health information apps. Thirty students from National United University and their family members were recruited to participate in the formal test. All respondents completed and submitted written informed consent prior to the test. Among the participants, 13 were men (43.3%) and 17 were women (56.7%). Three were aged 20–29 years, seven were aged 30–39 years, seven were aged 40–49 years, 11 were aged 50–65 years, and two were aged over 65 years. For the statistical analysis, respondents aged between 20 and 49 years (17 respondents) were classified as younger users, and those aged 50 years and above (13 respondents) were classified as older users.

*3.2. Materials*

A number of studies were reviewed to analyze relevant design principles. The four design graduates from the National United University assisted the researchers in collecting 60 health information display interfaces on the market during the time of research. Then, several of these interfaces for blood pressure information were redesigned by using Adobe Illustrator and printed out on paper for the pretest. Following the pretest, an expert discussion was organized, after which the four graduate students discussed and revised the interfaces. They considered the interfacing approach, amount of information displayed, degree of abstraction, and level of dynamics, finally retaining four test samples. The pretest also showed that the respondents were biased by color. Therefore, a standard color palette was developed for all the interface samples. The samples used in the formal test were text, diagram, image, and animation interfaces. The selection process also accounted for these four interface formats presented in previous studies on display design [33,46]. Since animation has become a factor influencing users' attention and usability perceptions in recent years [32], an animation sample was also included in the sample lineup to enhance research integrity. Animations were created using Adobe Flash. In the formal survey, the main questionnaires were on paper, and all interface samples were embedded in Adobe Flash Player and presented on a 15" portable computer.

Normal value ranges for SYS and DIA on the text interface were between 90 and 140 mmHg and 60 and 90 mmHg, respectively. A value above or below these ranges indicated abnormal blood pressure. The diagram interface also followed the preceding principles. However, values were expressed as bar charts. In the image interface, a circle denoted normal blood pressure and a cross denoted abnormal blood pressure. In the animation interface, a smiley face denoted normal blood pressure and a sad face denoted an abnormal blood pressure. The eyes and mouth repeatedly moved every one second to enhance facial expressions of emotion. The sample designs and characteristics are displayed in Table 2.

**Table 2.** Sample design and interface characteristics.

| Sample Name | Text | Diagram | Image | Animation |
|---|---|---|---|---|
| Healthy | | | | |
| Unhealthy | | | | |
| Interfacing approach | Text, number | Diagram, bar chart | Image, metaphor | Animation, personification |
| Information scale | Rate | Rate | Type | Type |
| Information type | Detailed numbers | Data range | Status | Status |
| Level of abstraction | Random | Random | Random | Portrait |

*3.3. Questionnaire Design*

A quantitative design was adopted to develop a three-part questionnaire (Table 3). The first part focused on respondents' demographics (gender, age, and product experience) and health awareness. The health awareness section consisted of a health value scale and a health knowledge scale, which were revised from the questionnaire used in the Survey on Knowledge, Attitude, and Practice of Health Promotion in Taiwan [47]. The scales surveyed the respondents' feelings toward their health, perceived value of their health, understanding of health information, and health examination knowledge (including blood pressure knowledge).

Table 3. Questionnaire content.

| Items | Number of Items | Items | Content |
|---|---|---|---|
| 1. Basic information and background | 12 | Multiple choice | Respondents' backgrounds, health values, and health knowledge |
| 2. Information correctness | 20 | True or false/converted to five points | Respondents' accuracy in interpreting the health information |
| 3.1. Comprehension Preference Information adequacy | 3 | Five-point Likert scale | Understandability of the four interfaces Respondents' preferences Adequacy of the content displayed |
| 3.2. SAM | 2 | Nine-point Likert scale | Respondents' affective valence and arousal |
| 3.3. SUS | 10 | Five-point Likert scale/converted to 1–100 scale | Perceived interface usability |
| 3.4. QUIS | 11 | Seven-point SD scale | Respondents' satisfaction |

The second part tested the respondents' interface interpretation performance. The respondents were presented with health information on one of the four interfaces for 5 s to measure the accuracy of their interpretation of the information. To facilitate statistical analysis, the respondents' scores were converted to a five-point scale.

The third part was the main questionnaire. (1) A five-point Likert scale was adopted to measure the respondents' comprehension, preferences, and perceived information adequacy. (2) The nine-point SAM was adopted to measure the respondents' affective valence and arousal. (3) The five-point SUS was used to measure perceived usability. Respondents' scores were converted to a scale of 1–100. (4) The revised seven-point QUIS (containing 11 items after revision) was adopted to measure the respondents' interface usability satisfaction.

In addition to the formal survey, a semistructured interview was conducted to explore the explanations for the survey results. The interview consisted of three parts: (1) the respondents' consideration in preferences (Item 3.1 in questionnaire content) towards these four types of interfaces; (2) the respondents' suggestions to revise the interface and their reasons; and (3) the respondents' opinions to the comprehension, adequacy, and usability towards these four types of interfaces.

## 4. Results and Discussion

In this study, the perceived usability and affective valence of the younger and older users concerning the four interface formats were analyzed. The variables were interpretation accuracy, comprehension, preference, affective valence and arousal (SAM), usability (SUS and QUIS), and semistructured interviews.

*4.1. Subjects' Backgrounds*

Thirty subjects were recruited to participate in the formal test. The first part of the questionnaire focused on respondents' backgrounds and health awareness. Regarding the experiences of using smart products, eight of the respondents were very experienced users, nine were experienced, 10 were inexperienced, and three were very inexperienced. Regarding various computer products, two were very experienced users, four were experienced, 11 were average, seven were inexperienced, and six were very inexperienced. Regarding health apps, one of the respondents was a frequent user, two were occasional users, 10 were infrequent users, and 17 were nonusers (Table 4). The background questionnaire showed that, regarding participants' demand for health information, a consolidation of the data (marked "moderate" or above for this item) revealed that 90% of the respondents concerning their desire to receive health information. Regarding respondents' willingness and usage frequency of healthcare apps, 72.5% of the respondents expressing a moderate desire to use healthcare apps; however, few respondents (3.3%) used them frequently.

Table 4. Respondents' experiences and usage frequency for relative products and apps.

| Item | Experience | | | | |
|---|---|---|---|---|---|
| | Very Experienced | Experienced | Average | Inexperienced | Very Inexperienced |
| smart products | 8 (26.7%) | 9 (30.0%) | 0 (0%) | 10 (33.3%) | 3 (10.0%) |
| computer products | 2 (6.7%) | 4 (13.3%) | 11 (36.7%) | 7 (23.3%) | 6 (20.0%) |
| | Usage Frequency | | | | |
| Item | Frequent | | Occasional | Infrequent | Nonusers |
| health apps | 1 (3.3%) | | 2 (6.7%) | 10 (33.3%) | 17 (56.7%) |

Only a few younger users (2.5%) were in the habit of measuring chronic illnesses, with 97.5% expressing that they seldom did so. This was attributed to how younger users youngerly perceived themselves to be healthy. Moreover, the younger users generally led a substandard lifestyle, but showed increased awareness of blood pressure. This knowledge was attributed to successful health education.

*4.2. Analysis of Interpretation Accuracy, Comprehension, Preference, and Information Adequacy*

The overall means and standard deviations for interpretation accuracy, comprehension, preference, and information adequacy are tabulated in Table 5. The results of the one-way ANOVA revealed that text, diagrams, images, and animation achieved significant statistical differences (<0.05). A comparison of the interpretation accuracy, comprehension, and preference for the four interfaces is illustrated in Figure 7. The results of the post-hoc test are provided in Table 6.

Table 5. Average mean and standard deviation values for interpretation accuracy, comprehension, preference, and information adequacy (standard deviation in parentheses; unit: points; five-point Likert scale).

| Category | Text | Diagram | Image | Animation |
|---|---|---|---|---|
| Interpretation accuracy | 4.37(0.96) | 2.80(0.66) | 4.80(0.66) | 4.73(0.64) |
| Comprehension | 3.63(1.189) | 2.87(0.90) | 3.87(1.14) | 4.07((0.94) |
| Preference | 3.33(0.88) | 2.77(0.93) | 3.27(1.20) | 3.80(0.96) |
| Information adequacy | 3.30(0.95) | 3.03(1.03) | 3.23(1.30) | 3.53(1.17) |

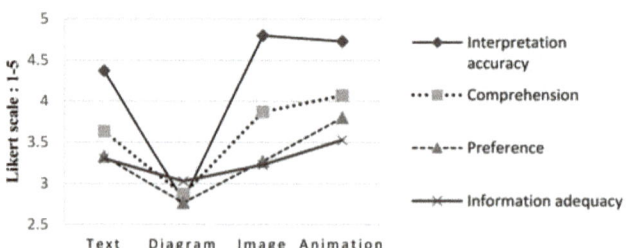

Figure 7. Comparison of interpretation accuracy, comprehension, preference, and information adequacy (unit: points; five-point Likert scale).

Each variable is discussed individually as follows.

**Interpretation accuracy:** The respondents achieved the highest interpretation accuracy for the image interface, followed by the animation, text, and diagram interfaces. The ANOVA results indicated that the data achieved statistical significance. Post-hoc test results showed that the interpretation accuracy for the diagram interface was significantly lower than those for the text, image, and animation interfaces ($p = 0.000$ *). The other results failed to achieve statistical significance. Therefore, information interpretation accuracy is a key factor to consider when designing diagram interfaces.

**Comprehension:** The animation interface was the easiest for the respondents to understand, followed by the image, text, and diagram interfaces. ANOVA results indicated that the data achieved statistical significance. Post-hoc test results showed that the diagram interface achieved significant differences with the image ($p = 0.005$ *) and animation ($p = 0.000$ *) interfaces. The other results failed to achieve statistical significance. This suggests that animation and image interfaces are preferable for information presentation.

**Preference:** The respondents preferred the animation interface the most, followed by the text, image, and diagram interfaces. The ANOVA results indicated that the data achieved statistical significance. Post-hoc test results showed that the preferences for the animation interface were significantly greater than those for the diagrams ($p = 0.002$ *). These results suggest that respondents preferred animation interfaces to image interfaces.

**Information Adequacy:** The mean adequacy values of the four interfaces were compared to determine respondents' perceived information adequacy. The results showed that the animation interface demonstrated the highest information adequacy, followed by the text, image, and diagram interfaces. However, these results failed to achieve statistical significance.

**Table 6.** Post-hoc test: interpretation accuracy, comprehension, and preference.

| | Interpretation Accuracy | | | |
|---|---|---|---|---|
| Significance | Text | Diagram | Image | Animation |
| Text |  | 0.000 * | 0.173 | 0.309 |
| Diagram | 0.000 * |  | 0.000 * | 0.000 * |
| Image | 0.173 | 0.000 * |  | 0.989 |
| Animation | 0.309 | 0.000 * | 0.989 |  |
| | Comprehension | | | |
| Significance | Text | Diagram | Image | Animation |
| Text |  | 0.051 | 0.863 | 0.468 |
| Diagram | 0.051 |  | 0.005 * | 0.000 * |
| Image | 0.863 | 0.005 * |  | 0.909 |
| Animation | 0.468 | 0.000 * | 0.909 |  |
| | Preference | | | |
| Significance | Text | Diagram | Image | Animation |
| Text |  | 0.194 | 0.996 | 0.359 |
| Diagram | 0.194 |  | 0.298 | 0.002 * |
| Image | 0.996 | 0.298 |  | 0.242 |
| Animation | 0.359 | 0.002 * | 0.242 |  |

* represents statistical difference; $p < 0.05$.

*4.3. Affective Valence and Arousal*

The SAM was adopted to measure the respondents' affective valence and arousal concerning the four interface formats. A one-way ANOVA was used to analyze the data. The means (and standard deviations, presented in parentheses) are tabulated in Table 7.

**Table 7.** Means and standard deviations for affective valence and arousal (standard deviation in parentheses; unit: points; nine-point Likert scale).

| Group | Text | Diagram | Image | Animation |
|---|---|---|---|---|
| Affective valence | 6.10(1.97) | 4.77(1.61) | 6.07(1.80) | 7.03(1.65) |
| Arousal | 4.30(1.80) | 4.20(1.79) | 4.73(1.60) | 4.80(1.97) |

**Affective valence:** A high score denoted high affective valence for health information. A review of the means showed that the respondents had the highest affective valence for the animation interface, followed by the text, image, and diagram interfaces (Figure 8). Analysis results showed that on average, respondents gave scores of less than five for the diagram interface, suggesting that they disliked it. By comparison, the other interfaces scored an average of six or higher, suggesting that the respondents found these interfaces to be more pleasing. ANOVA results indicated that the data achieved statistical significance. Post-hoc test results showed that the diagram interface scored significantly lower than the other three interfaces ($p = 0.040$ *, $p = 0.048$ *, $p = 0.000$ *). The results of the text, image, and animation interfaces failed to achieve significant differences (Table 8). The findings of this study indicated that diagram interfaces are less able than other interfaces to incite affective valence among users.

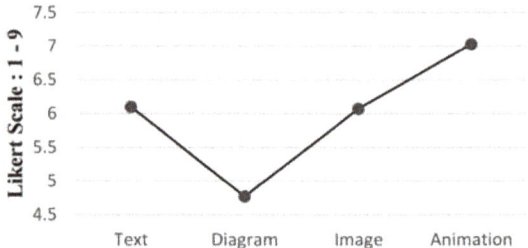

**Figure 8.** Comparison of affective valences (unit: points; nine-point Likert scale).

**Table 8.** Post-hoc test of affective valence: significance of the four interfaces.

| Significance | Text | Diagram | Image | Animation |
|---|---|---|---|---|
| Text |  | 0.040 * | 1.000 | 0.246 |
| Diagram | 0.040 * |  | 0.048 * | 0.000 * |
| Image | 1.000 | 0.048 * |  | 0.218 |
| Animation | 0.246 | 0.000 * | 0.218 |  |

* represents statistical difference; $p < 0.05$.

**Arousal:** The respondents displayed the most evident emotional arousal when interpreting health information on the animation interface, followed by the image, text, and diagram interfaces. The means were between 4 and 5. ANOVA results indicated that the data failed to achieve statistical significance.

### 4.4. Usability

**SUS**

The SUS was adopted to measure the respondents' perceived usability of the four interfaces. The overall means and standard deviations are shown in Table 9. A comparison of the results is illustrated in Figure 9. The one-way ANOVA results demonstrate that the interfaces achieved significant differences ($p < 0.05$).

**Table 9.** Average means and standard deviations of the four interfaces according to the SUS results (standard deviation in parentheses; full score = 100).

| Group | Text | Diagram | Image | Animation |
|---|---|---|---|---|
| SUS | 72.1(25.28) | 47.7(27.60) | 70(23.58) | 80(23.55) |

Regarding usability, the text, image, and animation interfaces received scores of over 70. The ANOVA and post-hoc test results indicated that the perceived usability of the diagram interface was significantly lower than the other interfaces ($p = 0.004$ *, $p = 0.007$ *, $p = 0.000$ *). The perceived usability of the text, image, and animation interfaces failed to achieve significant differences (Table 10). The findings showed that the performance of only the diagram interface was considered unacceptable.

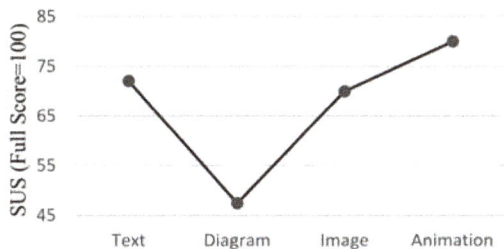

**Figure 9.** Comparison of SUS results (full score = 100).

**Table 10.** Post-hoc test of usability: significance of the four interfaces.

|  | Text | Diagram | Image | Animation |
|---|---|---|---|---|
| Text |  | 0.004 * | 0.998 | 0.672 |
| Diagram | 0.004 * |  | 0.007 * | 0.000 * |
| Image | 0.998 | 0.007 * |  | 0.561 |
| Animation | 0.672 | 0.000 * | 0.561 |  |

* represents statistical difference; $p < 0.05$.

## QUIS

The items in the "overall reaction" and "screen" sections of the QUIS were used to elucidate the respondents' satisfaction with the four interface formats. The overall means and standard deviations are tabulated in Table 11. A comparison chart is illustrated in Figure 10.

**Table 11.** Average means and standard deviations according to the QUIS (standard deviation in parentheses; unit: points; seven-point Likert scale).

| Group | Text | Diagram | Image | Animation |
|---|---|---|---|---|
| Overall reaction | 4.83(1.61) | 3.53(1.62) | 5.00(1.49) | 5.13(1.49) |
| Screen | 5.39(1.21) | 3.82(1.72) | 5.12(1.52) | 5.53(1.47) |

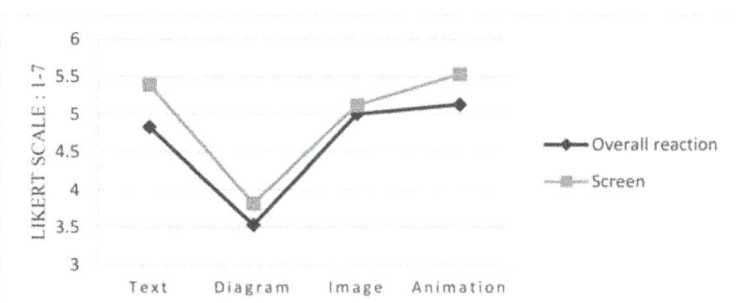

**Figure 10.** Overall reaction comparison (unit: points; seven-point Likert scale).

The respondents scored the "overall reaction" section greater than 4 and the "screen" section greater than 5, on average, for the text, image, and animation interfaces, suggesting that they responded positively, aside from the diagram interface. ANOVA results indicated that the data achieved statistical significance. Post-hoc test results for the "overall reaction" and "screen" sections indicate that the values for the diagram interface were significantly lower than those for the text, image, and animation interfaces. No significant differences were exhibited between the values of the text, image, and animation interfaces (Table 12). The findings indicated that diagram interface designs have poor overall reaction and screen performance.

**Table 12.** Post-hoc test of "overall reaction" and "screen": significance of the four interfaces.

| Overall Reaction | | | | |
|---|---|---|---|---|
| Significance | Text | Diagram | Image | Animation |
| Text |  | 0.018 * | 0.982 | 0.418 |
| Diagram | 0.018 * |  | 0.005 * | 0.000 * |
| Image | 0.982 | 0.005 * |  | 0.654 |
| Animation | 0.418 | 0.000 * | 0.654 |  |
| Screen | | | | |
| Significance | Text | Diagram | Image | Animation |
| Text |  | 0.001 * | 0.924 | 0.988 |
| Diagram | 0.001 * |  | 0.012 * | 0.000 * |
| Image | 0.924 | 0.012 * |  | 0.778 |
| Animation | 0.988 | 0.000 * | 0.778 |  |

\* represents statistical difference; $p < 0.05$.

*4.5. Comparison of Younger and Older Users*

**Comprehension**

The mean and standard deviation values concerning the younger and older respondents' comprehension of the four interfaces are tabulated in Table 13. A comparison chart is illustrated in Figure 11.

**Table 13.** Means and standard deviations for comprehension (standard deviation in parentheses, unit: points; five-point Likert scale).

| Group | Text | Diagram | Image | Animation |
|---|---|---|---|---|
| Younger users | 3.29(1.16) | 2.76(0.90) | 3.94(1.20) | 4.24(1.03) |
| Older users | 4.08(1.12) | 3(0.91) | 3.77(1.09) | 3.85(0.80) |

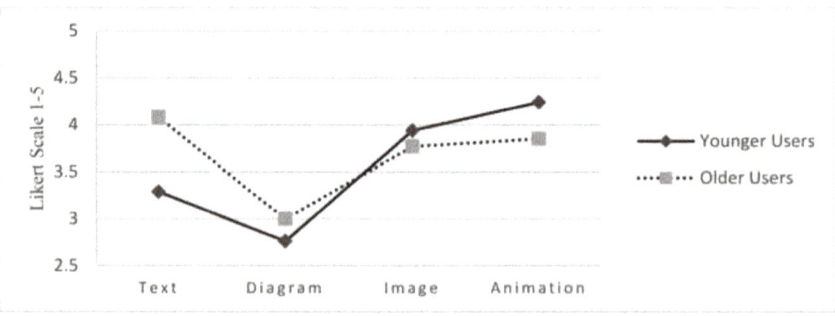

**Figure 11.** Comprehension comparison of the four interfaces.

ANOVA results indicated that the data achieved statistical significance. Post-hoc test results (Table 14) indicated that (1) the younger respondents' comprehension of the animation interface was significantly different from that of the diagram and text interfaces ($p = 0.010$ * and $p = 0.000$ *), suggesting that they more fully understood the animation interface; (2) the older respondents' comprehension of the diagram interface was significantly different from that of the text and animation interfaces ($p = 0.010$ * and $p = 0.041$ *), suggesting that they found it more difficult to interpret the health information on the diagram interface than that on the text or animation interfaces; and (3) a comparison of comprehension in the two groups for all four interfaces showed that the text interface achieves statistical differences ($p = 0.044$ *), suggesting that the older respondents were more capable of understanding the information on the text interface than the younger respondents.

**Table 14.** Post-hoc comparison of younger and older users' comprehension of the four interfaces.

|  |  | Younger Users | | | | Older Users | | | |
| --- | --- | --- | --- | --- | --- | --- | --- | --- | --- |
|  |  | Text | Diagram | Image | Animation | Text | Diagram | Image | Animation |
| Younger users | Text |  | 0.141 | 0.073 | 0.010 * | 0.044 * | 0.445 | 0.218 | 0.153 |
|  | Diagram | 0.141 |  | 0.001 * | 0.000 * | 0.001 * | 0.541 | 0.010 * | 0.006 * |
|  | Image | 0.073 | 0.001 * |  | 0.412 | 0.724 | 0.016 * | 0.655 | 0.805 |
|  | Animation | 0.010 * | 0.000 * | 0.412 |  | 0.681 | 0.002 * | 0.227 | 0.313 |
| Older users | Text | 0.044 * | 0.001 * | 0.724 | 0.681 |  | 0.010 * | 0.453 | 0.573 |
|  | Diagram | 0.445 | 0.541 | 0.016 * | 0.002 * | 0.010 * |  | 0.062 | 0.041 * |
|  | Image | 0.218 | 0.010 * | 0.655 | 0.227 | 0.453 | 0.062 |  | 0.851 |
|  | Animation | 0.153 | 0.006 * | 0.805 | 0.313 | 0.573 | 0.041 * | 0.851 |  |

* represents statistical difference; $p < 0.05$.

### SAM: Affective Valence

The means and standard deviations concerning the younger and older respondents' affective valences of the four interfaces are tabulated in Table 15, with the standard deviations in parentheses. A comparison chart is illustrated in Figure 12.

**Table 15.** Means and standard deviations for affective valence (standard deviation in parentheses, unit: points; nine-point Likert scale).

| Group | Text | Diagram | Image | Animation |
| --- | --- | --- | --- | --- |
| Younger Users | 5.41(1.77) | 4.94(1.39) | 6.00(1.90) | 7.24(1.64) |
| Older Users | 7(1.91) | 4.54(1.89) | 6.15(1.72) | 6.77(1.69) |

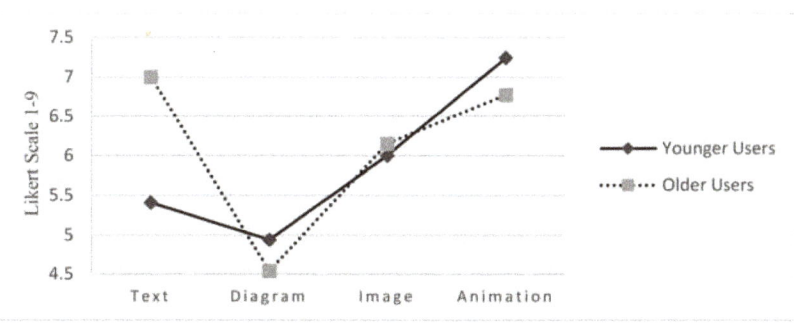

**Figure 12.** Comparison of affective valences of the four interfaces.

ANOVA results indicated that the data achieved statistical significance. Post-hoc test results (Table 16) indicated that (1) the younger respondents had a higher affective valence for the animation interface than the other three interfaces ($p = 0.003$ *, $p = 0.000$ *, $p = 0.041$ *), suggesting that the animation interface produced the highest affective valence, consistent with general expert and design principals; (2) the older respondents had a significantly lower valence for the diagram interface than the other three interfaces ($p = 0.000$ *, $p = 0.020$ *, $p = 0.001$ *); and (3) a comparison of the affective valence in the two groups for all four interfaces showed that the text interface achieved significant differences ($p = 0.015$ *), suggesting that younger respondents had a lower affective valence for the text interface.

**Table 16.** Post-hoc comparison of younger and older users concerning affective valences.

|  |  | Younger Users | | | | Older Users | | | |
| --- | --- | --- | --- | --- | --- | --- | --- | --- | --- |
|  |  | Text | Diagram | Image | Animation | Text | Diagram | Image | Animation |
| Younger users | Text |  | 0.432 | 0.327 | 0.003 * | 0.015 * | 0.176 | 0.250 | 0.037 |
|  | Diagrams | 0.432 |  | 0.079 | 0.000 * | 0.002 * | 0.531 | 0.061 | 0.005 * |
|  | Images | 0.327 | 0.079 |  | 0.041 * | 0.122 | 0.025 * | 0.811 | 0.233 |
|  | Animation | 0.003 * | 0.000 * | 0.041 * |  | 0.714 | 0.000 * | 0.095 | 0.469 |
| Older users | Text | 0.015 * | 0.002 * | 0.122 | 0.714 |  | 0.000 * | 0.218 | 0.736 |
|  | Diagrams | 0.176 | 0.531 | 0.025 * | 0.000 * | 0.000 * |  | 0.020 * | 0.001 * |
|  | Images | 0.250 | 0.061 | 0.811 | 0.095 | 0.218 | 0.020 * |  | 0.369 |
|  | Animation | 0.037 * | 0.005 * | 0.233 | 0.469 | 0.736 | 0.001 * | 0.369 |  |

* represents statistical difference; $p < 0.05$.

**SUS: Usability**

The means and standard deviations concerning the younger and older respondents' perceived usability of the four interfaces are tabulated in Table 17. A comparison chart is illustrated in Figure 13.

**Table 17.** Means and standard deviations for SUS (standard deviation in parentheses; full score = 100).

| Group | Text | Diagram | Image | Animation |
| --- | --- | --- | --- | --- |
| Younger Users | 63.23(25.25) | 44.41(24.67) | 68.38(25.10) | 80.08(27.78) |
| Older Users | 83.84(20.83) | 52.11(31.52) | 74.23(21.97) | 80.38(17.64) |

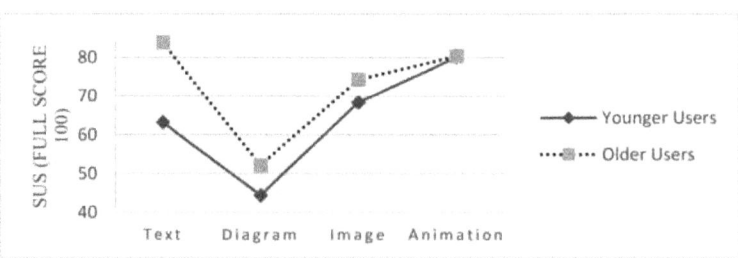

**Figure 13.** Comparison of the SUS results of the younger and older users.

ANOVA results indicated that the data achieved statistical significance. Post-hoc test results (Table 18) indicated that (1) the SUS scores (perceived usability) for the diagram interface were significantly lower than the other interfaces in both groups, suggesting that the diagram interfaces had the least favorable performance in terms of usability; and (2) a comparison between the two groups showed that older respondents largely perceived the text interface to have the highest usability, indicating that the older respondents' scores for the text interface were significantly higher than those of the younger respondents ($p = 0.026$ *), and thereby suggesting that the two groups had different opinions on the text interface.

**Table 18.** Post-hoc comparison of younger and older users' SUS results.

|  |  | Younger Users | | | | Older Users | | | |
| --- | --- | --- | --- | --- | --- | --- | --- | --- | --- |
|  |  | Text | Diagram | Image | Animation | Text | Diagram | Image | Animation |
| Younger users | Text |  | 0.029 * | 0.547 | 0.05 | 0.026 * | 0.227 | 0.232 | 0.063 |
|  | Diagrams | 0.029 * |  | 0.006 * | 0.000 * | 0.000 * | 0.402 | 0.001 * | 0.000 * |
|  | Images | 0.547 | 0.006 * |  | 0.172 | 0.094 | 0.078 | 0.524 | 0.192 |
|  | Animation | 0.05 | 0.000 * | 0.172 |  | 0.682 | 0.003 * | 0.523 | 0.974 |
| Older users | Text | 0.026 * | 0.000 * | 0.094 | 0.682 |  | 0.001 * | 0.326 | 0.723 |
|  | Diagrams | 0.227 | 0.402 | 0.078 | 0.003 * | 0.001 * |  | 0.025 * | 0.004 * |
|  | Images | 0.232 | 0.001 * | 0.524 | 0.523 | 0.326 | 0.025 * |  | 0.529 |
|  | Animation | 0.063 | 0.000 * | 0.192 | 0.974 | 0.723 | 0.004 * | 0.529 |  |

\* represents statistical difference; $p < 0.05$.

## QUIS: Overall Reaction and Screen

The means and standard deviations of the younger and older respondents' overall reactions to the four interfaces are tabulated in Table 19. A comparison chart is illustrated in Figure 14.

**Table 19.** Means and standard deviations for overall reactions (standard deviation in parentheses, unit: points; seven-point Likert scale).

| Group | Text | Diagram | Image | Animation |
| --- | --- | --- | --- | --- |
| Younger Users | 4.22(1.53) | 3.43(1.59) | 5.04(1.55) | 5.67(1.63) |
| Older Users | 5.63(1.38) | 3.66(1.72) | 4.93(1.46) | 5.30(1.31) |

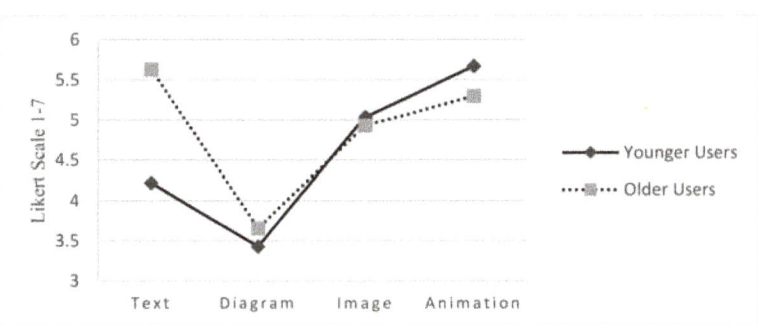

**Figure 14.** Comparison of overall reactions to the four interfaces.

The means and standard deviations of the younger and older respondents' comprehension of the four interfaces are tabulated in Table 20. A comparison chart is depicted in Figure 15.

**Table 20.** Means and standard deviations for screen. (standard deviation in parentheses, unit: points; seven-point Likert scale).

| Group | Text | Diagram | Image | Animation |
| --- | --- | --- | --- | --- |
| Younger Users | 5.01(1.29) | 3.74(1.72) | 5.22(1.65) | 5.62(1.61) |
| Older Users | 5.89(0.92) | 3.92(1.78) | 5.00(1.38) | 5.41(1.32) |

ANOVA results indicated that both the "overall reaction" and "screen" sections of the QUIS achieved significance. The post-hoc test results for the Overall Reaction section are tabulated in Table 21, and those for the "screen" section are tabulated in Table 22.

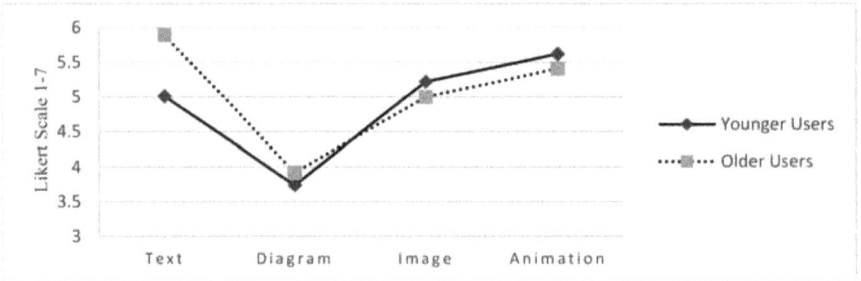

**Figure 15.** Comparison of the screen results of younger and older users.

**Table 21.** Post-hoc test of younger and older users' overall reactions to the four interfaces.

|  |  | Younger Users |  |  |  | Older Users |  |  |  |
|---|---|---|---|---|---|---|---|---|---|
|  |  | Text | Diagram | Image | Animation | Text | Diagram | Image | Animation |
| Younger users | Text |  | 0.138 | 0.122 | 0.007 * | 0.015 * | 0.324 | 0.210 | 0.059 |
|  | Diagrams | 0.138 |  | 0.003 * | 0.000 * | 0.000 * | 0.691 | 0.009 * | 0.001 * |
|  | Images | 0.122 | 0.003 * |  | 0.240 | 0.306 | 0.016 * | 0.849 | 0.647 |
|  | Animation | 0.007 * | 0.000 * | 0.240 |  | 0.944 | 0.001 * | 0.200 | 0.524 |
| Older users | Text | 0.015 * | 0.000 * | 0.306 | 0.944 |  | 0.001 * | 0.254 | 0.594 |
|  | Diagrams | 0.324 | 0.691 | 0.016 * | 0.001 * | 0.001 * |  | 0.037 * | 0.007 * |
|  | Images | 0.210 | 0.009 * | 0.849 | 0.200 | 0.254 | 0.037 * |  | 0.542 |
|  | Animation | 0.059 | 0.001 * | 0.647 | 0.524 | 0.594 | 0.007 * | 0.542 |  |

* represents statistical difference; $p < 0.05$.

**Table 22.** Post-hoc screen test of younger and older users.

|  |  | Younger Users |  |  |  | Older Users |  |  |  |
|---|---|---|---|---|---|---|---|---|---|
|  |  | Text | Diagram | Image | Animation | Text | Diagram | Image | Animation |
| Younger users | Text |  | 0.015 * | 0.678 | 0.235 | 0.112 | 0.052 | 0.986 | 0.472 |
|  | Diagrams | 0.015 * |  | 0.005 * | 0.000 * | 0.000 * | 0.746 | 0.025 * | 0.003 * |
|  | Images | 0.678 | 0.005 * |  | 0.438 | 0.227 | 0.020 * | 0.686 | 0.739 |
|  | Animation | 0.235 | 0.000 * | 0.438 |  | 0.625 | 0.003 * | 0.261 | 0.697 |
| Older users | Text | 0.112 | 0.000 * | 0.227 | 0.625 |  | 0.001 * | 0.131 | 0.410 |
|  | Diagrams | 0.052 | 0.746 | 0.020 * | 0.003 * | 0.001 * |  | 0.070 | 0.013 * |
|  | Images | 0.986 | 0.025 * | 0.686 | 0.261 | 0.131 | 0.070 |  | 0.489 |
|  | Animation | 0.472 | 0.003 * | 0.739 | 0.697 | 0.410 | 0.013 * | 0.489 |  |

* represents statistical difference; $p < 0.05$.

According to the preceding tables, the younger respondents' "overall reaction" results for the animation interface were significantly higher than those for the text and diagram interfaces ($p = 0.007$ * and p = 0.000*). Their "screen" results for the animation interface were significantly higher than those for the diagram interface ($p = 0.000$ *), suggesting that the younger respondents were most satisfied with the animation interface. The younger respondents' "screen" results for the diagram interfaces were significantly lower than those for the other three interfaces ($p = 0.015$ *, $p = 0.005$ *, $p = 0.000$ *). Their "overall reaction" results for the diagram interface were significantly lower than those for the image and animation interfaces ($p = 0.003$ *, $p = 0.000$ *), suggesting that the younger respondents were least satisfied with the diagram interface. The older respondents' "overall reaction" results for the diagram interface was significantly lower than the other three interfaces ($p = 0.001$ *, $p = 0.037$ *, $p = 0.007$ *). Their "screen" results for the diagram interface were significantly lower than those for the text and animation interfaces ($p = 0.001$ *, $p = 0.013$ *), suggesting that the older adults were dissatisfied with the diagram interface. A comparison of the results of the younger and older respondents showed that only the text interface achieved significant differences in the "overall reaction" section of the QUIS ($p = 0.015$ *), suggesting that the older respondents had a more positive perception of the text interface.

*4.6. Summary of Unstructured Interviews*

A series of unstructured interviews were conducted after the tests. The results were as follows:

**Information Comprehension, Information Adequacy, and Usability**

In the interviews, the respondents expressed that the animation and image interfaces provided less health information (normal and abnormal) than the other two interfaces. Less time was required to interpret the information, improving the respondents' perceived usability. The characteristics of these interfaces are useful for users who wish to track simple health results and less suitable for users who require detailed health information and data changes. The respondents expressed that the text and diagram interfaces contained more information, but more effort was required to interpret the information (e.g., blood pressure levels and value changes), reducing their perceived usability. These interfaces were more suitable for users suffering from specific illnesses who must monitor their health on a daily basis. Therefore, interface designers should consider the content and volume of the information presented to the users to select a suitable design that can facilitate information interpretation. A simple comparison chart with summary and suggestion is depicted in Figure 16.

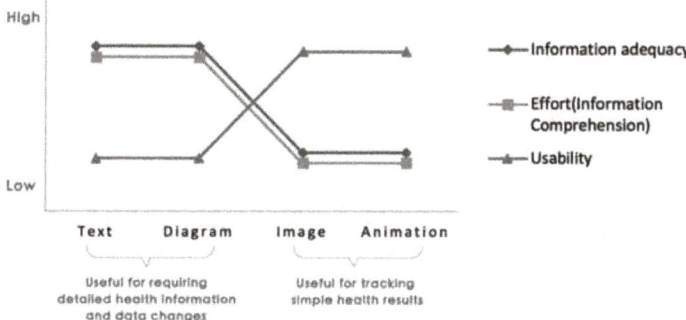

**Figure 16.** Simple comparison of information comprehension, information adequacy, and usability of the four interfaces.

**Younger and Older Users**

The results of the post-hoc tests showed that for the younger respondents, the animation interface incited the highest affective valence (pleasure). The respondents responded positively to the image interface but negatively to the diagram interface. Interview results showed that the animation interface had excellent emotional expression, making respondents feel like they were interacting with the interface, which was enjoyable. Although the diagram interface was easier to interpret than the text interface, the respondents felt that it contained too much information, making it intimidating. They also expressed that they needed more time to interpret the information. The respondents found the animation and image interfaces to be more interesting in general than the diagram interface. These results were consistent with the statistical findings.

Furthermore, the older respondents had higher information comprehension, affective valence, and perceived usability evaluations for the text interface. Interview results suggested that the older respondents were more accustomed to the traditional text-based interfaces. The newer and more complicated interfaces were comparatively unpopular among the older respondents.

*4.7. Discussion*

In summary, all respondents responded poorly to the diagram interface, as reflected in the respondents' interpretation accuracy, affective valence, SUS, and QUIS results. The pleasure, SUS, and QUIS results of the older respondents also showed that they disliked the diagram interface the most of the four interfaces. Interview results indicated that a possible reason for this was that too much information was packed into it, making it difficult to interpret the information and consequently reducing their perceived usability and increasing their negative emotions.

Most of the respondents preferred the animation interface. For the younger respondents, the comprehension aspect of the animation interface was more favorable than that of the diagram and text interfaces. The animation interfaces also incited strong affective valence in the younger respondents. QUIS results showed that the overall reaction of the younger respondents was significantly higher for the animation interface than the text or diagram interfaces. In the "screen" section, the animation interface was also higher than the diagram interface. Their results show that the animation interface was popular all-around and incited positive responses, which was consistent with expert views and extant design principals.

A comparison of the younger respondents and older respondents indicated that the older respondents scored higher in comprehension, perceived usability (SUS), and overall reaction (QUIS) than the younger respondents for the text interface. The younger respondents expressed negative emotions toward the text interface. A generation gap can be observed between the responses of the younger and older respondents.

## 5. Conclusions

The findings of this study showed that different interfaces produced different usability perceptions and emotions and validated that responses differed between older and younger users. In conclusion, the diagram interface underperformed compared with the other interfaces. The animation interface was popular among the respondents and generated positive emotions. The text interface was accepted by the older users but generated negative emotions among younger users. These results can serve as a reference for designing interfaces for older users.

There are two major limitations in this study that could be addressed in future research. First, as mentioned above, to avoid excessive variables, this research only focuses on the visual interface without the consideration of providing sound feedback and applying the technology of voice user interfaces. Second, diagram interfaces can convey health changes or compare data. However, the health information on such interfaces may be difficult to interpret when applied to wearable devices, inciting negative perceptions of such interfaces. In this study, the capacity issues of wearable devices were observed. Users typically desire large interfaces but are unable to accept the reduced mobility that accompanies larger interfaces.

Finally, future scholars can consider investigating the balance between information volume and display size on wearable devices. Designers can also apply the results obtained in this study, particularly those concerning the usability and affective valence of different interfaces and the special requirements of older users, as a reference for future designs.

**Author Contributions:** Conceptualization, Y.-M.F.; Data curation, L.C.; Formal analysis, L.C. and B.-C.C.; Funding acquisition, Y.-M.F.; Investigation, L.C. and B.-C.C.; Methodology, Y.-M.F.; Project administration, Y.-M.F.

**Funding:** This research was funded by the Ministry of Science and Technology of Taiwan, grant number MOST 106-2410-H-239-009-.

**Conflicts of Interest:** The author(s) declared no potential conflicts of interest with respect to the research, authorship, and/or publication of this article.

## References

1. Cluff, L. The Role of Technology in Long-Term Care. In *The Future of Long Term Care*; Binstock, R., Cluff, L., von Meerin, O., Eds.; Johns Hopkins University Press: Baltimore, MD, USA, 1996; p. 103.
2. Faetti, T.; Paradiso, R. A Novel Wearable System for Elderly Monitoring. *Adv. Sci. Technol.* **2013**, *85*, 17–22. [CrossRef]
3. Fang, Y.M.; Chang, C.C. Users' Psychological Perception and Perceived Readability of Wearable Devices for Elderly People. *Behav. Inf. Technol.* **2016**, *35*, 225–232. [CrossRef]

4. Jiang, F.; Jiang, Y.; Zhi, H.; Dong, Y.; Li, H.; Ma, S.; Wang, Y.; Dong, Q.; Shen, H.; Wang, Y. Artificial intelligence in healthcare: Past, present and future. *Stroke Vasc. Neurol.* **2017**, *2*, 230–243. [CrossRef] [PubMed]
5. Panch, T.; Szolovits, P.; Atun, R. Artificial intelligence, machine learning and health systems. *J. Glob Health* **2018**, *8*, 1–8. [CrossRef] [PubMed]
6. Pyrkov, T.V.; Slipensky, K.; Barg, M.; Kondrashin, A.; Zhurov, B.; Zenin, A.; Fedichev, P.O. Extracting biological age from biomedical data via deep learning: Too much of a good thing? *Sci. Rep.* **2018**, *8*, 5210. [CrossRef] [PubMed]
7. Bharadwaj, R. Will Doctors Fear Being Replaced by AI in the Hospital Settling? *Emerj Artificial Intelligence Research (formerly TechEmergence)*. 2019. Available online: https://www.techemergence.com/will-doctors-fear-being-replaced-by-ai-in-the-hospital-settling/ (accessed on 28 December 2018).
8. Arnold, D.; Wilson, T. *Why AI and Robotics Will Define New Health*; PwC: London, UK, June 2017.
9. Haghi, M.; Thurow, K.; Stoll, R. Wearable Devices in Medical Internet of Things: Scientific Research and Commercially Available Devices. *Healthc. Inform. Res.* **2017**, *23*, 4–15. [CrossRef] [PubMed]
10. Metcalf, D.; Milliard, S.T.J.; Gomez, M.; Schwartz, M. Wearables and the Internet of Things for Health: Wearable, Interconnected Devices Promise More Efficient and Comprehensive Health Care. *IEEE Pulse* **2016**, *7*, 35–39. [CrossRef] [PubMed]
11. Gartner Inc. *Forecast: Wearable Electronic Devices, Worldwide*; Gartner Inc.: Egham, UK, August 2017.
12. Research and Markets Inc. *Wearable Medical Devices Market by Device (Diagnostic (Heart, Pulse, BP, Sleep), Therapeutic), Application (Sport, Fitness, RPM), Type (Smartwatch, Patch), Distribution Channel (Pharmacy, Online)—Global Forecast to 2022*; MarketsandMarkets Research Private Ltd.: Northbrook, IL, USA, 2018.
13. Kulkarni, A.; Kalburgi, D.; Ghuli, P. Design of Predictive Model for Healthcare Assistance Using Voice Recognition. In Proceedings of the 2017 2nd International Conference on Computational Systems and Information Technology for Sustainable Solution (CSITSS), Bangalore, India, 21–23 December 2017; pp. 1–5.
14. Sun, O.; Chen, J.; Magrabi, F. Using Voice-Activated Conversational Interfaces for Reporting Patient Safety Incidents: A Technical Feasibility and Pilot Usability Study. *Stud. Health Technol. Inform.* **2018**, *252*, 139–144. [PubMed]
15. Alsaleh, D.A. *A Social Model for the Consumer Acceptance of Technology Innovation*; Southern Illinois University at Carbondale: Carbondale, IL, USA, 2010.
16. Lee, W.; Xiong, L.; Hu, C. The effect of Facebook users' arousal and valence on intention to go to the festival: Applying an extension of the technology acceptance model. *Int. J. Hosp. Manag.* **2012**, *31*, 819–827. [CrossRef]
17. Saariluoma, P.; Cañas, J.J.; Leikas, J. Emotions, Motives, Individuals, and Cultures in Interaction. In *Designing for Life*; Palgrave Macmillan: London, UK, 2016.
18. Feldman, S.S.; Yalcin, O.N.; DiPaola, S. Engagement with artificial intelligence through natural interaction models. In Proceedings of the Conference on Electronic Visualisation and the Arts, London, UK, 11–13 July 2017; pp. 296–303.
19. Luxton, D. *Artificial Intelligence in Behavioral and Mental Health Care*; Academic Press: Cambridge, MA, USA, 2015.
20. Tehrani, K.; Michael, A. Wearable Technology and Wearable Devices: Everything You Need to Know. *Wearable Devices Mag.* WearableDevices.com. March 2014. Available online: http://www.wearabledevices.com/what-is-a-wearable-device/ (accessed on 28 December 2018).
21. Wu, J.; Li, H.; Lin, Z.; Zheng, H. Competition in wearable device market: The effect of network externality and product compatibility. *J. Electron. Commer. Res.* **2017**, *17*, 335–359. [CrossRef]
22. Department of Economic and Social Affairs, United Nations Population Division. *World Population Aging 1950–2050*; WHO, Department of Economic and Social Affairs Population Division: Geneva, Switzerland, 2002.
23. Upkar, V. Pervasive healthcare and wireless health monitoring. *Mob. Netw. Appl.* **2007**, *12*, 113–127.
24. Chan, M.; Estève, D.; Fourniols, J.Y.; Escriba, C.; Campo, E. Smart wearable systems: Current status and future challenges. *Artif. Intell. Med.* **2012**, *56*, 137–156. [CrossRef] [PubMed]
25. Morris, J.M. User interface design for older adults. *Interact. Comput.* **1994**, *6*, 373–393. [CrossRef]
26. Kobayashi, M.; Hiyama, A.; Miura, T.; Asakawa, C.; Hirose, M.; Ifukube, T. Elderly user evaluation of mobile touchscreen interactions. In Proceedings of the Human-Computer Interaction–INTERACT, Lisbon, Portugal, 5–9 September 2011; pp. 83–99.

27. Bai, Y.W.; Chan, C.C.; Yu, C.H. Design and implementation of a simple user interface of a smartphone for the elderly. In Proceedings of the 2014 IEEE 3rd Global Conference on Consumer Electronics (GCCE), Tokyo, Japan, 7–10 October 2014; pp. 753–754.
28. Marcus, A. Universal, Ubiquitous, User-Interface Design for the Disabled and Elderly. In *HCI and User-Experience Design*; Springer: London, UK, 2015; pp. 47–52.
29. Bederson, B.; Shneiderman, B. (Eds.) *The Craft of Information Visualization: Readings and Reflections*; Morgan Kaufmann: Burlington, MA, USA, 2003.
30. Cook, K.A.; Thomas, J.J. *Illuminating the path: The research and development agenda for visual analytics 2005*; IEEE Computer Society: Los Alamitos, CA, USA, 2005.
31. Pousman, Z.; Stasko, J. A taxonomy of ambient information systems: Four patterns of design. In Proceedings of the Working Conference on Advanced Visual Interfaces, Venezia, Italy, 23–26 May 2006; ACM: New York, NY, USA, 2006; pp. 67–74.
32. Fang, Y.M.; Sun, M.S. Applying Eco-Visualisations of Different Iinterface Formats to Evoke Sustainable Behaviours towards Household Water Saving. *Behav. Inf. Technol.* **2016**, *35*, 748–757. [CrossRef]
33. Tullis, T.S. Screen Design. In *Handbook of Human-Computer Interaction*, 2nd ed.; Helander, M.G., Landauer, T.K., Prabhu, P.V., Eds.; Elsevier: Amsterdam, The Netherlands, 2014; pp. 503–532.
34. Rogers, Y.; Sharp, H.; Preece, J. *Interaction Design: Beyond Human-Computer Interaction*; John Wiley and Sons: Hoboken, NJ, USA, 2011.
35. Chiang, T.; Natarajan, S.; Walker, I. A laboratory test of the efficacy of energy display interface design. *Energy Build.* **2012**, *55*, 471–480. [CrossRef]
36. Harada, H. *UI Design Textbook in Web Design for Multi-Device Era—From Aarchitecture to UX*; Shoeisha Co. Ltd.: Tokyo, Japan, 2013.
37. Google Inc. Material Design Guidelines. Available online: https://material.io (accessed on 31 August 2017).
38. Mehrabian, A.; Russell, J.A. *Approach to Environmental Psychology*; The MIT Press: Cambridg, UK, 1974; pp. 8–26.
39. Bradley, M.M.; Lang, P.J. Measuring emotion: The self-assessment manikin and the semantic differential. *J. Behav. Therapy Exp. Psychiatry* **1994**, *25*, 49–59. [CrossRef]
40. Brooke, J. SUS: A "Quick and Dirty" Usability Scale. In *Usability Evaluation in Industry*; Jordan, P.W., Thomas, B., We-erdmeester, B.A., McClelland, A.L., Eds.; Taylor and Francis: London, UK, 1996; pp. 189–194.
41. Bangor, A.; Kortum, P.T.; Miller, J.A. An empirical evaluation of the System Usability Scale (SUS). *Int. J. Hum. Comput. Interact.* **2008**, *24*, 574–594. [CrossRef]
42. Chin, J.P.; Diehl, V.A.; Norman, K.L. Development of an instrument measuring user satisfaction of the human-computer interface. In Proceedings of the SIGCHI Conference on Human Factors in Computing Systems, Washington, DC, USA, 15–19 May 1988; ACM: New York, NY, USA, 1988; pp. 213–218.
43. Harper, B.D.; Norman, K.L. Improving Us-er Satisfaction: The Questionnaire for User In-teraction Satisfaction. In Proceedings of the 1st Annual Mid-Atlantic Human Factors Conference, Virginia Beach, VA, USA, 25–26 February 1993; pp. 224–228.
44. Tullis, T.S.; Stetson, J.N. A Comparison of Questionnaires for Assessing Website Usability. In Proceedings of the Usability Professionals Association (UPA) 2004 Conference, Minneapolis, MN, USA, 7–11 June 2004.
45. Tullis, T.S.; Albert, W. *Measuring the User Experience: Collecting Analyzing, and Presenting Usability*; Morgan Kaufmann Publishers Inc.: San Francisco, CA, USA, 2008.
46. Preece, J. *A Guide to Usability—Human Factors in Computing*; Addison Wesley: Boston, MA, USA, 1993.
47. Bureau of Health Promotion, Department of Health, Taiwan. *National Survey on Knowledge, Attitude, Practice of Health Promotion*; Available from Survey Research Data Archive; Academia Sinica: Taipei, Taiwan, 2010.

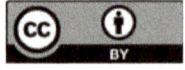

© 2019 by the authors. Licensee MDPI, Basel, Switzerland. This article is an open access article distributed under the terms and conditions of the Creative Commons Attribution (CC BY) license (http://creativecommons.org/licenses/by/4.0/).

Article

# Photoplethysmography-Based Continuous Systolic Blood Pressure Estimation Method for Low Processing Power Wearable Devices

Rolandas Gircys [1], Agnius Liutkevicius [1,\*], Egidijus Kazanavicius [1], Vita Lesauskaite [2], Gyte Damuleviciene [2] and Audrone Janaviciute [1]

[1] Centre of Real Time Computer Systems, Kaunas University of Technology, Barsausko str. 59-A316, LT-51423 Kaunas, Lithuania; rolandas.gircys@ktu.lt (R.G.); egidijus.kazanavicius@ktu.lt (E.K.); audrone.janaviciute@ktu.lt (A.J.)
[2] Clinical Department of Geriatrics, Lithuanian University of Health Sciences, Josvainiu str. 2, LT-47144 Kaunas, Lithuania; vita.lesauskaite@lsmuni.lt (V.L.); gytedamu@gmail.com (G.D.)
\* Correspondence: agnius.liutkevicius@ktu.lt

Received: 13 April 2019; Accepted: 28 May 2019; Published: 30 May 2019

**Abstract:** Regardless of age, it is always important to detect deviations in long-term blood pressure from normal levels. Continuous monitoring of blood pressure throughout the day is even more important for elderly people with cardiovascular diseases or a high risk of stroke. The traditional cuff-based method for blood pressure measurements is not suitable for continuous real-time applications and is very uncomfortable. To address this problem, continuous blood pressure measurement methods based on photoplethysmogram (PPG) have been developed. However, these methods use specialized high-performance hardware and sensors, which are not available for common users. This paper proposes the continuous systolic blood pressure (SBP) estimation method based on PPG pulse wave steepness for low processing power wearable devices and evaluates its suitability using the commercially available CMS50FW Pulse Oximeter. The SBP estimation is done based on the PPG pulse wave steepness (rising edge angle) because it is highly correlated with systolic blood pressure. The SBP estimation based on this single feature allows us to significantly reduce the amount of data processed and avoid errors, due to PPG pulse wave amplitude changes resulting from physiological or external factors. The experimental evaluation shows that the proposed SBP estimation method allows the use of off-the-shelf wearable PPG measurement devices with a low sampling rate (up to 60 Hz) and low resolution (up to 8-bit) for precise SBP measurements (mean difference MD = −0.043 and standard deviation SD = 6.79). In contrast, the known methods for continuous SBP estimation are based on equipment with a much higher sampling rate and better resolution characteristics.

**Keywords:** blood pressure estimation; photoplethysmogram; pulse wave; pulse oximeter; wearable device

## 1. Introduction

It is very important to be able to determine the moment when physiological parameters deviate from normal levels in order to prevent chronic diseases. The dynamics of observed physiological parameters are more important over the long-run than accurate instant values, which are used in an emergency or cases of critical health disorders. It is important to detect the degree of a physiological parameter's deviation from normal during a day, week, month or even a year, as well as the length of such a deviation. If deviation persists for a long time, this can suggest the risk of irreversible changes. Timely detection of such dangerous deviations from normal and an immediate start of treatment can help to avoid negative and irreversible health changes.

Therefore, the long-term constant observation of physiological parameters, such as blood pressure allows us to reduce the healthcare costs, as discussed in Reference [1], minimizes the risk of visiting secondary healthcare institutions, and ensures a better quality of life for a longer period. Blood pressure measurements made at home indicate the state of the cardiovascular system better than those obtained during regular visits to a doctor, as discussed in Reference [2]. A very significant proportion of chronic diseases are cardiovascular diseases. Atherosclerosis and endothelial function changes are accompanied by a rise in blood pressure. As suggested in Reference [3], increasing blood pressure values, measured at home, can be considered as a prognostic sign of atherosclerosis or endothelial dysfunction. Long-term blood pressure variability, obtained during daily home blood pressure measurement (HBP), can show internal organ damage or risk of cardiovascular events, as reported in Reference [4]. The authors of [5] show that increased blood pressure is a potential dementia illness risk factor; thus, registering the dynamics of blood pressure for elderly people can serve as a preventive mental health disorder measure. Hence, the continuous monitoring of blood pressure is critical for the prevention and diagnosis of hypertension and cardiovascular diseases.

Both SBP and diastolic blood pressure (DBP) are important to assess the state of the cardiovascular system, but according to References [6–8], systolic hypertension is much more common than diastolic hypertension, and systolic blood pressure contributes more to the huge global disease burden attributable to hypertension than diastolic pressure. Systolic blood pressure is much more important for elderly people and their health state evaluation, as discussed in References [9–12]. Since elderly people are the major group of geriatrics patients, which are subjects of this study, the estimation of systolic blood pressure is the main focus of this paper.

The traditional auscultatory blood pressure measurement method is not continuous and is quite uncomfortable, because it uses a cuff wrapped around the arm which is inflated repeatedly. To address this problem, continuous blood pressure measurement methods have been developed recently. The most popular methods for continuous and cuffless blood pressure monitoring are based on pulse transit time (PTT) [13–18]. However, PTT is calculated using two signals (usually electrocardiogram and pulse wave), which is quite difficult to implement in wearable devices for daily use.

Blood pressure estimation methods which are based on one-channel pulse wave measurements are less complex and allow us to create wearable devices which are more comfortable for the end users. A pulse wave is often obtained using the photoplethysmogram (PPG) optical measurement method. Blood pressure measurement methods based on one-channel PPG are implemented using stationary medical devices [10,19–22], original PPG measurement devices, such as those in References [23–25], or even smartphones [26,27]. The smartphone approach is not truly continuous, since the user does not wear a PPG sensor. Meanwhile, stationary medical devices or devices created in laboratories are hardly wearable or are available only for a very small group of potential users.

Therefore, this research investigates the possibility of using commercial-off-the-shelf wrist pulse oximeters for continuous cuffless blood pressure measurement, since they are certified, quite cheap, and, most importantly, accessible to everyone (see Figure 1).

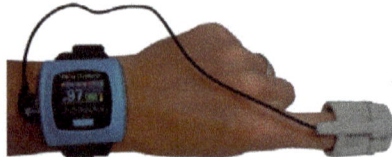

**Figure 1.** The CMS50FW wearable oxygen saturation (SpO2) and pulse rate device with wireless communication for real-time vital-sign monitoring.

If a pulse oximeter is capable of PPG signal transmission over Bluetooth or Wi-Fi, then it is possible to send PPG values to a mobile phone or another device for further SBP estimation and SBP value recording. This allows us to implement a 24/7 system for SBP monitoring.

Other authors usually obtain PPG signal values using a 125–1000 Hz sampling rate and 8–12-bit resolution analog digital converter (ADC) [10,13,15,19–25]. However, energy consumption is the key feature of wearable devices, and a lower sampling rate and resolution allow us to significantly reduce ADC energy consumption, as discussed in Reference [28]. Moreover, the energy used for the data transmission is lower as well, because of the lower number of bytes per sample and the samples per second rate.

This paper proposes a novel approach for the estimation of SBP, using a much lower PPG sampling rate and resolution than other authors and analyzing not all of the PPG pulse wave, but its rising edge only, thereby reducing the number of calculations (and energy consumption) to obtain a result. Experimental evaluation is done using a CMS50FW wrist pulse oximeter with a 60 Hz sampling frequency and 8-bit resolution, which is widely available, quite cheap and is capable of transmitting PPG values over Bluetooth.

## 2. Materials and Methods

The methodology proposed in this paper is depicted in Figure 2.

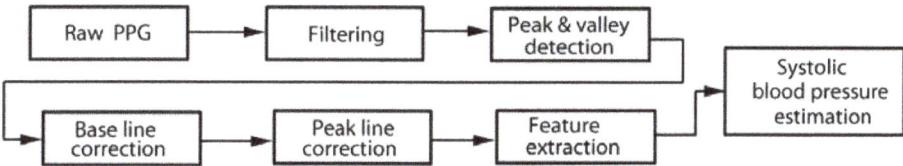

**Figure 2.** The block diagram of the proposed methodology. PPG: Photoplethysmogram.

The PPG signal preprocessing is performed, including normalization and filtering, pulse wave peak and valley point detection, as well as base line correction and peak line correction, as described in the following sections. The systolic blood pressure values are estimated from PPG according to the mathematical model proposed in our previous work [29].

### 2.1. Systolic Blood Pressure Estimation Model

The mathematical–physical model for SBP estimation proposed in Reference [29] is based on Hook's law as defined in Equation (1):

$$\sigma = E \cdot \varepsilon \cdot h / (1 - \theta^2), \tag{1}$$

where $d$ is the diameter of the artery, $d_0$ is the initial diameter of the artery, $h$ is the thickness of the artery wall, $\varepsilon = d/d_0$ is strain, $\sigma$ is stress, $E$ is the Young's modulus, and $\theta$ is Poisson's ratio.

Although pressure ($p$), stress and Young's modulus are different physical quantities, they have the same dimensions $dim(p) = dim(\sigma) = dim(E) - L^{-1}MT^{-2}$, where $L$ is length, $M$ is mass, and $T$ is time; hence, an equals sign can be written between them: $p \equiv E \equiv \sigma$. Hence, Young's modulus in Equation (1) can be changed with pressure without losing physical meaning. Changing one physical quantity to another when their dimensions are equal is quite common practice, which can be seen by comparing the Bramwell–Hill and Moens–Korteweg equations describing pulse wave velocity. The Moens–Korteweg equation uses Young's modulus, while Bramwell–Hill uses pressure.

Let us change stress in Equation (1) to pressure as defined in Equation (2):

$$p = E \cdot \varepsilon \cdot h / (1 - \theta^2). \tag{2}$$

When blood pressure $p(t)$ changes during the cardiac cycle, the diameter of artery $d(t)$ changes as well; therefore, Equation (2) can be re-written as a time function as given by Equation (3):

$$p(t) = E \cdot \frac{d(t)}{d_0} \cdot \frac{h}{(1-\theta^2)}, \qquad (3)$$

where $p(t)$ is the blood pressure change function during the cardiac cycle (blood pressure pulse wave). Function $p(t)$ is called the pressure pulse wave (PPW) in the remainder of this paper, while relative deformation variation $d(t)/d_0$ is the deformation pulse wave (DPW), where $d_0$ is the artery diameter at the beginning of the cardiac cycle. Let us denote DPW as $D(t) = d(t)/d_0$, and the remainder of Equation (3) as a constant $K = E(h/(1-\theta^2))$, leading to the following Equation (4):

$$p(t) = K \cdot D(t). \qquad (4)$$

If the stress–strain characteristic is linear, i.e., $E = const.$, then, if $K$ is known, $p(t)$ values can be calculated for the whole cardiac cycle interval. Usually, we are interested in finding the maximum PPW value, systolic blood pressure value $p_i = max(p(t))$, which is achieved during time period $t_s$ at the $i$-th cardiac cycle.

If $K = const.$ in Equation (4), then the DPW steepness $tan(\gamma)_i = DPW(t)/t$ during $i$-th cardiac cycle is $tan(\gamma)_i = const.$, while the systolic blood pressure value $p_i = max(p(t))$, when $0 \leq t \leq t_s$, can be obtained as following Equation (5):

$$p_i = K \cdot tan(\gamma) \cdot t_s, \qquad (5)$$

where $p_i$ and $tan(\gamma)_i$ change equally during each cardiac cycle.

The DPW form depends on the stress–strain characteristic, which is not linear in the case of blood vessels. Because of this, pressure and deformation pulse waveforms are different, while $K \neq const.$ The authors of [30–32] show that in the part where PPW and DPW are changing most rapidly, their trajectories concur (see Figure 3).

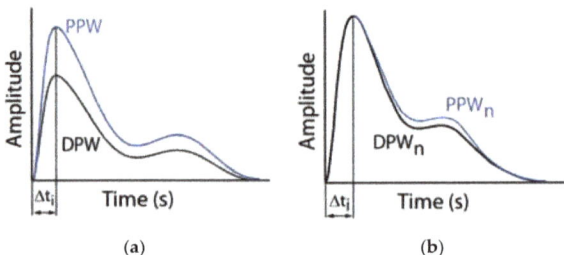

**Figure 3.** (a) PPW and DPW trajectories; (b) normalized $PPW_n = PPW/max(PPW)$ and $DPW_n = DPW/max(DPW)$ trajectories coincide.

Hence, $tan(\gamma)_{max\_i}$ correlates with the systolic blood pressure value of the $i$-th cardiac cycle, and this SBP value can be calculated using Equation (5) and taking the steepest part of the DPW rising edge: $tan(\gamma)_{max\_i} = max(tan(\gamma_j))$, $1 \leq j \leq M - 1$, where M is the number of sampled points of DPW rising edge, $\gamma_j$ is the angle between the base line and the line drawn through the $j$-th and $(j + 1)$-th points of rising edge, and $i$ is the pulse wave number.

## 2.2. Signal Preprocessing

SBP is estimated in two steps. The initial step includes the calculation of systolic blood pressure values as an average value obtained from 15 pulse waves. Later medians of these values are averaged once more (see the "Systolic blood pressure estimation algorithm" subsection and Equation (6) for details) to get the final result. Averaging is common practice to reduce variability. In order to get a mean value, which reflects the real value with a probability higher than $p = 0.5$, more than 10 values should be taken for averaging. The time period of the PPG record, which contains at least 15 pulse waves, is called the blood pressure estimation window (BPEW) (see Figure 4). The time span for BPEW is based on the minimum possible heart rate of elderly patients with bradycardia, which can fall to 40 bpm. In such a case, one pulse wave fits in 60/40 = 1.5 s (the time interval between two heartbeats). Therefore, BPEW should not be less than $15 \times 1.5 \approx 23$ s (we used a 25 s BPEW for better results). The BPEW duration remains constant during the whole PPG recording time.

The signal being recorded is influenced by various noise sources: Breath, PPG sensor motion noise, high voltage lines' induced noise, low amplitude PPG signal, and premature ventricular contraction, as reported in Reference [33]. This can lead to a situation where BPEW does not contain 15 pulse waves suitable for processing. In such a case, BPEW is dropped, and the next 25 s BPEW is taken for further calculations (non-overlapping moving window principle). This is completely acceptable for soft real-time self-measured blood pressure (SMBP) monitoring, since the final SBP value is estimated from several BPEW (in our case, one SBP value is obtained in a 5-min period, as explained later). Additionally, to reduce such cases, PPG sensor motion noise is eliminated using common signal processing methods.

The width of the signal preprocessing window (SPW) is chosen according to the breath period, because it is the lowest-frequency noise in the signal. The inhalation phase in the PPG signal gives a rising/falling trend. Normally, in a calm state, a person performs around 10–20 breath cycles per minute, while inspiration takes approximately 5 s, as discussed in References [34–37]. Therefore, SPW = 5 s is chosen for signal preprocessing in BPEW (see Figure 4).

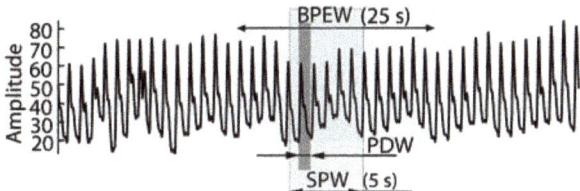

**Figure 4.** PPG with signal preprocessing window (SPW), blood pressure estimation window (BPEW) and peak detection window (PDW).

The following steps are performed for PPG signal preprocessing:

(1) *Normalization*: The PPG signal in SPW is replaced by a signal with a zero mean and variability equal to one.

(2) *Filtering*: Although the power of the high-frequency harmonics is small compared to the harmonics in low and mid-frequency bands (see Figure 5b), their influence on the form of the signal in the time domain is still obvious (see Figure 5a).

Various algorithms are proposed for noise filtering: Empirical mode decomposition [38], discrete wavelet transform [39–41], infinite impulse response (IIR) [10] and fast Fourier transform [26]. The FFT technique is chosen in this work, the output of which is shown in Figure 6.

The largest part of the energy of the PPG signal is accumulated in the frequency band up to 16 Hz. In this frequency band, the average frequencies describe the pulse wave structure, while the high frequencies define the details of the pulse waveform, as discussed in Reference [42]. The FFT filter is implemented by zeroing the frequency band above 16 Hz according to Reference [43]. The filtered signal (see Figure 7) is obtained by reverse FFT; then, the signal is normalized, making its average equal zero.

(3) *Eliminating the rising/falling trend of the signal*: As mentioned before, the inspiration phase takes approximately 5 s, and therefore SPW contains PPG, which is influenced by breathing (see Figure 4), resulting in a rising/falling signal trend. To eliminate this linear trend in SPW, the least squares method is used to find the straight line (see Figure 8a) of this trend. Then, each PPG signal value is decreased

by the corresponding value of this straight line, resulting in a detrended PPG signal, as depicted in Figure 8b.

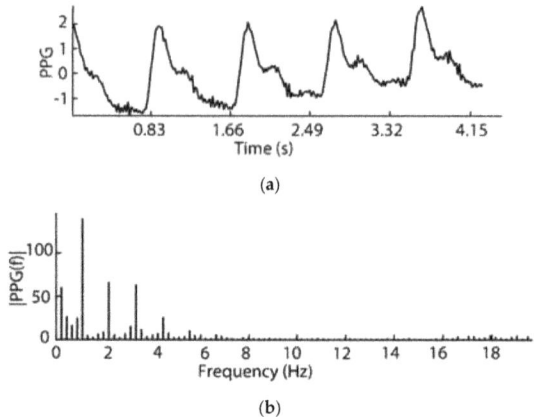

**Figure 5.** (**a**) Normalized PPG signal in SPW and (**b**) its spectrum.

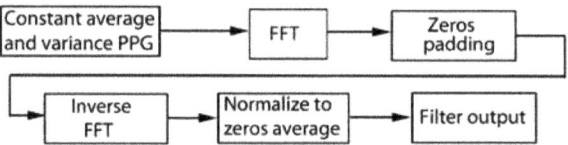

**Figure 6.** The block diagram of signal fast Fourier transform (FFT) filtering algorithm.

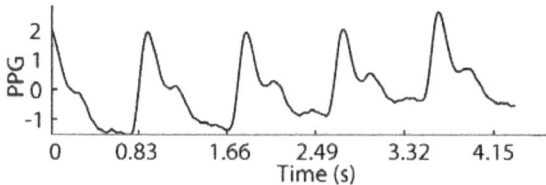

**Figure 7.** Filtered signal in SPW.

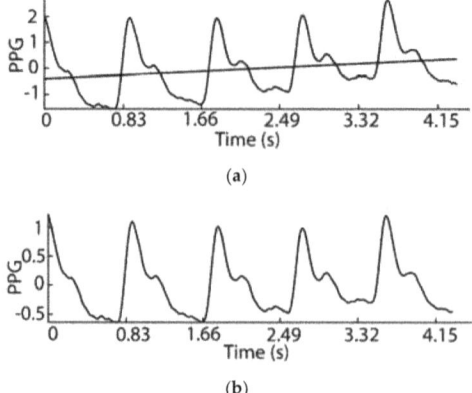

**Figure 8.** (**a**) PPG signal in SPW with the linear trend; (**b**) detrended PPG signal.

(4) *Pulse wave peak point detection* is performed using the adaptive peak detection window (PDW) method [44], which starts by setting PDW as the minimum heart contraction period. Then, PDW is divided into three parts, and according to the proposed algorithm, the heart rate is calculated. PDW is increased, divided into three parts and the heart rate is calculated again. This process is repeated until the PDW width reaches its maximum possible period. The histogram is constructed from the obtained heart rates, and the period corresponding to the most commonly found heart rate is used as optimal PDW.

Such an algorithm sometimes gives incorrect results when more than two pulse waves fall into PDW; for example, if a heart rate is 200 bpm and PDW width reaches 1.5 s (40 bpm), then 5 pulse waves will fall into the PDW. Besides, if the heart rate is low, this algorithm is not efficient in terms of calculation time.

We modified this method by changing the PDW definition rules. These rules are applied for each SPW separately, as defined in Algorithm 1.

**Algorithm 1. PDW size calculation**

| | |
|---|---|
| 1 | **procedure** *pdw* (*p1, p2*) ∇A: Input Signal |
| | ∇ *mHR*: min Heart Rate |
| 2 | $T_{min} = (1/mHR)*1/2; L = round(T_{min}/F_s)$; |
| 3 | $i = 1; N = length(A)/L$; |
| 4 | **while** $(i+1)*L <= N$ **do** |
| 5 | $[k1, c] = linaprox(A(i*L-L+1: i*L))$ |
| 6 | $[k2, c] = linaprox(A(i*L:(i+1)*L))$ |
| 7 | **if** $k1 > 0$ **and** $k2 < 0$ |
| 8 | **then** $p1 = i*L-L+1; p2 = (i+1)*L$; |
| 9 | **goto** *16 line* |
| 10 | **end** |
| 11 | **if** $(k1 < 0$ **and** $k2 < 0)$ **or** $(k1 < 0$ **and** $k2 > 0)$ |
| 12 | **then** $i = i + 1$; **goto** *15 line* |
| 13 | **if** $(k1 > 0$ **and** $k2 > 0)$ |
| 14 | **then** $L = L + 0.1*L$; |
| 15 | **end** /*While*/ |
| 16 | **end** |

The first part of PDW can contain a pulse wave falling edge (or part of it), while the rising edge of the wave appears at the end of PDW. In such a case, the pulse wave peak will not fall into PDW. To detect the beginning of PDW ($p_1$) and its end ($p_2$), PDW = 2L signal values are taken from SPW, where L is number of values fitting in half of the minimum period $T_{min}$.

The least squares method is used to derive straight lines through A(p1:L) and A(L:p2). If the slopes of these lines are negative ($k_1 < 0, k_2 < 0$), then the values belong to the falling edge of the pulse wave (see Figure 9a), and PDW is shifted to the right by the L values. If the slope coefficients are positive ($k_1 > 0, k_2 > 0$), then the values belong mostly to the rising edge, but they do not contain peak values (see Figure 9c). In this case, L is increased by 1/10 and new slope coefficients are found.

When $k_1 < 0$ and $k_2 > 0$ values belong to the rising and falling edges of the pulse wave, but do not contain a peak (see Figure 9b), the PDW is shifted to the right by the L values. Only when $k_1 > 0$ and $k_2 < 0$ does the PDW contain a peak value (see Figure 9d).

(5) *Pulse wave valley point detection* is performed using the algorithm proposed in Reference [45].

(6) *Base line correction*: This step is performed when the starting points of pulse waves in BPEW are found. When a PPG signal is filtered, the unwanted harmonics are eliminated, while base line corrections give a signal whose values vary about a constant value. However, the line connecting the starting points of each pulse waveform a piecewise linear curve. This means that the amplitude values of the pulse wave's starting and ending points are different. For this reason, incorrect start

points, peak points, and rising edge slopes of the pulse wave can be found; thus, base line correction is implemented as explained in Reference [46] (see Figure 10a).

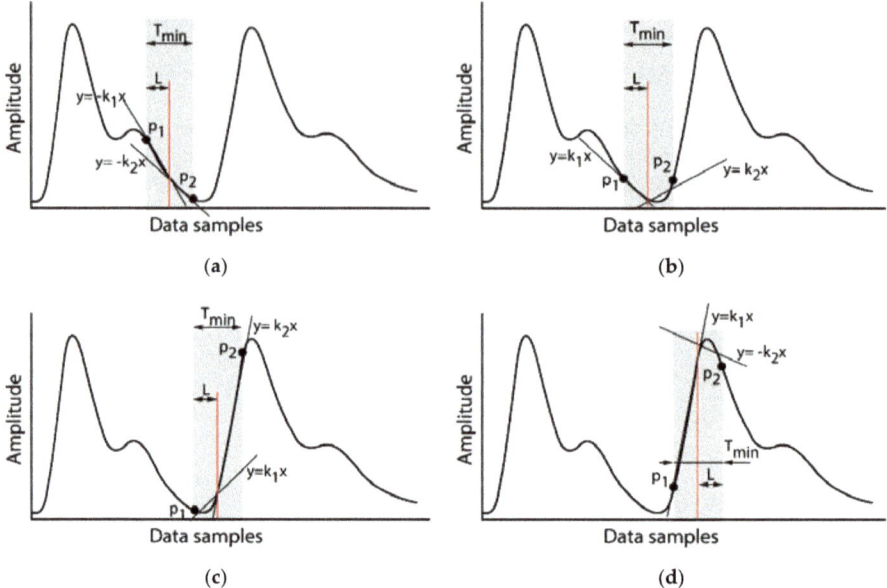

**Figure 9.** (a) PPG signal's falling edge in PDW; (b, c) PPG signal's falling and rising edge without a peak point in PDW; (d) PPG signal with a peak point in PDW. PDW: Peak detection window.

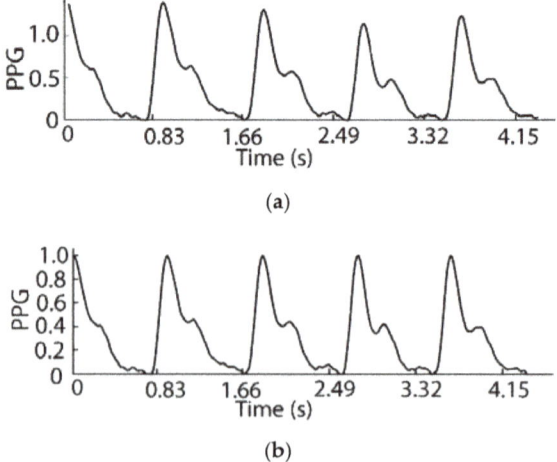

**Figure 10.** (a) PPG signal after base line correction; (b) PPG signal after peak line correction.

(7) *Peak line correction*: This correction is performed when pulse wave peaks are found in BPEW. The form of the DPW rising edge trajectory (not the amplitude) carries information about systolic blood pressure as explained in Reference [29]. Therefore, it is important to ensure uniform time-amplitude proportions of all DPW rising edges. When the DPW sampling rate is 60 Hz, the variability of duration of the rising edge is low, as reported in Reference [47], which results in a constant value of abscissa

(time) and does not affect the time–amplitude proportions. The motion of the arms or body of the patient (with sensors put on them) results in an uneven amplitude fluctuation during PPG registration and distorts the rising edge trajectory time–amplitude proportions. Therefore, the peak line (connecting pulse wave peak points) correction helps to eliminate random amplitude changes (see Figure 10b), without influencing the form of the pulse wave.

This correction is done for each pulse wave (when base line correction is performed, and all pulse wave starting point values become zero) by dividing its values by maximum value, as explained in Reference [48].

### 2.3. Systolic Blood Pressure Estimation Algorithm

Systolic blood pressure is estimated using Equation (5). Coefficient $K$ is found for each subject experimentally from one 5 min duration *training period* and later is used for all *testing periods*. Coefficient $K$ is determined using Equation (5) in such a way that the difference between estimated (from PPG record) and measured (using a conventional cuff-based meter) blood pressure values would be minimal. $SBP_{ei}$ ($0 \leq i \leq length\ (BPEW)$, $i$—value number) is estimated for each pulse wave rising edge in BPEW as described in Figure 11.

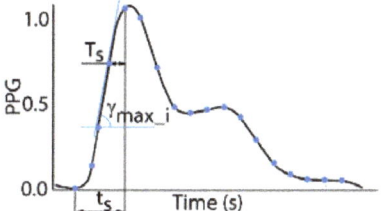

**Figure 11.** Estimation of $SBP_{ei} = K \cdot tan(g_{max\_i}) \cdot t_s$, where $t_s$ is the duration of the rising edge, $T_s$ is the sampling period, $g_{max\_i}$ is the maximum steepness of the rising edge, $K = SBP_m/tan(g_{max\_i}) \cdot t_s$, and $SBP_m$ is the systolic blood pressure which is measured using a conventional cuff-based meter during the initial training session.

Since estimated values are very scattered—i.e., standard deviation $SD_{SBPei} = \pm 10.6$—$SBP_{ei}$ values in BPEW are replaced by their median values $SBP_{mdj}$ (see Figure 12).

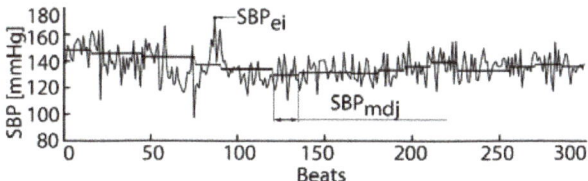

**Figure 12.** Estimated $SBP_{ei}$ blood pressure values (curved line) and $SBP_{mdj}$ median values (stepwise line), calculated from $SBP_{ei}$ in BPEW.

When blood pressure is measured a few times per day at home or in the hospital, it is assumed that it remains constant between measurements.

$$SBP_e = \frac{1}{M} \sum_{j=1}^{M} SBP_{mdj}. \tag{6}$$

Therefore, in this work, for a 5-min PPG period, we calculate one $SBP_e$ value using Equation (6), which is equal to the mean of the medians (see Figure 13):

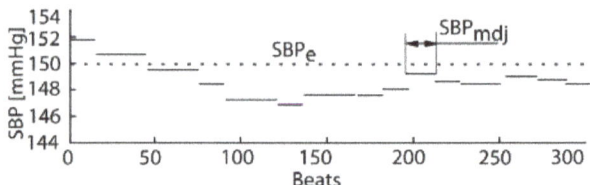

**Figure 13.** Estimated $SBP_e$ blood pressure value (dot line) and $SBP_{mdj}$ in BPEW (stepwise line).

*2.4. Experiment Setup*

A commercial blood pressure meter with a cuff (OMRON M1) was used as the gold standard in this work to measure SBP on the left brachial artery. The PPG signal was collected using the CMS50FW Pulse Oximeter without automatic gain control (AGC) function. The PPG signal sampling rate was 60 Hz and the quantization resolution was 8 bits. The optical sensor with both red (wavelength 660 nm) and infrared (wavelength 880 nm) light sources were used. The collected signal was sent via Bluetooth to a PC, where SBP estimations were performed.

This study was performed at the Clinical Department of Geriatrics of the Lithuanian University of Health Sciences. Nineteen subjects took part in the research (12 women and 7 men), including 6 persons aged 70–77, 11 persons aged 82–85, and 2 persons aged 88 years old with body mass index BMI = 22.4 ± 1.3. All subjects, but two, used blood pressure-regulating drugs. Five subjects had ischemic heart disease.

SBP measurements and PPG records were done for each subject 5 days in a row (one per day), at any convenient time for the subject. The subjects sat with their left hand placed on a support and a PPG sensor placed on their left-hand finger, as shown in Figure 14a. The PPG signal recording was always done first using the pulse oximeter. This procedure took 5 min. The SBP measurements were done immediately after that, using the blood pressure meter, as shown in Figure 14b. Standard cuff type for an arm circumference ranging from 220 to 320 mm was used. Since measurements were performed in a calm state, the records are without movement artefacts.

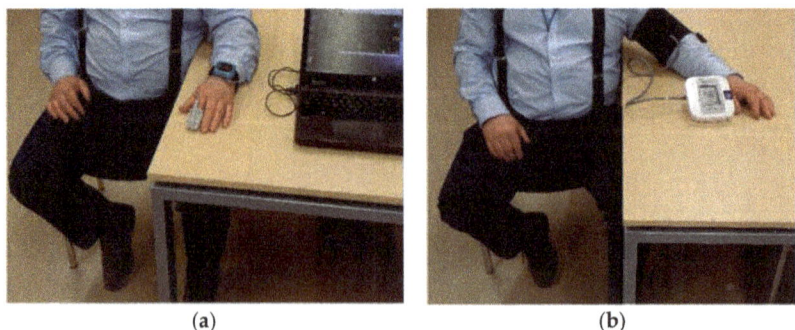

**Figure 14.** (a) PPG signal recording posture; (b) SBP measurements posture.

The experimental protocol of the study was approved by the Kaunas Regional Biomedical Research Ethics Committee (permission No. BE-2-53), allowing the use of a pulse oximeter CMS50FW at the Clinical Department of Geriatrics. According to the Association for the Advancement of Medical Instrumentation (AAMI) protocol [49], the blood pressure values were measured by experienced medical staff.

All subjects were informed about the performed research and their written consent was obtained.

## 3. Results

Nineteen subjects took part in the research. For each of them, 5 SBP values were measured using the oscillometric technique, and 5 SBP values were estimated using the proposed method. Therefore, the measured values vector $x$ and estimated values vector $y$ contains N = 95 values.

The difference between measured and estimated SBP was calculated for each examination, including the mean difference (MD), the standard deviation (SD), and the relative error ($e_r$), in order to evaluate the performance of the proposed method (Table 1):

**Table 1.** Performance of the proposed method.

| r (p < 0.001) | MD | SD | $e_r$, % |
|---|---|---|---|
| 0.86 | −0.043 | 6.79 | 0.025 ± 5.44 |

A Pearson's correlation value shows that the estimated and measured SBP values correlated well (r = 0.86, p < 0.001). This statistically significant tight correlation shows that the proposed method is suitable for continuous systolic blood pressure estimation using PPG recording devices with a low sampling rate (up to 60 Hz) and low resolution (up to 8 bits).

The measured MD and SD values are within the requirements of the AAMI standard (MD = ±5 mmHg and SD = ±8 mmHg) [49], since the mean difference MD = −0.043 and standard deviation SD = 6.79, though the study does not comply with the AAMI protocol, which requires more subjects with different blood pressures and auscultatory technique as a reference method to evaluate the accuracy of the proposed method.

The Bland–Altman plot, as discussed in Reference [50], is commonly used for the comparison of clinical results obtained by using different methods. In Figure 15, we present the agreements of the measured and estimated blood pressure values. The horizontal part of the plot corresponds to the mean values of the measured and estimated SBP, while the vertical axis shows the difference between these values. The mean difference of all the subjects is calculated and represented as a horizontal line, and this horizontal line means better results if it is closer to zero.

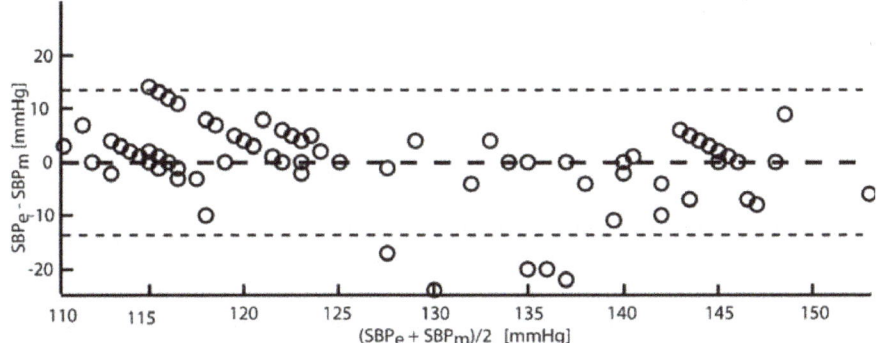

**Figure 15.** Bland–Altman plot presenting the values of the difference ($SBP_e$–$SBP_m$) as a function of the mean of $SBP_m$ and $SBP_e$.

The comparison of estimated and measured values in Figure 15 shows that the error bias, −0.043 mmHg between the gold standard and measured SBP values, is close to zero, while the values of the SD of bias 6.79 mmHg for SBP are very similar to the results of other authors. The systematic trends in Figure 15 show, that there are some errors caused by the method itself, most likely due to rounding procedures.

Table 2 shows the comparison of the proposed SBP estimation method with other authors' results:

**Table 2.** Evaluation of the performance of the systolic blood pressure estimation methods (MD—mean difference, SD—standard deviation, SPS—samples per second).

| Methods | | Systolic Blood Pressure Method Performance | | |
|---|---|---|---|---|
| | | MD | SD | SPS |
| Proposed method | | −0.043 | 6.79 | 60 Hz |
| Ding [15] | | 0.37 | 5.21 | 1 KHz |
| Lin [13] | | 3.22 | 8.02 | 1 KHz |
| Yan [25] | | −0.37 | 4.3 | 200 Hz |
| Kurylyak [22] | | 3.24 | 3.47 | 125 Hz |
| Choudhury [20] | | 0.78 | 13.1 | 100 Hz |
| Khalid [19] | | −1.1 | 5.7 | 100 Hz |
| Xing [21] | | −1.67 | 2.46 | 100 Hz |
| Mousavi [10] | Method 1 | 0.25 | 6.7 | 125 Hz |
| | Method 2 | 0.66 | 7.5 | 125 Hz |
| | Method 3 | 0.19 | 4.17 | 125 Hz |
| | Method 4 | 0.2 | 4.73 | 125 Hz |

As can be seen in Table 2, the proposed SBP estimation method gives similar or better results even when the sampling rate is almost two times lower.

## 4. Discussion

### 4.1. Advantage

The original PPG based method for the continuous estimation of systolic blood pressure using ADC with a 60 Hz sampling rate and 8-bit resolution is proposed in this paper. The main advantage of the method is its high accuracy, which is achieved using lower sampling rates and less capable hardware than other methods.

Since the resolution of SBP estimation is not linear (because the dependency between DPW and SBP is not linear, as explained in "Systolic Blood Pressure Estimation Model" section), the mean difference MD and standard deviation SD is used to evaluate the accuracy of the proposed method. The mean difference MD = −0.043 and standard deviation SD = 6.79 matches, or even improve, the results of the known methods (see Table 2). Though the proposed method does not meet the accuracy requirements of the AAMI standard (due to protocol violations), the MD and SD values are within the requirements of this standard (MD = ±5 mmHg and SD = ±8 mmHg). This shows the great potential of the method and additional experiments are planned in the future work to evaluate full compliance with the AAMI standard.

There are many authors performing state-of-the-art research activities in the field of continuous and cuffless blood pressure monitoring. They admit that continuous blood pressure monitoring is a very important activity and propose various non-invasive PPG based methods to solve this problem. However, the main attention is given to the verification of the accuracy of the proposed methods and comparison with related works, while very little or no attention is paid to the possibilities to implement these methods in wearable systems [10,13,15,19,20,22,25]. There are known wearable (portable) blood pressure measurement systems based on smartphones [26,27], allowing to make measurements at any selected moment. But it is not continuous monitoring, since the idea of the continuous monitoring of physiological parameters (including blood pressure) is that the user does not need to pay any attention to registering those parameters.

Therefore, the main distinction of the proposed method in comparison with other state-of-the-art approaches is that this method can be successfully applied for the implementation of a real life wearable continuous SBP monitoring systems. The method is successfully tested using a prototype system based on the widely available and quite cheap CMS50FW Pulse Oximeter, which is capable of transferring PPG values via Bluetooth to a mobile phone or any other remote device. In order to reduce the number and complexity of calculations (and energy consumption), the proposed method analyzes the rising edge of the PPG pulse wave only. The rising edge is less than 1/3 of the duration of the PPG pulse wave; therefore, this significantly reduces the calculations compared to the methods which process the entire PPG pulse wave. This is relevant for the development of wearable monitoring systems which have very limited processing and energy resources.

*4.2. Limitation*

The proposed method allows us to estimate systolic blood pressure only, and this can be done when subjects are in a calm state. Ideally, wearable devices should allow us to record systolic and diastolic blood pressure in different situations (sitting, walking, driving, etc.) without distracting from daily activities. In order to make such systems, the proposed method should be upgraded by adding an additional processing stage, which would allow us to eliminate movement-induced noise, as well as noise caused by a raised or lowered arm.

## 5. Conclusions

The possibility of estimating systolic blood pressure using a PPG collecting device with a low sampling rate and resolution was investigated in this paper. We believe that such a wearable estimation system will enable the on-demand home monitoring of systolic blood pressure as an important vital sign, resulting in an overall reduction in cardiovascular morbidity and mortality.

Our results show that PPG recording devices with a low sampling rate (60 Hz) and low resolution (8-bit) ADC can be successfully applied for systolic blood pressure estimation using the proposed systolic blood pressure estimation method based on the pulse wave rising edge steepness.

**Author Contributions:** Conceptualization, R.G.; Formal analysis, R.G.; Investigation, R.G., V.L. and G.D.; Methodology, R.G. and A.L.; Project administration, E.K. and A.J.; Resources, G.D. and A.J.; Supervision, E.K. and V.L.; Validation, A.L.; Writing—original draft, A.L. and A.J.

**Funding:** This research was funded by the Research Council of Lithuania, grant number SEN-06/2016.

**Conflicts of Interest:** The authors declare no conflict of interest.

## References

1. Jacob, V.; Chattopadhyay, S.K.; Proia, K.K.; Hopkins, D.P.; Reynolds, J.; Thota, A.B.; Jones, C.D.; Lackland, D.T.; Rask, K.J.; Pronk, N.P.; et al. Economics of self-measured blood pressure monitoring: A community guide systematic review. *Am. J. Prev. Med.* **2017**, *53*, e105–e113. [CrossRef] [PubMed]
2. Sankar, J.; Mahesh, N.; Sharma, P.; Sankar, L.; Balasubramanian, A. Role of ambulatory blood pressure monitoring in chronic hypertensive patients on antihypertensive therapy-a cross-sectional study. *J. Clin. Diagn. Res.* **2018**, *12*, OC01–OC04. [CrossRef]
3. Liu, Z.; Zhao, Y.; Lu, F.; Zhang, H.; Diao, Y. Day-by-day variability in self-measured blood pressure at home: Effects on carotid artery atherosclerosis, brachial flow-mediated dilation, and endothelin-1 in normotensive and mild–moderate hypertensive individuals. *Blood Press. Monit.* **2013**, *18*, 316–325. [CrossRef]
4. Toriumi, S.; Hoshide, S.; Nagai, M.; Kario, K. Day-to-day blood pressure variability as a phenotype in a high-risk patient: Letters to the Editor. *Geriatr. Gerontol. Int.* **2014**, *14*, 1005–1006. [CrossRef]
5. Pan, J.; Zhang, Y. Improved blood pressure estimation using photoplethysmography based on ensemble method. In Proceedings of the 2017 14th International Symposium on Pervasive Systems, Algorithms and Networks & 2017 11th International Conference on Frontier of Computer Science and Technology & 2017 Third International Symposium of Creative Computing (ISPAN-FCST-ISCC), Exeter, UK, 21–23 June 2017; pp. 105–111.
6. Lewington, S.L.; Clarke, R.; Qizilbash, N.; Peto, R.; Collins, R. Age-specific relevance of usual blood pressure to vascular mortality: A meta-analysis of individual data for one million adults in 61 prospective studies. *Lancet* **2002**, *360*, 1903–1913. [PubMed]
7. Asia Pacific Cohort Studies Collaboration. Blood pressure indices and cardiovascular disease in the asia pacific region: A pooled analysis. *Hypertension* **2003**, *42*, 69–75. [CrossRef]

8. Lawes, C.M.; Hoorn, S.V.; Rodgers, A. Global burden of blood-pressure-related disease, 2001. *Lancet* **2008**, *371*, 1513–1518. [CrossRef]
9. Bose, S.S.N.; Kandaswamy, A. Sparse representation of photoplethysmogram using K-SVD for cuffless estimation of arterial blood pressure. In Proceedings of the 2017 4th International Conference on Advanced Computing and Communication Systems (ICACCS), Coimbatore, India, 6–7 January 2017; pp. 1–5.
10. Mousavi, S.S.; Firouzmand, M.; Charmi, M.; Hemmati, M.; Moghadam, M.; Ghorbani, Y. Blood pressure estimation from appropriate and inappropriate PPG signals using A whole-based method. *Biomed. Signal Process. Control* **2019**, *47*, 196–206. [CrossRef]
11. Taylor, B.C.; Wilt, T.J.; Welch, H.G. Impact of diastolic and systolic blood pressure on mortality: Implications for the definition of "normal". *J. Gen. Intern. Med.* **2011**, *26*, 685–690. [CrossRef] [PubMed]
12. Rothwell, P.M.; Howard, S.C.; Dolan, E.; O'Brien, E.; Dobson, J.E.; Dahlöf, B.; Sever, P.S.; Poulter, N.R. Prognostic significance of visit-to-visit variability, maximum systolic blood pressure, and episodic hypertension. *Lancet* **2010**, *375*, 895–905. [CrossRef]
13. Lin, W.-H.; Wang, H.; Samuel, O.W.; Li, G. Using a new PPG indicator to increase the accuracy of PTT-based continuous cuffless blood pressure estimation. In Proceedings of the 2017 39th Annual International Conference of the IEEE Engineering in Medicine and Biology Society (EMBC), Seogwipo, Korea, 11–15 July 2017; pp. 738–741.
14. Khan, N.; Mikael Eklund, J. A Highly integrated computing platform for continuous, non-invasive bp estimation. In Proceedings of the 2018 IEEE Canadian Conference on Electrical & Computer Engineering (CCECE), Quebec City, QC, Canada, 13–16 May 2018; pp. 1–5.
15. Ding, X.-R.; Zhang, Y.-T.; Liu, J.; Dai, W.-X.; Tsang, H.K. Continuous cuffless blood pressure estimation using pulse transit time and photoplethysmogram intensity ratio. *IEEE Trans. Biomed. Eng.* **2016**, *63*, 964–972. [CrossRef]
16. Zhang, J.M.; Wei, P.F.; Li, Y. A LabVIEW based measure system for pulse wave transit time. In Proceedings of the 2008 International Conference on Technology and Applications in Biomedicine, Shenzhen, China, 18 July 2008; pp. 477–480.
17. Liu, S.-H.; Cheng, D.-C.; Su, C.-H. A cuffless blood pressure measurement based on the impedance plethysmography technique. *Sensors* **2017**, *17*, 1176. [CrossRef]
18. Liu, H.; Ivanov, K.; Wang, Y.; Wang, L. Toward a smartphone application for estimation of pulse transit time. *Sensors* **2015**, *15*, 27303–27321. [CrossRef]
19. Khalid, S.G.; Zhang, J.; Chen, F.; Zheng, D. Blood pressure estimation using photoplethysmography only: comparison between different machine learning approaches. *J. Healthc. Eng.* **2018**, *2018*, 1–13. [CrossRef]
20. Choudhury, A.D.; Banerjee, R.; Sinha, A.; Kundu, S. Estimating blood pressure using Windkessel model on photoplethysmogram. In Proceedings of the 2014 36th Annual International Conference of the IEEE Engineering in Medicine and Biology Society, Chicago, IL, USA, 26–30 August 2014; pp. 4567–4570.
21. Xing, X.; Sun, M. Optical blood pressure estimation with photoplethysmography and FFT-based neural networks. *Biomed. Opt. Express* **2016**, *7*, 3007–3020. [CrossRef]
22. Kurylyak, Y.; Barbe, K.; Lamonaca, F.; Grimaldi, D.; Van Moer, W. Photoplethysmogram-based Blood pressure evaluation using Kalman filtering and Neural Networks. In Proceedings of the 2013 IEEE International Symposium on Medical Measurements and Applications (MeMeA), Gatineau, QC, Canada, 4–5 May 2013; pp. 170–174.
23. Kao, Y.-H.; Chao, P.C.-P.; Tu, T.-Y.; Chiang, K.-Y.; Wey, C.-L. A new cuffless optical sensor for blood pressure measuring with self-adaptive signal processing. In Proceedings of the 2016 IEEE SENSORS, Orlando, FL, USA, 30 October–3 November 2016; pp. 1–3.
24. Cohen, Z.; Haxha, S. Optical-based sensor prototype for continuous monitoring of the blood pressure. *IEEE Sens. J.* **2017**, *17*, 4258–4268. [CrossRef]
25. Yan, Y.S.; Zhang, Y.T. Noninvasive estimation of blood pressure using photoplethysmographic signals in the period domain. In Proceedings of the 2005 IEEE Engineering in Medicine and Biology 27th Annual Conference, Shanghai, China, 17–18 January 2006; pp. 3583–3584.
26. Gaurav, A.; Maheedhar, M.; Tiwari, V.N.; Narayanan, R. Cuff-less PPG based continuous blood pressure monitoring—A smartphone based approach. In Proceedings of the 2016 38th Annual International Conference of the IEEE Engineering in Medicine and Biology Society (EMBC), Orlando, FL, USA, 16–20 August 2016; pp. 607–610.

27. Matsumura, K.; Rolfe, P.; Toda, S.; Yamakoshi, T. Cuffless blood pressure estimation using only a smartphone. *Sci. Rep.* **2018**, *8*, 7298. [CrossRef]
28. Tobola, A.; Streit, F.J.; Espig, C.; Korpok, O.; Sauter, C.; Lang, N.; Schmitz, B.; Hofmann, C.; Struck, M.; Weigand, C.; et al. Sampling rate impact on energy consumption of biomedical signal processing systems. In Proceedings of the 2015 IEEE 12th International Conference on Wearable and Implantable Body Sensor Networks (BSN), Cambridge, MA, USA, 9–12 June 2015; pp. 1–6.
29. Gircys, R.; Liutkevicius, A.; Vrubliauskas, A.; Kazanavicius, E. Blood pressure estimation accoording to photoplethysmographic signal steepness. *Inf. Technol. Control* **2015**, *44*, 443–450. [CrossRef]
30. Harada, A.; Okada, T.; Niki, K.; Chang, D.; Sugawara, M. On-line noninvasive one-point measurements of pulse wave velocity. *Heart Vessel.* **2002**, *17*, 61–68. [CrossRef] [PubMed]
31. Diourté, B.; Siché, J.-P.; Comparat, V.; Baguet, J.-P.; Mallion, J.-M. Study of arterial blood pressure by a Windkessel-type model: Influence of arterial functional properties. *Comput. Methods Programs Biomed.* **1999**, *60*, 11–22. [CrossRef]
32. Sugawara, M.; Niki, K.; Furuhata, H.; Ohnishi, S.; Suzuki, S. Relationship between the pressure and diameter of the carotid artery in humans. *Heart Vessel.* **2000**, *15*, 49–51. [CrossRef]
33. Elgendi, M. Detection of c, d, and e waves in the acceleration photoplethysmogram. *Comput. Methods Programs Biomed.* **2014**, *117*, 125–136. [CrossRef] [PubMed]
34. Song, H.-S.; Lehrer, P.M. The effects of specific respiratory rates on heart rate and heart rate variability. *Appl. Psychophysiol. Biofeedback* **2003**, *28*, 13–23. [CrossRef] [PubMed]
35. AL-Khalidi, F.Q.; Saatchi, R.; Burke, D.; Elphick, H.; Tan, S. Respiration rate monitoring methods: A review. *Pediatric Pulmonol.* **2011**, *46*, 523–529. [CrossRef] [PubMed]
36. Charlton, P.H.; Villarroel, M.; Salguiero, F. Waveform analysis to estimate respiratory rate. In *Secondary Analysis of Electronic Health Records*; Springer International Publishing: Cham, Switzerland, 2016; pp. 377–390. ISBN 978-3-319-43740-8.
37. Jennings, J.R.; McKnight, J.D.; Molen, M. Phase-sensitive interaction of cardiac and respiratory timing in humans. *Psychophysiology* **1996**, *33*, 514–521. [CrossRef]
38. Sadrawi, M.; Shieh, J.-S.; Fan, S.Z.; Lin, C.H.; Haraikawa, K.; Chien, J.C.; Abbod, M.F. Intermittent blood pressure prediction via multiscale entropy and ensemble artificial neural networks. In Proceedings of the 2016 IEEE EMBS Conference on Biomedical Engineering and Sciences (IECBES), Kuala Lumpur, Malaysia, 4–8 December 2016; pp. 356–359.
39. Bhoi, A.K.; Sarkar, S.; Mishra, P.; Savita, G. Pre-processing of PPG signal with performance based methods. *Int. J. Comput. Appl.* **2012**, *4*, 251–256.
40. Lee, C.M.; Zhang, Y.T. Reduction of motion artifacts from photoplethysmographic recordings using a wavelet denoising approach. In Proceedings of the IEEE EMBS Asian-Pacific Conference on Biomedical Engineering, Kyoto, Japan, 20–22 October 2003; pp. 194–195.
41. Boloursaz Mashhadi, M.; Asadi, E.; Eskandari, M.; Kiani, S.; Marvasti, F. Heart rate tracking using wrist-type photoplethysmographic (PPG) signals during physical exercise with simultaneous accelerometry. *IEEE Signal Process. Lett.* **2016**, *23*, 227–231. [CrossRef]
42. Wang, D.; Zhang, D.; Lu, G. A robust signal preprocessing framework for wrist pulse analysis. *Biomed. Signal Process. Control* **2016**, *23*, 62–75. [CrossRef]
43. Alian, A.A.; Shelley, K.H. Photoplethysmography: Analysis of the pulse oximeter waveform. In *Monitoring Technologies in Acute Care Environments*; Ehrenfeld, J.M., Cannesson, M., Eds.; Springer: New York, NY, USA, 2014; pp. 165–178. ISBN 978-1-4614-8556-8.
44. Kavsaoğlu, A.R.; Polat, K.; Bozkurt, M.R. An innovative peak detection algorithm for photoplethysmography signals: An adaptive segmentation method. *Turk. J. Electr. Eng. Comput. Sci.* **2016**, *24*, 1782–1796. [CrossRef]
45. Kazanavicius, E.; Gircys, R.; Vrubliauskas, A.; Lugin, S. Mathematical methods for determining the foot point of the arterial pulse wave and evaluation of proposed methods. *Inf. Technol. Control* **2005**, *34*, 29–36.
46. Banerjee, R.; Ghose, A.; Dutta Choudhury, A.; Sinha, A.; Pal, A. Noise cleaning and Gaussian modeling of smart phone photoplethysmogram to improve blood pressure estimation. In Proceedings of the 2015 IEEE International Conference on Acoustics, Speech and Signal Processing (ICASSP), South Brisbane, Queensland, Australia, 19–24 April 2015; pp. 967–971.
47. Akl, T.J.; Wilson, M.A.; Ericson, M.N.; Coté, G.L. Quantifying tissue mechanical properties using photoplethysmography. *Biomed. Opt. Express* **2014**, *5*, 2362–2375. [CrossRef] [PubMed]

48. Datta, S.; Banerjee, R.; Choudhury, A.D.; Sinha, A.; Pal, A. Blood pressure estimation from photoplethysmogram using latent parameters. In Proceedings of the 2016 IEEE International Conference on Communications (ICC), Kuala Lumpur, Malaysia, 22–27 May 2016; pp. 1–7.
49. White, W.B.; Berson, A.S.; Robbins, C.; Jamieson, M.J.; Prisant, L.M.; Roccella, E.; Sheps, S.G. National standard for measurement of resting and ambulatory blood pressures with automated sphygmomanometers. *Hypertension* **1993**, *21*, 504–509. [CrossRef] [PubMed]
50. Bland, J.M.; Altman, D.G. Statistical methods for assessing agreement between two methods of clinical measurement. *Int. J. Nurs. Stud.* **2010**, *47*, 931–936. [CrossRef]

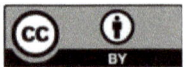

© 2019 by the authors. Licensee MDPI, Basel, Switzerland. This article is an open access article distributed under the terms and conditions of the Creative Commons Attribution (CC BY) license (http://creativecommons.org/licenses/by/4.0/).

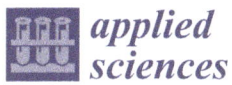 

Article

# Thermal-Performance Evaluation of Bicycle Helmets for Convective and Evaporative Heat Loss at Low and Moderate Cycling Speeds

Shriram Mukunthan [1,*], Jochen Vleugels [1], Toon Huysmans [2,3], Kalev Kuklane [4], Tiago Sotto Mayor [5] and Guido De Bruyne [1,6,*]

1. Product Development, Faculty of Design Sciences, University of Antwerp, Ambtmanstraat, 2000 Antwerp 1, Belgium
2. Applied Ergonomics and Design, Department of Industrial Design, Delft University of Technology, Landbergstraat 15, 2628 CE Delft, The Netherlands
3. Vision Lab, Department of Physics, University of Antwerp (CDE), Universiteitsplein, 2610 Antwerp 1, Belgium
4. Division of Ergonomics and Aerosol Technology, Department of Design Sciences, Lund University, 221 00 Lund, Sweden
5. SIMTECH Laboratory, Transport Phenomena Research Centre, Engineering Faculty of Porto University, Rua Dr. Roberto Frias, 4200-465 Porto, Portugal
6. Lazer Sport NV, Lamorinierestraat 33-37 bus D, 2018 Antwerp, Belgium
* Correspondence: shriram.mukunthan@uantwerpen.be (S.M.); guido.debruyne@uantwerpen.be (G.D.B.)

Received: 10 July 2019; Accepted: 29 August 2019; Published: 5 September 2019

**Featured Application:** Authors are encouraged to provide a concise description of the specific application or a potential application of the work. This section is not mandatory.

**Abstract:** The main objective of the study was to investigate the thermal performance of five (open and closed) bicycle helmets for convective and evaporative heat transfer using a nine-zone thermal manikin. The shape of the thermal manikin was obtained by averaging the 3D-point coordinates of the head over a sample of 85 head scans of human subjects, obtained through magnetic resonance imaging (MRI) and 3D-printed. Experiments were carried out in two stages, (i) a convective test and (ii) an evaporative test, with ambient temperature maintained at 20.5 ± 0.5 °C and manikin skin temperature at 30.5 ± 0.5 °C for both the tests. Results showed that the evaporative heat transfer contributed up to 51%–53% of the total heat loss from the nude head. For the convective tests, the open helmet A1 having the highest number of vents among tested helmets showed the highest cooling efficiency at 3 m/s (100.9%) and at 6 m/s (101.6%) and the closed helmet (A2) with fewer inlets and outlets and limited internal channels showed the lowest cooling efficiency at 3 m/s (75.6%) and at 6 m/s (84.4%). For the evaporative tests, the open helmet A1 showed the highest cooling efficiency at 3 m/s (97.8%), the open helmet A4 showed the highest cooling efficiency at 6 m/s (96.7%) and the closed helmet A2 showed the lowest cooling efficiency at 3 m/s (79.8%) and at 6 m/s (89.9%). Two-way analysis of variance (ANOVA) showed that the zonal heat-flux values for the two tested velocities were significantly different ($p < 0.05$) for both the modes of heat transfer. For the convective tests, at 3 m/s, the frontal zone (256–283 W/m$^2$) recorded the highest heat flux for open helmets, the facial zone (210–212 W/m$^2$) recorded the highest heat flux for closed helmets and the parietal zone (54–123 W/m$^2$) recorded the lowest heat flux values for all helmets. At 6 m/s, the frontal zone (233–310 W/m$^2$) recorded the highest heat flux for open helmets and the closed helmet H1, the facial zone (266 W/m$^2$) recorded the highest heat flux for the closed helmet A2 and the parietal zone (65–123 W/m$^2$) recorded the lowest heat flux for all the helmets. For evaporative tests, at 3 m/s, the frontal zone (547–615 W/m$^2$) recorded the highest heat flux for all open helmets and the closed helmet H1, the facial zone (469 W/m$^2$) recorded the highest heat flux for the closed helmet A2 and the parietal zone (61–204 W/m$^2$) recorded the lowest heat flux for all helmets. At 6 m/s, the frontal zone

(564–621 W/m$^2$) recorded highest heat flux for all the helmets and the parietal zone (97–260 W/m$^2$) recorded the lowest heat flux for all helmets.

**Keywords:** bicycle helmets; thermal manikin; convective and evaporative heat loss; zonal performance characteristics

## 1. Introduction

Cycling is popular, healthy, and environment-friendly. However, cycling is reported to be the third most dangerous mode of transport, resulting in injuries and mortalities. Head injuries are the most typical injuries observed among fatalities reported [1–3]. Studies have shown that these head-related injuries can be significantly reduced by the usage of helmets [4–6]. Emphasis on user safety has resulted in significant increase in research pertaining to safety [7–9]. However, these developments have not resulted in an increased number of helmet users among cyclists. This finding points to the existence of different influencing parameters when it comes to helmet usage by cyclists. Further research indicates that the reluctance of users to wear helmets stems from thermal discomfort [10–12]. For instance, helmet usage in northern and southern Italy during the summer months ranged from 93% and 60%, respectively [13], which indicated that environmental temperature may play an important role in thermal comfort or discomfort, and thus impact helmet usage.

Thermal comfort is the condition of the mind that expresses satisfaction with the thermal environment and is assessed by subjective evaluation [14]. This perception of thermal comfort widely depends on the extent to which the clothing or, in this case, the helmet ensemble allows for heat transfer between head and the environment. Therefore, the heat transfer characteristics of the helmet design that has a major influence on the user comfort must be evaluated. The heat transfer characteristics of the helmet design and the influencing parameters, has been evaluated using subject studies or objective studies. Subject studies used human participants to assess helmet-wearing effects, and focused mainly on physiology, comfort, and thermal sensation. Various studies include analyzing body heat storage using controlled chambers [15], water-perfused suits [16], or water immersion [17] to understand heat transfer between body and environment. Although subject studies provided realistic results, testing using subjects is time consuming and individual differences between subjects result in repeatability issues [18,19]. Objective studies or biophysical methods deploy anatomically correct head-forms or thermal manikins to simulate heat and mass transfer from the head and thereby evaluate the helmet performance. Thermal manikins are based on constant surface-temperature methodology to study heat and mass transfer between head and environment. The surface of the manikin was set to a constant temperature and the total power needed to maintain this temperature over a steady period of time was recorded. Total power accounts for combined heat loss by convection, radiation, and evaporation, depending on the modes of transfer being studied.

Several manikins have been developed and used to evaluate thermal performance for different applications [19–28]. Among the developed head-forms, some are commercially available for testing and experiments, such as head-forms from Thermetrics—Measurement Technology Northwest (Seattle, WA, USA) and UCS d.o.o (Ljubljana, Slovenia). The developed head-forms differ in terms of the number of measurement segments, sweating technique, local heat-transfer data, testing duration, and measurement methodology [29]. However, there is little to no information on the shape and size of the manikin that have been developed and used in the studies and hence it can be assumed that the manikins were developed from a standard window manikin [19] or may be from a head-scan of an individual and thus may not represent the average head shape of the user population. The shape and size of the manikin controls the fitment between the head and the helmet and thereby the gaps and contact zones between the head and the helmet and thus influences the heat transfer between the head and the environment. Since the user can feel even small difference in heat loss as less as 1 W [30], it is paramount that the manikin used in evaluation of helmet performance represents the actual human head-shape as close as possible such that a realistic performance validation can be performed. Hence, a need for an anthropometrically developed biofidelic thermal manikin was identified. The developed biofidelic thermal manikin should provide more segmentation and high spatial resolution [31] such that the zonal heat-transfer characteristics can be studied in detail, which could be more useful in understanding the heat-transfer mechanisms specific to local zones. Hence, as suggested by this study [31], the manikin used in this study was modelled with nine measurement zones representing nine zones of human head.

Thermal manikins have been consistently used to analyze different heat-transfer modes. The convective characteristics of helmets have been studied in detail using manikins: To assess the influence of comfort-angle on helmet ventilation [30], to evaluate the global and local characteristics of bicycle helmets [31], to evaluate helmet-design parameters [32], to understand rowing head-gear characteristics [33], for local ventilation-efficiency quantification [34], to quantify variation among helmets and helmet-ventilation efficiency [35], convective characteristics of cricket helmets [36], and ventilation changes in full-face motorcycle helmets [37] and industrial helmets [23,27]. Thermal manikins were also used in evaluating the radiant heat-transfer characteristics of rowing head gear [33] and bicycle helmets [38] in combination with forced convection. Evaporative heat-transfer helmet characteristics were also studied using thermal manikins in pure evaporation studies for cricket helmets [36], and in combination with convection for industrial helmets [23,27]. However, combined convective and evaporative heat-transfer studies using a biofidelic thermal manikin have not been performed. Hence, the focus of this study was to perform both a convective, and a combined convective and evaporative heat-transfer study to evaluate the influence of evaporation on helmet thermal performance.

Most of the studies mentioned in this section dealt with evaluating different kinds of headgear, such as rowing headgear [33], motorcycle helmets [37], industrial helmets [23,27], and the convective characteristics of bicycle helmets [31–35,38]. In this study, the focus is on bicycle helmets, since helmet thermal performance plays a vital role in aiding users' decision-making process on whether to wear a helmet or not. Hence, in this research, we aimed to evaluate the combined convective and evaporative performance of bicycle helmets using an anthropometrically developed nine-zone biofidelic thermal manikin depicting an average European head shape. Results from this study can be used to establish the heat- and mass-transfer properties of helmet ensembles that could result in improved bicycle helmets for thermal comfort.

## 2. Materials and Methods

### 2.1. Helmets

Five bicycle-helmet designs, listed in Table 1, were tested in this study. These helmet designs were selected to understand the heat transfer characteristics of helmets with maximum and minimum vent openings, and with and without internal channels. A1-Z1, A2-Armor, A3-Blade, and A4-Century are commercial bicycle helmets from the Lazer brand. The tested helmets were classified into open (A1-Z1, A3-Blade and A4-Century) and closed (A2-Armor and H1) based on the design characteristics. A1-Z1 was considered as an open helmet in this study because of the presence of many vent openings on the helmet surface and internal channels underneath the interior surface resulting in large exposure to incoming air flow. A3-Blade and A4-Century are similar to open helmet A1-Z1, but differ in terms of vent number and location, and the presence of prominent internal channels. H1 is not a commercial helmet and was used in this study to evaluate a closed helmet design with prominent internal channels and no vents in the front and sides. A2-Armor has fewer inlet/outlet openings and limited internal channels compared to the other three Lazer helmets.

Table 1. Helmets tested in the study and their properties.

| No. | | A1-Z1 | A2-Armor | A3-Blade | A4-Century | H1 |
|---|---|---|---|---|---|---|
| | Type/Size | Open/M | Closed/M | Open/M | Open/M | Closed |
| 1 | Weight (g) | 190 | 250 | 230 | 277 | 150 |
| 2 | Material | Polycarbonate outer shell with expanded polystyrene (EPS) foam inner layer and padding | | | | Plaster shell with padding |
| 3 | No. of vents | 31 | 16 | 22 | 18 | 4 |
| 4 | Surface area (m$^2$) | 0.270 | 0.263 | 0.255 | 0.240 | 0.196 |
| 5 | Remarks | Padding: 5 × 3 mm. | Padding: 8 mm thick on the sides | Multidirectional impact protection system (MIPS) layer below inner layer | Twist cap technology for better aerodynamics and ventilation | Prototype design, 3 mm thick padding [39] |
| 6 | Homologation | EN 1078 | | | | Not available |

## 2.2. Thermal Manikin

The convective and evaporative performance of the 5 bicycle helmets (Table 1) were measured using a sweating thermal manikin (Figure 1d) that was electrically heated such that the manikin surface-temperature remained constant in an environmental chamber. The thermal manikin used for this purpose was developed in-house based on an average head shape (Figure 1b), obtained by averaging the 3D point coordinates of the head over a population sample.

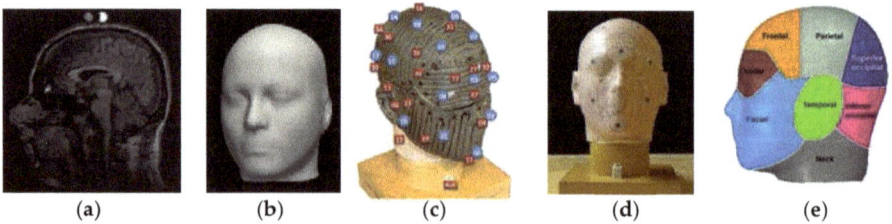

(a) (b) (c) (d) (e)

**Figure 1.** (a) Slice of head scan [32]; (b) average head shape obtained from magnetic resonance imaging (MRI) scans using shape-modeling approach; (c) manikin inner layer with marked thermal-sensor locations and sweat openings; (d) thermal manikin; (e) manikin measurement zones.

The 3D point coordinates were acquired from 85 magnetic resonance imaging (MRI) T1-weighted fast field echo (FFE) scans (male and female (Figure 1a) from the International Consortium for Brain Mapping (ICBM) database) [40]. The population average was obtained in two steps. In the first step, a correspondence was built between the surfaces in the population by registering a template surface via elastic-surface deformation to each individual head, thereby representing it with a fixed number of (semi)landmarks that were at the corresponding locations. In the second step, a population average was derived from the corresponded surfaces by averaging the location of each landmark over the set of surfaces [40]. The ear shape obtained from the scans was distorted due to fixtures used while scanning, so the ears on the final head shape were reconstructed using standard ear shapes available in meshmixer.

The average head-form shape was 3D-printed in a VisiJet PXL core on a ProJet CJP 660Pro and strengthened with Colorbond infiltrate. The manikin was constructed with two layers (Figure 1c), a 2 mm thick outer layer for zone visualization and sweat-duct placement, and a 2.5 mm thick inner layer for heating elements and the installation of 0.5 mm thick thermal sensors. The inner layer was lined with heating elements (Figure 1c) (Cu–Ni alloy) connected to a power source to simulate different metabolic heat-output rates. In addition to the heating elements, 40 NTC 10 k coated temperature-measurement sensors were installed in every measurement-zone location, as marked in Figure 1c. The temperature sensors provide zonal-temperature feedback that allows to control power input to maintain a constant zone temperature. The heating and feedback system were controlled using a dedicated proportional integral derivative (PID) controller for each zone.

The outer layer of the thermal manikin head was provided with 16 openings (Figure 1c) on the surface to simulate sweat. These openings were connected to an automated pumping mechanism that was programmed to pump sweat/fluid at a defined sweat rate to simulate sweating. Although a mixture of salt and water can be used to simulate realistic sweat, the fluid used in this study was water at room temperature to prevent scale formation during evaporation on the manikin surface that could inhibit heat transfer. The surface-heat loss of individual zones was determined through zonal power output over time. The surface temperature and power reading for each zone were measured at a frequency of 1 Hz for 60 min. The manikin included nine measurement regions (Figure 1e), in line with the test requirements, namely: Frontal (scalp1), parietal (scalp2), superior occipital (scalp-rear1), inferior occipital (scalp-rear2), facial (face), ocular (forehead), ears (left and right temporal), and neck. The surface area of the measurement zones is listed in Table 2.

Table 2. Manikin measurement zone and surface area.

| S. No. | Zone | Surface Area (m$^2$) |
|---|---|---|
| 1 | Frontal (scalp1) | 0.017 |
| 2 | Parietal (scalp2) | 0.017 |
| 3 | Superior occipital (scalp-rear1) | 0.015 |
| 4 | Inferior occipital (scalp-rear2) | 0.015 |
| 5 | Ocular (forehead) | 0.010 |
| 6 | Facial (face) | 0.026 |
| 7 | Left temporal (ear–left) | 0.007 |
| 8 | Right temporal (ear–right) | 0.007 |
| 9 | Neck | 0.030 |
|  | Total | 0.144 |

*2.3. Experiment Procedure*

The tests were conducted in controlled laboratory conditions as specified in the test standard [41,42]. Convective-heat-transfer and evaporative-heat-transfer tests were conducted with a nude manikin (Figure 1d), and five helmets at two different velocities to evaluate helmet convective and evaporative performance, and the influence of air velocity on helmet resistance and heat-transfer characteristics. The experiments were conducted in an open-loop wind tunnel (Figure 2a) enclosed in a climate chamber at air velocities $3 \pm 0.1$ m/s (10.8 km/h) and $6 \pm 0.1$ m/s (21.6 km/h) to simulate low and moderate cycling speeds. These two air velocities were selected to simulate the studies from previous research for low [32,43] and moderate speeds [30]. A flowchart depicting the process flow and the test setup is shown in Figure 2b.

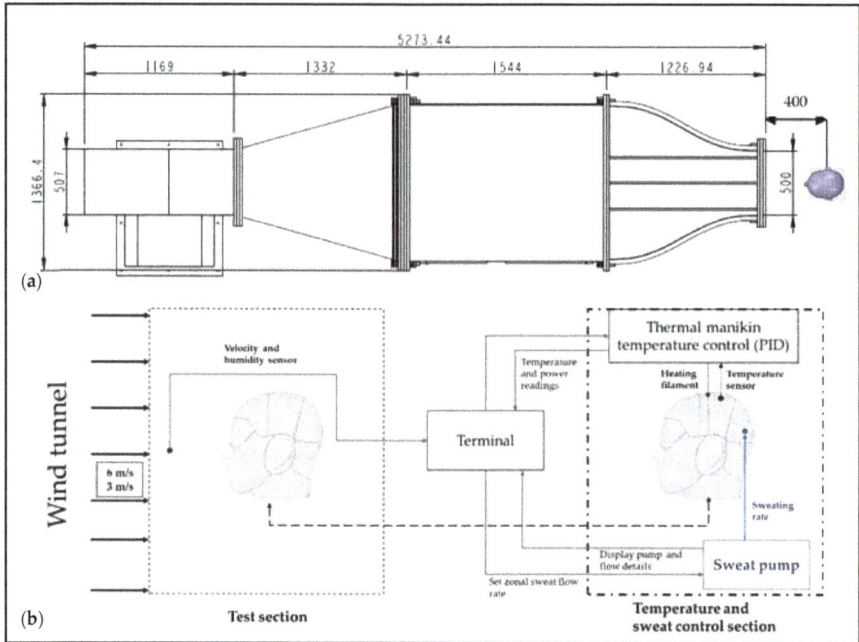

**Figure 2.** (**a**) Schematic of open-loop wind tunnel used for simulating tested velocities with thermal manikin; (**b**) schematic and process flow of convective and evaporative testing.

2.3.1. Convective Heat-Loss Tests

Convective (or dry) heat-transfer testing was done to evaluate the heat-transfer characteristics of selected bicycle helmets for convective heat-transfer mode. Tests were carried out as specified in the test standard [41] except for the temperature setting. The manikin surface was maintained at 30.5 ± 0.5 °C instead of 35 °C, to maintain a temperature difference ($\Delta T$) of 10 °C, as done in the previous studies [19,43] as well as to mimic the thermal responses of the human head during cycling [28]. In dry tests, the manikin was covered with a skin suit (Figure 3). The skin suit covering the head was made from 80% polyamide and 20% Lycra. The dry conditions were simulated by maintaining the environmental temperature at 20.5 ± 0.5 °C. For every test set, heat loss from the nude manikin was measured and used in the calculation of heat fluxes and thermal resistance.

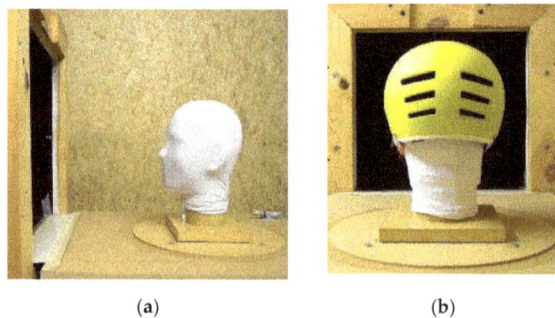

**Figure 3.** (**a**) Manikin head with skin suit at wind-tunnel exit; (**b**) thermal manikin with skin suit and helmet ensemble.

The surface temperature of the manikin zones measured using temperature sensors during the entire test duration is plotted in Figure 4. Head-surface temperature reached a steady state approximately 20 min after the start, after which temperature was in the range of 30.5 °C, with a standard deviation of ± 0.5°C for the remaining duration of the test.

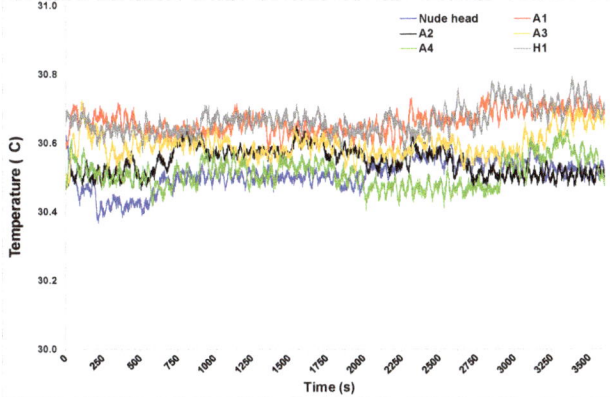

**Figure 4.** Surface temperature of thermal manikin measured at 39 locations (locations shown in Figure 1c) by temperature sensors during test.

2.3.2. Latent Heat-Loss Tests

Latent heat-loss testing was carried out as per the standard [42] to determine the combined convective and evaporative heat-transfer characteristics of the helmets under the influence of sweating at different air velocities. Manikin surface temperature ($T_{sk}$) and ambient temperature ($T_a$) were maintained as for the convective tests. The skin fabric that covered the head was pre-wetted by spraying water before the start of every test to ensure reasonably homogeneous water distribution on the fabric. During testing, perspiration rate was set to 550 g/(m$^2$·h) [18,44] through a pumping mechanism that was controlled through an independent controller that pumped water onto the manikin surface every three min to simulate continuous sweating.

*2.4. Methods—Theoretical Background*

2.4.1. Body and Environment

Thermal discomfort that arises while using helmets is directly related with body thermoregulation. The head plays an important role in human-body thermoregulation. Studies show that the human head shows high heat sensitivity [45] and unique biology due to which, under forced convection, the head can contribute up to one-third of total metabolic body-heat dissipation [29]. Helmets are constructed from high-strength materials like polymers such as plastics or composites and inner foam material to protect users from impact-related injuries. However, helmet shells made from high-strength materials act as an insulating layer for heat and moisture transfer from the head, resulting in thermal discomfort. Hence it is vital to understand the influence of helmet design on the thermoregulation of the human head.

To understand the thermal factors influencing thermal comfort, the thermophysiological response of the human body must be understood. The core temperature of the human body is maintained at approximately 37 °C, which indicates that there exist heat-transfer mechanisms between body and environment such that heat is dissipated when in surplus and retained when in deficit. The relationship between heat generation in the body and transfer to the environment is dynamic, resulting in a heat balance that is described by the heat-balance equation [46]:

$$S = M - W - (E_{res} + C_{res} + E_{sk} + C_{sk} + K + R), \tag{1}$$

where M (W) is the body metabolic rate and W (W) is work rate, quantifying the rate of heat production. Heat loss/gain is the result of evaporation (E) (W), convection (C) (W), conduction (K) (W), and radiation (R) (W). Evaporation and convection occur through respiration (res) (W) and skin (sk) (W), and S (W) is heat storage in the human body. Heat storage/dissipation by the human body plays a vital role in maintaining energy balance in the body. However, the rate of heat production is not always equal to the rate of heat dissipation, resulting in changes in thermal balance. A basic understanding of what this concept would be, if heat storage S = 0 or S ~ 0, i.e., generated heat is approximately equal to dissipated heat (M = W + heat-transfer modes), energy balance is attained, which results in thermal balance and vice versa. Heat transfer through conduction (K) is studied in combination with convective components since heat-transfer-through-conduction mode is relatively small due to little or no direct contact between head and helmet, and because of the much bigger contributions from evaporation, convection, and radiant exchange.

Researchers have often used dry (or sensible) heat transfer and wet (or evaporative) heat transfer when describing the heat-transfer mechanisms between head and environment. Dry heat transfer is the combination of heat transfer by convection (natural and forced) and radiation. The convective component is primarily influenced by the ΔT that exists between head surface and environment. Convective heat transfer is defined by [47]

$$\dot{Q}_{cs} = h_c A (T_{sk} - T_a), \tag{2}$$

where, $\dot{Q}_{cs}$ (W) is the convective heat transfer per unit of time, A (m$^2$) is the surface area of the object, $h_c$ (W/m$^2$.K) is the convective heat-transfer coefficient, $T_{sk}$ (K) is the temperature of head surface and $T_a$ (K) is the temperature of air/fluid. Wet or evaporative heat transfer is related with heat transfer because of sweat evaporation and is primarily influenced by the difference in partial vapor pressure between skin surface and environment, and is defined as [48]

$$\dot{Q}_{ls} = h_e A (P_{sk} - P_a), \tag{3}$$

where, $\dot{Q}_{ls}$ (W) is evaporative heat transfer per unit of time, A (m$^2$) is the surface area of the object, $h_e$ (W/m$^2$.Pa) is the evaporative heat-transfer coefficient, $P_{sk}$ (Pa) is the partial vapor pressure of skin and $P_a$ (Pa) is the partial vapor pressure of the surrounding air/fluid. $\dot{Q}_{cs}$ (W) is the value measured in convective tests and ($\dot{Q}_{cs} + \dot{Q}_{ls}$) (W) is the value measured in combined convective and evaporative tests.

The cooling efficiency (%) of a helmet informs about the ability of a helmet to dissipate heat from the head to the environment, relative to a nude head. It can be calculated as follows:

$$\text{Cooling efficiency (\%)} = \frac{\text{Heat transfer with helmet}}{\text{Heat transfer (nude head)}} \times 100, \tag{4}$$

The main helmet property that influences convective heat transfer between head and environment is the helmet thermal resistance ($R_{ct}$) [49].

2.4.2. Thermal Resistance ($R_{ct}$)

In dry heat-transfer conditions, the total thermal resistance of the helmet ensemble, i.e., between head surface and the environment (thus including the effect of the air layer around the manikin surface) is quantified using thermal resistance ($R_{ct}$) (m$^2$ °C/W), and is calculated using the following formula [49]:

$$R_{ct} = \frac{(T_{sk} - T_a)}{(Q/A)}, \tag{5}$$

where $T_{sk}$ (°C) is the zone average skin temperature, $T_a$ (°C) is the ambient environment temperature, and Q/A (W/m$^2$) is the area-weighted heat flux.

2.4.3. Statistical Analysis

Statistical analysis was carried out on the test results using two-way analysis of variance (ANOVA) to determine if the differences between the heat-flux values for each variable (measurement zones, helmets) were significant. Null hypothesis stated that there exists no significant difference ($p > 0.05$), and the alternative hypothesis stated there existed significant difference ($p < 0.05$). Post hoc analysis was performed (Bonferroni) to identify zones and helmets with statistically significant variation. The above-mentioned statistical analyses were carried out for a 95% confidence interval.

*2.5. Limitations and Considerations*

To the best knowledge of the authors, experimental methodology to determine the combined convective and evaporative thermal-performance characteristics of bicycle helmets using an anthropometrically developed biofidelic thermal manikin has not yet been published. Aiming to address this limitation, the present study was based on available standard experimental methodologies [41,42] to quantify factors affecting the dry and wet thermal performance of several different helmets. However, the study also has some limitations that are discussed in this section.

The test standards [41,42] followed in this study prescribe ambient room temperature ($T_a$) of 23 °C and manikin surface temperature ($T_{sk}$) of 35 °C. However, in this study, ambient temperature ($T_a$) was maintained at 20.5 ± 0.5 °C, and surface temperature ($T_{sk}$) at 30.5 ± 0.5 °C. This change was done to enable the comparison with results from previous studies [19,43]. Testing was carried out at two velocities (3 m/s and 6 m/s) that are different from the air velocity prescribed in the test standards (0.08 m/s). This study considered higher velocities in order to investigate the effects of low and moderate velocities on the thermal and evaporative characteristics of bicycle helmets. Several works in the literature [50–52] show the effect of air flow on heat transfer between body and environment, and its importance in understanding thermal performance. The chosen conditions are a closer representation of the real-use conditions of helmets because, as indicated in another study [36], resistance values obtained in static conditions are likely overestimations of actual resistances surrounding a rider's head during normal bicycle use.

## 3. Results and Discussion

*3.1. Convective Heat-Transfer Characteristics of Head-Helmet Ensembles*

The convective loss from the nude manikin and the manikin with the helmets at 3 m/s and 6 m/s are shown in Figure 5. The convective heat loss increased from 16.6–22.1 W at 3 m/s to 20.8–25.1 W at 6 m/s, showing that heat transfer is strongly influenced by air velocity. Convective heat flux for the nude head-form was 192 ± 2.5 W/m$^2$ at 3 m/s and 216 ± 2.5 W/m$^2$ at 6 m/s. These values are approximately 25% lower than the theoretical heat flux calculated using heat-transfer coefficient values obtained from this study [53] for low ($h_{c(3)}$ = 24.8 W/m$^2$.K) and moderate ($h_{c(6)}$ = 28.5 W/m$^2$.K) velocities in Equation (2). Further investigation indicated that temperature-measurement sensors in the manikin were placed between the two layers, and the reported measurements are the temperature readings between the inner layer and outer layer plus fabric. The outer layer (thickness: 2 mm) acts as an insulation skin resulting in the external fabric layer temperature (measured using an IR thermometer) 2–2.5° C lower than the temperature measured by the sensors resulting in reduction in heat flux values recorded in the tests. The heat flux from nude head (216 ± 2.5 W/m$^2$) recorded at 6 m/s is comparable with the heat flux values recorded in these studies [31,35].

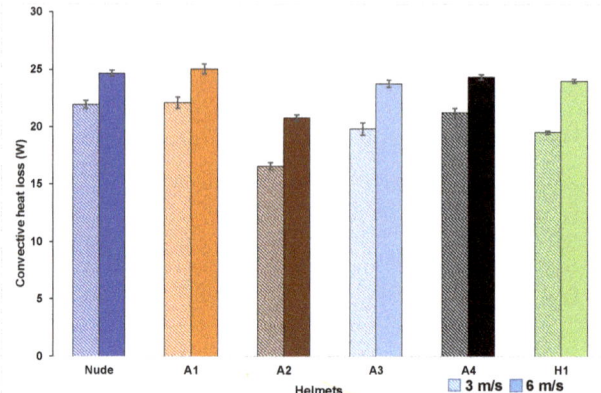

**Figure 5.** Convective heat loss of helmet ensembles at tested velocities (confidence intervals obtained for a 95% confidence level and a sample size of three).

Dry heat losses with the tested helmet ensembles (Table 3) were 11%–25% lower than those of the nude head for all helmets except A1, indicating that most helmets hampered heat transfer from the head by serving as a thermal resistance to heat transfers. The cooling efficiency of the helmets (Table 3) ranged 75%–101% at 3 m/s and 84%–101% at 6 m/s, with Helmets A1 and A2, showing the highest and the lowest efficiency, respectively, for the two tested velocities. Total heat transfer from Helmet A1 was recorded to be higher than the nude head. To understand the reason behind this behavior a zonal heat flux investigation using two-way ANOVA was carried out on total heat flux values. The analysis of the total heat fluxes obtained with the different helmets at two tested velocities showed that all obtained heat fluxes were statistically different ($p < 0.05$) from those obtained with the nude head except for Helmet A1 ($p = 1.0$) thus indicating that the heat flux values of helmet A1 and nude head are comparable. Hence, analysis of zonal heat-flux values was performed using two-way ANOVA combined with post hoc (Bonferroni) analysis since helmet classification based on total heat flux may not correspond to classification based on the heat fluxes of the individual zones, as indicated in [31].

Zonal Heat Transfer Characteristics

*Frontal zone*: Frontal-zone heat fluxes when wearing helmets were statistically different from values obtained for the same zone without a helmet except for Helmet A1 ($p = 1.0$). From the plots (Figure 6), it was inferred that Helmets A1, A3, and A4 depicted similar frontal heat-transfer behavior due to design features. Results also showed that heat flux from the frontal zones decreased for closed helmets.

*Parietal zone*: For parietal zones, no significant difference was observed between the nude head and Helmets A3 and H1 but heat-flux values for the nude head and Helmet A1 were significantly different ($p < 0.05$). Further investigation showed that the parietal zone of the manikin head with Helmet A1 recorded higher heat transfer than the nude head. This is because, at the parietal zones under Helmet A1, the gap between head and helmet at the vent outlet was smaller than the inlet, resulting in the Venturi effect, as observed in this study [54], causing higher local velocity profiles, which, in turn resulted in higher heat transfer from that zone. A similar effect was observed in helmet A4, which has a similar profile as helmet A1 resulting in helmets A1 and A4 dissipating 28%–39% more heat than from parietal zone the nude head. The parietal zone showed minimal difference in the measured heat flux for 3 and 6 m/s (Figure 6).

Table 3. (a) Convective heat-loss values at 3 m/s. (b) Convective heat-loss values at 6 m/s.

(a)

| Helmet | Convective Heat Loss (W) | | Thermal Resistance $R_{ct}$ (°C.m²/W) | Cooling Efficiency (%) |
|---|---|---|---|---|
| | Mean | SD | | |
| Nude | 21.9 | 0.30 | 0.052 | |
| A1 | 22.1 | 0.42 | 0.051 | 100.9 |
| A2 | 16.6 | 0.28 | 0.069 | 75.6 |
| A3 | 19.8 | 0.48 | 0.057 | 90.5 |
| A4 | 21.3 | 0.35 | 0.054 | 96.9 |
| H1 | 19.5 | 0.12 | 0.058 | 89.0 |

(b)

| Helmet | Convective Heat Loss (W) | | Thermal Resistance $R_{ct}$ (°C.m²/W) | Cooling Efficiency (%) |
|---|---|---|---|---|
| | Mean | SD | | |
| Nude | 24.7 | 0.3 | 0.046 | |
| A1 | 25.1 | 0.4 | 0.046 | 101.6 |
| A2 | 20.8 | 0.2 | 0.055 | 84.4 |
| A3 | 23.8 | 0.3 | 0.049 | 96.4 |
| A4 | 24.4 | 0.2 | 0.047 | 98.7 |
| H1 | 24.0 | 0.2 | 0.048 | 97.3 |

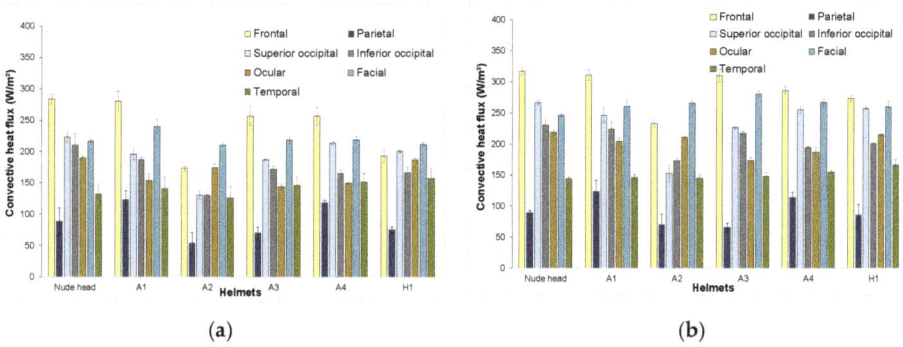

Figure 6. Zonal convective heat-flux distribution at (a) 3 m/s; (b) 6 m/s.

*Occipital zones:* The superior occipital zone of the helmets when compared to the nude head showed that all helmets were significantly different ($p < 0.05$). Helmets H1 and A4 showed the highest cooling efficiency for this zone. Helmet H1 had outlet vent openings at occipital zones resulting in unrestricted air flow. Moreover, there was no retention system interacting with the occipital region of the head during helmet H1 usage. Hence, resistance to heat transfer in this region was lower. The retention system of Helmet A4 was present but did not block air flow in the mentioned zone, as observed in other helmets. It is important to note that Helmet A1, with the highest overall cooling efficiency (slightly above 100%), transferred only 87%–93% of heat from the superior occipital region due to the retention system blocking air flow in that zone. When compared to the nude head, the inferior occipital zone of the helmets showed that all helmets were significantly different ($p < 0.05$) except for A1. The cooling efficiency of Helmet A1 for the inferior occipital zone was the highest among the tested helmets. Helmet A4, which showed 97%–98% overall cooling efficiency for the tested velocities, dissipated 73%–82% of heat from the inferior occipital zone due to the presence of a retention system blocking air flow in that zone. Helmet A2 performed poorly between the tested helmets because of the helmet design that reduced air flow into the helmet.

Ocular, Facial and Temporal zone characteristics: The ocular region of the helmets, when compared to the nude thermal manikin, showed no significant difference for Helmet H1 ($p = 1.0$). For this particular region, Helmet H1 also showed the highest heat loss among the tested helmets for both tested velocities. This is because the design of the helmet H1 favors the air flow in the ocular region. The gap between ocular region and the inner side of Helmet H1 was also found to be bigger when compared to the other helmets. It was also observed in all helmets that the gap between ocular region and helmet inner side was directly proportional to heat loss in the region, i.e., the higher the gap was, the higher the heat loss would be, and vice versa. The facial and temporal regions of the manikin with the helmets showed no significant difference when compared to the facial and temporal regions of the nude manikin for both velocities, which is logical since the helmets did not cover these regions of the head. However, the facial zone under helmet A1 recorded higher heat transfer from facial zone (Figure 6) than the nude head. This is due to the helmet front profile that directs more air flow onto the facial region as observed in this study [35], where some helmets showed more heat transfer from the facial zone than the mean value of the facial zone heat transfer from the nude head.

*Thermal Resistance:* Dry thermal resistances were obtained for the nude manikin and the manikin with the helmet ensembles in steady-state conditions at 3 m/s and 6 m/s as shown in Table 3a,b, respectively. From the resistance values, it is evident that Helmet A2 exhibited high resistance to heat transfer and helmet A1 recorded the lowest. Between the $R_{ct}$ values of the tested helmets, A2 recorded the highest resistances at both 3 m/s and 6 m/s, resulting in the lowest heat dissipation and cooling efficiency among the tested helmets.

Although the range of the obtained total thermal resistances was found to be narrow, results indicated that even a small change in resistance values could impact heat-transfer values. For example, $R_{ct}$ at 6 m/s for Helmets A2 and A3 was 0.055 and 0.048 (°C.m²/W), respectively. This shows that a reduction of about 14% in the total thermal resistance of the mentioned helmets implied an increase in cooling efficiency, from 85% (A2) to 96% (A3).

### 3.2. Evaporative-Heat-Transfer Characteristics of Helmet Ensembles

Heat losses registered by the manikin with and without helmets during the combined convective-evaporative tests at 3 m/s and 6 m/s are shown in Figure 7. Apparent evaporative heat loss was in the range of 37.8–47.4 W at 3 m/s and 44.6–50.5 W at 6 m/s (Table 4). From the test results, it is evident that convection combined with evaporation results in 51–54% higher heat transfer than pure convection demonstrating the importance of evaporation mode in heat transfer between head and helmet. The apparent evaporative heat flux value recorded in this study for nude head at 3 m/s is comparable to that reported in this study [27]. A comparison of cooling efficiency of helmets (Table 4) indicated that, at 3 m/s, helmet A1 recorded the highest (97.3%) and helmet A2 recorded the lowest (79.8%). At 6 m/s, helmet A4 recorded the highest (96.7%) and helmet A2 recorded the lowest (89.9%). Furthermore, a global analysis on the total heat flux values was carried out using two-way ANOVA that showed, in comparison with the nude head, Helmets A1, A4, and H1 were statistically not different ($p > 0.05$). However, as indicated in this study [31], classification based on overall heat transfer is not sufficient and, hence, zonal heat-transfer characteristics were also studied.

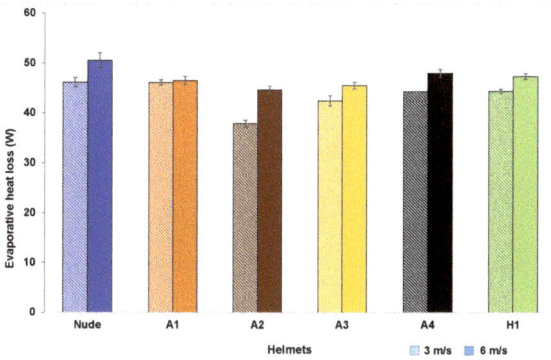

**Figure 7.** Apparent evaporative heat loss of helmet ensembles at tested velocities (confidence intervals obtained for a 95% confidence level and a sample size of three).

**Table 4.** (a) Apparent evaporative-heat-loss values at 3 m/s. (b) Apparent evaporative-heat-loss values at 6 m/s.

| (a) | | | |
|---|---|---|---|
| Helmet | Apparent Evaporative Heat Loss (W) | | Cooling Efficiency (%) |
| | Mean | SD | |
| Nude | 47.4 | 2.2 | |
| A1 | 46.1 | 0.6 | 97.3 |
| A2 | 37.8 | 0.7 | 79.8 |
| A3 | 42.4 | 1.0 | 89.5 |
| A4 | 44.3 | 0.0 | 93.4 |
| H1 | 44.3 | 0.4 | 93.5 |
| (b) | | | |
| Helmet | Apparent Evaporative Heat Loss (W) | | Cooling Efficiency (%) |
| | Mean | SD | |
| Nude | 50.4 | 0.5 | |
| A1 | 47.3 | 0.8 | 95.4 |
| A2 | 44.6 | 0.8 | 89.9 |
| A3 | 45.5 | 0.7 | 91.7 |
| A4 | 48.0 | 0.8 | 96.7 |
| H1 | 47.4 | 0.6 | 95.4 |

Zonal Heat Transfer Characteristics

*Frontal zone*: In comparison with the evaporative heat losses of the nude manikin, losses from the frontal zone of Helmets A1, A4 and H1 were not statistically different ($p > 0.05$). However, plots indicate that the heat flux from the frontal zone of nude head at 3 m/s was, surprisingly, 2% higher than the heat flux from the frontal zone at 6 m/s (Figure 8). During the experiments, it was observed that, at 6 m/s, the fabric used to retain the fluid simulating sweat had dry spots in the frontal zone, which implied a lower surface area with evaporation, and thus lower heat losses in the zone in question. In opposition, at 3 m/s, the fabric was relatively wet, and hence implied more evaporation and higher heat losses than for 6 m/s. The same effect was observed on the fabric for Helmet A1 tests, resulting in higher frontal-region heat fluxes at the lower velocity.

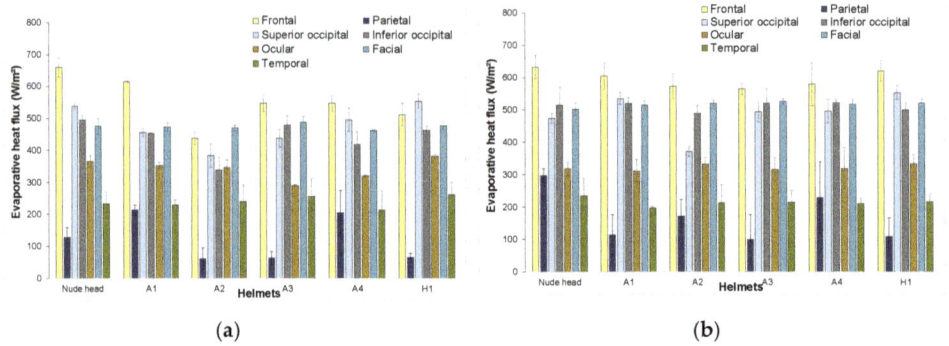

**Figure 8.** Zonal apparent evaporative heat-flux distribution at (**a**) 3 m/s; (**b**) 6 m/s.

*Parietal zone:* When covered with helmet, the parietal zone had 2–15% lower evaporative losses when compared to nude manikin. Statistical analysis showed that the parietal region of Helmets A1, A2 and A4 was not statistically different when compared to that of the nude manikin. Heat-flux transfer from the parietal region at 3 m/s was lower than heat flux at 6 m/s for all helmets except for A1 (Figure 8). It could be considered that the high parietal cooling efficiency of Helmet A1 caused the 'dry-fabric effect' as observed in frontal zone resulted in lower power consumption at 6 m/s than at 3 m/s.

*Occipital zones:* The occipital region of Helmets A1, A3, A4 and H1 shows no significant difference when compared to the nude head ($p > 0.05$). The occipital regions are located on the leeward side of the air flow. Hence, the effect of air speed on this region was not very pronounced, as shown in statistical analysis. However, Helmet A2 showed the lowest heat transfer from the occipital region (8%–31% lower than nude head) for both velocities, and this can be attributed to helmet design (which implies a snug fit in the occipital region).

*Ocular, facial and temporal zone characteristics:* The facial region of the nude manikin with and without helmets showed no significant difference for both velocities ($p > 0.05$). Interaction between facial region and the helmets was minimal during helmet usage; hence, no difference was observed. Heat-flux values from the ocular region of the thermal manikin with and without helmets showed no significant difference ($p > 0.05$). However, heat flux values for low air velocity (3 m/s) were found to be 4–12% higher than the heat-flux values for moderate speed (6 m/s). It was assumed that the existence of dry spots in the fabric during the tests at moderate speeds (6 m/s) resulted in low power consumption, as observed in parietal region. The temporal region showed no significant difference when compared to the nude head for both tested velocities.

From the frontal zonal evaporative-heat-loss plots (Figure 8), it can be observed that the helmets transmitted 70%–85% of the evaporative heat at 3 m/s and 88–98% at 6 m/s (as compared to nude manikin). These values are comparable with the evaporative-heat-transfer results from a study [36] on cricket helmets that showed helmets dissipated 68–78% of the evaporative heat. Considering that the study [36] was carried out at a very low velocity (0.2 m/s) for cricket helmets (different from bicycle helmets), it can be presumed that high evaporative-heat-dissipation values recorded in the current study from the scalp and face zones are due to higher air velocities used in testing.

## 4. Conclusions

The thermal performance of five bicycle helmets for convective and evaporative heat transfer was studied using an anthropometrically developed nine-zone biofidelic thermal manikin for low (3 m/s) and moderate velocities (6 m/s). In-depth analysis of helmet-design effectiveness was done using zonal heat-transfer values obtained from thermal-manikin experiments. The results showed that evaporative heat transfer plays a vital role in helmet performance. The combined convective and evaporative helmet performance can be different from that of convective performance, as shown by the overall cooling-efficiency values of helmets for different air velocities. It was also observed that global heat transfer characteristics and zonal heat transfer characteristics differed significantly and this difference in characteristics was influenced by zone position with respect to incoming air flow and helmet design features. The major findings of this study are as follows:

1. Evaporative heat-transfer mode accounts for 51%–53% of total heat transferred from the nude head, demonstrating the significant role played by sweat in heat transfer and thermal performance.
2. At low velocity (3 m/s), open Helmet A1 showed the highest overall cooling efficiency due to high heat transfer from parietal and facial zones and closed Helmet A2 showed the lowest overall cooling efficiency due to low heat transfer from all the zones for both convective and evaporative heat transfer.
3. At moderate velocity (6 m/s), for convection, open Helmet A1 recorded the highest cooling efficiency due to high heat transfer from parietal zone and closed Helmet A2 showed lowest cooling efficiency due to low heat transfer from all the zones as a result of it shell-like design. For evaporation, open Helmet A4 recorded the highest cooling efficiency as a result of high parietal zone heat transfer.
4. Overall cooling efficiency of closed helmet with prominent internal channels and outlets (H1) was better than the closed helmets with inlets and outlets (A2) depicting the influence of internal channels on heat transfer.
5. Among the zonal heat flux values for the zones under the helmet, frontal zones recorded the highest heat transfer and the parietal zone recorded the lowest heat transfer for all the tested helmets. Further research into the parameters influencing these zonal heat transfer characteristics would provide valuable insight on improving the zonal thermal performance of helmets.

This research provides a description of combined convective and evaporative helmet characteristics tested using a sweating thermal-manikin head and confirms the need for evaporative-heat-transfer tests and their influence on the cooling efficiency of bicycle helmets. It is recommended that the future research on this topic should study/examine zonal design parameters affecting the evaporative heat transfer characteristics of helmets. The results of this study could be complemented by conducting real field trials or subject studies using the same helmets to investigate both the thermal and physiological aspects of bicycle helmets.

**Author Contributions:** S.M., K.K., and G.D.B. developed the experimental methodology. S.M., J.V., and T.H. developed the thermal manikin used in the experiments. T.S.M., G.D.B., K.K., and T.H. helped to review and edit the original draft.

**Funding:** This research was funded by European Union's Horizon 2020 research and innovation program under the Marie Skłodowska-Curie Grant Agreement No. 645770, SmartHELMET: Intersectoral Network for Innovation on Smart Thermal Solutions for Bicycle Helmets and Flanders Innovation and Entrepreneurship (VLAIO) under Grant Agreement 140881, Phyt: Physical and thermal comfort of helmets. The APC was funded by the product development research group.

**Acknowledgments:** We acknowledge the support from the European Union's Horizon 2020 research and innovation program under the Marie Skłodowska-Curie Grant Agreement No. 645770, SmartHELMET: Intersectoral Network for Innovation on Smart Thermal Solutions for Bicycle Helmets. Additionally, we acknowledge the support from Flanders Innovation and Entrepreneurship (VLAIO) under Grant Agreement 140881, Phyt: Physical and thermal comfort of helmets. The authors express their gratitude to Werner Coppieters for his invaluable time and help with the statistical analysis study.

**Conflicts of Interest:** The authors declare no conflict of interest.

## References

1. Wood, T.; Milne, P. Head-injuries to pedal cyclists and the promotion of helmet use in Victoria, Australia. *Accid. Anal. Prev.* **1988**, *20*, 177–185. [CrossRef]
2. Hoye, A. Bicycle helmets—To wear or not to wear? A meta-analysis of the effects of bicycle helmets on injuries. *Accid. Anal. Prev.* **2018**, *117*, 85–97. [CrossRef] [PubMed]

3. Joseph, B.; Azim, A.; Haider, A.A.; Kulvatunyou, N.; O'Keeffe, T.; Hassan, A.; Gries, L.; Tran, E.; Latifi, R.; Rhee, P. Bicycle helmets work when it matters the most. *Am. J. Surg.* **2017**, *213*, 413–417. [CrossRef]
4. Burke, E.R. Safety standards for bicycle helmets. *Physician Sportsmed.* **1988**, *16*, 148–153. [CrossRef] [PubMed]
5. Olivier, J.; Creighton, P. Bicycle injuries and helmet use: A systematic review and meta-analysis. *Int. J. Epidemiol.* **2017**, *46*, 372. [CrossRef] [PubMed]
6. Cripton, P.A.; Dressler, D.M.; Stuart, C.A.; Dennison, C.R.; Richards, D. Bicycle helmets are highly effective at preventing head injury during head impact: Head-form accelerations and injury criteria for helmeted and unhelmeted impacts. *Accid. Anal. Prev.* **2014**, *70*, 1–7. [CrossRef] [PubMed]
7. Mills, N.J.; Gilchrist, A. Oblique impact testing of bicycle helmets. *Int. J. Impact Eng.* **2008**, *35*, 1075–1086. [CrossRef]
8. Bliven, E.; Rouhier, A.; Tsai, S.; Willinger, R.; Bourdet, N.; Deck, C.; Madey, S.M.; Bottlang, M. Evaluation of a novel bicycle helmet concept in oblique impact testing. *Accid. Anal. Prev.* **2019**, *124*, 58–65. [CrossRef] [PubMed]
9. Hansen, K.; Dau, N.; Feist, F.; Deck, C.; Willinger, R.; Madey, S.M.; Bottlang, M. Angular Impact Mitigation system for bicycle helmets to reduce head acceleration and risk of traumatic brain injury. *Accid. Anal. Prev.* **2013**, *59*, 109–117. [CrossRef] [PubMed]
10. Patel, R.; Mohan, D. An improved motorcycle helmet design for tropical climates. *Appl. Ergon.* **1993**, *24*, 427–431. [CrossRef]
11. Li, G.-L.; Li, L.-P.; Cai, Q.-E. Motorcycle helmet use in southern china: An observational study. *Traffic Inj. Prev.* **2008**, *9*, 125–128. [CrossRef]
12. Skalkidou, A.; Petridou, E.; Papadopoulos, F.C.; Dessypris, N.; Trichopoulos, D. Factors affecting motorcycle helmet use in the population of Greater Athens, Greece. *Inj. Prev.* **1999**, *5*, 264–267. [CrossRef] [PubMed]
13. Servadei, F.; Begliomini, C.; Gardini, E.; Giustini, M.; Taggi, F.; Kraus, J. Effect of Italy's motorcycle helmet law on traumatic brain injuries. *Inj. Prev.* **2003**, *9*, 257–260. [CrossRef] [PubMed]
14. ASHRAE. *ANSI/ASHRAE Standard 55 2010—Thermal Environmental Conditions for Human Occupancy*; ASHRAE: Atlanta, GA, USA, 2010.
15. Reardon, F.D.; Leppik, K.E.; Wegmann, R.; Webb, P.; Ducharme, M.B.; Kenny, G.P. The Snellen human calorimeter revisited, re-engineered and upgraded: Design and performance characteristics. *Med. Biol. Eng. Comput.* **2006**, *44*, 721–728. [CrossRef] [PubMed]
16. Hambraeus, L.; Sjodin, A.; Webb, P.; Forslund, A.; Hambraeus, K.; Hambraeus, T. A suit calorimeter for energy-balance studies on humans during heavy exercise. *Eur. J. Appl. Physiol. Occup. Physiol.* **1994**, *68*, 68–73. [CrossRef] [PubMed]
17. Hartley, G.L.; Flouris, A.D.; Plyley, M.J.; Cheung, S.S. The effect of a covert manipulation of ambient temperature on heat storage and voluntary exercise intensity. *Physiol. Behav.* **2012**, *105*, 1194–1201. [CrossRef] [PubMed]
18. De Bruyne, G.; Aerts, J.M.; Van Der Perre, G.; Goffin, J.; Verpoest, I.; Berckmans, D. Spatial differences in sensible and latent heat losses under a bicycle helmet. *Eur. J. Appl. Physiol.* **2008**, *104*, 719–726. [CrossRef]
19. Bruhwiler, P.A. Heated, perspiring manikin headform for the measurement of headgear ventilation characteristics. *Meas. Sci. Technol.* **2003**, *14*, 217–227. [CrossRef]
20. Hsu, Y.; Tai, C.; Chen, T. Improving thermal properties of industrial safety helmets. *Int. J. Ind. Ergon.* **2000**, *26*, 109–117. [CrossRef]
21. Abeysekera, J.D.A.; Holmer, I.; Dupuis, C. Heat-transfer characteristics of industrial safety helmets. In *Towards Human Work. Solutions to Problems in Occupational Health and Safety*; Taylor and Francis Group: London, UK, 1991; pp. 297–303.
22. Osczevski, R.J. *Design and Evaluation of a Three-Zone Thermal Manikin Head*; Defense and Civil Institute of Environmental Medicine: Toronto, ON, Canada, 1996; p. 20.
23. Liu, X.X.; Holmer, I. Evaporative heat-transfer characteristics of industrial safety helmets. *Appl. Ergon.* **1995**, *26*, 135–140. [CrossRef]
24. Reid, J.; Wang, E.L. A system for quantifying the cooling effectiveness of bicycle helmets. *J. Biomech. Eng.-Trans. Asme* **2000**, *122*, 457–460. [CrossRef] [PubMed]
25. Ghani, S.; Elbialy, E.M.A.A.; Bakochristou, F.; Gamaledin, S.M.A.; Rashwan, M.M. The effect of forced convection and PCM on helmets' thermal performance in hot and arid environments. *Appl. Therm. Eng.* **2017**, *111*, 624–637. [CrossRef]

26. Martinez, N.; Psikuta, A.; Corberan, J.M.; Rossi, R.M.; Annaheim, S. Multi-sector thermo-physiological head simulator for headgear research. *Int. J. Biometeorol.* **2017**, *61*, 273–285. [CrossRef] [PubMed]
27. Ueno, S.; Sawada, S. Effects of ventilation openings in industrial safety helmets on evaporative heat dissipation. *J. Occup. Health* **2019**, *61*, 157–164. [CrossRef] [PubMed]
28. Underwood, L.; Vircondelet, C.; Jermy, M. Thermal comfort and drag of a streamlined cycling helmet as a function of ventilation hole placement. *Proc. Inst. Mech. Eng. Part P-J. Sports Eng. Technol.* **2018**, *232*, 15–21. [CrossRef]
29. Bogerd, C.P.; Aerts, J.-M.; Annaheim, S.; Bröde, P.; De Bruyne, G.; Flouris, A.D.; Kuklane, K.; Sotto Mayor, T.; Rossi, R.M. A review on ergonomics of headgear: Thermal effects. *Int. J. Ind. Ergon.* **2015**, *45*, 1–12. [CrossRef]
30. Bruhwiler, P.A.; Ducas, C.; Huber, R.; Bishop, P.A. Bicycle helmet ventilation and comfort angle dependence. *Eur. J. Appl. Physiol.* **2004**, *92*, 698–701. [CrossRef]
31. Martinez, N.; Psikuta, A.; Rossi, R.M.; Corberan, J.M.; Annaheim, S. Global and local heat transfer analysis for bicycle helmets using thermal head manikins. *Int. J. Ind. Ergon.* **2016**, *53*, 157–166. [CrossRef]
32. Bruhwiler, P.A. Role of the visor in forced convective heat loss with bicycle helmets. *Int. J. Ind. Ergon.* **2009**, *39*, 255–259. [CrossRef]
33. Bogerd, C.P.; Bruhwiler, P.A.; Heus, R. The effect of rowing headgear on forced convective heat loss and radiant heat gain on a thermal manikin headform. *J. Sport Sci.* **2008**, *26*, 733–741. [CrossRef]
34. De Bruyne, G.; Aerts, J.M.; Vander Sloten, J.; Goffin, J.; Verpoest, I.; Berckmans, D. Quantification of local ventilation efficiency under bicycle helmets. *Int. J. Ind. Ergon.* **2012**, *42*, 278–286. [CrossRef]
35. Bruhwiler, P.A.; Buyan, M.; Huber, R.; Bogerd, C.P.; Sznitman, J.; Graf, S.F.; Rosgen, T. Heat transfer variations of bicycle helmets. *J. Sport Sci.* **2006**, *24*, 999–1011. [CrossRef] [PubMed]
36. Pang, T.Y.; Subic, A.; Takla, M.; Pang, T.Y.; Subic, A.; Takla, M. Evaluation of thermal and evaporative resistances in cricket helmets using a sweating manikin. *Appl. Ergon.* **2014**, *45*, 300–307. [CrossRef] [PubMed]
37. Bogerd, C.P.; Bruhwiler, P.A. Heat loss variations of full-face motorcycle helmets. *Appl. Ergon.* **2009**, *40*, 161–164. [CrossRef] [PubMed]
38. Bruhwiler, P.A. Radiant heat transfer of bicycle helmets and visors. *J. Sport Sci.* **2008**, *26*, 1025–1031. [CrossRef] [PubMed]
39. Aljaste, H.; Kuklane, K.; Heidmets, S. Better bicycle helmets for commuters—Evaluation of ventilation. In Proceedings of the International Cycling Safety Conference 2014, Gothenburg, Sweden, 18–19 November 2014.
40. Danckaers, F.; Lacko, D.; Verwulgen, S.; De Bruyne, G.; Huysmans, T.; Sijbers, J. A combined statistical shape model of the scalp and skull of the human head. *Adv. Intell. Syst.* **2018**, *591*, 538–548.
41. ASTM. *ASTM F1291-16. Standard Test Method for Measuring the Thermal Insulation of Clothing Using a Heated Manikin*; ASTM: West Conshohocken, PA, USA, 2015.
42. ASTM. *ASTM F2370-16. Standard Test Method for Measuring the Evaporative Resistance of Clothing Using a Sweating Manikin*; ASTM: West Conshohocken, PA, USA, 2016.
43. Mukunthan, S.; Kuklane, K.; Huysmans, T.; De Bruyne, G. A comparison between physical and virtual experiments of convective heat transfer between head and bicycle helmet. *Adv. Intell. Syst.* **2018**, *591*, 517–527.
44. Weiner, J.S. The regional distribution of sweating. *J. Physiol.* **1945**, *104*, 32–40. [CrossRef] [PubMed]
45. Nadel, E.R.; Mitchell, J.W.; Stolwijk, J.A.J. Control of local and total sweating during exercise transients. *Int. J. Biometeorol.* **1971**, *15*, 201–206. [CrossRef] [PubMed]
46. IUPS. Glossary of terms for thermal physiology. *Jpn. J. Physiol.* **2001**, *51*, 245–280.
47. Fanger, P.O. *Thermal Comfort: Analysis and Applications in Environmental Engineering*; McGraw-Hill Book Co.: New York, NY, USA, 1972.
48. Clark, R.E.; Edholm, O.G. Man and his thermal environment. *J. Am. Soc. Nav. Eng.* **1958**, *70*, 331–340.
49. Song, G.W.; Paskaluk, S.; Sati, R.; Crown, E.M.; Dale, J.D.; Ackerman, M. Thermal protective performance of protective clothing used for low radiant heat protection. *Text. Res. J.* **2011**, *81*, 311–323. [CrossRef]
50. Mccullough, E.A. Factors Affecting the resistance to heat-transfer provided by clothing. *J. Therm. Biol.* **1993**, *18*, 405–407. [CrossRef]
51. Havenith, G.; Holmer, I.; Parsons, K. Personal factors in thermal comfort assessment: Clothing properties and metabolic heat production. *Energy Build.* **2002**, *34*, 581–591. [CrossRef]
52. Qian, X.M.; Fan, J.T. Interactions of the surface heat and moisture transfer from the human body under varying climatic conditions and walking speeds. *Appl. Ergon.* **2006**, *37*, 685–693. [CrossRef] [PubMed]

53. Osczevski, R.J. The Basis of Wind Chill. *Arctic* **1995**, *48*, 313–405. [CrossRef]
54. Shishodia, B.S.; Sanghi, S.; Mahajan, P. Computational and subjective assessment of ventilated helmet with venturi effect and backvent. *Int. J. Ind. Ergon.* **2018**, *68*, 186–198. [CrossRef]

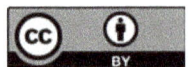 © 2019 by the authors. Licensee MDPI, Basel, Switzerland. This article is an open access article distributed under the terms and conditions of the Creative Commons Attribution (CC BY) license (http://creativecommons.org/licenses/by/4.0/).

Article

# Squat Lifting Imposes Higher Peak Joint and Muscle Loading Compared to Stoop Lifting

Arthur van der Have *, Sam Van Rossom and Ilse Jonkers

Human Movement Biomechanics Research Group, Department of Kinesiology, Katholieke Universiteit Leuven, 3001 Leuven, Belgium; sam.vanrossom@kuleuven.be (S.V.R.); ilse.jonkers@kuleuven.be (I.J.)
* Correspondence: tuur.vanderhave@kuleuven.be

Received: 20 July 2019; Accepted: 8 September 2019; Published: 10 September 2019

**Featured Application: This framework provides a biomechanics-based reference data set for the development of new ergonomic guidelines to successfully decrease the number of work-related musculoskeletal disorders (WMSDs) due to spine overloading.**

**Abstract:** (1) Background: Yearly, more than 40% of the European employees suffer from work-related musculoskeletal disorders. Still, ergonomic guidelines defining optimal lifting techniques to decrease work-related musculoskeletal disorders (WMSDs) has not been unambiguously defined. Therefore, this study investigates if recommended squat lifting imposes lower musculoskeletal loading than stoop lifting while using a complex full body musculoskeletal OpenSim model. (2) Methods: Ten healthy participants lifted two different weights using both lifting techniques. 3D marker trajectories and ground reaction forces were used as input to calculate joint angles, moments and power using a full body musculoskeletal model with articulated lumbar spine. In addition, the muscle activity of nine different muscles was measured to investigate muscle effort when lifting. (3) Results: Peak moments and peak joint power in L5S1 were not different between the squat and the stoop, but higher peak moments and peak power in the hip, knee, elbow and shoulder were found during squat lifting. Moment impulses in L5S1 were higher during stoop lifting. This is reflected in higher peak electromyography (EMG) but lower muscle effort in prior described muscles during the squat. (4) Conclusions: Squat lifting imposes higher peak full body musculoskeletal loading but similar low back loading compared to stoop lifting, as reflected in peak moments, peak power, and peak EMG.

**Keywords:** lifting technique; stoop; squat; work-related musculoskeletal disorders; musculoskeletal modeling; spine; shoulder; back loading

## 1. Introduction

Annually, more than 40% of all employees in Europe suffer from work-related musculoskeletal disorders (WMSDs), such as low back, neck or shoulder pain, despite ongoing efforts to improve the working conditions [1]. These WMSDs result from excessive physical workloads due to repetitive movements (61%), non-neutral posture (44%) and heavy material handlings (31%) [1]. They are responsible for the absence of 3%–6% of the working time, causing an average cost of 2.5% of the gross domestic product across Europe [2]. Of all these WMSDs, 52% are due to overloading during lifting tasks, of which 65% affect the back [3]. It is assumed that by reducing excessive physical workloads, the amount of WMSDs can be reduced, as can the concomitant costs. For this, ergonomic guidelines, such as the ISO standards, can be used. The ISO standards, more specifically ISO standard 11228 Part 1, advises a reference mass for two handed lifting under ideal conditions. Ideal conditions are characterized by having a symmetric standing, one's trunk in a neutral position, a horizontal distance to the object center of mass less than 25 cm, and a grip height of less than 25 cm above knuckle height, thereby allowing a firm grip. Lifting duration should not exceed 1 h per day, with a frequency less or equal than 0.2 lifts per minute. In addition, favorable environmental conditions are assumed, i.e., not too warm/cold and humid. Under ideal conditions, the reference loads are 25 and 15 kg for 95% of men and women, respectively. It is assumed that when the lift situation is in accordance with the above-mentioned guidelines, the lifting technique is more ergonomic and thus reduces the risk of developing WMSDs. The action mechanism potentially reduces the compressive and shear forces between the vertebras. This is important, as high compressive forces on the vertebral discs have been related to low back injury [4].

Two standard lifting techniques, the stoop and the squat, are well-described in literature [5–11]. In general, squatting is advised to lift heavy objects, as this technique is thought to result in lower disc compression and shear forces compared to the stoop. On the other hand, stoop lifting should be restricted to lifting light objects because stoop lifting causes higher disc compression and shear forces compared to the squat [8]. The high disc compression observed during stoop lifting results from a high flexion moment around the L5S1 joint, causing high muscle forces delivered by the back extensor muscles (i.e., m. erector spinae) to overcome the external flexion moment. Indeed, it is known that the muscle forces of the extensor muscle are the main contributors to the compression of the vertebral joints [6].

To estimate joint moments, shear and compression forces, different biomechanical models (like static models [12], electromyography (EMG)-assisted models [6,13–15], finite element models [9,12], 2D dynamic linked segment models in combination with an EMG-assisted models [14] and a full-body musculoskeletal OpenSim model [16]) have been used. These studies found lower moments in the lower back with lower disc compression and shear forces during squat lifting compared to the stoop, and they thereby advised using the squat technique for lifting. However, most studies have only focused on the L5S1 joint in isolation and have neglected loading on the other joints within the human body, which are also likely to be affected by lifting techniques. Squatting results in lower lumbar extensor moments, but to our knowledge, the effect on the shoulder or other joints has not yet been investigated during these lifting techniques. This is highly relevant given the comparable prevalence of shoulder and low back injuries in industry [1].

When muscle loading associated with different lifting techniques has been studied based on EMG, most studies [8,17–20] have only focused on a limited number of muscles that span the fifth lumbar vertebrae joint (i.e., m. erector spinae illiocostalis). Despite the small number of muscles analyzed, these studies have confirmed the relationship between chronic low back pain and increased trunk muscle activity during squat lifting [8,17].

Nevertheless, muscle activations only present localized and therefore partial information on musculoskeletal loading. Other kinematic and kinetic measures are therefore being considered in ergonomic risk analysis. Joint moments that combine kinematic and kinetic movement and which represent the resultant joint action and joint power, thus providing an estimate of energy absorption or generation by the musculoskeletal system, may serve as alternative indicators of musculoskeletal function and loading. Though joint moments and power are often reported parameters in clinical gait research, they are less frequently used within an ergonomic research context [21,22].

The use of a full body musculoskeletal model, multiple EMG-based muscle analyses and the introduction of joint power tackles the single-joint-analyses-problem in this research field. Therefore, the aim of this study was to investigate the effect of squat and stoop lifting techniques on full body musculoskeletal loading, as assessed by joint power and moments calculated using a detailed full body musculoskeletal OpenSim model with a complex definition of the back and the shoulder. In addition, the effect of lifting technique on muscle activity of nine different muscles was studied. We hypothesized that squat lifting would shift the power and moment contribution to the extremities compared to stoop lifting, thereby redistributing the muscle activity away from the lumbar region to the limbs.

## 2. Materials and Methods

Ten healthy participants (7 men; age: 31.5 years (± 12.7), body mass index (BMI): 22.19 kg/m$^2$ (±3.98)) participated in this study. Participants were excluded when suffering from musculoskeletal disorders or were experiencing pain that could affect activities of daily living. All participants provided written informed consent prior to the start of the study, and all study procedures were approved by the local ethics committee (Universitair Ziekenhuis Leuven, S61611).

Participants executed two standard lifting techniques: Stoop and squat. The two lifting techniques were verbally explained, and a small demo was performed before the actual measurements. During stoop lifting, participants were instructed to fully extend their knees and incline their trunk to lift the box from the ground to the upright position; the squat was performed with fully flexed knees, a heel lift-off, and the trunk close to erect (Figure 1) [8].

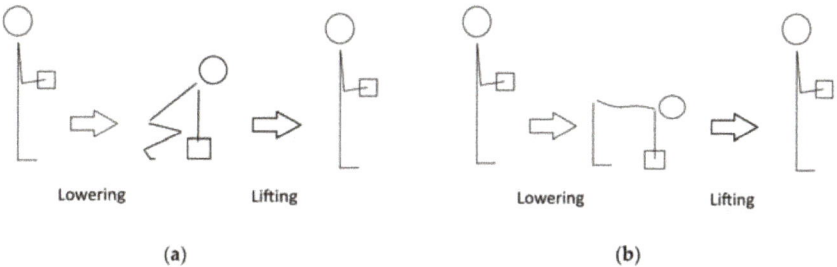

**Figure 1.** (**a**) Squat lifting and (**b**) stoop lifting.

Participants had to lift a standard weight of ten kilograms as well as a weight equal to 40% of the arm lifting strength test (ALST) [23], performed before the start of the measurement.

Ten infrared cameras (100 Hz, VICON, Oxford Metrics, Oxford, UK) captured 3D-marker trajectories during the lifting tasks. Retroflective markers were placed on the participants according to the plug-in gait marker model [24] extended with a spine marker model [25], and the single markers on the upper and lower arms and legs were replaced by three marker clusters. Two ground-embedded force plates synchronously recorded the ground reaction forces (1000 Hz, AMTI, Watertown, MA, USA). In addition, the unilateral (right side) muscle activation of 9 muscles was recorded, (more specifically, m. rectus femoris, m. biceps femoris, m. trapezius descendens, m. deltoideus anterior, m. deltoideus medius, m. triceps brachii, m. biceps brachii, m. erector spinae illiocostalis, and m. erector spinae longissimus) using surface electromyography (1000 Hz, Cometa, Bareggio, Italy) according to the Surface ElectroMyoGraphy for the Non-Invasive Assessment of Muscles (SENIAM)-guidelines.

Measured data were processed using a standard musculoskeletal modelling workflow implemented in OpenSim 3.3 [26] to calculate joint angles and moments. Three validated musculoskeletal models were combined: A modified model of the fully articulated thoracolumbar spine and rib cage model [27], a modified model of an upper extremity model [28], and the gait2354 lower extremity model [29]. To simplify the model, the joints between the five lumbar vertebrae were described as 3 degrees of freedom joints, and the thorax was defined as one rigid segment linked as a weld joint with L1. In addition, the kinematics of L4–L5 and L2–L3 were defined using a coupled coordinate function using the joint angle of L5–S1 and L3–L4 as an independent variable. The weight of the box was accounted for by adding half of the weight of the box to the mass of metacarpal III on the right and left hand.

Firstly, the generic model was scaled to the subjects' anthropometry based on the weight and the marker positions measured during a calibration trial. Secondly, joint angles (Appendix A) were calculated using inverse kinematics [30]. Thirdly joint moments were calculated using the Inverse Dynamics Tool implemented in OpenSim and normalized to body weight to account for differences in body mass. Joint power was then calculated based on the angular velocity and the normalized joint moment. Lastly, the moment impulse was calculated as the area under the normalized moment curve to estimate the cumulative loading over the whole lifting or lowering phase. Raw EMG signals were band pass filtered (20–400 Hz) and full-wave rectified. Then, the rectified signal was filtered with a 6 Hz low pass filter and normalized to the maximal muscle activity obtained during maximal voluntary contractions (MVC) measured during isolated tests before the lifting tests. Next, muscle effort was determined as the area under the MVC-normalized curve.

Subsequently, peak joint moments, powers, and muscle activities were determined during the lowering and lifting part of each trial, and the three were averaged over three trials per participant. The lifting and lowering phase started when the velocity of the box exceeded 0.25 cm/s and ended when the velocity was below 0.25 cm/s.

A general linear mixed model was used to identify statistically significant differences between techniques, weights and handling phases, i.e., lowering and lifting (MATLAB 2018a, The MathWorks, Inc., Natick, MA, United States). In this statistical model, the parameters (i.e., peak moment, peak power, peak muscle activity, moment impulse and muscle effort) are the different response variables; the technique, weights and handling phase are the predictor variables; and the subject is the grouping variable. As the distance between the load and L5 while handling 10 kg was significantly higher during the squat than during the stoop (36.49 ± 4.87 and 31.60 ± 3.09 cm for the squat and the stoop, respectively), the distance between the load and L5 was used as a covariate. Differences were interpreted as significantly different when $\alpha < 0.05$.

## 3. Results

The weight equal to 40% of the arm lifting strength test (ALST) was, on average, 12 ± 4 kg. The results of the 10 kg condition are shown in Appendix B. In general, the differences between the two conditions, the 10 kg and 40% ALST tests, were rather small, and differences in the 10 kg condition are in line with the differences observed in the 40% ALST condition. The 40% ALST condition is described in this section because this weight is relative to the strength of the participant and therefore did not influence the results between the male and female participants [31], as three women and seven men were included in this study.

Joint moments during squat and stoop lifting are presented in Figure 2, and joint power is presented in Figure 3. For all lifting conditions and both techniques, the highest joint moments during lifting and lowering were observed in L5S1, followed by the hip and knee (Figure 2). Joint power generation was highest at the hip for both techniques, with knee power generation being equal to hip power during squat lifting (Figure 3). During squat lifting, power was mainly generated by the hip and knee extensors (Figure 3a). On the other hand, during stoop lifting, knee flexors mainly absorbed power throughout the movement (Figure 3b). Power generation and absorption when lifting were inverted during lowering to absorption and generation, respectively. When lowering while using the squat technique, power was mainly absorbed at the hip and knee, whereas when lowering while using the stoop technique, power was mainly absorbed at the hip.

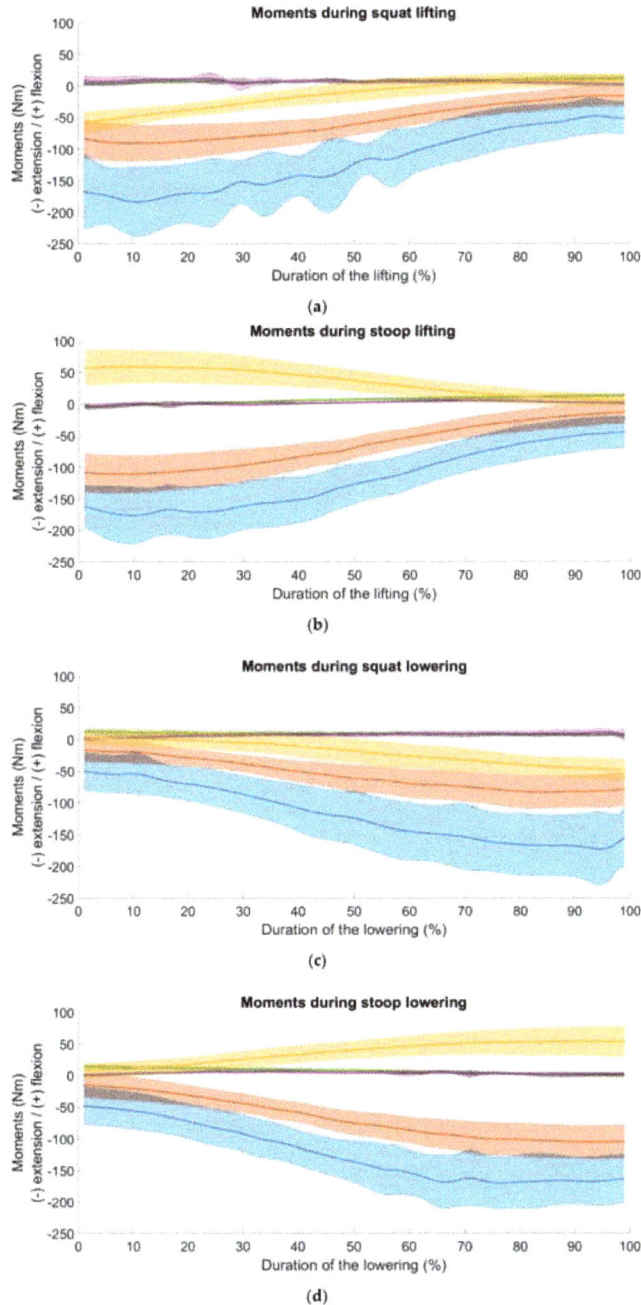

**Figure 2.** Moments of the five different joints (L5S1 (blue), hip (red), knee (yellow), shoulder (purple) and elbow (green)) during the two different lifting techniques (stoop and squat) with a load equal to 40% of the arm lifting strength test (40% ALST). Shaded areas indicate standard deviations. (**a**) Joint moments during squat lifting; (**b**) joint moments during stoop lifting; (**c**) joint moments during squat lowering; (**d**) joint moments during stoop lowering.

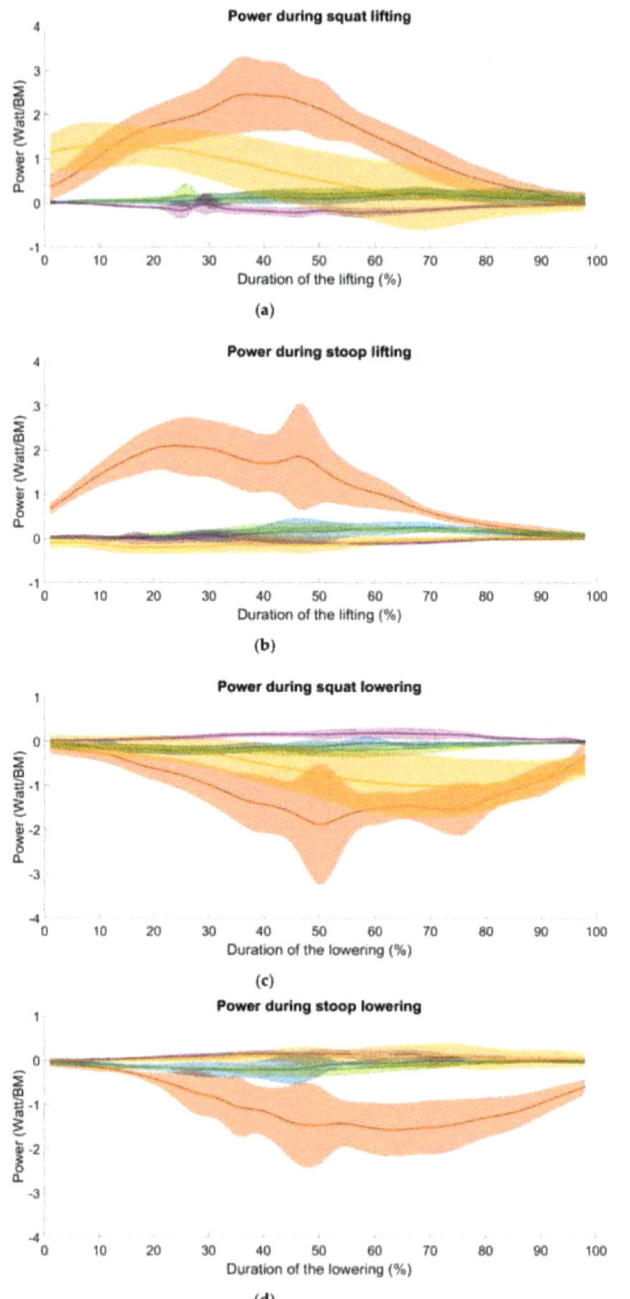

**Figure 3.** Joint power of the five different joints (L5S1 (blue), hip (red), knee (yellow), shoulder (purple) and elbow (green)) during the two different lifting techniques (stoop and squat) with a load equal to 40% ALST. Shaded areas indicate standard deviations. (**a**) Joint power during squat lifting; (**b**) joint power during stoop lifting; (**c**) joint power during squat lowering; (**d**) joint power during stoop lowering.

## 3.1. Peak Moments

Between lifting techniques, no significant differences in L5S1 peak moments were found, hip extension moments were significantly lower during squat lifting than during stoop lifting, and extension moments were significantly higher for the shoulder and the elbow flexion moment (Figure 4a,b). During squat lifting, a peak knee extension moment was observed in contrast to a knee flexion moment during stoop lifting (Figure 4a).

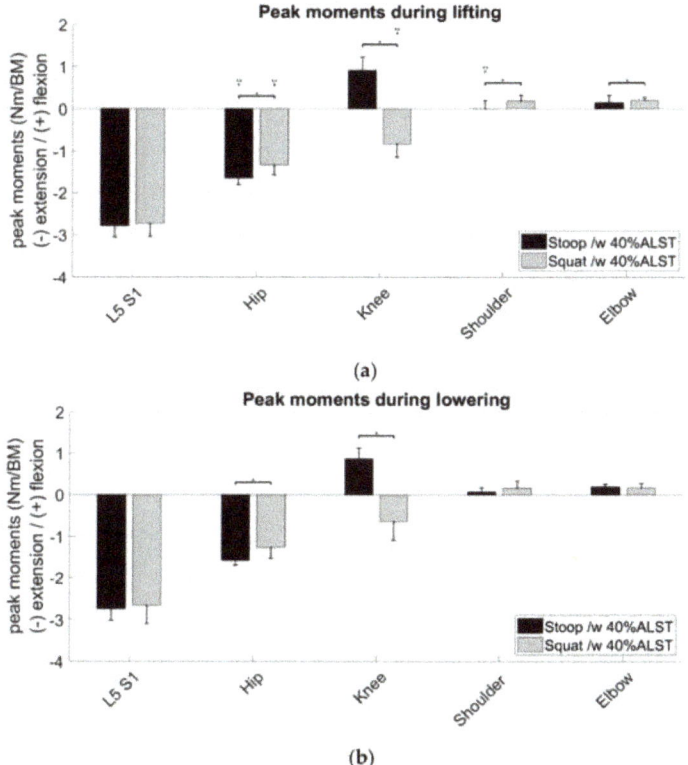

**Figure 4.** Peak moments normalized to body mass during the two different lifting techniques (stoop and squat) with a load equal to 40% of the arm lifting strength test. Statistical significant differences ($\alpha < 0.05$) between the handling phases are indicated with three dots, and statistical meaningful differences between technique and loads are indicated with one dot. Error bars indicate standard deviations. (**a**) Peak moments during the lifting phase in the five different joints (L5S1, hip, knee, shoulder and elbow); (**b**) peak moments during the lowering phase in the five different joints.

Peak hip extension moments were significantly higher during lifting than during lowering, whereas the opposite was observed for the shoulder flexion moments during stoop lifting. During squat lifting, peak knee extension moments were higher during lifting than during lowering.

## 3.2. Peak Power

Between lifting techniques, no significant differences in power generation nor absorption in L5S1 were found (Figure 5a). Hip and elbow peak power generation and absorption were significantly higher during the squat than during stoop lifting. Power generation and absorption in the knee were opposed during the squat compared to the stoop but were significantly higher during the squat than during the stoop.

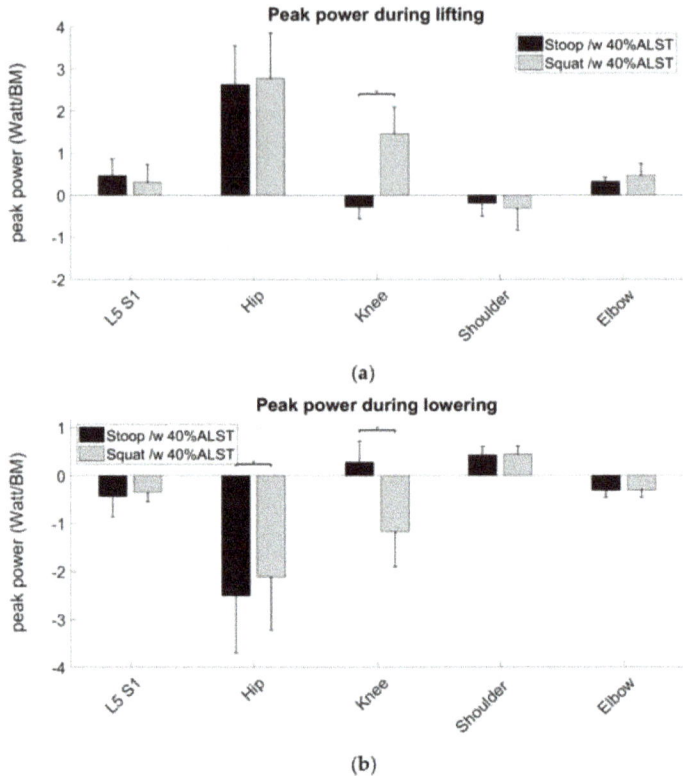

**Figure 5.** Peak power normalized to body mass during the two different lifting techniques (stoop and squat) with the load equal to 40% of the arm lifting strength test. Statistical significant differences ($\alpha < 0.05$) between the handling phases are not indicated because the handling phase affected peak power by inverting power generation and absorption in all conditions. Statistical meaningful differences between technique and loads are indicated with one dot. Error bars indicate standard deviations. (a) Peak power during the lifting phase in the five different joints (L5S1, hip, knee, shoulder and elbow); (b) peak power during the lowering phase in the five different joints.

Power generation and absorption during lifting were inverted during lowering. However, this did not affect the differences between lifting techniques.

The 40% ALST-condition resulted in significantly higher peak power generation and absorption in the hip and the elbow during stoop lifting and significantly higher peak power generation in the shoulder during the lowering phase of the stoop lift technique. In general, the results for peak moments and power were similar while handling a box of 10 kg. These results are shown in Appendix B (Figures A4 and A5).

*3.3. Moment Impulse*

Between lifting techniques, significantly lower moment impulses were observed in L5S1, hip and knee, but significantly higher moment impulses were observed in the shoulder and elbow during the squat than during the stoop (Figure 6). In general, moment impulses were significantly lower in all joints, except the elbow during the lifting stoop compared to lowering. The 40% ALST-condition resulted in a significantly lower moment impulse in the knee when lifting while using the stoop technique compared to the 10 kg-condition (Appendix B Figure A3).

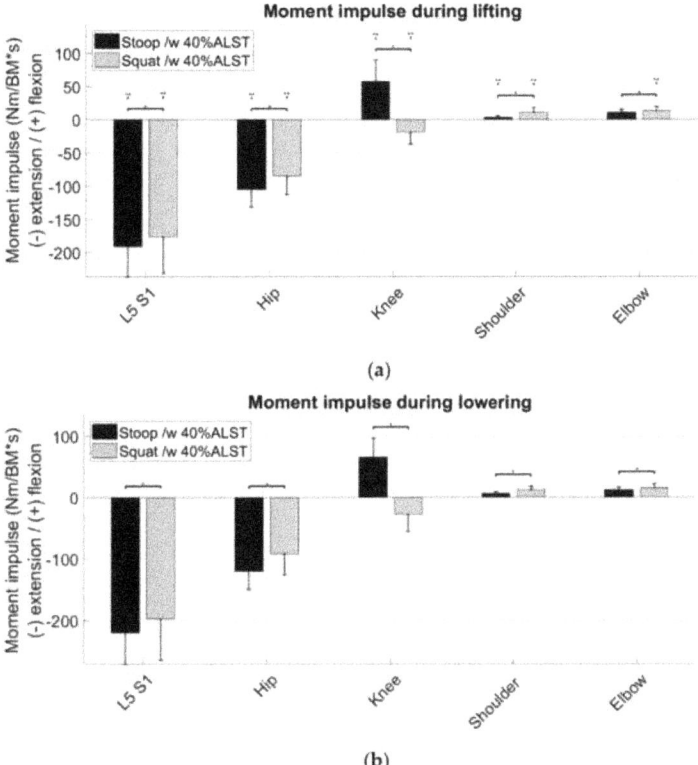

**Figure 6.** Moment impulse normalized to body mass during the two different lifting techniques (stoop and squat) with a load equal to 40% of the arm lifting strength test. Statistical significant differences ($\alpha < 0.05$) between the handling phases are indicated with three dots, and statistical meaningful differences between technique and loads are indicated with one dot. Error bars indicate standard deviations. (**a**) Moment impulse during the lifting phase in the five different joints (L5S1, hip, knee, shoulder and elbow); (**b**) moment impulse during the lowering phase in the five different joints.

*3.4. Peak Muscle Activity*

Between lifting techniques, significantly higher muscle activity for the back extensors (i.e., erector spinae longissimus and iliocostalis), leg extensor (i.e., m. rectus femoris), and shoulder muscles (i.e., m. trapezius descendens, m. deltoideus anterior and medius) was observed during the squat than during the stoop. Significantly lower muscle activity of the leg flexor (i.e., m. biceps femoris) was observed during the squat than during the stoop (Figure 7).

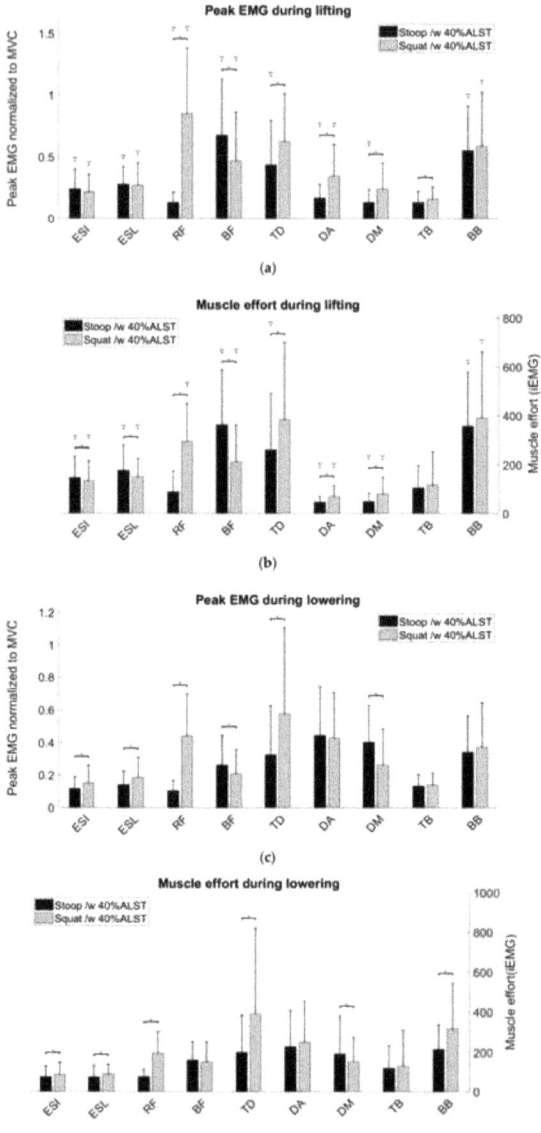

**Figure 7.** Peak electromyography (EMG) normalized to maximal voluntary contractions (MVC) during the two different lifting techniques (stoop and squat) for a load equal to 40% of the arm lifting strength test. Statistical significant differences ($\alpha < 0.05$) between the handling phases are indicated with three dots, and statistical meaningful differences between technique and loads are indicated with one dot. Error bars indicate standard deviations. (**a**) Peak measured EMG during the lifting phase in the nine muscles (erector spinae illiocostalis (ESI), erector spinae longissimus (ESL), rectus femoris (RF), biceps femoris (BF), trapezius descendens (TD), deltoideus anterior (DA), deltoideus medius (DM), triceps brachii (TB), and biceps brachii (BB)); (**b**) muscle effort during lifting for the same nine muscles.; (**c**) peak EMG during the lowering phase for the nine muscles; (**d**) muscle effort during the lowering phase for the same nine muscles.

Muscle activity was significantly higher for the back extensors, arm flexor, leg extensor and flexor muscle but significantly lower for the shoulder muscles during lifting than during lowering. The handling phase had no effect on the m. triceps brachii activity.

The 40% ALST-condition resulted in lower muscle activity for the back muscles when lifting while using the squat technique and lower muscle activity of the shoulder muscles when lifting while using the stoop technique compared to the 10 kg condition (Figure 7a—Appendix B Figure A2a). The 40% ALST-condition had significantly lower muscle activity for the arm muscles and the m. deltoideus medius during lowering using the squat technique (Figure 7c—Appendix B Figure A2c).

*3.5. Muscle Effort*

Between techniques, the muscle effort of m. rectus femoris and shoulder muscles was significantly higher during the squat than during the stoop (Figure 7c,d). Muscle effort of the back muscles and m. biceps femoris was significantly lower during the squat than during the stoop in the lifting phase. Muscle effort was significantly higher for almost all muscles except m. deltoideus anterior and medius during lifting than during lowering.

## 4. Discussion

This study compared whole body loading during two frequently used lifting techniques—squat and stoop lifting—based on joint moments, joint power and muscle activity. In general, squat lifting is the advised method to lift heavy objects because it reduces low back loading. However, it is likely that lifting technique affects joints other than L5S1 and could therefore contribute in the development of WMSDs. Indeed, the present results indicate that lifting technique has no significant effect on the peak moments and power generation in L5S1, but it does significantly increases musculoskeletal demand on the other joints. Furthermore, for the tested weights, the differences between lifting strategies were more pronounced than the effect of the weight lifted.

In line with our hypothesis, squat lifting was found to shift musculoskeletal loading merely to the extremities, potentially to safeguard the lower back. However, joint moments and powers in the back were found not to be significantly different between lifting techniques, therefore imposing similar musculoskeletal loading on the back during squat and stoop lifting. Squat lifting was found to be mainly executed by additional active work of the knee extensors compared to stoop lifting. This was further confirmed by the increased muscle activity of the rectus femoris muscle. Furthermore, squat lifting increased musculoskeletal loading in the shoulder and elbow. This could potentially explain the similar prevalence of WMSDs in the shoulder to low back pain in persons exposed to frequent lifting [1].

Previously, squat lifting was advised to be used over stoop lifting to lift heavy objects because lower moments and compressive forces at the back were reported [6,8,9,20,32]. This is in contrast to the findings of the present study, as similar joint moments were found in the L5S1 joint even when taking the distance between L5 and the object into account. Given the fact that muscle force is the dominant contributor to compressive forces on L5S1 and high muscle force results from high moments around L5S1 [6], we could not conclude that the squat imposes lower compressive forces on L5S1 than the stoop [6]. Based on the assumption that high flexion moments in L5S1 result in high compressive forces, we could assume (as we did not calculate compression and shear forces in this study) that compressive forces are similar between both techniques because both techniques resulted in similar moments around L5S1. Future research should focus on validating biomechanical models in order to calculate compression and shear forces at L5S1. Moreover, based on the L5S1 moment and power, we could not favor squat lifting over stoop lifting in contrast to current literature [6,9]. On the other hand, van Dieen et al. 1999 [32] concluded that there is no evidence of advising squat over stoop lifting in their comprehensive review of 27 studies, which is in line with our results.

Task characteristics, i.e., initial lifting height and dimensions object lift, influence back loading [33], which makes comparisons with literature delicate. Even small adjustments to the squatting technique such as rotating the knees outwards already reduces back loading [14], which was not controlled in this study. However, the handled weights during this experiment were fairly light, and the box was rather small (width: 21 cm; height: 14 cm; length: 36 cm) compared to other studies [6,9]. Potentially, the effect of the lifting technique will be more pronounced when heavier weights are handled. On the other hand, Kingma et al. 2004 concluded that squat lifting a box of 10.5 kg results in higher net moments and higher compression forces in L5S1 compared to the stoop. Our results, with similar moments in L5S1 during the squat and the stoop, can be explained by the higher upper body acceleration during the squat, as suggested by Kingma et al. 2004. This statement is supported by the fact that higher hip and knee joint powers are combined with lower hip and knee moments during the squat compared to the stoop.

However, when accounting for the execution time, i.e., based on the moment impulse on L5S1, squat lifting may still be preferred over stoop lifting. In addition to the slightly longer duration of the stoop lifting task, the longer persistence of the L5S1 extension moment during the stoop than during squat lifting may contribute to this finding (Figure 2). As a result, the cumulative loading during the whole movement is lower during squat lifting. Considering that low back pain is a result of cumulative damage in the lower back [4,11,31,34–36], the squat should be recommend when lifting frequently to prevent back injury. This finding is also supported by the lower muscle effort in the back muscles during the squat. On the other hand, cumulative loading is higher in the shoulder and elbow during the squat compared to the stoop based on the higher moment impulse in shoulder and elbow. In addition, the higher muscle effort of the m. biceps brachii and trapezius descendens, especially during the lowering phase, support this statement, allowing us to conclude that there is an increased injury risk for the shoulder and elbow during repetitive squat lifting.

The handling phase had only a minor effect on musculoskeletal loading in terms of the peak moments, powers and moment impulses, but it had a major effect on muscle activity. In general, muscle activity was higher during lifting than during lowering. This is in line with previous work that has investigated extensor muscle activations during the stoop [9]. The peak EMG of the back extensor muscles were lower during the lowering phase compared to the lifting phase (Figure 7a,c) as back extensor muscles activation peaks twice during the stoop: One small peak during the lowering phase and a larger one during the lifting phase [9]. Our results can be explained by the fact that the muscles have to overcome the moment generated by gravity during the lifting phase, whereas the muscles can cooperate with gravity to perform the required movement during lowering. This can be seen in the higher extensor muscles activity with the squat compared to the stoop while lowering the box, where the moment exerted by gravity can be used advantageous, resulting in higher muscle activation during squat lowering than during stoop lowering.

Interestingly, the findings based on the maximal loading (i.e., peak moment and power) differ from those that account for the movement duration (i.e., moment impulse and muscle effort). The most striking example is that the maximal loading in L5S1 did not differ between techniques, whereas moment impulse in L5S1 and muscle effort of the back muscles did differ between lifting techniques. This suggests that future risk assessment tools should also account for the duration of the lifting task instead of only focusing on the peak moments, as is currently typically done in practice. This is in line with a recently formulated fatigue-failure theorem [37] that relates the pathomechanics of WMSDs to both repetition and force magnitude. Combined with our results, this suggests that ergonomic analysis should use a more holistic approach when analyzing the risk for WMSDs in work situations rather than focusing on the musculoskeletal loading of the target region. Moreover, our results indicate that multiple techniques (i.e., moment estimation and electromyography) should be combined when assessing ergonomic risk and evaluating the effectiveness of ergonomic interventions. This is, in particular, illustrated by the difference in elbow moment between the two different lifting techniques, whereas there was no difference in peak EMG or muscle effort for the m. biceps brachii and triceps brachii.

Though our results indicate that squat lifting imposes similar peak musculoskeletal loading compared to stoop lifting, our results should be interpreted in the context of some limitations. First, although the musculoskeletal model used in the present study has a detailed description of the shoulder and lumbar back region, the thorax is defined as one rigid segment. Furthermore, not all degrees of freedom in the shoulder were modelled (i.e., pro- and retraction of the shoulder griddle). Secondly, healthy volunteers whose lifting dynamics are likely to be different compared to experienced blue-collar workers were studied. It was previously found that experienced blue-collar workers have adopted a more efficient method for lifting over the years [13]. However, we assume that the effect of experience on performance during isolated, well-standardized lifting tasks is minimal. Thirdly, the tasks performed in the lab might be difficult to generalize to real-world situations. According the National Institute for Occupational Safety and Health (NIOSH) [38] equations, the task in the lab could be classified as heavy; however, the set-up in the lab mostly conformed the guidelines reported in ISO 11228 part 1, whereas in the industry, ideal circumstances are not likely to be present the whole time and the weight of the object to lift often exceeds the weight that was used in the present study. Future research should focus on differentiating more between weights and investigate the effect of weight on lifting techniques and musculoskeletal loading.

In summary, peak moments in L5S1, a well-recognized risk factor for developing WMSDs, is not different between the two techniques while lifting a box of approximately 10 kg, although the moment impulse is higher in L5S1, hip and knee during the stoop. In contrast to these findings, ergonomic guidelines suggest using squat lifting as much as possible during materials handling, and for that reason, a reevaluation of the ergonomic guidelines is needed. Therefore, we suggest to adopt a more holistic framework that combines different measurement modalities as used in the present study when analyzing working tasks and to evaluate the effect of an intervention on the WMSDs risk.

**Author Contributions:** Conceptualization, A.v.d.H., S.V.R., and I.J.; methodology, A.v.d.H.; investigation, A.v.d.H., S.V.R., and I.J.; resources, I.J.; writing—original draft preparation, A.v.d.H.; writing—review and editing, S.V.R. and I.J.; visualization, A.v.d.H.; supervision, S.V.R. and I.J.

**Funding:** This research was funded by Exo4Work, SBO-E—S000118N.

**Conflicts of Interest:** The authors declare no conflict of interest.

## Appendix A

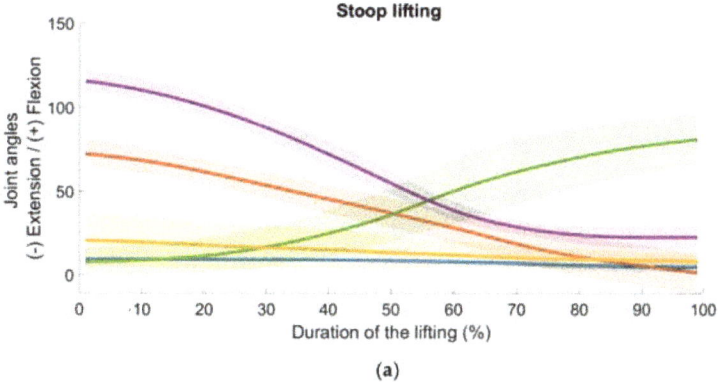

(a)

**Figure A1.** *Cont.*

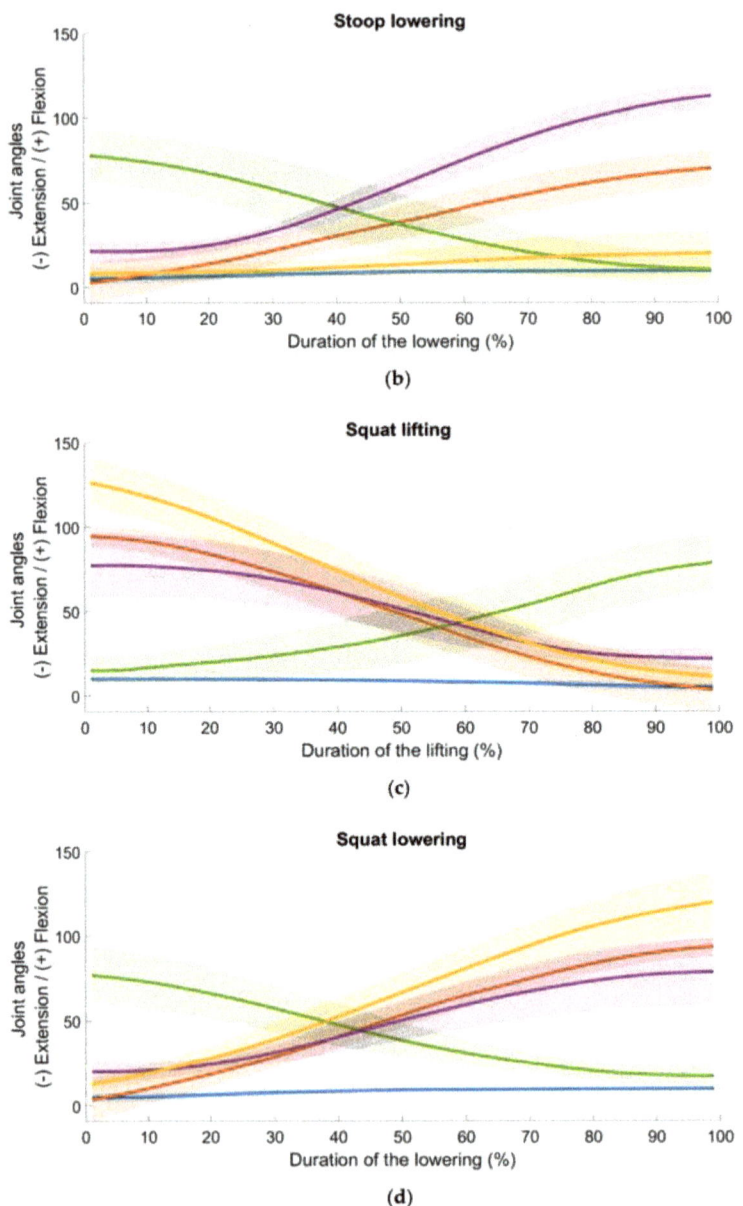

**Figure A1.** Kinematics of the five different joints (L5S1 (blue), hip (red), knee (yellow), shoulder (purple) and elbow (green)) during the two different lifting techniques (stoop and squat) with a load equal to 40% ALST. Shaded areas indicate standard deviations. (**a**) Joint angles during stoop lifting; (**b**) joint angles during stoop lowering; (**c**) joint angles during squat lifting; (**d**) joint angles during squat lowering.

## Appendix B

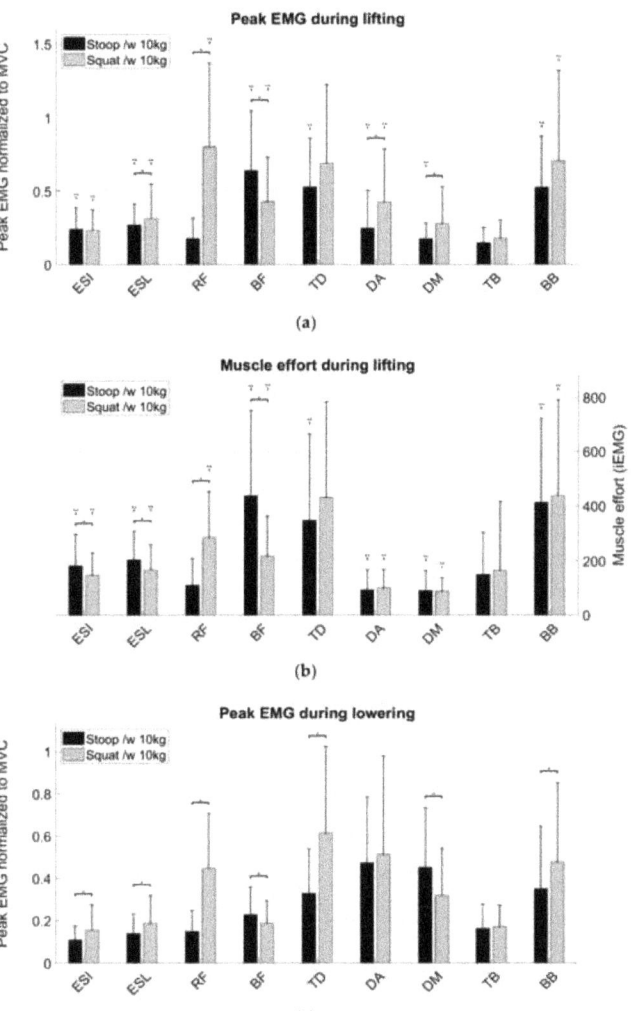

**Figure A2.** *Cont.*

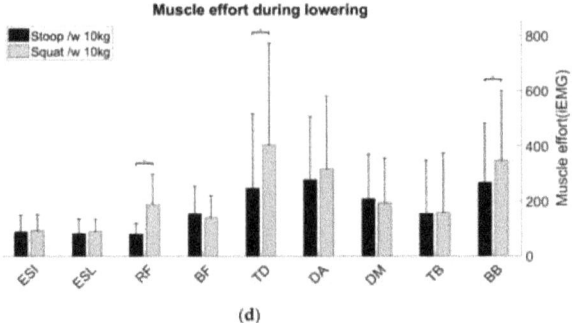

**Figure A2.** Peak EMG normalized to MVC during the two different lifting techniques (stoop and squat) for the 10 kg box. Statistical significant differences ($\alpha < 0.05$) between the handling phases are indicated with three dots, and statistical meaningful differences between technique and loads are indicated with one dot. Error bars indicate standard deviations. (**a**) Peak measured EMG during the lifting phase in the nine muscles (erector spinae illiocostalis (ESI), erector spinae longissimus (ESL), rectus femoris (RF), biceps femoris (BF), trapezius descendens (TD), deltoideus anterior (DA), deltoideus medius (DM), triceps brachii (TB), and biceps brachii (BB)); (**b**) muscle effort during lifting for the same nine muscles.; (**c**) peak EMG during the lowering phase for the nine muscles; (**d**) muscle effort during the lowering phase for the same nine muscles.

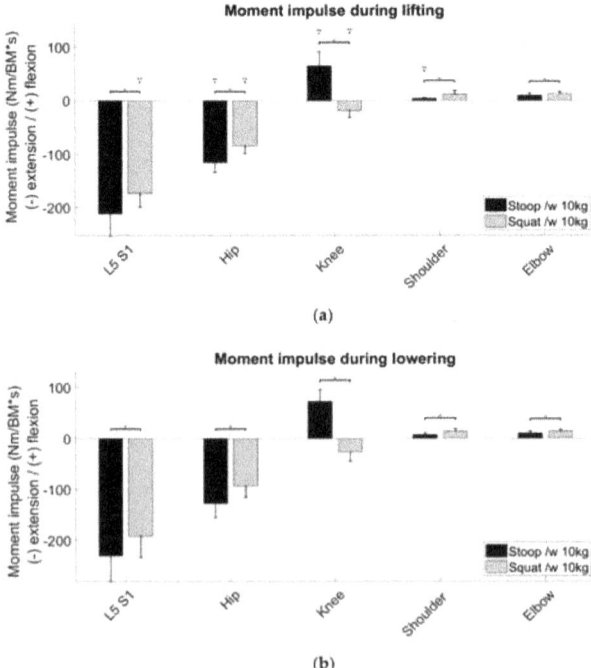

**Figure A3.** Moment impulse normalized to body mass during the two different lifting techniques (stoop and squat) with the 10 kg box. Statistical significant differences ($\alpha < 0.05$) between the handling phases are indicated with three dots, and statistical meaningful differences between techniques and loads are indicated with one dot. Error bars indicate standard deviations. (**a**) Moment impulse during the lifting phase in the five different joints (L5S1, hip, knee, shoulder and elbow); (**b**) moment impulse during the lowering phase in the five different joints.

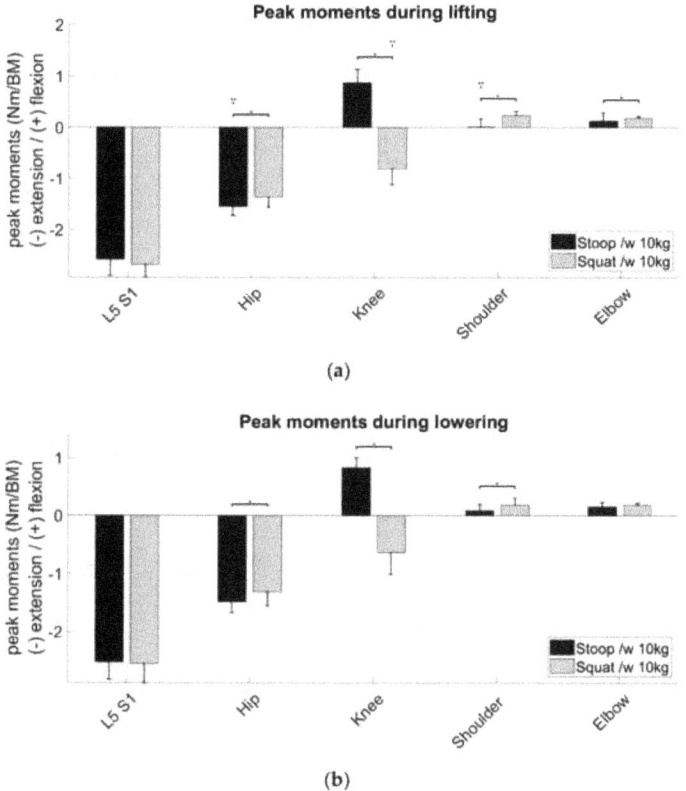

**Figure A4.** Moment impulse normalized to body mass during the two different lifting techniques (stoop and squat) with the 10 kg box. Statistical significant differences ($\alpha < 0.05$) between the handling phases are indicated with three dots, and statistical meaningful differences between technique and loads are indicated with one dot. Error bars indicate standard deviations. (**a**) Moment impulse during the lifting phase in the five different joints (L5S1, hip, knee, shoulder and elbow); (**b**) moment impulse during the lowering phase in the five different joints.

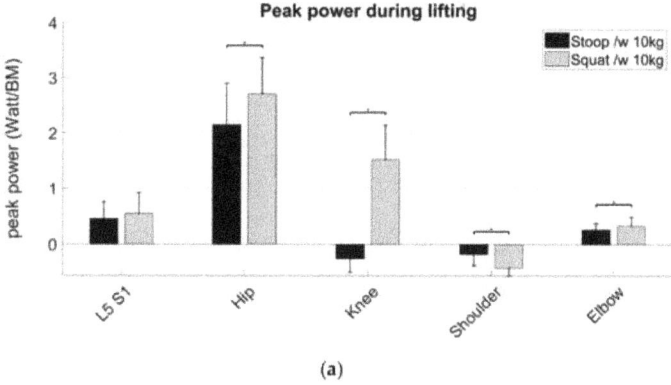

**Figure A5.** *Cont.*

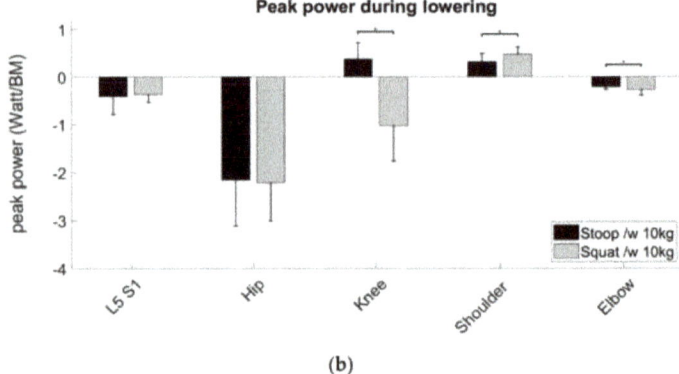

(b)

**Figure A5.** Peak power normalized to body mass during the two different lifting techniques (stoop and squat) with the 10 kg box. Statistical significant differences ($\alpha < 0.05$) between the handling phases are not indicated, as handling phase affected peak power by inverting power generation and absorption in all conditions. Statistical meaningful differences between technique and loads are indicated with one dot. Error bars indicate standard deviations. (**a**) Peak power during the lifting phase in the five different joints (L5S1, hip, knee, shoulder and elbow); (**b**) peak power during the lowering phase in the five different joints. In the 10 kg condition only, peak power absorption and generation in the shoulder were significantly higher during the squat than during the stoop, which is in contrast to the 40% ALST-condition.

## References

1. EU-OSHA European Agency for Safety and Health at Work. *Sixth European Working Conditions Survey—Overview Report (2017 Update)*; EU-OSHA European Agency for Safety and Health at Work: Bilbao, Spain, 2017; ISBN 978-9-28-971596-6.
2. European Foundation for the Improvement of Living and Working Conditions (Eurofound). Absence from work. *Eurofound* **2010**, *2*, 314.
3. Putz-Anderson, V.; Bernard, B.P.; Burt, S.E.; Cole, L.L.; Fairfield-Estill, C.; Fine, L.J.; Grant, K.A.; Gjessing, C.; Jenkins, L.; Hurrell, J.J.; et al. *Musculoskeletal Disorders and Workplace Factors: A Critical Review of Epidemiologic Evidence for Work-Related Musculoskeletal Disorders of the Neck, Upper Extremity, and Low Back*; US Department of Health and Human Services, Public Health Service, Centers for Disease Control and Prevention, National Institute for Occupational Safety and Health: Cincinnati, OH, USA, 1997.
4. Norman, R.; Neumann, P.; Wells, R.; Shannon, H.; Frank, J.; Kerr, M. A comparison of peak vs cumulative physical work exposure risk factors for the reporting of low back pain in the automotive industry. *Clin. Biomech.* **1998**, *13*, 561–573. [CrossRef]
5. Dreischarf, M.; Rohlmann, A.; Graichen, F.; Bergmann, G.; Schmidt, H. In vivo loads on a vertebral body replacement during different lifting techniques. *J. Biomech.* **2016**, *49*, 890–895. [CrossRef] [PubMed]
6. Kingma, I.; Faber, G.S.; van Dieën, J.H. How to lift a box that is too large to fit between the knees. *Ergonomics* **2010**, *53*, 1228–1238. [CrossRef] [PubMed]
7. Revuelta, N.; Dauphin, A.; Kowslowski, O.; Dubois, D.; Thevenon, A. Heart rate response to two lifting techniques. *Arch. Phys. Med. Rehabil.* **2000**, *81*, 958–959. [CrossRef] [PubMed]
8. Wang, Z.; Wu, L.; Sun, J.; He, L.; Wang, S.; Yang, L. Squat, stoop, or semi-squat: A comparative experiment on lifting technique. *J. Huazhong Univ. Sci. Technol. Med. Sci.* **2012**, *32*, 630–636. [CrossRef] [PubMed]
9. Bazrgari, B.; Shirazi-Adl, A.; Arjmand, N. Analysis of squat and stoop dynamic liftings: Muscle forces and internal spinal loads. *Eur. Spine J.* **2007**, *16*, 687–699. [CrossRef]
10. Burgess-Limerick, R. Squat, stoop, or something in between? *Int. J. Ind. Ergon.* **2003**, *31*, 143–148. [CrossRef]
11. Antwi-Afari, M.F.; Li, H.; Edwards, D.J.; Pärn, E.A.; Seo, J.; Wong, A.Y.L. Biomechanical analysis of risk factors for work-related musculoskeletal disorders during repetitive lifting task in construction workers. *Autom. Constr.* **2017**, *83*, 41–47. [CrossRef]

12. Arjmand, N.; Shirazi-Adl, A. Sensitivity of kinematics-based model predictions to optimization criteria in static lifting tasks. *Med. Eng. Phys.* **2006**, *28*, 504–514. [CrossRef]
13. Gagnon, D.; Plamondon, A.; Larivière, C. A biomechanical comparison between expert and novice manual materials handlers using a multi-joint EMG-assisted optimization musculoskeletal model of the lumbar spine. *J. Biomech.* **2016**, *49*, 2938–2945. [CrossRef] [PubMed]
14. Kingma, I.; Bosch, T.; Bruins, L.; van Dieën, J.H. Foot positioning instruction, initial vertical load position and lifting technique: Effects on low back loading. *Ergonomics* **2004**, *47*, 1365–1385. [CrossRef] [PubMed]
15. Marras, W.S.; Parakkat, J.; Chany, A.M.; Yang, G.; Burr, D.; Lavender, S.A. Spine loading as a function of lift frequency, exposure duration, and work experience. *Clin. Biomech.* **2006**, *21*, 345–352. [CrossRef] [PubMed]
16. Kim, H.; Zhang, Y. Estimation of lumbar spinal loading and trunk muscle forces during asymmetric lifting tasks: Application of whole-body musculoskeletal modelling in OpenSim. *Ergonomics* **2017**, *60*, 563–576. [CrossRef]
17. Larivière, C.; Gagnon, D.; Loisel, P. The comparison of trunk muscles EMG activation between subjects with and without chronic low back pain during flexion-extension and lateral bending tasks. *J. Electromyogr. Kinesiol.* **2000**, *10*, 79–91. [CrossRef]
18. Graham, R.B.; Agnew, M.J.; Stevenson, J.M. Effectiveness of an on-body lifting aid at reducing low back physical demands during an automotive assembly task: Assessment of EMG response and user acceptability. *Appl. Ergon.* **2009**, *40*, 936–942. [CrossRef]
19. Shair, E.F.; Ahmad, S.A.; Marhaban, M.H.; Mohd Tamrin, S.B.; Abdullah, A.R. EMG Processing Based Measures of Fatigue Assessment during Manual Lifting. *BioMed Res. Int.* **2017**, *2017*, 1–12. [CrossRef]
20. Kingma, I.; Faber, G.S.; van Dieën, J.H. Supporting the upper body with the hand on the thigh reduces back loading during lifting. *J. Biomech.* **2016**, *49*, 881–889. [CrossRef]
21. Zelik, K.E.; Honert, E.C. Ankle and foot power in gait analysis: Implications for science, technology and clinical assessment. *J. Biomech.* **2018**, *75*, 1–12. [CrossRef]
22. Tenenbaum, S.; Bariteau, J.; Coleman, S.; Brodsky, J. Functional and clinical outcomes of total ankle arthroplasty in elderly compared to younger patients. *Foot Ankle Surg.* **2017**, *23*, 102–107. [CrossRef]
23. Chaffin, D.B.; Herrin, G.D.; Keyserling, W.M. Pre-employment strength testing. An updated position. *J. Occup. Med.* **1978**, *20*, 403–408. [PubMed]
24. Davis, B.R.; Õunpuu, S.; Tyburski, D.; Gage, J.R. A gait analysis collection and reduction technique. *Hum. Mov. Sci.* **1991**, *10*, 575–587. [CrossRef]
25. Leardini, A.; Biagi, F.; Merlo, A.; Belvedere, C.; Benedetti, M.G. Multi-segment trunk kinematics during locomotion and elementary exercises. *Clin. Biomech.* **2011**, *26*, 562–571. [CrossRef] [PubMed]
26. Delp, S.L.; Anderson, F.C.; Arnold, A.S.; Loan, P.; Habib, A.; John, C.T.; Guendelman, E.; Thelen, D.G. OpenSim: Open source to create and analyze dynamic simulations of movement. *IEEE Trans. Biomed. Eng.* **2007**, *54*, 1940–1950. [CrossRef] [PubMed]
27. Bruno, A.G.; Bouxsein, M.L.; Anderson, D.E. Development and Validation of a Musculoskeletal Model of the Fully Articulated Thoracolumbar Spine and Rib Cage. *J. Biomech. Eng.* **2015**, *137*, 081003. [CrossRef] [PubMed]
28. Holzbaur, K.R.S.; Murray, W.M.; Delp, S.L. A model of the upper extremity for simulating musculoskeletal surgery and analyzing neuromuscular control. *Ann. Biomed. Eng.* **2005**, *33*, 829–840. [CrossRef] [PubMed]
29. Delp, S.L.; Loan, J.P.; Hoy, M.G.; Zajac, F.E.; Topp, E.L.; Rosen, J.M. An interactive graphics-based model of the lower extremity to study orthopaedic surgical procedures. *IEEE Trans. Biomed. Eng.* **1990**, *37*, 757–767. [CrossRef] [PubMed]
30. Lu, T.-W.; O'Connor, J.J. Bone position estimation from skin marker co-ordinates using global optimisation with joint constraints. *J. Biomech.* **1999**, *32*, 129–134. [CrossRef]
31. Plamondon, A.; Larivière, C.; Denis, D.; Mecheri, H.; Nastasia, I. Difference between male and female workers lifting the same relative load when palletizing boxes. *Appl. Ergon.* **2017**, *60*, 93–102. [CrossRef]
32. Van Dieën, J.H.; Hoozemans, M.J.M.; Toussaint, H.M. Stoop or squat: A review of biomechanical studies on lifting technique. *Clin. Biomech.* **1999**, *14*, 685–696. [CrossRef]
33. Kingma, I.; Faber, G.S.; Bakker, A.J.M.; van Dieen, J.H. Can low back loading during lifting be reduced by placing one leg beside the object to be lifted? *Phys. Ther.* **2006**, *86*, 1091–1105. [PubMed]
34. Gallagher, S.; Schall, M.C. Musculoskeletal disorders as a fatigue failure process: Evidence, implications and research needs. *Ergonomics* **2017**, *60*, 255–269. [CrossRef] [PubMed]

35. Ma, L.; Chablat, D.; Bennis, F.; Zhang, W.; Guillaume, F. A new muscle fatigue and recovery model and its ergonomics application in human simulation. *Virtual Phys. Prototyp.* **2010**, *5*, 123–137. [CrossRef]
36. Zehr, J.D.; Tennant, L.M.; Callaghan, J.P. Examining endplate fatigue failure during cyclic compression loading with variable and consistent peak magnitudes using a force weighting adjustment approach: An in vitro study. *Ergonomics* **2019**, 1–10. [CrossRef] [PubMed]
37. Gallagher, S.; Heberger, J.R. Examining the interaction of force and repetition on musculoskeletal disorder risk: A systematic literature review. *Hum. Factors* **2013**, *55*, 108–124. [CrossRef] [PubMed]
38. Waters, T.; Putz-Anderson, V.; Garg, A. *Work Practices Guide for Manual Lifting*; The National Institute for Occupational Safety and Health (NIOSH): Cincinnati, OH, USA, 1981.

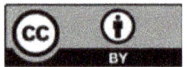
© 2019 by the authors. Licensee MDPI, Basel, Switzerland. This article is an open access article distributed under the terms and conditions of the Creative Commons Attribution (CC BY) license (http://creativecommons.org/licenses/by/4.0/).

Article

# Effect of In-Shoe Foot Orthosis Contours on Heel Pain Due to Calcaneal Spurs

**Dwi Basuki Wibowo [1],\*, Achmad Widodo [1], Gunawan Dwi Haryadi [1], Wahyu Caesarendra [1,2] and Rudiansyah Harahap [3]**

[1] Mechanical Engineering Department, Diponegoro University, Jl. Prof. Soedharto, SH, Tembalang, Semarang 50275, Indonesia; awidodo2010@gmail.com (A.W.); gunawan_dh@ft.undip.ac.id (G.D.H.); wahyu.caesarendra@ubd.edu.bn (W.C.)
[2] Faculty of Integrated Technologies, Universiti Brunei Darussalam, Jalan Tungku Link, BE1410, Brunei Darussalam
[3] Department of Orthopedic, RSUD Tugurejo Semarang, Semarang 50185, Indonesia; rudiansyahrsutugurejo@gmail.com
\* Correspondence: ir.dwibasuki.ms@gmail.com; Tel.: +62-812-298-9124

Received: 27 November 2018; Accepted: 25 January 2019; Published: 31 January 2019

**Featured Application:** The proposed method for easily obtaining contoured insoles from the variation of the insole foot area together with the pain pressure threshold could potentially be applied to orthotic shoe designers for reducing pain in calcaneal spur patients.

**Abstract:** The objective of this study is to investigate the effect of contouring the shoe insole on calcaneal pressure and heel pain in calcaneal spur patients. Calcaneal pressure was measured using three force sensors from 13 patients including three males and 10 females. These patients have plantar heel pain due to calcaneal spurs, and we examined five customized contour insole foot areas (0–100%). Sensors were attached at the central heel (CH), lateral heel (LH) and medial heel (MH) of the foot. The pain was measured using an algometer and evaluated by the pain minimum compressive pressure (PMCP). In this study, it was observed that the calcaneal pressure decreased with increasing insole foot area. In addition, increasing the insole foot area from 25% to 50% can reduce the calcaneal pressure approximately 17.4% at the LH and 30.9% at the MH, which are smaller than the PMCP, while at the MH, pressure reduced 6.9%, which is greater than the PMCP. Therefore, to reduce pain, one can use 50% insole foot area, even though at MH it is still 19.3% greater than the PMCP. Excellent pain relief was observed when using 100% insole foot area, as the pressures in those three areas are lower than the PMCPs, but it is not recommended because it requires large production costs.

**Keywords:** calcaneal spur; pain minimum compressive pressure; contour of shoe insole; insole foot area

## 1. Introduction

Plantar heel pain is one of the most common musculoskeletal conditions affecting the foot in adults, with a highest incidence at the age of 40 to 60 years [1,2]. There are many causes of pain in the plantar heel area, and one of them is due to a calcaneal/heel spur [3].

A calcaneal spur is a condition where a calcium deposit grows between the heel and arch of the foot [4]. Generally, this does not affect a person's daily life, but repetitive stress from activities may result in the spur breaking into sharp pieces and pressing the nerves of the plantar fascia [5–7]. This condition causes plantar fasciitis, in which patients experience pain and tenderness at the heel [8,9]. People who are obese, individuals with either flat feet or high arches, and individuals who engage in prolonged standing or walking are very vulnerable to this disease [6].

Heel pain treatment (including pain caused by a calcaneal spur) is listed in the document of the Clinical Practice Guideline (CPG) developed by the heel pain committee of the American College of Foot and Ankle Surgeons (ACFAS), which recommends quick procedures in assessment and management of heel pain [10]. The authors classify treatments into three phases for heel pain treatments, and the use of orthotic shoes is recommended in phase II.

Orthotic shoes for calcaneal spur patients are specially designed to reduce pain when used for walking activity by modifying pressure in the heel region [11,12]. Pressure reduction using orthotic shoes requires knowledge of the location and dimensions of the spur, and typically the minimum pressure that causes pain in the patient's heel area. A large-dimension spur ($\geq$6 mm) causes high pain level compared to a small spur (1–2 mm) [13]. Determining the area in the heel where the spur growth is plays a major role in knowing the level of the pain. The research on pressure pain threshold (PPT) in patients experiencing plantar heel pain syndrome using a pressure algometer was presented by Saban et al. [14]. To measure PPT, the heel was divided into five regions. The results indicated that PPT levels at posterior/medial, anterior/medial and central regions were significantly lower than at anterior/lateral and posterior/lateral regions.

Various types of shoe soles have been studied to reduce pain in the heel area. Shoes with thick soles and extra cushioning can reduce pain while standing and walking [15,16]. High-heel shoes can shift pressure away from the heel to the mid-foot and fore-foot [17]. Contoured insoles are better than flat insoles in reducing local peak pressures [18–20]. A number of methods have been carried out to estimate the contact pressures or pressure distribution patterns in both feet for each subject during standing and/or walking activity. The methods applied the finite element method (FEM) [15], used a pressure sensor, that is, the Force Sensing Resistor (FSR) [16,17], were based on a weighting scale method [18], used a flexible F-Scan® insole sensing system [19], or used capacitance sensor/transducers (the PEDAR® pressure measurement system) [20].

Commonly, to obtain a contour-customized in-shoe foot orthotics is done by taking a plaster cast of the patient's foot plantar surface (the negative cast) and then moulding this negative cast on a plaster casting board to obtain the positive cast [21]. Tsung et al. [18] made the positive cast with full-weight-bearing and semi-weight-bearing by directly printing the plantar foot on the casting board placed on top of the electronic balance. Another method to obtain the patient's foot plantar surface is to use 3D scanning, which is the latest technology that has been widely used by many researchers [22,23]. This study aims to determine the effect of contouring of an in-shoe foot orthosis on heel pressure while standing, and its relationship to the pain in the heel area.

## 2. Materials and Methods

Thirteen patients (3 male and 10 female) at the local public hospital Tugurejo Semarang with plantar heel pain due to a calcaneal spur from June 2017 to August 2018 were involved in the experimental work of the study. The ethical clearance has been approved and issued by the Ethics Committee of the Tugurejo Hospital. All subjects have also signed and provided their written informed consent before participating in this study. The diagnosis of plantar heel pain of the patients was based on pain upon palpation. The mean age of the subjects was 56.5 $\pm$ 9.9 years (range between 38–73 years), mean height was 155.6 $\pm$ 7.6 cm (range from 144 to 172 cm) and mean weight was 63.3 $\pm$ 9.4 kg (range between 50–84.6 kg). The location and dimension of each patient's spur were obtained from lateral X-rays [17]. The length of the spur is classified into 3 types: small (1–2 mm), medium (3–5 mm) and large ($\geq$6 mm) [13]. There were 7 patients with a calcaneal spur on both feet, but in this study, only the longest spur was evaluated because there is a significant correlation between the length of spur and the pain minimum compressive pressure (PMCP) [17].

In order to obtain an exact location and dimension of the spur in the plantar view as shown in Figure 1 up, each patient was requested to do a two-dimensional footprint using a digital footprint scanner (LSR 2D Laser Foot Scanner, Vismach Technology Ltd., China). This scanner is equipped with software to measure foot length (FL) and foot width (FW) to determine the shoe size and heel width

(HW) of each patient [24]. The spur is assumed to be located in the heel center line, which is a line drawn from the center of the heel (CH) to the tip of the second toe [25].

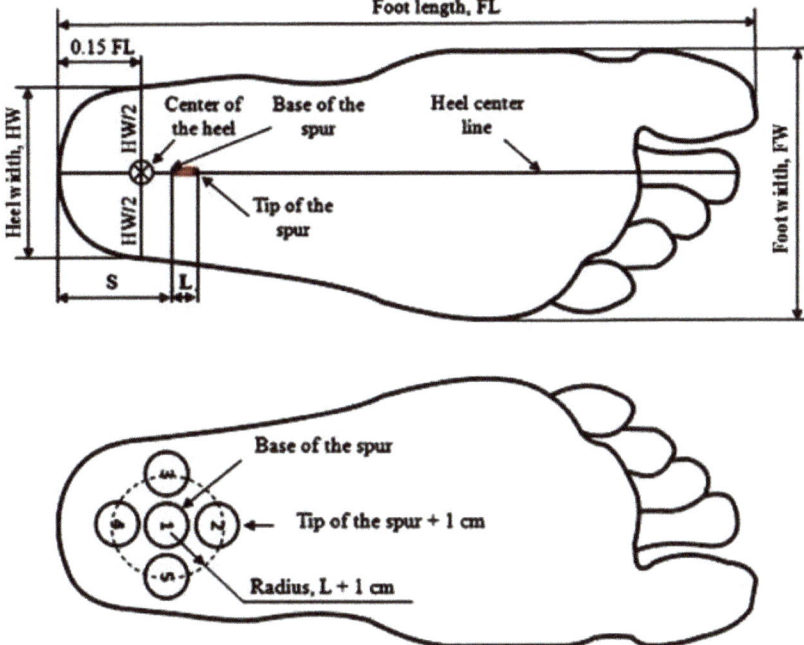

**Figure 1.** (**up**) Location and dimension of the spur in the plantar view; (**down**) Five locations of the pressure pain threshold (PPT) around spur growth.

The pain in the heel area was measured using an FDIX 25 algometer (Wagner Instruments, Greenwich CT, USA), which consists of a flat rubber tip probe 1.0 cm in diameter [26]. This instrument can display the compression force in either Newtons or kilograms and also can measure the pressure which is calculated from the force divided by the probe area. The region of the pain pressure threshold (PPT) was determined around the spur growth which is divided into five points: point 1 at the base of the spur, and the next compressive test points at the anterior site (point 2), the lateral site (point 3), the posterior site (point 4), and the medial site (point 5), made circular with radius of spur length, L plus 1 cm as presented in Figure 1 down. The addition of 1 cm is needed to compensate for the diameter of the algometer probe. The calculation method of PPT region in this paper is similar to the study conducted by Saban et al., but the exact location of pain suppression was not specified and the patients recruited were not specifically recruited due to the calcaneal spur [14].

To measure PPT, the patient was requested to lay supine in a relaxed position and press the algometer probe at point 1 as shown in Figure 1 down. S is the distance from the tip of the heel to the base of the spur and L is the length of the spur. We increased the pressure gradually until the patient complained of pain. We recorded the pressure value and applied a similar procedure to others points. From the recorded data, the PMCP and the point location in each patient can be monitored [17].

*2.1. Determining the Contour of the Shoe Insole*

In this study, the negative cast of the custom insole foot contour is made from a 3D foot scanner (ScanPod 3D, Vismach Technology Ltd., Hongkong, China). The accuracy of this scanner is ± 1.0 mm and the output is in the standard language (dxf/stl/wrl/obj/ply/asc). These formats are associated with any 3D software, for example, AutoCAD. The output can be in the form of the 3D plantar the of foot in difference of colors as presented in Figure 2a, where the red color indicates where the foot has the largest convex (largest z-coordinates), the 3D foam negative impression to make a negative cast of the foot as shown in Figure 2b, and the 3D positive model of the footprint in the form of a foam impression as shown in Figure 2c [27].

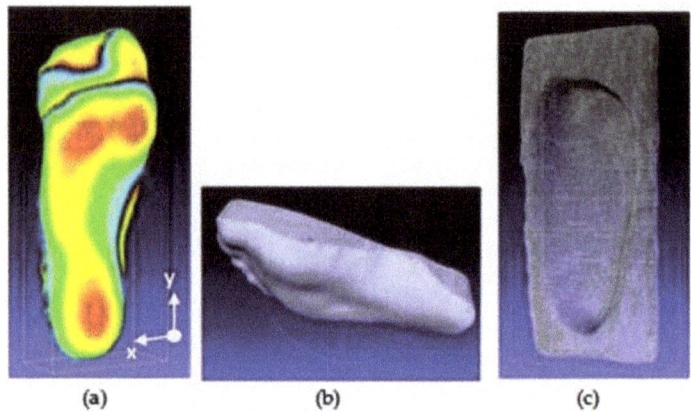

**Figure 2.** Example outputs of 3D scanning: (**a**) footprint depth in difference of colors; (**b**) 3D foam negative impression; (**c**) footprint 3D positive model.

This technique has been used previously by Telfer et al. [22] and Stankovic et al. [23]. The difference between the technique proposed in this paper and the above-mentioned published papers is in the variation of the shape of the foot that was evaluated. In this study, the shoe insole foot contours are distinguished by the insole foot area, where the largest area is equal to the contour of the unloaded foot (100% A) and the smallest is the same as the flat insole (0% A). This is based on the fact that the sole of the foot will follow the contour of the shoe insole as long as it does not exceed the contour of the unloaded foot. There were 5 variations of shoe insole foot area, that is, (1) 100% A, (2) 75% A, (3) 50% A, (4) 25% A, and (5) 0% A. One hundred percent and zero percent areas express the contour and projection areas of the 3D scanning result of the foot evaluated using Rhinoceros software, respectively. The other shoe insole area is calculated as follows:

$$n\% \ A = n\% \times \Delta A + 0\% \ A, \tag{1}$$

where n are 75, 50 and 25 and $\Delta A = 100\% \ A - 0\% \ A$.

Varying the area of shoe insole means changing the z-coordinates at 100% A until it reaches z-coordinates at 75% A to 25% A. The procedure for determining variations of the shoe insole area is presented in detail in Figure 3a. The following steps are conducted in the experimental work:

Scan the foot in 3D format and import this 3D scanned image file into AutoCAD.

(1) Evaluate the area 100% A and 0% A using Rhinoceros software.
(2) Generate the xyz-coordinates of 100%_A by using Microsoft Excel which integrated with AutoCAD software as presented in Figure 3b.
(3) Adjust the z-coordinates of 100% A to 75% A; initially specify a reduced percentage of 5% (reduced percentage z-coordinates of 100% A and 0% A are 0% and 100%, respectively) and display the coordinates in AutoCAD to evaluate its area using Rhinoceros software.
(4) If the area is still much greater than 5 mm$^2$ [28] compared with Equation (1), repeat the procedure four times by increasing the percentage of 5% reduction.
(5) If the difference of area approaches 5 mm$^2$, increase the percentage reduction to 1–2%.

A similar procedure (step 4 to 6) is conducted to obtain shoe insole area of 50% A and 25% A by initially determining that the deduction percentage is slightly greater than the deduction percentage of 75% and 50%, respectively. The z-coordinates for every n% A can then be calculated using Equation (2), where z, $z_{max}$ and $z_{min}$ express the z-coordinates at 100% A ($z_{100\%\_A}$) and the largest and smallest z-coordinates at 100% A, respectively.

$$z_{n\%A} = z - \left(\frac{2z - (z_{max} + z_{min})}{2}\right) \times \% \text{ deduction} \quad (2)$$

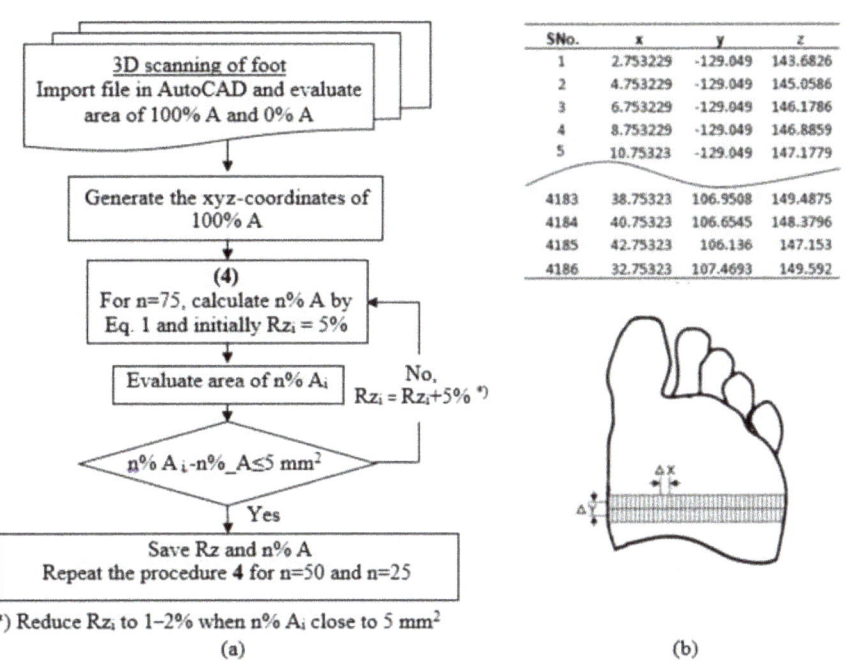

Figure 3. (a) Flowchart evaluation of n% insole foot area; (b) Table of 3D coordinates (x, y, and z axis) generated from AutoCAD with the visualization of the increment of x- and y-axis.

## 2.2. Measuring Pressure in Heel Area

To measure the burden of its own weight, we used three force sensing resistors (FSR 402, Interlink Electronics) which are attached to the calcaneal area of the feet with double tape. Determination of the location of each sensor was performed using an unloaded foot scan around the area that was estimated to receive a large burden when standing, as shown in Figure 2a. For this purpose, sensor 2 is placed at CH (0.15 FL) [29] and sensors 1 and 3 are placed arbitrarily at the lateral heel (LH) and medial heel (MH), in line above sensor 2, under the boundary between the heel and mid foot area (0.31 FL) [30], as shown in Figure 4.

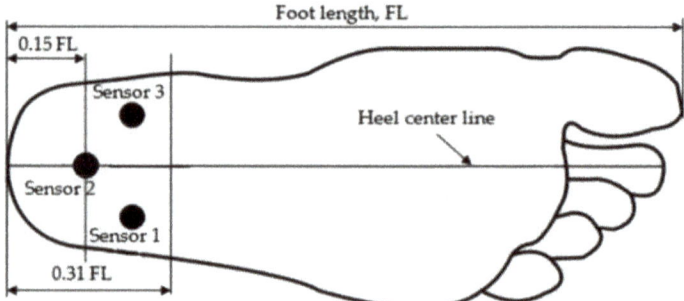

**Figure 4.** Illustration of the Force Sensing Resistor (FSR) sensor locations.

The FSR is a polymer thick-film device which exhibits a decrease in resistance with an increase in the force applied to the active surface. Its force sensitivity is optimized for use in human touch control of electronic devices. FSRs are not a load cell or strain gauge, though they have similar properties. The FSR 402 has active area of 0.5" (12.7 mm) diameter, the nominal thickness of 0.018" (0.46 mm), force sensitivity range of 100 g to 10 kg, and pressure sensitivity range of 1.5 to 150 psi. The relationship between the load L (grams) and the voltage V (volts) can be expressed by polynomial regression, as presented in Equation (3). Each sensor is connected to one resistor. The output voltage of the FSR sensor is read by the Arduino MEGA 2560 microcontroller using 10 pin analog input bits [31]. Then, the voltage is sent to DAQ software LabVIEW via serial USB to be converted into load using Equation (3).

$$L = 927.7\ V^3 - 1643.9\ V^2 + 1083.5\ V - 31.02 \qquad (3)$$

Each patient was requested to stand upright using the appropriate test shoe size for each shoe insole area. The outsole material is made of Microcell Puff EVA foam and the insole made of Poron cushioning [32]. Initially, each patient is requested to wear the shoe with 0% A, and three pressure datapoints from CH, MH and LH areas are recorded. A similar procedure is carried out for the 25% A, 50% A and 100% A, and the results are compared to the value of PMCP which is measured using an algometer. The patient will feel pain if the pressure in the heel region is greater than the PMCP.

## 3. Results

Among the 13 patients, seven patients had symptomatic heel spurs on two feet. Since the longest spur was used in this study, a total of 20 feet were evaluated. The length of spur (L) ranged between 1.5 and 7 mm, as presented in detail in Table 1. According to Table 1, three classifications are determined: (1) there are two patients with small length of spur, with average L of 1.75 ± 0.35 mm; (2) there are seven patients with medium length of spur, with average L of 3.93 ± 0.73 mm; and (3) there are four patients with large length of spur, with average L of 6.50 ± 0.58 mm. Based on data of FL and FW, we can obtain the shoe size of each patient [33]; one patient has shoe size 37; four patients have shoe size 38; one patient has shoe size 39; four patients have shoe size 40; two patients have shoe size 42; and one patient has shoe size 43. Thus, we summarize a total of six shoe sizes of 37–40 and 42–43. Each size is not made in the shoe form, but in the form of a foam impression (Figure 2c), and for variation in the shoe insole area of 0% A to 100% A, a total of 30 foam impressions were made. The distance measurements of the center of the heel (used for pressure measurement of sensor 2, Figure 1 up) and the base of the spur (used for PPT measurement of point 1, Figure 1 down) are not coincident. The distance from the center of the heel (CH) ranged between 35.1–41.4 mm, and the distance from the base of spur (S) ranged between 30–41 mm, where there were seven patients with the base of spur location on the right CH and six other patients at the left CH (the farthest distance of S and CH is 7 mm, and the closest is 0.4 mm).

Table 1. A detailed description of each subject.

| Subject Number | 1 | 2 | 3 | 4 | 5 | 6 | 7 | 8 | 9 | 10 | 11 | 12 | 13 |
|---|---|---|---|---|---|---|---|---|---|---|---|---|---|
| Height, cm | 155 | 157 | 151 | 153 | 153 | 172 | 150 | 156 | 146 | 159 | 164 | 163 | 144 |
| Weight, kg | 57.2 | 60 | 50 | 52 | 70 | 63.8 | 59 | 68.6 | 55.3 | 84.6 | 62.7 | 72 | 67.6 |
| FL, mm | 249 | 266 | 237 | 240 | 252 | 276 | 237 | 251 | 240 | 240 | 270 | 273 | 234 |
| FW, mm | 98 | 118 | 106 | 91 | 100 | 108 | 96 | 102 | 94 | 100 | 100 | 99 | 90 |
| Shoe size | 40 | 42 | 38 | 38 | 40 | 43 | 38 | 40 | 38 | 39 | 40 | 42 | 37 |
| L, mm | 4.5 | 3.0 | 1.5 | 4.0 | 5.0 | 3.0 | 4.0 | 7.0 | 6.0 | 7.0 | 2.0 | 4.0 | 6.0 |
| CH, mm | 37.4 | 39.9 | 35.6 | 36.0 | 37.8 | 41.4 | 35.6 | 37.7 | 36.0 | 36.0 | 40.5 | 41.0 | 35.1 |
| S, mm | 38.0 | 34.0 | 36.0 | 38.0 | 39.0 | 41.0 | 35.0 | 39.0 | 30.0 | 38.0 | 34.0 | 34.0 | 36.0 |
| (CH-S), mm | −0.6 | 5.9 | −0.5 | −2.0 | −1.2 | 0.4 | 0.5 | −1.4 | 6.0 | −2.0 | 6.5 | 7.0 | −0.9 |

The information on the results of PMCP measurements at each heel site is very important to know which sites have the smallest PMCP value. Table 2 shows the pressure pain sensitivity in patients with plantar heel pain due to a calcaneal spur at each heel site, where the PMCP ranged between 1.24–3.3 kg/cm$^2$ and averaged 2.09 ± 0.63 kg/cm$^2$. The result shows that the smallest PMCP occurs at the anterior site, and the PMCP at the medial site was significantly lower than at the lateral site.

Table 2. The pain minimum compressive pressure (PMCP) values at each heel site.

| Heel Site | Number of Feet | PMCP (kg/cm$^2$) | PMCP Related to the Length of Spur Types (kg/cm$^2$) | | |
|---|---|---|---|---|---|
| | | | Mean ± SD (Number of Feet) | | |
| | | Mean ± SD (Range) | Small | Medium | Large |
| 1 | 1 | 1.32 | 1.32 (1) | - | - |
| 2 | 5 | 1.63 ± 0.25 (1.24–1.87) | - | 1.24 (1) | 1.73 ± 0.13 (4) |
| 3 | 2 | 3.13 ± 0.25 (2.95–3.3) | 2.95 (1) | 3.3 (1) | - |
| 4 | 2 | 2.38 ± 0.37 (2.11–2.64) | - | 2.38 ± 0.37 (2) | - |
| 5 | 3 | 2.25 ± 0.41 (1.92–2.71) | - | 2.25 ± 0.41 (3) | - |

The procedure to obtain n% insole foot area (Figure 3) produces the values of percentage deductions that can be applied to all of the shoe insoles (Table 3). The contour results of the foot of the shoe insole area of 0% A to 100% A from one of the study subjects are shown in Figure 5.

Table 3. The deduction percentage and area of shoe insole result of modification of z-coordinate and calculation using Equation (1) from one of the study subjects.

| % Shoe Insole Area | % Deduction | Shoe Insole Area (mm$^2$) | |
|---|---|---|---|
| | | From Modification of z-Coordinates | From Equation (1) |
| 100 | 0 | 17,972 | 17,972 |
| 75 | 16.5 | 17,063 | 17,071 |
| 50 | 34.5 | 16,169 | 16,170 |
| 25 | 56 | 15,266 | 15,269 |
| 0 | 100 | 14,368 | 14,368 |

According to the body weight (BW), there was a relationship between BW and the pressure in the calcaneal region. As the BW increases, the pressure at MH, LH and CH will increase as well [6]. There was a significant increase in pressure for the MH area, except at 100% A, with an average correlation coefficient of 0.74. At LH, a significant increase in pressure is seen at 0–50% A with an average correlation coefficient of 0.85. Furthermore, at CH, a significant increase in pressure is seen at 0–25% A with an average correlation coefficient of 0.85. To find the effect of area of shoe insole on the pressure of each pressure sensor in detail, it is easier to use a comparison of the pressure of each sensor to the BW or the total pressure of all sensors. Table 4 shows the distribution of pressure on the calcaneal region of one foot (assumed to be the same between left and right feet), expressed as a proportion of BW and the percentage of each sensor to the total pressure of all of the sensors. In comparison to the BW, it is seen that the percentage area of the shoe insole is increased. However, the peak pressure is decreased for the MH, LH and CH. The significant decreases are seen at the MH of 75% to 100% A and at the LH of 50% to 75% A and 75% to 100% A, respectively. In comparison to the total pressure of all sensors seen, there is a significant increase at the MH of 50% to 75%. In contrast, the pressure at the LH shows a significant decrease at the same percentage areas of shoe insole.

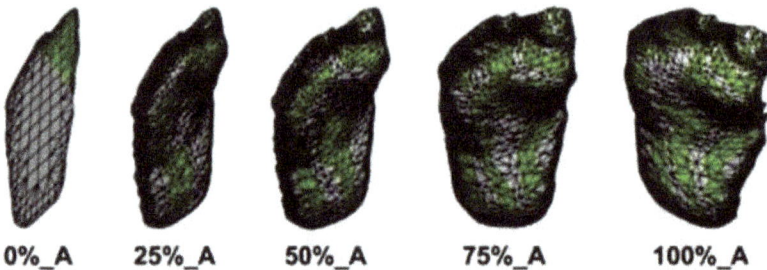

**Figure 5.** Example of negative casts of the foot from one subject.

**Table 4.** Comparison of load of each sensor to the BW and all sensors (%).

| Percentage Area of Shoe Insole | 0% | 25% | 50% | 75% | 100% |
| --- | --- | --- | --- | --- | --- |
| Calcaneal region | Comparison to the BW (mean ± SD) | | | | |
| MH | 10.14 ± 1.46 | 8.93 ± 1.16 | 8.26 ± 1.65 | 7.01 ± 1.09 | 3.64 ± 0.60 |
| LH | 7.46 ± 1.28 | 6.70 ± 1.06 | 5.53 ± 0.91 | 2.23 ± 0.52 | 0.93 ± 0.16 |
| CH | 1.44 ± 0.20 | 1.05 ± 0.21 | 0.73 ± 0.09 | 0.59 ± 0.09 | 0.24 ± 0.06 |
| Calcaneal region | Comparison to all sensors (mean ± SD) | | | | |
| MH | 53.31 ± 0.82 | 53.60 ± 1.55 | 56.69 ± 1.26 | 71.49 ± 2.36 | 75.47 ± 3.04 |
| LH | 39.11 ± 1.01 | 40.11 ± 1.04 | 38.20 ± 0.78 | 22.44 ± 2.55 | 19.44 ± 2.41 |
| CH | 7.58 ± 0.18 | 6.29 ± 0.51 | 5.11 ± 0.48 | 6.07 ± 0.20 | 5.09 ± 1.03 |

The distribution of loading at the MH, LH and CH for the five percentage areas of shoe insole is shown in Figure 6. The pressure applied at the CH is lower than the PMCP for all percentage areas of the shoe insole, while the pressure at the LH is lower than the PMCP with increasing percentage area of shoe insole from 25%. The magnitude of pressure is significantly greater than PMCP at the MH of 0% to 50% A (that is, 34.07%, 25.09% and 19.30% of PMCP, respectively). In relation to the length of spur, the pressures applied at the MH, LH and CH for five percentage areas of shoe insole are shown in Table 5 and Figure 7. As percentage area of shoe insole increased, the pressure in the calcaneal region decreased for all lengths of the spur. For the small and medium lengths of spur, the pressure at MH is greater than PMCP at percentage area of shoe insole 0–50%, while for the large length of spur, the pressure at MH is greater than PMCP at percentage area of shoe insole 0–75%. At LH, the pressure is slightly higher than PMCP at small length of spur only in the 0% A, while at the medium length of spur, the pressure is lower than PMCP for all percentage areas of shoe insole. For large lengths of spur, the pressure at the LH is greater than the PMCP in the percentage area of shoe insole 0–50%. The significant lowered pressure is seen at the CH for all lengths of spur and percentage areas of the shoe insole, compared to the PMCP.

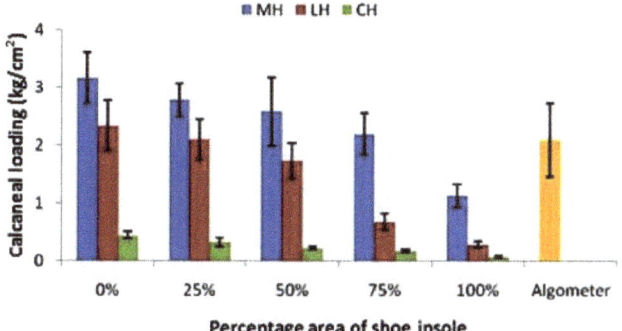

**Figure 6.** Calcaneal loading during standing for the five percentage areas of shoe insole, compared to the PMCP measured using the algometer (mean ± SD).

**Table 5.** The distribution of pressure at the MH, LH and CH for each length of spur.

| Spur Length | PMCP (kg/cm²) | Calcaneal Region | Calcaneal Loading for Each Percentage Area of Shoe Insole (kg/cm²) | | | | |
|---|---|---|---|---|---|---|---|
| | | | 0% | 25% | 50% | 75% | 100% |
| Small | 2.14 ± 1.15 | MH | 3.00 ± 0.34 | 2.67 ± 0.22 | 2.37 ± 0.45 | 2.06 ± 0.27 | 1.02 ± 0.10 |
| | | LH | 2.17 ± 0.34 | 1.96 ± 0.27 | 1.61 ± 0.24 | 0.69 ± 0.15 | 0.27 ± 0.04 |
| | | CH | 0.43 ± 0.05 | 0.30 ± 0.06 | 0.22 ± 0.02 | 0.17 ± 0.02 | 0.05 ± 0.00 |
| Medium | 2.29 ± 0.66 | MH | 3.11 ± 0.33 | 2.75 ± 0.21 | 2.52 ± 0.43 | 2.15 ± 0.26 | 1.18 ± 0.22 |
| | | LH | 2.28 ± 0.32 | 2.06 ± 0.26 | 1.70 ± 0.23 | 0.68 ± 0.11 | 0.29 ± 0.04 |
| | | CH | 0.44 ± 0.04 | 0.32 ± 0.06 | 0.23 ± 0.02 | 0.18 ± 0.02 | 0.08 ± 0.01 |
| Large | 1.73 ± 0.13 | MH | 3.35 ± 0.69 | 2.91 ± 0.45 | 2.84 ± 0.91 | 2.34 ± 0.56 | 1.13 ± 0.18 |
| | | LH | 2.52 ± 0.68 | 2.24 ± 0.54 | 1.86 ± 0.48 | 0.71 ± 0.22 | 0.31 ± 0.08 |
| | | CH | 0.47 ± 0.09 | 0.36 ± 0.12 | 0.24 ± 0.03 | 0.20 ± 0.04 | 0.09 ± 0.03 |

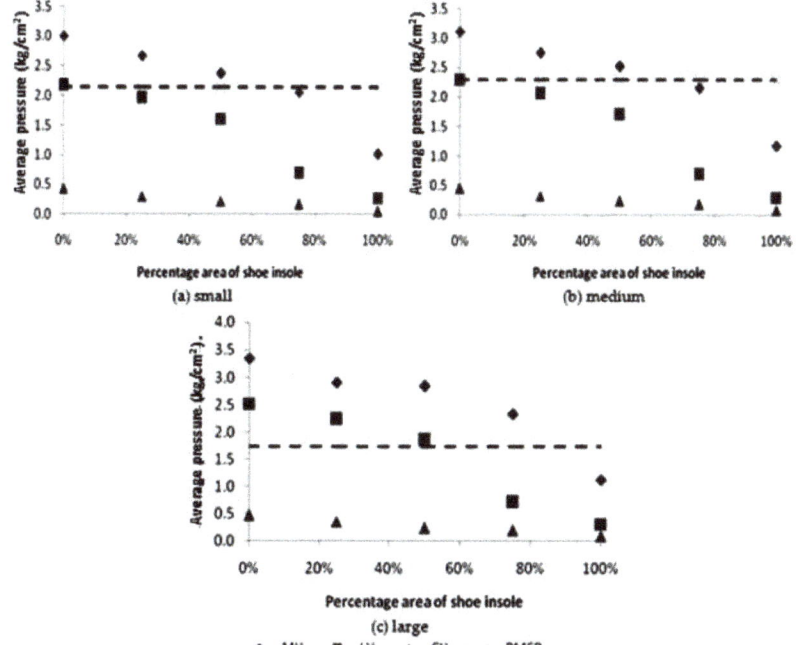

**Figure 7.** The pressure at the MH, LH and CH for the five percentage areas of shoe insole and each length of spur, as presented in Table 5.

## 4. Discussion

The determination of PPT location as a function of base and length of spur (Figure 1 down) is necessary for obtaining an accurate PMCP value and the point location in each patient. The results of PPT from 13 patients, as shown in Table 2, showed that the PMCP occurs mostly at the anterior site (that is, 38.5%). This result is similar to previously published work reported by Goff et al. [6] and Wibowo et al. [17]. These PPT results are also in accordance with the study of Saban et al. [14], which indicated that the average PMCP at the medial site was significantly lower than the one at the lateral site (that is, 2.25 and 3.13 kg/cm$^2$, respectively).

The research for obtaining the contour of the sole by varying the contact area of the foot using 3D scanners is a novelty. By using a 3D foot scanner [22,23,27], it is easier to obtain a form of a shoe insole mold (foot impression cast) than previously, which involved placing the sole of a foot on a gypsum mold for any different bearing conditions [18,19]. The procedure that is described in Figure 3a can be applied to determine any foot impression cast shape of the shoe insole area. For example, it is desirable to get a foot impression cast shape shoe insole area of 70%; the initial value of the percentage of z deduction can be set to 10% (Table 3). The generating xyz-coordinates obtained from Equation (2) can be made into a 3D negative cast model from wood (Figure 5) by using Computer Numerical Control (CNC) milling.

Table 4 is used to check the validity of load measurements and the position of the foot during standing. In comparison to the BW, at 0% A, it shows that the subjects' feet support a total load of 19.04% of BW in the calcaneal region. This result is similar to the previous study of 19.32% BW presented in Ref. [34]. In comparison to the total pressure of all sensors, the pressure at MH is larger than at LH for all insole foot areas, which indicates that most of the patients' heels tend to pronation while standing [35,36]. The pronation tendency occurs very clearly in 75% A and 100% A, and are possibly caused by the sensor mounted at the LH shifting to the heel center line for holding pain, seen from the significant decrease in load to only 22.44% and 19.44%, respectively, compared to MH.

This study proved that contoured insoles are better than flat insoles in reducing local peak pressures [18–20], but in relation to pressure relieving pain, are only 100% A at MH and 50–100% A at LH, which are lower pressures than the PMCPs. The pressures at CH are all lower than PMCP for the all insole foot areas (Figure 6). These results are corresponding to the research conducted by Chia et al. [16] and Bonanno et al. [37], and prove that the contoured insole increases foot area contact and reduces pain pressure in the calcaneal region. To find the percentage of insole foot areas suitable for each patient without causing pain in detail, we can examine the evaluation of pressure in the calcaneal region associated with the types of spur length (Table 5). For large spur lengths there are four patients requiring a 100% A; for the medium spur lengths there is one patient requiring 50% A, five patients requiring 75% A, and one patient requiring 100% A; while for small spur lengths there are two patients requiring 50% A and 100% A, respectively.

The average difference between the location of the base of the spur (S) and the location of the center of the heel (CH) was 1.37 mm (Table 1). Therefore, the position of the CH as the basis for the measurement of pressure using the FSR sensor was relatively accurate, since the area of the sensor was still able to compress the base of the spur.

## 5. Conclusions

The main criterion for the use of a contoured orthotic shoe insole for heel pain sufferers due to a calcaneal spur depends on how well it can reduce pain when used for standing. Therefore, the information on how the shape of the contour of the foot changes with weight bearing, which results in the smallest pain at the heel area, is essential in shoe design. This quantitative study shows that it is easy to obtain a variety of shoe insole foot contours by varying the contact area of the shoe insole, compared to directly printing the plantar foot on the casting board for any weight bearing condition. The use of larger insole areas could reduce local peak pressure. Contoured insoles were significantly better than flat insoles.

To reduce pain in patients with a calcaneal spur while standing, we can use 50–100% insole foot area. The average pressures at CH and LH for a 50% insole foot area are 0.23 kg/cm$^2$ and 1.73 kg/cm$^2$, respectively, which are significantly lower than the average PMCPs (89.0% and 17.1%, respectively), while the average pressures at 75% insole foot area are 0.19 kg/cm$^2$ and 0.69 kg/cm$^2$, respectively, which are also significantly lower than the average PMCPs (91.1% and 67.0%, respectively). On the other hand, the average pressures at MH for a 50% and 75% insole foot area are 2.59 kg/cm$^2$ and 2.20 kg/cm$^2$, respectively, which are still greater than the average PMCPs (19.3% and 4.7%, respectively). One hundred percent insole foot area can also be used, but is not recommended—even though the average pressure in all regions and the percentage of insole foot area are smaller than the average PMCP—because it requires large production costs.

**Author Contributions:** Conceptualization, D.B.W.; methodology, D.B.W.; software, D.B.W. and W.C.; validation, A.W. and G.D.H.; formal analysis, D.B.W. and A.W.; investigation, G.D.H.; resources, G.D.H. and R.H.; data curation, W.C. and R.H.; writing—original draft preparation, D.B.W.; writing—review and editing, A.W. and W.C.; visualization, D.B.W., A.W. and W.C.; supervision, R.H.; project administration, G.D.H.; funding acquisition, D.B.W. and G.D.H.

**Acknowledgments:** This work was supported by the Superior Applied Research in higher education Directorate of Research and Community Service, Directorate General of Research and Development Strengthening, Indonesian Ministry of Research, Technology and Higher Education. Contract No: 101-155/UN7.P4.3/PP/2018.

**Conflicts of Interest:** The authors declare that there are no known conflicts of interest related to this project that could have influenced this manuscript.

## References

1. Buchbinder, R. Clinical practice: Plantar fasciitis. *N. Engl. J. Med.* **2004**, *350*, 2159–2166. [CrossRef] [PubMed]
2. McCarthy, D.J.; Gorecki, G.E. The anatomical basis of inferior calcaneal lesions: A cryomicrotomy study. *J. Am. Podiatry Assoc.* **1979**, *69*, 527–536. [CrossRef] [PubMed]
3. Bartold, S.J. The Plantar Fascia as a Source of Pain – Biomechanics, Presentation and Treatment. *J. Bodyw. Mov. Ther.* **2004**, *8*, 214–226. [CrossRef]
4. Barrett, S.L.; O'Malley, R. Plantar Fasciitis and Other Causes of Heel Pain. *Am. Fam. Physician* **1999**, *59*, 2200–2206. [PubMed]
5. Smith, S.; Tinley, P.; Gilheany, M.; Grills, B. The inferior calcaneal spur-anatomical and histological considerations. *Foot* **2007**, *17*, 25–31. [CrossRef]
6. Goff, J.D.; Crawford, R. Diagnosis and treatment of plantar fasciitis. *Am. Fam.* **2011**, *84*, 676–682.
7. Zhou, B.; Zhou, Y.; Tao, X.; Yuan, C.; Tang, K. Classification of calcaneal spurs and their relationship with plantar fasciitis. *J. Foot Ankle Surg.* **2015**, *54*, 594–600. [CrossRef] [PubMed]
8. Roberts, S. Scott's Book on Plantar Fasciitis, Heel Spurs, and Heel Pain. Available online: http://heelspurs.com/_intro.html.
9. Hyland, M.R.; Gaffney, A.; Cohen, L.; Lichtman, S.W. Randomized control trial of calcaneal taping, sham taping, and plantar fascia stretching for short-term management of plantar heel pain. *J. Orthop. Sports Phys. Ther.* **2006**, *36*, 364–371. [CrossRef]
10. Thomas, J.L.; Christensen, J.C.; Kravitz, S.R.; Mendicino, R.W.; Schuberth, J.M.; Vanore, J.V.; Weil, L.S., Sr.; Zlotoff, H.J.; Bouché, R.; Baker, J. The Diagnosis and Treatment of Heel Pain: A Clinical Practice Guideline—Revision 2010. *J. Foot Ankle Surg.* **2010**, *49*, S1–S19. [CrossRef]
11. Kogler, G.; Solomonidis, S.E.; Paul, P.J. Biomechanics of longitudinal arch support mechanics in foot orthoses and their effect on plantar aponeurosis strain. *Clin. Biomech.* **1998**, *11*, 243–252. [CrossRef]
12. Kogler, G.; Veer, F.; Solomonidis, S.E.; Paul, PJ. The influence of medial and lateral placement of orthotic wedges on loading of the plantar aponeurosis. *J. Bone Jt. Surg. Am.* **1999**, *81*, 1403–1413. [CrossRef]
13. Ozdemir, H.; Soyuncu, Y.; Ozgorgen, M.; Dabak, K. Effects of changes in heel fat pad thickness and elasticity on heel pain. *J. Am. Podiatr. Med. Assoc.* **2004**, *94*, 47–52. [CrossRef] [PubMed]
14. Saban, B.; Masharawi, Y. Pain threshold tests in patients with heel pain syndrome. *Foot Ankle Int.* **2016**, *37*, 730–736. [CrossRef] [PubMed]
15. Cheung, J.; Zhang, M. A 3-dimensional finite element model of the human foot and ankle insole design. *Arch. Phys. Med. Rehabil.* **2005**, *86*, 353–358. [CrossRef]

16. Chia, J.K.; Suresh, S.; Kuah, A.; Ong, J.L.; Phua, J.M.; Seah, A.L. Comparative trial of the foot pressure patterns between corrective orthotics, formthotics, bone spur and flat insoles in patients with chronic plantar fasciitis. *Ann. Acad. Med. Sing.* **2009**, *38*, 869–875.
17. Wibowo, D.B.; Harahap, R.; Widodo, A.; Haryadi, G.D.; Ariyanto, M. The effectiveness of raising the heel height of shoes to reduce heel pain in patients with calcaneal spurs. *J. Phys. Ther. Sci.* **2017**, *29*, 2068–2074. [CrossRef] [PubMed]
18. Tsung, B.Y.S.; Zhang, M.; Fan, Y.B.; Boone, D.A. Quantitative comparison of plantar foot shapes under different weight-bearing conditions. *J. Rehabil. Res. Dev.* **2003**, *40*, 517–526. [CrossRef] [PubMed]
19. Tsung, B.Y.S.; Zhang, M.; Mak, A.F.T.; Wong, M.W.N. Effectiveness of insoles on plantar pressure redistribution. *JRRD* **2004**, *41*, 6A. [CrossRef]
20. Bousie, J.A.; Blanch, P.; McPoil, T.G.; Vicenzino, B. Contoured in-shoe foot orthoses increase mid-foot plantar contact area when compared with a flat insert during cycling. *J. Sci. Med. Sport* **2013**, *16*, 60–64. [CrossRef]
21. Losito, J.M. Impression casting techniques. In *Clinical Biomechanics of the Lower Extremity*; Valmassy, R., Ed.; Mosby: St. Louis, MO, USA, 1996.
22. Telfer, S.; Woodburn, J. The use of 3D surface scanning for the measurement and assessment of the human foot. *J. Foot Ankle Res.* **2010**, *3*, 19. [CrossRef]
23. Stanković, K.; Booth, B.G.; Danckaers, F.; Burg, F.; Vermaelen, P.; Duerinck, S.; Sijbers, J.; Huysmans, T. Three-dimensional quantitative analysis of healthy foot shape: A proof of concept study. *J. Foot Ankle Res.* **2018**, *11*, 8. [CrossRef] [PubMed]
24. Lee, Y.C.; Lin, G.; Wang, M.J. Comparing 3D foot scanning with conventional measurement methods. *J. Foot Ankle Res.* **2014**, *7*, 44. [CrossRef]
25. Cavanagh, P.R.; Rodgers, M. The Arch index: A useful measure from footprints. *J. Biomech.* **1987**, *20*, 547–551. [CrossRef]
26. Wagner Instruments. *Wagner FPTX Series Economy Manual Pain Threshold Testers*; PAIN TEST™ ALGOMETER: Greenwich, CT, USA; Available online: http://www.wagnerinstruments.com/products/pain-test-algometer/fpk-fpn (accessed on 1 February 2019).
27. Wibowo, D.B.; Haryadi, G.D.; Priambodo, A. Estimation of foot pressure from human footprint depths using 3D scanner. *AIP Conf. Proc.* **2016**, *1717*, 040008. [CrossRef]
28. Robinette, K.; Daanen, H. Precision of the CAESAR scan-extracted measurements. *ApplErgon* **2006**, *37*, 259–265. [CrossRef]
29. Wibowo, D.B.; Haryadi, G.D.; Widodo, A.; Rahayu, S.P. Estimation of calcaneal loading during standing from human footprint depths using 3D scanner. *AIP Conf. Proc.* **2017**, *1788*, 030063. [CrossRef]
30. Yung-Hui, L.; Wei-Hsein, H. Effects of shoe inserts and heel height on foot pressure, impact force, and perceived comfort during walking. *Appl. Ergon.* **2005**, *36*, 335–362. [CrossRef] [PubMed]
31. Druga, C.; Serban, I. Study of foot pressure-sole pressure sensor. In Proceedings of the 7th International Conference on Computational Mechanics and Virtual Engineering (COMEC) 2017, Brasov, Rumania, 16–17 November 2017.
32. Goske, S.; Erdemir, A.; Petre, M.; Budhabhatti, S. Reduction of plantar heel pressure: Insole design using finite element analysis. *J. Biomech.* **2006**, *39*, 2363–2370. [CrossRef] [PubMed]
33. Boehm, R. *The Foot & the Shoe: Measurement & Size*; DARCO (Europe) GmbH: Raisting, Germany, 2015.
34. Maiwald, C.; Grau, S.; Krauss, I.; Mauch, M.; Axmann, D.; Horstmann, T. Reproducibility of plantar pressure distribution data in barefoot running. *J. Appl. Biomech.* **2008**, *24*, 14–23. [CrossRef]
35. Cavanagh, P.R.; Rodgers, M.; Liboshi, A. Pressure distribution under symptom-free feet during barefoot standing. *Foot Ankle Int.* **1987**, *7*, 262. [CrossRef]
36. Shimizu, M.; Andrew, P.D. Effect of heel height on the foot in unilateral standing. *J. Phys. Ther. Sci.* **1999**, *11*, 95–100. [CrossRef]
37. Bonanno, D.R.; Landorf, K.B.; Menz, H.B. Pressure-relieving properties of various shoe inserts in older people with plantar heel pain. *Gait Posture* **2011**, *33*, 385–389. [CrossRef] [PubMed]

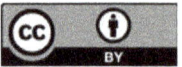

© 2019 by the authors. Licensee MDPI, Basel, Switzerland. This article is an open access article distributed under the terms and conditions of the Creative Commons Attribution (CC BY) license (http://creativecommons.org/licenses/by/4.0/).

*Article*

# Development of the Dyskinesia Impairment Mobility Scale to Measure Presence and Severity of Dystonia and Choreoathetosis during Powered Mobility in Dyskinetic Cerebral Palsy

Saranda Bekteshi [1,*], Marco Konings [1], Ioana Gabriela Nica [2], Sotirios Gakopoulos [3], Inti Vanmechelen [1], Jean-Marie Aerts [2], Hans Hallez [3] and Elegast Monbaliu [1]

[1] KU Leuven, Bruges Campus, Department of Rehabilitation Sciences, Research Group for Neurorehabilitation, 8200 Bruges, Belgium
[2] KU Leuven, Department of Biosystems, Division of Animal and Human Health Engineering, Measure, Model and Manage Bioresponse (M3–BIORES), 3001 Leuven, Belgium
[3] KU Leuven, Bruges Campus, Department of Computer Science, Mechatronics Research Group, 8200 Bruges, Belgium
* Correspondence: saranda.bekteshi@kuleuven.be; Tel.: +32-5066-4992

Received: 20 July 2019; Accepted: 20 August 2019; Published: 23 August 2019

**Featured Application:** The Dyskinesia Impairment Mobility Scale (DIMS) is a reliable tool to measure presence and severity of dystonia and choreoathetosis during powered mobility in dyskinetic cerebral palsy. In clinical practice, the DIMS can assist a better structure of the mobility training programs to shorten learning curves and a better evaluation of mobility training progress. In research, the DIMS can be used to explore clinical patterns during powered mobility and evaluate future mobility intervention studies.

**Abstract:** The majority of individuals with dyskinetic cerebral palsy cannot use powered mobility with a joystick, due to the lack of manual abilities by the severe presence of dystonia and choreoathetosis. Reliable measurements of these movement disorders is indispensable for good evaluation towards evidence–based insights during powered mobility. This study aimed to develop and assess the Dyskinesia Impairment Mobility Scale (DIMS), a video–based tool to measure presence and severity of dystonia and choreoathetosis during powered mobility. DIMS was measured for the neck and arms region during five mobility tasks. Interrater reliability, test–retest reliability, internal consistency and concurrent validity of the DIMS were assessed. Interrater reliability coefficients ranged between 0.68 and 0.87 for the total DIMS, and the dystonia and choreoathetosis subscales. Test–retest reliability was moderate to excellent (range 0.51–0.93) while Cronbach's alpha was good (range 0.69–0.81) for the total scale and subscale scores. Concurrent validity showed during mobility tasks significant correlations with rest postures in the arm region, and with requested but voluntary activity in the neck region. The DIMS reliably measures the presence and severity of the movement disorders during powered mobility, increasing insights into the underlying mechanisms of independent mobility. This scale may therefore be a promising tool to evaluate mobility training.

**Keywords:** powered mobility; dyskinetic cerebral palsy; dystonia; choreoathetosis; mobility scale; movement disorder; children; youth; reliability; validity

## 1. Introduction

Impaired mobility is the leading cause of reduced functionality, restricted participation levels and decreased activity levels in children and youth with severe movement disabilities, resulting in, among others, social isolation, anxiety and depression [1–3]. Introducing powered mobility wheelchairs to children with severe motor limitations has shown to improve their psychosocial and cognitive skills while increasing independence, self–exploration and intuition without any negative impact on their motor development [4]. Therefore, mobility training is of major importance starting at a young age [5].

In the child-population, cerebral palsy is the most common neuromotor disability, with a prevalence of 1.7 per 1000 livebirths [6] and is categorized into three groups: Spastic, dyskinetic and ataxic [7]. Dyskinetic cerebral palsy (DCP) is the second largest and most limiting CP group [8]. DCP is characterized by two complex movement disorders: Dystonia (i.e., involuntary movements, distorted voluntary movements and abnormal postures due to sustained muscle contractions) and choreoathetosis (i.e., chorea defined as rapid, involuntary, often fragmented movements and athetosis defined as slower and constantly changing movements) [8]. In DCP, dystonia and choreoathetosis are also present as overflow movements, defined as unintentional contractions of muscles different from the ones used during a goal–directed movement [9]. More than 70% of the DCP population presents with the highest levels of severity in gross motor functioning and fine manual abilities [10]. As a result, children with DCP are unable to use powered mobility wheelchairs with a conventional joystick, hence leaving them heavily dependent on caregivers' assistance [4,8,11].

Alternate steering methods such as switches or head arrays for powered mobility are proposed in literature as a way to achieve independence for children with severe gross and manual limitations [12]. In this respect, in DCP, the basal movements of the head and the feet are better controlled than the movements of the arms [8]. Therefore, clinical practice widely supports the use of a head/foot steering system as the best option to promote independent powered mobility for children with DCP, where the head movements are used to steer the wheelchair to the right and left and the feet are used to drive the wheelchair forward and backward. In general, there is little evidence supporting the best methods to train children to use a powered wheelchair and a lack of comprehensive training results in longer, time–consuming and unstructured motor learning and skill acquisition processes [4,13].

Thus, evidence–based knowledge into the different stages of powered mobility, from learning towards self–exploration remains scarce in DCP and mobility training so far is based only on clinical expertise. To increase insights into the potential use and learning process of powered mobility wheelchairs for children with DCP, the process of learning to use it, operation of the system, the impact of movement disorders and environmental factors need to be further explored. These insights would contribute to a better understanding of the mobility limitations in this population, and assist in tailoring of better powered mobility training programs to shorten learning curves.

Whereas the characterizing dystonia and choreoathetosis movement disorders seem to be the biggest limiting concepts of powered mobility in DCP [8], it is important to be able to assess the presence and severity of these movement disorders during powered mobility tasks. That is, it is stipulated that an increase in severity causes higher distortion of voluntary movements and higher presence of involuntary/overflow movements, which might result in longer and more difficult powered mobility skills training. Thereby, increased insights in the severity of dystonia and choreoathetosis during powered mobility may generate knowledge to develop more straightforward mobility training guidelines and assist powered mobility training by shortening learning curves.

To date, presence and severity of dystonia and choreoathetosis are measured using the Dyskinesia Impairment Scale (DIS) [9,14–16], a video–based tool which measures the movement disorders during requested but voluntary activities and rest postures. The DIS measures requested but voluntary activities in a controlled environment and may, therefore, not provide information about the occurrence of the movement disorders in a more real–life context, such as steering a powered wheelchair using a head/foot steering system. This implies that there is a necessity for a reliable and valid assessment tool that will generate insights on the presence and severity of movement disorders during daily–life activities. The DIS has shown high reliability and validity in measuring dystonia and choreoathetosis in DCP [14,15]. Thereby, an adapted protocol of the DIS which will reliably measure the movement disorders during powered mobility could be the solution to fill in the gap in the current existing assessment tools.

Therefore, this study aimed to (1) develop an adapted standardized protocol of the DIS which will measure presence and severity of dystonia and choreoathetosis during powered mobility tasks in individuals with DCP, and (2) to assess the reliability and validity of this protocol. Serving that purpose, the new scale will be named the Dyskinesia Impairment Mobility Scale (DIMS).

## 2. Materials and Methods

*2.1. Development of the Dyskinesia Impairment Mobility Scale (DIMS)*

In the first step towards developing the adapted DIMS protocol, the DIS was examined thoroughly for dystonia and choreoathetosis characteristics which would be relevant to be included in the DIMS [9,14–16]. The DIS measures the presence and severity of dystonia and choreoathetosis over 12 body regions; i.e., central body (eyes, mouth, neck and trunk) and limbs (upper and lower, proximal and distal limbs) [14]. Dystonia and choreoathetosis are assessed at rest and during two requested voluntary activities, both for duration (i.e., the amount of time that dyskinesia is present) and amplitude (i.e., the maximum range of motion (ROM) achieved due to dyskinesia) [14]. Duration and amplitude are scored on a five–point ordinal scale ranging from 0 to 4. Summation of region scores gives a total rest score, ranging 0–96, and a total action score, ranging 0–192. A total dystonia subscale score and total choreoathetosis score is obtained by the sum of the total rest and action score with a range from 0–288. A diagram of the DIS protocol is shown in Appendix A, Figure A1.

For the DIMS, a similar protocol as for the DIS was adopted (Figure 1). The final DIMS protocol is a video–based protocol which consists of the dystonia subscale (DIMS-D) and choreoathetosis subscale (DIMS-CA). Both subscales measure duration (i.e., the amount of time that dystonia and choreoathetosis were present during the powered mobility task) and amplitude (i.e., the maximum ROM achieved due to dystonia and choreoathetosis) during five different powered mobility tasks. Scoring of duration and amplitude ranges from 0 to 4 (Table 1). For the duration factor, score 0 means the movement disorder is absent during powered mobility, score 1 means occasionally present (i.e., less than 10%), score 2 means frequently present (i.e., between 10 and 50% of the time), score 3 means mostly present (i.e., between 50 and 90% of the time) and score 4 means always present (more than 90% of the time). For the amplitude factor, the range of percentages is the same as for the duration factor with score 0 assigned when the movement disorder is absent during powered mobility, score 1 when the movement disorder is present in a small ROM, score 2 when present in moderate ROM, score 3 when present in submaximal ROM and score 4 when present in maximal ROM. The DIMS is comprised of the neck region, representing the voluntary movements used to steer the wheelchair to the right and to the left, and the arm region, representing the dystonia and choreoathetosis overflow movements during mobility tasks. For the arm region, a distinction is made between left and right and proximal and distal parts. As such, the DIMS is comprised of five body regions: neck, right arm proximal (i.e., arm RP), left arm proximal (i.e., arm LP), right arm distal (i.e., arm RD), and left arm distal (i.e., arm LD). Even though the feet are used to accelerate and brake with the wheelchair, they are strapped during powered mobility manifesting minimal movement, and were therefore excluded from the final DIMS protocol.

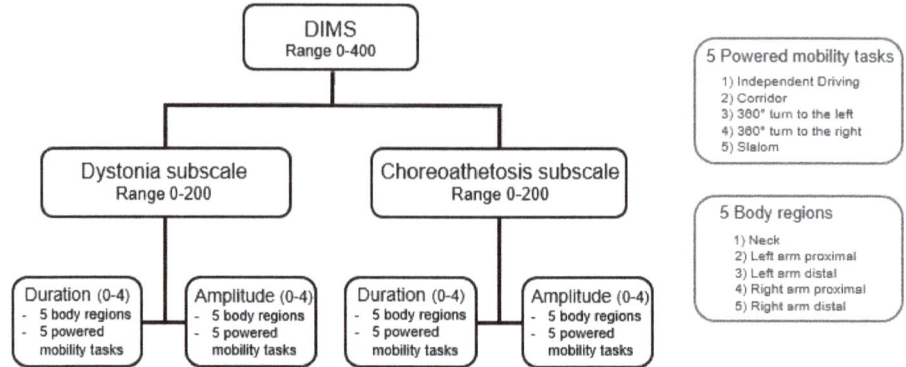

**Figure 1.** Diagram of the Dyskinesia Impairment Mobility Scale (DIMS) protocol.

**Table 1.** Scoring protocol of the Dyskinesia Impairment Mobility Scale (DIMS) duration and amplitude during powered mobility.

|  | Duration | Amplitude |
| --- | --- | --- |
| Score 0 | D/CA is absent | D/CA is absent |
| Score 1 (<10%) | D/CA is occasionally present | D/CA is present in small ROM |
| Score 2 (≥10 <50%) | D/CA is frequently present | D/CA is present in moderate ROM |
| Score 3 (≥50 <90%) | D/CA is mostly present | D/CA is present in submaximal ROM |
| Score 4 (>90%) | D/CA is always present | D/CA is present in maximal ROM |

DIMS, Dyskinesia Impairment Mobility Scale; D/CA, dystonia/choreoathetosis; ROM, range of motion; <, lower than; ≥, higher than or equal; >, higher than; %, percentage.

## 2.2. Reliability and Validity

### 2.2.1. Participants

This study included five participants aged 6–21 years old, recruited from four Flemish special education schools for children with motor disorders. Included were (1) participants with DCP diagnosed by a pediatric neurologist, (2) level IV–V for both gross motor abilities classified with the Gross Motor Function Classification System—extended and revised (GMFCS E&R) [17] and fine manual abilities classified with the Manual Abilities Classification System—extended and revised (MACS E&R) [17] who owned a head/foot steering wheelchair (Table A1). Excluded were individuals who (1) showed difficulties to understand and follow instructions, (2) had severe visual impairments or who (3) underwent an orthopedic or neurosurgical intervention within the last 12 months. The study was conducted in accordance with the Declaration of Helsinki, and the protocol was approved by the Medical Ethics Committee UZ KU Leuven. Informed assent and/or consent forms were signed by all participants and/or their parents.

### 2.2.2. Data Collection

Data to assess the reliability and validity of the DIMS was collected in the special education schools of the five participants, in a standardized set–up using their own head/foot steering wheelchair. Participants performed five powered mobility tasks, which were video–recorded for future scoring of the DIMS. The videos were recorded using a commercially available Sony Handycam HDR–CX405 (Sony Corporation, Tokyo, Japan) placed on a tripod on both sides of the powered mobility tasks set–up. The video recording was started manually by the researchers at the beginning of the data collection and was stopped at the end of it. The sample rate of the videos was 29 frames per second. This video–recording procedure was repeated for the powered mobility performance of each participant.

The included tasks [18] were independent driving (i.e., T1), driving through a created corridor (i.e., T2), a 360 degree turn to the left (i.e., T3), a 360 degree turn to the right (i.e., T4) and a slalom (i.e., T5) (Figure A2). The set–up of T1, T2 and T5 was ten meters in length. The width of the corridor (T2) and the distance between cones (T5) were calculated separately per participant by measuring the length of their wheelchair and adding 50% of this length to ensure fairness in set–up, as well as comfort and safety. To meet the aims of this study, each participant was recorded twice, (i.e., Week 1 (W1) and Week 2 (W2) with two weeks' break in–between). To assess the concurrent validity of the DIMS, all five participants were additionally recorded following the standardized protocol of the existing DIS.

2.2.3. Procedure of Scoring and Analyzing data

The videos were independently assessed by three raters who underwent a DIS training session by the developer of the DIS (EM). Training consisted of definitions and video explanations on how to discriminate between dystonia and choreoathetosis in DCP. After the training session, the three raters independently scored ten training videos of the existing DIS to assess if they are reliable to score the DIMS videos (see Table A2).

The videos of each powered mobility task (i.e., T1, T2, T3, T4 and T5) during the two measuring weeks (W1 and W2) were scored by the three raters independently. Kinovea motion analysis software, version 0.8.15 (Kinovea, Bordeaux, France) [19] was used to cut and view the videos. Both the dystonia and choreoathetosis subscale are evaluated for duration and amplitude in five body regions. All body regions are scored during the five powered mobility tasks. Summation of the region scores gives a total score for the DIMS-D subscale and DIMS-CA subscale, each with a range from 0 to 200. The total DIMS score is the sum of the DIMS-D and DIMS-CA subscale (range 0 to 400; see Figure 1). In the current study, missing values were only 4.2% of all collected data. To account for these missing values, the summed region and subscale scores were each separately converted into percentage scores relative to their maximum score. The maximum score was accordingly adjusted (i.e., decreased) for the region or subscale scores which had missing values.

To assess the interrater reliability of the total scores of the DIMS, the DIMS-D and the DIMS-CA subscale, the scores of three raters were compared. First, all scores of W1 and W2 were converted into percentage scores. Then, the percentage scores of W1 and W2 for each rater were averaged and the obtained final score was used for the interrater reliability analysis.

To determine test–retest reliability of the DIMS, the total score of the DIMS, DIMS-D, DIMS-CA and region scores were compared between W1 and W2. The final percentage scores used for this comparison were obtained by averaging the scores of all three raters.

The internal consistency analysis was performed to assess the consistency of measuring the presence and severity of dystonia and choreoathetosis over time during powered mobility.

For the concurrent validity, neck scores of the DIMS were compared with the neck scores of the DIS for two requested voluntary activities and one rest posture. In the DIS, the first neck requested voluntary activity is neck lateroflexion and the second neck requested voluntary activity is neck rotation. The arms scores (i.e., left proximal, left distal, right proximal and right distal) of the DIMS were compared with overflow movements (scoring the contralateral side of the arm which does the required activity [9]) and rest postures scores of the DIS. The DIS and the W1 data collection of the DIMS were administered during the same week, thereby only data of W1 was used for this analysis.

2.2.4. Statistical Analysis

In accordance with Rigby's statistical recommendations, the intraclass correlation coefficients (ICCs) and 95% confidence intervals (CIs) were used for the total scores and item scores of the DIMS to evaluate the interrater– and test–retest reliability [20]. To interpret the ICCs, recommendations by Monbaliu et al. were considered, with ICCs higher than 0.90 as excellent, between 0.75 and 0.90 as good, between 0.60 and 0.74 as moderately high and between 0.40 and 0.59 as moderate. ICCs less than 0.40 were indicative of low reliability [15]. Spearman's rank correlation coefficients ($r_s$) were used to determine concurrent validity where 0.00–0.19 was considered very weak/no correlation, 0.20–0.39 weak, 0.40–0.59 moderate, 0.60–0.79 strong and 0.80 to 1.00 very strong [21]. Internal consistency was calculated by Cronbach's alpha with α = 0.00 meaning no internal consistency and α = 1.00 perfect internal consistency [21]. All statistics were calculated using IBM SPSS Statistics 25 (SPSS Inc., Chicago, IL, USA).

## 3. Results

*3.1. Interrater Reliability of the DIMS*

The ICCs and 95% CIs of the total scale, subscale and region scores are shown in Table 2.

Moderately high to good interrater reliability was obtained for the total score of the DIMS with ICC 0.87 (95% CI 0.35–0.99; $p = 0.011$), for the total DIMS-D with ICC 0.68 (95% CI 0.00–0.98; $p = 0.098$) and for the total DIMS-CA with ICC 0.79 (95% CI 0.07–0.98; $p = 0.000$). Similar interrater reliability was found for the total score of the DIMS duration factor and amplitude factor with ICC 0.62 and 0.87 respectively.

For the DIMS-D subscale, interrater reliability of the duration factor, amplitude factor and the summation of both factors were low to good, with ICCs 0.22, 0.85 and 0.68 respectively. For the DIMS-D subscale of the neck region, good interrater reliability was found for the total score with ICC 0.83 while for the DIMS-D subscale of the arm regions, ICCs ranged between 0.04 and 0.73.

For the DIMS-CA subscale, interrater reliability of the duration factor, amplitude factor and summation of both factors were good with ICCs 0.83, 0.73 and 0.79 respectively. The interrater reliability of the total DIMS-CA for the neck was excellent with ICC 0.96. Good to excellent interrater reliability was found for the total DIMS-CA subscale of the arm regions with ICCs ranging between 0.79 and 0.96.

**Table 2.** Interrater reliability: Intraclass correlation coefficients (ICC) with 95% confidence intervals (CI) between three raters for the Dyskinesia Impairment Mobility Scale (DIMS).

| | | Duration | | Amplitude | | $\sum(D + A)$ | |
|---|---|---|---|---|---|---|---|
| | | ICC | 95% CI; $p$–value | ICC | 95% CI; $p$–value | ICC | 95% CI; $p$–value |
| | **DIMS** | | | | | | |
| | Total score | 0.62 | 0.00–0.96; 0.131 | 0.87 | 0.41–0.99; 0.001 | 0.87 | 0.35–0.99; 0.011 |
| | **DIMS-D SUBSCALE** | | | | | | |
| 1 | Neck | 0.60 | 0.00–0.96; 0.131 | 0.89 | 0.40–0.99; 0.000 | 0.83 | 0.27–0.98; 0.015 |
| 2 | Arm RP | 0.04 | 0.00–0.90; 0.443 | 0.88 | 0.36–0.99; 0.009 | 0.67 | 0.00–0.96; 0.099 |
| 3 | Arm LP | 0.15 | 0.00–0.91; 0.391 | 0.87 | 0.37–0.99; 0.010 | 0.67 | 0.00–0.96; 0.093 |
| 4 | Arm RD | 0.73 | 0.00–0.97; 0.074 | 0.78 | 0.13–0.97; 0.006 | 0.86 | 0.39–0.98; 0.005 |
| 5 | Arm LD | 0.57 | 0.00–0.96; 0.171 | 0.97 | 0.87–0.99; 0.000 | 0.89 | 0.37–0.99; 0.009 |
| | Total score | 0.22 | 0.00–0.93; 0.370 | 0.85 | 0.35–0.98; 0.008 | 0.68 | 0.00–0.98; 0.098 |
| | **DIMS-CA SUBSCALE** | | | | | | |
| 1 | Neck | 0.96 | 0.55–0.99; 0.000 | 0.97 | 0.75–0.99; 0.000 | 0.96 | 0.63–0.99; 0.000 |
| 2 | Arm RP | 0.96 | 0.79–0.99; 0.000 | 0.80 | 0.20–0.98; 0.011 | 0.79 | 0.09–0.98; 0.001 |
| 3 | Arm LP | 0.98 | 0.88–0.99; 0.000 | 0.90 | 0.25–0.99; 0.000 | 0.96 | 0.65–0.99; 0.000 |
| 4 | Arm RD | 0.92 | 0.33–0.99; 0.000 | 0.81 | 0.16–0.98; 0.000 | 0.87 | 0.24–0.99; 0.000 |
| 5 | Arm LD | 0.92 | 0.45–0.99; 0.000 | 0.83 | 0.13–0.98; 0.000 | 0.88 | 0.23–0.99; 0.000 |
| | Total score | 0.83 | 0.13–0.98; 0.000 | 0.73 | 0.04–0.97; 0.000 | 0.79 | 0.07–0.98; 0.000 |

DIMS, Dyskinesia Impairment Mobility Scale; $\sum(D + A)$, summation of duration and amplitude factors; ICC, intraclass correlation coefficient; CI, confidence interval; RP, right proximal; LP, left proximal; RD, right distal; LD, left distal; %, percentage.

*3.2. Test-Retest Reliability of the DIMS*

The ICCs and 95% CIs of the total scale, subscale and region scores are shown in Table 3.

Moderate to excellent test–retest reliability was found for the total score of the DIMS, DIMS-D and DIMS-CA with ICCs 0.80 (95% CI 0.00–0.98; $p = 0.079$), 0.93 (95% CI 0.42–0.99; $p = 0.000$) and 0.51 (95% CI 0.00–0.95; $p = 0.283$). Good test–retest reliability was found for the total DIMS duration factor and amplitude factor with ICCs 0.76 and 0.84 respectively.

For the DIMS-D subscale, excellent test-retest reliability was found for the duration factor, amplitude factor and summation of both, having ICCs of 0.90, 0.94, and 0.93 respectively. For the DIMS-D subscale of the neck region, excellent test–retest reliability was found for the total score with ICC 0.92 while for the DIMS-D subscale of the arm regions, ICCs ranged between 0.69 and 0.96.

For the DIMS-CA subscale, the ICCs for the total duration factor, amplitude factor and summation of both were 0.38, 0.61 and 0.51 respectively. The ICC of the total DIMS-CA subscale for the neck region was 0.96 whereas for the arm regions, ICCs ranged between 0.00* and 0.83. SPSS reported negative ICC scores, most likely related to the relatively small between-subject variation compared to within-subject variation, however as negative ICCs are not theoretically possible [22], (the ICC score was changed to 0.00*) [23]. For this reason, an additional analysis was performed excluding the DIMS-CA arm LP scores. DIMS-CA subscale ICC scores varied from moderately high to good when excluding left proximal arm scores (see Appendix C, Table A3).

Table 3. Test-retest reliability: Intraclass Correlation Coefficients (ICC) with 95% Confidence Interval (CI) between two measuring weeks for the Dyskinesia Impairment Mobility Scale (DIMS).

|   |   | Duration | | Amplitude | | $\sum(D + A)$ | |
|---|---|---|---|---|---|---|---|
|   |   | ICC | 95% CI; p-value | ICC | 95% CI; p-value | ICC | 95% CI; p-value |
|   | **DIMS** | | | | | | |
|   | Total score | 0.76 | 0.00–0.98; 0.112 | 0.84 | 0.00–0.98; 0.058 | 0.80 | 0.00–0.98; 0.079 |
|   | **DIMS-D SUBSCALE** | | | | | | |
| 1 | Neck | 0.82 | 0.00–198; 0.072 | 0.97 | 0.78–0.99; 0.001 | 0.92 | 0.37–0.99; 0.018 |
| 2 | Arm RP | 0.94 | 0.43–0.99; 0.005 | 0.97 | 0.57–0.99; 0.001 | 0.96 | 0.45–0.99; 0.001 |
| 3 | Arm LP | 0.64 | 0.00–0.96; 0.070 | 0.75 | 0.00–0.97; 0.007 | 0.69 | 0.00–0.96; 0.023 |
| 4 | Arm RD | 0.87 | 0.00–0.99; 0.051 | 0.91 | 0.18–0.90; 0.026 | 0.89 | 0.00–0.99; 0.036 |
| 5 | Arm LD | 0.88 | 0.09–0.99; 0.016 | 0.83 | 0.00–0.98; 0.066 | 0.88 | 0.14–0.99; 0.030 |
|   | Total score | 0.90 | 0.26–0.99; 0.022 | 0.94 | 0.35–0.99; 0.004 | 0.93 | 0.42–0.99; 0.006 |
|   | **DIMS-CA SUBSCALE** | | | | | | |
| 1 | Neck | 0.96 | 0.66–0.99; 0.006 | 0.96 | 0.54–0.99; 0.008 | 0.96 | 0.63–0.99; 0.006 |
| 2 | Arm RP | 0.79 | 0.00–0.98; 0.087 | 0.86 | 0.04–0.98; 0.032 | 0.78 | 0.00–0.98; 0.084 |
| 3 | Arm LP | 0.00* | 0.00–0.86; 0.631 | 0.00* | 0.00–0.90; 0.518 | 0.00* | 0.00–0.88; 0.611 |
| 4 | Arm RD | 0.77 | 0.00–0.98; 0.115 | 0.87 | 0.00–0.99; 0.048 | 0.83 | 0.00–0.98; 0.073 |
| 5 | Arm LD | 0.50 | 0.00–0.95; 0.290 | 0.67 | 0.00–0.97; 0.177 | 0.60 | 0.00–0.96; 0.229 |
|   | Total score | 0.38 | 0.00–0.94; 0.353 | 0.61 | 0.00–0.96; 0.223 | 0.51 | 0.00–0.95; 0.283 |

DIMS, Dyskinesia Impairment Mobility Scale; $\sum(D + A)$, summation of duration and amplitude factors; ICC, intraclass correlation coefficient; CI, confidence interval; RP, right proximal; LP, left proximal; RD, right distal; LD, left distal; *, negative ICC; %, percentage.

### 3.3. Internal Consistency

Cronbach's alphas for the total DIMS, DIMS-D subscale and DIMS-CA subscale were $\alpha = 0.81$, $\alpha = 0.80$ and $\alpha = 0.69$ respectively. For the total DIMS-D subscale, $\alpha = 0.80$ was obtained for both duration factor and amplitude factor. For the total DIMS-CA subscale, $\alpha = 0.71$ was found for the duration factor and $\alpha = 0.66$ for the amplitude factor.

### 3.4. Concurrent Validity

For the concurrent validity of the neck region, DIMS-D subscale showed moderate correlation ($r_s = 0.41$ 95% CI,0.00–0.95, $p = 0.003$) while DIMS-CA subscale showed weak correlation ($r_s = 0.33$ 95% CI 0.00–0.94, $p = 0.018$) with the DIS scores of the second requested voluntary activity (i.e., neck rotation). No correlation was found with the first DIS requested voluntary activity (i.e., neck lateroflexion) or with DIS neck rest postures.

For the arm RP region, DIMS-D subscale showed strong correlations ($r_s = 0.63$ 95% CI 0.00–0.97, $p = 0.000$) and DIMS-CA showed moderate correlations ($r_s = 0.46$ (95% CI 0.00–0.95, $p = 0.001$) with arm RP rest postures of the DIS. No correlations were found with the DIS overflow movements.

For the arm RD region, DIMS-D subscale showed a strong correlation ($r_s = 0.63$ 95% CI 0.00–0.97, $p = 0.000$) with DIS rest postures and no correlation with DIS overflow movements. The DIMS-CA subscale showed weak correlation ($r_s$ = 0.29 95% CI 0.00–0.93, $p$ = 0.049) with DIS overflow movements and no correlation with DIS rest postures.

For the arm LP region, both the DIMS-D and the DIMS-CA subscale showed moderate correlations of $r_s$ = 0.45 (95% CI 0.00–0.95, $p$ = 0.001) and $r_s$=0.41 (95% CI 0.00–0.95, $p$ = 0.003) only with DIS rest postures.

For the arm LD region, both the DIMS-D ($r_s$ = 0.29 95% CI 0.00–0.93, $p$ = 0.057) and the DIMS-CA ($r_s$ = 0.37 95% CI 0.00–0.94, $p$ = 0.011) subscale showed weak correlations only with the DIS rest postures.

## 4. Discussion

This study aimed to develop the DIMS, a new tool to measure presence and severity of both dystonia and choreoathetosis during powered mobility tasks in DCP. The DIMS is an adapted standardized protocol of the DIS which is a reliable and valid tool to measure presence and severity of dystonia and choreoathetosis during requested but voluntary activities and rest postures. The outcomes of this study indicate that DIMS is a reliable and valid measurement tool to determine presence and severity of dystonia and choreoathetosis during powered mobility. A moderately high to good interrater reliability was found for the total score of the DIMS, the DIMS-D and the DIMS-CA with correlation coefficients of 0.87, 0.68 and 0.79 respectively. Good interrater reliability was found for the total DIMS duration factor and amplitude factor with coefficients of 0.83 and 0.73. In addition, internal consistency scores were moderately high to good. Finally, concurrent validity showed during mobility tasks significant correlations with rest postures in the arm region, and with voluntarily, requested activity in the neck region.

Interrater reliability scores are good, in particular for DIMS total and DIMS-CA. The reliability of DIMS total is in line with both the interrater reliability of junior and senior physiotherapists [15], implying that the DIMS can be reliably used in the future by all clinicians, regardless of their work experience. Interrater reliability scores of DIMS-D duration are relatively lower as is in line with previous literature [14,15]. Visual inspection of the raw data showed a much lower variability in the scores of the duration factor than the scores of the amplitude factor. In addition, low DIMS-D duration scores primarily occur in proximal arm regions, while scores in neck and distal arm regions are still moderate to moderately high. This might be because the visibility of the proximal arms is slightly lower due to the sitting position of the participants while driving the wheelchair in comparison to the distal arm region and neck region. Similarly, this may explain why scoring the duration of dystonia for the proximal arms is more difficult than scoring its amplitude, which is clinically easier to see and evaluate [14]. Interestingly, for the proximal arm regions, an excellent interrater reliability was found for the duration factor of the DIMS-CA. This is likely due to the hyperkinetic nature of choreoathetosis, which is easier to observe than the hypertonic nature of dystonia [8]. The summation of both factors revealed a good interrater reliability for the DIS-D region scores, implying a reliable measure of dystonia for both voluntary and overflow movements during powered mobility. In this respect, higher scores for the duration factor as opposed to the amplitude factor were obtained for the DIMS-CA subscale, which is in line with previous research [14,15]. The good to excellent interrater reliability of the DIMS-CA duration and amplitude factors shows that presence and severity of choreoathetosis can be reliably measured during powered mobility.

The current study of the DIMS is the first to assess test–retest reliability in measuring presence and severity of movement disorders in DCP. The test–retest reliability of the total DIMS score, DIMS-D subscale and DIMS-CA subscale was moderate to excellent, with correlation coefficients of 0.80, 0.93 and 0.51 respectively. The test–retest reliability for the total duration factor and amplitude factor of the DIMS was also good, with coefficients 0.76 and 0.84. Excellent test–retest reliability was obtained for the DIMS-D subscale both for the duration factor, amplitude factor and the summation of both factors. In–depth analysis of the DIMS-D region scores showed moderately high to excellent test–retest reliability for all constructs, which implies that the presence and severity of dystonia during powered mobility can be reliably measured over time, both for the voluntary and overflow movements.

Test–retest reliability was lower for the DIMS-CA subscale when compared to the DIMS-D subscale. These low test–retest coefficients of the DIMS-CA may be because of scores at the proximal part of the left arm (i.e., arm LP). This is most likely related to the relatively small between–subject variation compared to within–subject variation of the different independent raters [23]. To explore in more depth, the arm LP scores for the DIMS-CA subscale, the raw data of the arm LP was visually inspected. This informed that for two of the participants, the presence and severity of choreoathetosis indeed changed drastically when comparing one week to the other. For one participant, the presence and severity of choreoathetosis largely decreased, while for the other participant, a large increase was seen. This could be an explanation of the obtained ICCs for the arm LP. An additional test–retest statistical analysis for the DIMS-CA subscale was performed by excluding the scores of the arm LP (Table A2). Consequently, higher test–retest reliability coefficients were obtained for the total DIMS-CA subscale, total duration factor and amplitude factor, including higher test–retest coefficients of the total DIMS. The test–retest coefficients of the DIMS-CA for the remaining neck and arm regions (i.e., arm RP, arm RD and arm LD) were moderate to excellent, suggesting that the DIMS can reliably measure the presence and severity of choreoathetosis over time.

The internal consistency of the DIMS was good, with Cronbach's α ranging between 0.69 and 0.81 for the total score of the DIMS and the DIMS-D and DIMS-CA subscales. This indicates a stable rating construct in measuring the movement disorders during mobility tasks in children with DCP which is comparable with the internal consistency of the DIS scale [14,15]. Although the DIMS could potentially become a tool to use in longitudinal follow–ups or intervention studies, future research should also focus in assessing its responsiveness.

The concurrent validity was assessed between the DIMS scores and the DIS scores (i.e., requested voluntary activities, rest postures and overflow movements) of the same participants. Interestingly, for the neck region, both dystonia and choreoathetosis scores of the DIMS were correlated with the DIS neck rotation requested voluntary activity and no correlation was obtained with the DIS neck lateroflexion or DIS neck rest postures. The participants indeed use a rotation of the neck to be able to steer the wheelchair to the right or to the left; therefore, the obtained findings correspond with observations and knowledge from clinical practice. On the contrary, the DIMS scores of the arms region showed correlations with the arms rest postures of the DIS and not with overflow movements, except for the right distal arm. Research suggests that presence and severity of dystonia and choreoathetosis increase during requested voluntary activities as opposed to rest [24]. As the arms are not doing any goal–directed activity while operating with the head/foot steering wheelchair, it is highly likely that the presence and severity of the movement disorders in the arms during powered mobility corresponds more to the resting postures of the participants rather than requested voluntary activities which are challenging to perform.

This study is the first to present a tool that reliably measures presence and severity of dystonia and choreoathetosis during powered mobility in children and youth with DCP. The DIMS and generated insights from its use have the potential to inform and help clinicians set up more a more straightforward and efficient mobility training based on structured guidelines. As a first tool to measure movement disorders relevant for DCP during powered mobility tasks, future studies using the DIMS will yield important insights on powered mobility in DCP, which is of crucial importance and yet underexplored in the target population. Nevertheless, this study warrants some reflections to consider. First, the sample size of this study is small, considering the challenging inclusion criteria like the rare DCP diagnosis and the use of their own head/foot steering wheelchair. However, the number of tasks and regions scored by three independent raters gives confidence in the reported results. The low number of included participants has likely a relatively negative impact on the reliability scores in comparison to a higher number of participants. That is, it is plausible that with more scores included in the reliability statistical analysis, the obtained reliability coefficients would be higher. Still, given the reported outcomes in this study, the DIMS can be perceived a reliable and valid measurement tool to measure presence and severity of dystonia and choreoathetosis during powered mobility. Second, the age range of the participants and their years of experience in driving a head/foot steering system is large. Again, this could have negatively affected our outcomes in terms of the reliability scores and concurrent validity scores of the DIMS. Therefore, future studies are also advised to consider categorizing the sample based on their age and years of experience to explore any differences and generate more in–depth insights. Finally, due to the importance of the quality of the video recordings, we would like to strongly advise to use high–quality cameras with a high resolution and zoom–in function.

## 5. Conclusions

This study developed the Dyskinesia Impairment Mobility Scale (DIMS), an adapted protocol of the existing Dyskinesia Impairment Scale (DIS), to evaluate the presence and severity of dystonia and choreoathetosis during powered mobility tasks in individuals with DCP. The DIMS is a reliable and valid measurement tool to determine presence and severity of dystonia and choreoathetosis during powered mobility. The DIMS showed moderately high to good interrater reliability, good internal consistency and moderate to excellent test–retest reliability for the voluntary and overflow movements. Concurrent validity showed, during mobility tasks, significant correlations with rest postures in the arm region, and with requested voluntary activity in the neck region.

In clinical practice, the DIMS could be a promising tool to assess and evaluate the presence and severity of dystonia and choreoathetosis during powered mobility tasks, and assist in accelerating the learning process of using a powered mobility wheelchair by providing baseline profiles and a reliable longitudinal follow–up of the severity of the movement disorders which greatly impact mobility. Increased insights in clinical movement disorders during powered mobility may generate knowledge on the powered mobility driving patterns which can be used by the clinicians to tailor individualized mobility training programs. Furthermore, in future research, the DIMS can be used to explore clinical patterns of dystonia and choreoathetosis during steering and be used as an evaluation tool of future mobility intervention studies. Moreover, the DIMS could inform on the impact of factors such as fatigue, stress or emotional arousal on movement disorders during powered mobility, leading to increased insights that could assist in the development of more straightforward mobility training guidelines.

**Author Contributions:** Conceptualization, S.B., I.G.N., S.G., J.-M.A., H.H. and E.M; methodology, S.B., I.G.N., M.K., J.-M.A. and E.M.; validation, S.B.; formal analysis, S.B.; investigation, S.B., I.G.N., S.G. and I.V.; resources, S.B. and E.M.; data curation, S.B. and M.K.; writing—original draft preparation, S.B.; writing—review and editing, M.K., I.V., I.G.N., S.G., J.-M.A., H.H. and E.M.; visualization, S.B.; supervision, E.M., M.K., J.-M.A and H.H.; project administration, S.B. and E.M.; funding acquisition, E.M., J.-M.A. and H.H.

**Funding:** This research was funded by a C3 grant from the Research Council of KU Leuven, grant number C32/17/056.

**Acknowledgments:** The authors express immense gratitude to the participants who were included in this study and their supportive parents. A special thank you goes to the therapists of the participants for their invaluable help from the screening process to data collection: Bart Moerman, physical therapist, Dominiek Savio Institute, Gits, Belgium; Ms. Heleen Soens, physical therapist, Dominiek Savio Institute, Gits, Belgium; and Veerle Janssens, occupational therapist in Sint Jozef Institute (Heder), Antwerp. Acknowledged are the two master thesis students: Alice Di Berardino and Hannah Rooseleers for their help and hard work in scoring the participants as part of their master thesis project. The authors thank professor Jan Deklerck for the valuable feedback on the methodology and statistical analysis of this study.

**Conflicts of Interest:** The authors declare no conflict of interest. The funders had no role in the design of the study; in the collection, analyses, or interpretation of data; in the writing of the manuscript, or in the decision to publish the results.

## Appendix A

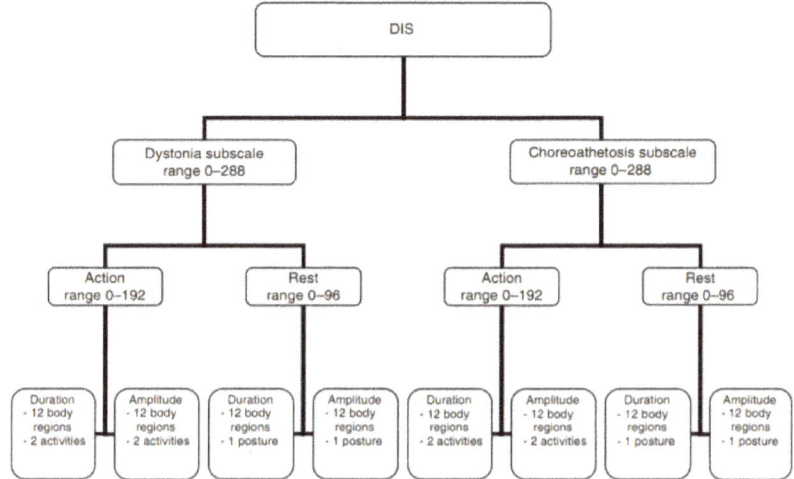

**Figure A1.** Diagram of the Dyskinesia Impairment Scale (DIS) protocol.

## Appendix B

**Table A1.** Participants' characteristics.

|     | Gender (M/F) | Age (yo) | GMFCS | MACS | Experience with Powered Mobility (Years) |
| --- | --- | --- | --- | --- | --- |
| P01 | M | 19 | 4 | 4 | 10 |
| P02 | M | 16 | 4 | 4 | 6 |
| P03 | F | 6 | 4 | 4 | 1.5 |
| P04 | F | 21 | 5 | 4 | 6 |
| P05 | F | 8 | 4 | 5 | 1 |

P, participant; M, male; F, female; yo, year old; GMFCS, Gross Motor Function Classification System; MACS, Manual Ability Classification Scale.

## Appendix C

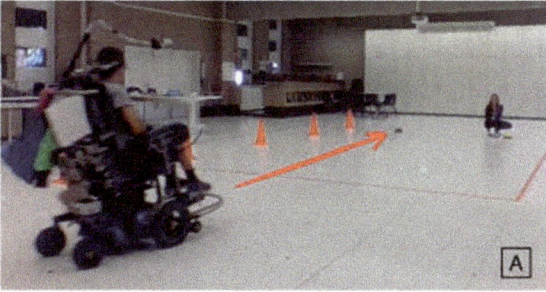

**Figure A2.** *Cont.*

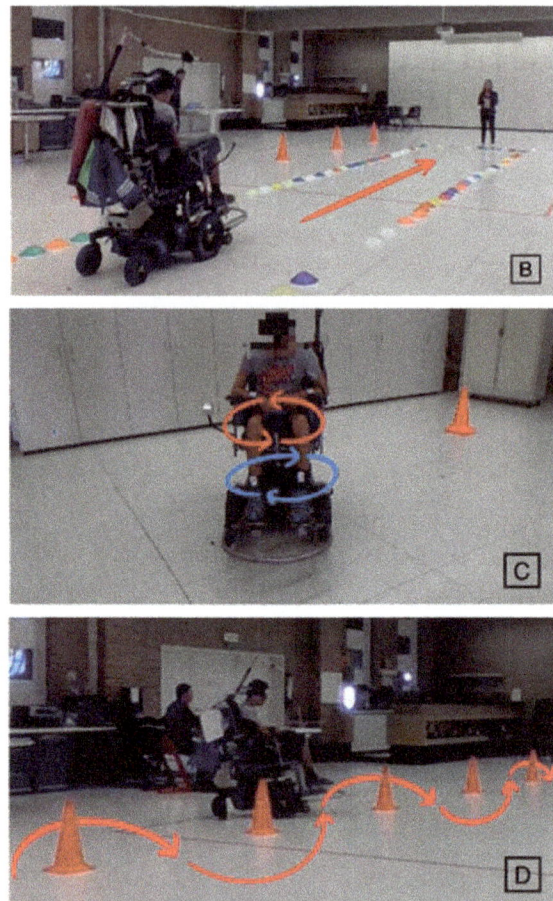

**Figure A2.** Data collection set–up with five standardized powered mobility tasks: (**A**) T1, Independent driving; (**B**) T2, driving through a created corridor; (**C**) T3, 360° turn to the left (red arrow); T4, 360° turn to the right (blue arrow); (**D**) T5, slalom.

## Appendix D

**Table A2.** Interrater reliability of DIS Training: Intraclass Correlation Coefficients (ICC) with 95% confidence interval (CI) between three raters for the total scores.

|  | Duration | | | Amplitude | | | $\sum(D + A)$ | | |
| --- | --- | --- | --- | --- | --- | --- | --- | --- | --- |
|  | ICC | 95% CI; $p$–value | | ICC | 95% CI; $p$–value | | ICC | 95% CI; $p$–value | |
| Dystonia | 0.91 | 0.74–0.98; 0.000 | | 0.89 | 0.69–0.97; 0.000 | | 0.89 | 0.70–0.97; 0.000 | |
| Choreoathetosis | 0.95 | 0.85–0.99; 0.000 | | 0.96 | 0.90–0.99; 0.000 | | 0.96 | 0.88–0.99; 0.000 | |
| DIS Training | 0.94 | 0.83–0.98; 0.000 | | 0.95 | 0.86–0.99; 0.000 | | 0.96 | 0.88–0.99; 0.000 | |

ICC, Intraclass Correlation Coefficient; CI, Confidence Interval; DIS, Dyskinesia Impairment Scale; $\sum(D + A)$, summation of duration and amplitude factors; %, percentage.

## Appendix E

**Table A3.** Test–retest reliability: Intraclass correlation coefficients (ICC) with 95% confidence interval (CI) between two measuring weeks for the Dyskinesia Impairment Mobility Scale, with excluded left arm proximal scores for the DIMS-CA subscale.

|   |   | Duration | | Amplitude | | $\sum(D + A)$ | |
|---|---|---|---|---|---|---|---|
|   |   | ICC | 95% CI; $p$-value | ICC | 95% CI; $p$-value | ICC | 95% CI; $p$-value |
|   | *DIMS* | | | | | | |
|   | Total score | 0.81 | 0.00–0.98; 0.059 | 0.88 | 0.17–0.99; 0.028 | 0.87 | 0.03–0.99; 0.037 |
|   | *DIMS-D SUBSCALE* | | | | | | |
| 1 | Neck | 0.82 | 0.00–198; 0.072 | 0.97 | 0.78–0.99; 0.001 | 0.92 | 0.37–0.99; 0.018 |
| 2 | Arm RP | 0.94 | 0.43–0.99; 0.005 | 0.97 | 0.57–0.99; 0.001 | 0.96 | 0.45–0.99; 0.001 |
| 3 | Arm LP | 0.64 | 0.00–0.96; 0.070 | 0.75 | 0.00–0.97; 0.007 | 0.69 | 0.00–0.96; 0.023 |
| 4 | Arm RD | 0.87 | 0.00–0.99; 0.051 | 0.91 | 0.18–0.90; 0.026 | 0.89 | 0.00–0.99; 0.036 |
| 5 | Arm LD | 0.88 | 0.09–0.99; 0.016 | 0.83 | 0.00–0.98; 0.066 | 0.88 | 0.14–0.99; 0.030 |
|   | Total score | 0.90 | 0.26–0.99; 0.022 | 0.94 | 0.35–0.99; 0.004 | 0.93 | 0.42–0.99; 0.006 |
|   | *DIMS-CA SUBSCALE* | | | | | | |
| 1 | Neck | 0.96 | 0.66–0.99; 0.006 | 0.96 | 0.54–0.99; 0.008 | 0.96 | 0.63–0.99; 0.006 |
| 2 | Arm RP | 0.79 | 0.00–0.98; 0.087 | 0.86 | 0.04–0.98; 0.032 | 0.78 | 0.00–0.98; 0.084 |
| 3 | Arm LP | * | * | * | * | * | * |
| 4 | Arm RD | 0.77 | 0.00–0.99; 0.115 | 0.87 | 0.00–0.99; 0.048 | 0.83 | 0.00–0.98; 0.073 |
| 5 | Arm LD | 0.50 | 0.00–0.95; 0.290 | 0.67 | 0.00–0.97; 0.177 | 0.60 | 0.00–0.96; 0.229 |
|   | Total score | 0.62 | 0.00–0.96; 0.217 | 0.75 | 0.00–0.98; 0.130 | 0.71 | 0.00–0.97; 0.160 |

DIMS, Dyskinesia Impairment Mobility Scale; $\sum(D + A)$, summation of duration and amplitude factors; ICC, Intraclass Correlation Coefficient; CI, Confidence Interval; RP, Right Proximal; L, Left Proximal; RD, Right Distal; LD, Left Distal; *, negative ICCs excluded from the analysis of DIMS-CA subscale; %, percentage.

## References

1. Livingstone, R.; Field, D. Systematic review of power mobility outcomes for infants, children and adolescents with mobility limitations. *Clin. Rehabil.* **2014**, *28*, 954–964. [CrossRef] [PubMed]
2. Casey, J.; Paleg, G.; Livingstone, R. Facilitating Child Participation through Power Mobility. *Br. J. Occup. Ther.* **2013**, *76*, 158–160. [CrossRef]
3. Livingstone, R.; Field, D. The child and family experience of power mobility: A qualitative synthesis. *Dev. Med. Child Neurol.* **2015**, *57*, 317–327. [CrossRef] [PubMed]
4. Livingstone, R. A critical review of powered mobility assessment and training for children. *Disabil. Rehabil. Assist. Technol.* **2010**, *5*, 392–400. [CrossRef] [PubMed]
5. Rodby–Bousquet, E.; Paleg, G.; Casey, J.; Wizert, A.; Livingstone, R. Physical risk factors influencing wheeled mobility in children with cerebral palsy: A cross-sectional study. *BMC Pediatr.* **2016**, *16*. [CrossRef]
6. Sellier, E.; Platt, M.J.; Andersen, G.L.; Krageloh-Mann, I.; De La Cruz, J.; Cans, C. Decreasing prevalence in cerebral palsy: A multi-site European population-based study, 1980 to 2003. *Dev. Med. Child Neurol.* **2016**, *58*, 85–92. [CrossRef] [PubMed]
7. Rosenbaum, P.; Paneth, N.; Leviton, A.; Goldstein, M.; Bax, M.; Damiano, D.; Dan, B.; Jacobsson, B. A report: The definition and classification of cerebral palsy April 2006. *Dev. Med. Child Neurol. Suppl.* **2007**, *109*, 8–14. [PubMed]
8. Monbaliu, E.; Himmelmann, K.; Lin, J.P.; Ortibus, E.; Bonouvrie, L.; Feys, H.; Vermeulen, R.J.; Dan, B. Clinical presentation and management of dyskinetic cerebral palsy. *Lancet Neurol.* **2017**, *16*, 741–749. [CrossRef]
9. Vanmechelen, I.; Bekteshi, S.; Bossier, K.; Feys, H.; Deklerck, J.; Monbaliu, E. Presence and severity of dystonia and choreoathetosis overflow movements in participants with dyskinetic cerebral palsy and their relation with functional classification scales. *Disabil.Rehabil* **2019**, 1–8. [CrossRef] [PubMed]
10. Monbaliu, E.; De La Pena, M.G.; Ortibus, E.; Molenaers, G.; Deklerck, J.; Feys, H. Functional outcomes in children and young people with dyskinetic cerebral palsy. *Dev. Med. Child Neurol.* **2017**, *59*, 634–640. [CrossRef] [PubMed]
11. Rodby-Bousquet, E.; Hägglund, G. Use of manual and powered wheelchair in children with cerebral palsy: A cross-sectional study. *BMC Pediatr.* **2010**, *10*, 59. [CrossRef] [PubMed]

12. Livingstone, R.; Paleg, G. Practice considerations for the introduction and use of power mobility for children. *Dev. Med. Child Neurol* **2014**, *56*, 210–221. [CrossRef] [PubMed]
13. Giesbrecht, E.M.; Wilson, N.; Schneider, A.; Bains, D.; Hall, J.; Miller, W.C. Preliminary Evidence to Support a "Boot Camp" Approach to Wheelchair Skills Training for Clinicians. *Arch. Phys. Med. Rehabil.* **2015**, *96*, 1158–1161. [CrossRef] [PubMed]
14. Monbaliu, E.; Ortibus, E.; De Cat, J.; Dan, B.; Heyrman, L.; Prinzie, P.; De Cock, P.; Feys, H. The Dyskinesia Impairment Scale: A new instrument to measure dystonia and choreoathetosis in dyskinetic cerebral palsy. *Dev. Med. Child Neurol* **2012**, *54*, 278–283. [CrossRef] [PubMed]
15. Monbaliu, E.; Ortibus, E.; Prinzie, P.; Dan, B.; De Cat, J.; De Cock, P.; Feys, H. Can the Dyskinesia Impairment Scale be used by inexperienced raters? A reliability study. *Eur. J. Paediatr. Neurol.* **2013**, *17*, 238–247. [CrossRef] [PubMed]
16. Vanmechelen, I.; Dan, B.; Feys, H.; Monbaliu, E. Test-retest reliability of the Dyskinesia Impairment Scale: Can dystonia and choreoathetosis be reliably measured over time in dyskinetic cerebral palsy? *Dev. Med. Child Neurol.* **2019**, under review.
17. Palisano, R.J.; Avery, L.; Gorter, J.W.; Galuppi, B.; McCoy, S.W. Stability of the Gross Motor Function Classification System, Manual Ability Classification System, and Communication Function Classification System. *Dev. Med. Child Neurol.* **2018**, *60*, 1026–1032. [CrossRef] [PubMed]
18. Kirby, R.L.; Smith, C.; Routhier, F.; Best, K.L.; Cowan, R.; Giesbrecht, E.; Koontz, A.; MacKenzie, D.; Mortenson, B.; Parker, K.; et al. The Wheelchair Skills Program Manual Version 5.0. Available online: www.wheelchairskillsprogram.ca/eng/manual.php (accessed on 15 February 2018).
19. Kinovea 0.8.15. Available online: www.kinovea.org (accessed on 10 September 2018).
20. RIGBY, A.S. Statistical recommendations for papers submitted to Developmental Medicine & Child Neurology. *Dev. Med. Child Neurol.* **2010**, *52*, 299–304. [CrossRef] [PubMed]
21. Portney, L.G.; Watkins, M.P. *Foundations of Clinical Research: Applications to Practice*, 3rd ed.; Pearson/Prentice Hall: Upper Saddle River, NJ, USA, 2014.
22. Gireaudeau, B. Negative Values of the Intraclass Correlation Coefficients Are Not Theoretically Possible. *J. Clin. Epidemiol.* **1996**, *49*, 1205–1206. [CrossRef]
23. London King's College. Available online: https://www.kcl.ac.uk/ioppn/depts/BiostatisticsHealthInformatics/SAS/faqs (accessed on 28 March 2019).
24. Monbaliu, E.; de Cock, P.; Ortibus, E.; Heyrman, L.; Klingels, K.; Feys, H. Clinical patterns of dystonia and choreoathetosis in participants with dyskinetic cerebral palsy. *Dev. Med. Child Neurol.* **2016**, *58*, 138–144. [CrossRef] [PubMed]

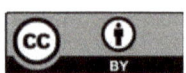

© 2019 by the authors. Licensee MDPI, Basel, Switzerland. This article is an open access article distributed under the terms and conditions of the Creative Commons Attribution (CC BY) license (http://creativecommons.org/licenses/by/4.0/).

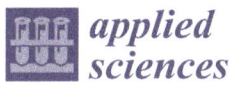 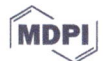

*Article*

# Determining Symptomatic Factors of Nomophobia in Peruvian Students from the National University of Engineering

Jimmy Aurelio Rosales-Huamani [1,*,†], Rita Rocio Guzman-Lopez [1,†], Eder Eliseo Aroni-Vilca [1,†], Carmen Rosalia Matos-Avalos [1,†] and Jose Luis Castillo-Sequera [2,†]

1. National University of Engineering, Lima 15333, Peru; rrguzman@uni.edu.pe (R.R.G.-L.); ederaronivilca@gmail.com (E.E.A.-V.); carmatos@uni.edu.pe (C.R.M.-A.)
2. Department of Computer Science, Higher Polytechnic School, University of Alcala, 28871 Alcalá de Henares, Spain; jluis.castillo@uah.es
* Correspondence: jrosales@uni.edu.pe; Tel.: +51-1-381-5630
† These authors contributed equally to this work.

Received: 1 February 2019; Accepted: 23 April 2019; Published: 1 May 2019

**Abstract:** The use of cell phones has increased worldwide in the past few decades, particularly in children and adolescents. Using these electronic devices provides personal benefits. Communicating through cell phones was a very important factor in the socioeconomic progress of developed countries. However, it is beyond doubt that its indiscriminate use can bring up certain psychiatric disorders or cause some disorder in a person, within the phobic group of anxiety disorders called nomophobia; basically associated with anxiety, nervousness, discomfort, and distress when contact with the smartphone is lost, mainly in the youngest users. This research proposal aims to identify symptoms that have not yet been detected by unceasing cell phone use, considering that in Peru there are few studies of human health engineering and the physical mental health. For that reason, we sought to identify the symptomatic factors of nomophobia presented by students at the National University of Engineering and its interference with their academic life. To accomplish this study, we designed a questionnaire according to our reality with the use of focus groups techniques when the test was taken in class. Three symptomatic factors of nomophobia were identified: feelings of anxiety, compulsive smartphone use, and feelings of anxiety and panic. The study included a representative sample of 461 students in different years of study engineering (21% women, 79% men, over 17 years of age). Finally, given the widespread adoption of smartphones and their integration into educational environments, the results of this study can help educators understand students' inclination to use their smartphones at all times.

**Keywords:** nomophobia; anxiety; smartphone; internet; cyberaddiction; new technologies

## 1. Introduction

Continuous technological developments have changed the way that human beings manage their daily activities. In particular, information and communication technologies have became an indispensable part of our social interactions, work activities, and education.

However, the appearance of smaller electronic devices with higher computing capabilities has enabled the proliferation of cheap mobile devices and smartphones are considered to be the latest Information and Communications Technology (ICT) development [1]. They are no longer just cell phones as, in addition to making calls or sending messages, they enable access to the Internet and thus a wide variety of services offered by the network [2]. Cell phone use is widespread, even surpassing the population in some countries [3], while 70% of young people (15–24 years old) in the world use the Internet through various means, including mobile devices [4]. They are used more widely among the youngest population. This is because young people have adopted new technologies quickly and because using a smartphone is a status symbol within the tech-culture [5]. At the end of 2017 in Peru, the number of mobile lines that access the Internet was 21.2 million, this means that two of every three people accessed the Internet through mobile services, which gives us an idea of the number of smartphones in Peru [4]. On the other hand, social networks have became one of the largest and most influential components on the web, providing an easy platform to everyone (young and the elderly alike). Many young people lose sight of the real world as they are absorbed by the virtual world and become slaves of technology [6].

Despite their considerable positive impacts, smartphones have a seemingly minor negative impact, called nomophobia, which in turn can be as serious as the positive side if these phones are not wisely used [7]. Nomophobia is an abbreviation of the English "no mobile phone phobia", which translates into the fear of not having a cell phone. Specific phobias are frequent anxiety disorders; at the same time, they precede other psychiatric disorders such as depression and abusive use of toxic substances. There have been problematic situations where people are too close to their smartphones, presenting symptoms of behavioral addiction that interferes with their daily activities.

Studies have also been conducted on the problem of indiscriminate cell phone use. In Walsh, White and Young presented a preliminary examination of the behavior of young Australians and their use of cell phones. This study explored the relationship between psychological predictors of the frequency of cell phone use and the participation of cell phones conceptualized as a cognitive and behavioral interaction of people with their cell phones. The participants in this study were young Australians between 15 and 24 years of age [8]. Independently, King et al. presented a study applied to individuals with panic disorder and agoraphobia because of dependence on their cell phones [9]. Then, Krajewska et al. examined the role of cell phones in the lives of Belorussian and Polish students. This study included the analysis of a sample of students from Belarus and Poland. Consequent to this study, they concluded that almost 20% of students in Poland and 10% in Belarus have symptoms of cell phone addiction [10]. Independently, Ouslasvirta et al. mentioned that smartphones may cause compulsive checking habits [1].

King et al. argued that studies on the relationships between individuals and new technologies are relevant with the justification that new technologies produce changes in behavior, as well as feelings and symptoms, that must be studied and monitored continuously in modern society [11]. Then, Castilla and Paez, among their research results, mentioned that the most used application among young people is "WhatsApp" for instant messaging and that they may feel social exclusion if they are not included in a group [12].

Billieux et al. mentioned that, despite the many positive results, cell phones when used excessively are now often associated with potentially harmful and/or disruptive behaviors [13]. Independently, Yildirim and Correia considered nomophobia to be the phobia of the modern age that has been introduced into our lives as a by-product of the interaction between people and mobile information and communication technologies, particularly smartphones. In their studies, the authors have identified and described the dimensions of nomophobia and developed a questionnaire to measure this nomophobia [14].

The definition of nomophobia is controversial [5]. Therefore, it is necessary to define the one that will be used for this study. We consider nomophobia to be a behavioral addiction to cell phones, which is manifested by psychological and physical symptoms of dependence. Yildirim and Correia mentioned that nomophobia is an abbreviated form of "no mobile phone phobia" and is thought to stem from the excessive use of a mobile phone [14]. Independently, Arpaci mentioned that nomophobia is a specific disorder caused by smartphone use [15]. Then, Dasgupta et al. mentioned that the purpose of their study is to find out the predominance of nomophobia among the smartphones used by undergraduates of West Bengal [16]. In their work, they used the Nomophobia Questionnaire (NMP-Q) developed by Yildirim and Correia [14].

The teaching of each course at the National University of Engineering requires on average 2 to 3 h; however, there are many factors that can cause distraction in the classroom. One factor is the excessive use of cell phones. Aguilera et al. presented a study to analyze the relationship between the level of nomophobia and the distraction associated with the use of smartphones. The study population were nursing students from the University of Almeria in Spain [17].

Froese et al. examined the impact of smartphone use in classroom learning; for this, they give a test to the students at the end of class, proving that those who had the lowest score were students that immediately answered the text messages from their cell phone with regard to who had kept their cell phone [18]. Independently, the studies of [19,20] mentioned that the ringing or notification of the cell phone, regardless of phone number, can be a distractor in the classroom. Then, Prasad et al. mentioned that the objective of the study is to evaluate the pattern of usage of mobile phones and its effects on the academic performance of dental students in India College. The authors concluded that there is an alarming indication of mobile phone addiction on the part of students, which affects their academic performance in a negative way [21]. Arpaci et al. presented a study that aims to investigate the mediating effect of mindfulness on the relationship between attachment and nomophobia. The study is also focused on gender differences in attachment, mindfulness, and nomophobia [22].

Mendoza et al. mentioned that the excessive use of cell phones has led researchers to focus on how the use of cell phones affects learning and memory in classroom. The participants were recruited from undergraduate psychology courses [23]. Independently, Bychkov and Young mentioned that there are symptoms of nomophobia from excessive use of the smartphone. Fortunately, these symptoms may be resolved through behavioral, as the technology itself may be useful tool for that very behavior therapy—for example, transmitting health ads published in radio, television, text messages, and mobile apps. From this research, the authors perform a review systematics of applications for mobiles for the decrease of the addiction to smartphones [24]. Lee et al. examined the relationship between the Nomophobia Questionnaire (NMP-Q) and the Obsessive Content Scale (OBS). This study helps to better understand personality disorders (e.g., obsessiveness) that are emerging from the excessive use of mobile phones or the excessive fear of losing a cell phone [25]. Independently, Balshan et al. developed and validated the Arabic version of the nomophobia questionnaire in university students of Kuwait. In their study, the authors concluded that more than half of the sample contained a moderate nomophobia and a quarter of the sample contained a serious level of nomophobia [26].

Then, Ahmed et al. carried out an online cross-sectional survey that was conducted by using the Google form platform. This research involved a total of 157 students in the course of physiotherapy at the University of North India, and used the questionnaire NMP-Q [27]. Ayar et al. analyzed levels of nomophobia in which the participants were undergraduate nursing students in a school located in western Turkey. In this study, the authors used several models to correlate the effect of problematic internet use, social appearance anxiety, and social media with the nomophobia [28]. Then, Gutierrez-Puertas et al. mentioned that the objective of this study was to compare the levels of nomophobia, experienced by nursing students at the University of Almeria, Spain and the Polytechnic Institute of Braganza, Portugal. The conclusions found by the authors indicate that the dimensions explored contain significant levels of nomophobia between both populations of nursing students [29].

On the other hand, the use of mobile phones causes alterations in the habits of daily life and perceptions of reality, which can be associated with negative results, such as deteriorated social interactions, social isolation, and mental health problems such as anxiety, depression, and stress. The present study discusses nomophobia in relation to the smartphone. In the absence of research information on nomophobia in our country, we believe that, by carrying out this study, we will be able to identify the main symptomatic factors that are presented by the National University of Engineering (UNI) students that are caused by indiscriminate cell phone usage, and that are not observable during the course of the students' daily lives. To identify these factors, our contribution has been to give viability to the test adapted with the objective of getting an answer according to our reality, and the use of focus group techniques. Consequently, we present three symptomatic factors of nomophobia in UNI students, which describe the need that students have for indiscriminate cell phone use.

The present study is described as follows: In Section 2, we explain the methodology to be used. In Section 3, we describe the results obtained. Finally, in Section 4, we show the conclusions and future studies.

## 2. Methodology

We have made a transversal, correlational, and factorial research methodology. It was carried out in 461 male and female students at the National University of Engineering. To carry out the proposal, we completed the following stages that are shown in Figure 1, trying to adapt a methodology that allows for covering the most relevant aspect of our study and following the recommendations of other authors.

- Test Adaptation. Currently, there is a wide variety of tools to identify dependency problems that are associated with smartphone use and the use of other information and communication technologies. However, in our study, we used the "Test of Mobile Phone Dependence (TMDbrief) Questionnaire" [30] as a main reference, which evaluates the main characteristics of cell phone dependence: tolerance, withdrawal syndrome, change of impulse control, excessive use, etc., using an intercultural approach. In our study, the test was improved through the methodology of focus group. This methodology was used as a tool to analyze the initial questionnaire and collect the general recommendations of many students from different careers. The meeting was moderated by the principal investigator. After the meeting, we concluded that some of the survey questions were improved in our research. There are several authors [31,32] who use the focus group techniques.
- Test Validation. In this stage, the questionnaire was validated using the Cronbach test [33].
- Sample Methodology. In this stage, the sample methodology was defined to calculate sample size in correlational studies and is proportional to the population of the faculties in the University.
- Factor Analysis Application. Taking into account the objective of this study, we are interested in finding out whether questions in part 2 (below) in the test is joined with some special feature or not. For this reason, we have decided to applicate factorial analyses. Thus, we looked for a smaller number of factors by reduction of variables. By the way, the minimum factors could be able to explain information inside data.
- Experimental Results. The results were processed using Statistical Package for the Social Sciences (SPSS) software for Windows (IBM Corp. Released 2013. IBM SPSS Statistics for Windows, Version 22.0. Armonk, NY, USA) to obtain the final reports and to be able to obtain the respective conclusions.

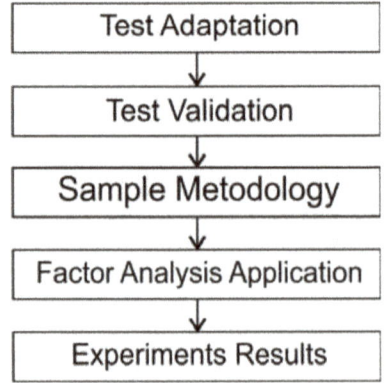

**Figure 1.** Methodology to carry out the proposal.

*2.1. Quantitative Instrument*

The test used was carefully adapted and translated from the Test of Mobile Phone Dependence (TMDbrief) [30] on the basis of previous recommendations and previous study experience [2]. Because of the multicultural approach of TMDbrief, it was not necessary to validate the translation.

Moreover, the test applied was objective and consists of two blocks. The first block corresponds to basic demographic data. The second block has 16 items, which show how UNI students relate to their smartphones, and each item proposes a statement that has seven response options, a Likert scale, with respect to students' level of agreement or disagreement with each sentence: 1 = Strongly disagree to 7 = Strongly agree. This is shown in the following survey.

---

NATIONAL UNIVERSITY OF ENGINEERING

We want to adapt and apply the following test to the UNI student population, with the goal of offering help to those who use their cell phones in an unhealthy manner. Thank you for your responses.

1. Age
2. Gender:    a. Female        b. Male
3. Department            4. Major
5. Cycle                 6. Origin

Answer or mark with "x", belongs to your opinion:

7. How long (in years) have you been use your smartphone or cell-phone:
   a) Lees one year
   b) More one year, but less two years    c) More two years, but less three years
   d) More three years, but less four years    e) More four years, but less five years
   f) More five years

8. Do you have a plan of mobile data that allows you to accessing to the internet through your smartphone or cell-phone?
   a. yes        b. not

9. Approximately, how much time during the day do you think that you use your cell phone or smartphone? .... hours.

10. More and less, how much time during the day do you check your smartphone or cell-phone? .... times.

11. How frequently do you think that you check your smartphone or cell-phone?
    a) Each 5 minutes
    b) Each 10 minutes                c) Each 20 minutes
    d) Each 30 minutes                e) Each hour
    f) Others (specify please)

---

Block 1

The following questions related to how you use your cell phone:

| Please indicate your level of agreement or disagreement with an "x" for the following statements in relation to smartphone or cell phone use | 1=strongly disagree | | | | 7=strongly agree | | |
|---|---|---|---|---|---|---|---|
| | 1 | 2 | 3 | 4 | 5 | 6 | 7 |
| 1. If my smartphone or cell phone wasn't working for a long time and it would take a long time to fix it, I would feel very bad. | | | | | | | |
| 2. If I don't have my smartphone or cell phone, I feel bad. | | | | | | | |
| 3. I don't think I could handle a week without my smartphone or cell phone. | | | | | | | |
| 4. If I couldn't check my smartphone or cell phone for a while, I would want to check it. | | | | | | | |
| 5. I spend more time than I should talking on my smartphone or cell phone, sending messages, and using other apps. | | | | | | | |
| 6. I go to bed later or have slept less to use my smartphone or phone cell. | | | | | | | |
| 7. I use my smartphone or cell phone (for calls, reading or sending messages, using WhatsApp, among other things) in situation that may not be dangerous but are not appropriate for smartphone use (such as while others are talking to me, etc). | | | | | | | |
| 8. I need to use my smartphone or cell phone more often. | | | | | | | |
| 9. I get angry or irritated when someone bothers me while I'm using my smartphone or cell phone. | | | | | | | |
| 10. If my smartphone or cell phone is with me, I can't stop using it. | | | | | | | |
| 11. Ever since I have had my smartphone or cell phone, I have increased sent messages. | | | | | | | |
| 12. As soon as I get up in the morning, the first thing I do is see who called up or whether anyone sent me a message. | | | | | | | |
| 13. When I feel lonely, I use my smartphone or cell phone to make calls, send messages, etc. | | | | | | | |
| 14. Right now, I would grab my smartphone or cell phone and send message, make a call, or check social networks. | | | | | | | |
| 15. I feel nervous if I do not receive messages, calls, and notifications from social networks on my smartphone or cell phone. | | | | | | | |
| 16. If I didn't have my smartphone or cell phone with me, I would feel bad because I wouldn't be able to check social networks. | | | | | | | |

Block 2

Validation of the Instrument

The reliability analysis was carried out to understand the internal consistency of the scale, i.e., the correlation between the items analyzed, as well as to assess the reliability or homogeneity of the questions [33] in block 2. Cronbach's alpha coefficient ($\alpha$) oscillates between 0 and 1, where 0 means a reliability assessment of null and 1 represents total reliability. In addition, internal consistency is considered high if it is between 0.70 and 0.90. Values below 0.70 indicate low internal consistency and those above 0.90 suggest that the scale has several items that measure exactly the same [34].

To calculate Cronbach's alpha coefficient, using the variance of the items and the variance of the total score, we use the following formula:

$$\alpha = \left[\frac{k}{k-1}\right]\left[1 - \frac{\sum_{i=1}^{k} S_i^2}{S_T^2}\right], \quad (1)$$

where:
$S_i^2$ : Is the variance of each item,
$S_T^2$ : Is the variance of all rows,
$k$ : Is the number of questions or items.

The calculation of the value of Cronbach's alpha was processed with the help of SPSS Software. Table 1 shows the results.

**Table 1.** Reliability statistics.

| Cronbach's Alpha | Cronbach's Alpha Based on the Categorized Elements | Number of Elements |
|---|---|---|
| 0.873 | 0.883 | 16 |

The value of Cronbach's alpha ($\alpha = 0.873$) shows that the questionnaire exhibits high internal consistency. The questionnaire was previously improved in focus group sessions to verify the interpretation and adequacy of the items.

Malhotra defined the pilot test as applying a questionnaire to a small sample of the units of analysis to identify and eliminate possible problems in the questionnaire's design [35]. The instrument in question was validated with a pilot sample of 30 students from the National University of Engineering to eliminate inconsistencies or questions within the questionnaire.

*2.2. Sample Size*

It is necessary to estimate the correlations, relationship, or association between the two variables–symptoms and indiscriminate smartphone use—hence, it is necessary to establish the calculation of the sample size using the following formula [36]:

$$n_0 = \left\{\frac{Z_{1-\alpha/2} + Z_{1-\beta}}{\frac{1}{2} \cdot \ln\frac{1+r}{1-r}}\right\}^2 + 3, \quad (2)$$

where:
$n_0$ : Sample size,
$\alpha$ : Level of significance, which is universally chosen as 5% (error type I),
$Z_{1-\alpha/2}$ : Value of the standard normal variable corresponding to a confidence level,
$\beta$ : Probability of accepting a false hypothesis, when this is really false (error type II), this value is fixed around 0.2 in a majority of cases, thus it will have a test power of 80%,
$Z_{1-\beta}$ : P-Normal variable value for a test power of 85%, the value of which in the normal table,
$r$ : is 1.04 Value of the correlation from which a relationship is considered in our study.

Assuming a 5% level of significance, a test power of 85%, and $r = 0.15$, a sample size of 397 students is reached. This size was increased to 16% of the size calculated to cover the non-response rate, culminating in the obtainment of a sample of 461 students to be used. In this way, we comply with evaluating a representative sample for our study, which guarantees valid results.

*2.3. Variable Classification*

Variables: Age, Gender, Department, and Major correspond to variables for the descriptive study of the sample (block 1). The dependent variables, i.e., the scores obtained from the 16 statements on how students relate to their smartphones (indiscriminate smartphone use), and the independent variable, symptoms, are detailed in 16 sentences in the second block of the previous survey.

*2.4. Data Collection Procedures*

The questionnaires were administered to the students on the National University of Engineering campus at different times and in areas near the university, the participants had 10 min to complete the test. We tried to consider different schedules because first semester students have classes in the mornings, while those in the last cycles usually have classes in the afternoon or evening. The respondents answered the questionnaire's questions freely and voluntarily. The recommendation was to respond truthfully and to try to answer as quickly as possible. No incentive was offered for participation. With this, it was possible to collect the data in an anonymous and reliable way, covering different types of students of the university.

### 3. Results and Discussion

*3.1. Descriptive Analysis*

A total of 461 completed questionnaires were processed from the database, using the SPSS software package for Windows (version 19.0, SPSS, Inc., Chicago, IL, USA). According to reports issued by SPSS, the sample consisted of 21% men and 79% women. With regard to the ages of the students in the sample, 35.8% were 17–19 years old; 30.4% were 20–21 years old; and 33.8% were 22 years old and above. The mean and standard deviation of age was $20.81 \pm 0.12$ with an age range of 17 to 32 years. See Table 2 for these results.

**Table 2.** Percentage distribution of respondents by age.

| Age | Frequency | Percentage (%) |
|---|---|---|
| [17, 19] | 165 | 35.8 |
| [20, 21] | 140 | 30.4 |
| [22, or more] | 156 | 33.8 |
| Total | 461 | 100 |

With regard to how long they had used a smartphone, 31.9% of students had one in use for more than five years; 30.2% had one in use for 3–4 years; and 37.9% had one in use for less than two years. See Table 3 for these results.

**Table 3.** How long the respondent has had a smartphone.

| | Frequency | Percentage (%) |
|---|---|---|
| Less than a year | 37 | 8 |
| More than 1 year but less than 2 | 72 | 15.6 |
| More than 2 years but less than 3 | 66 | 14.3 |
| More than 3 years but less than 4 | 77 | 16.7 |
| More than 4 years but less than 5 | 62 | 13.5 |
| More than 5 years | 147 | 31.9 |
| Total | 461 | 100 |

When asked whether the students had a data plan that would allow them to access the Internet, 68.3% of the respondents answered yes and 31.7% answered that they did not have a data plan.

With regard to the total time dedicated to smartphone use per day, 26.8% answered that they used their smartphones for a total of 1–3 h a day. The majority (34.1%) answered that they used their smartphones for 4–5 h; 19.1% answered saying 5–10 h; and 20% answered saying 10 or more hours a day. Table 4 shows these results.

Table 4. Time per day devoted to smartphone use.

| Time per Day | Frequency | Percentage (%) |
|---|---|---|
| 1 to 3 h | 124 | 26.8 |
| 4 to 5 h | 157 | 34.1 |
| 6 to 9 h | 88 | 19.1 |
| 10 or more | 92 | 20.0 |
| Total | 461 | 100 |

With regard to the number of times they usually checked their smartphones in a day, 25.8% of the respondents answered that they checked 1–8 times; 24.5% checked 9–16 times; 29.7% checked 17–30 times; and 20% checked 31 or more times. Table 5 shows these results.

Table 5. Frequency of checking smartphone or cell phone per day.

| Time per Day | Frequency | Percentage (%) |
|---|---|---|
| 1 to 8 times | 119 | 25.8 |
| 9 to 16 times | 113 | 24.5 |
| 17 to 30 times | 137 | 29.7 |
| 31 or more times | 92 | 20.0 |
| Total | 461 | 100 |

We can note that 7.6% of students responded to the survey stating that they checked their smartphones every 5 min; 33.2% checked every 10–20 min; 38.2% checked every 30–60 min; and 21% checked every 2 h or less. Table 6 shows these results.

Table 6. How often do you think you usually check your smartphone or cell phone?.

| Frequency | Frequency | Percentage (%) |
|---|---|---|
| Every 5 min | 35 | 7.6 |
| Every 10 min | 76 | 16.5 |
| Every 20 min | 77 | 16.7 |
| Every 30 min | 93 | 20.2 |
| Every hour | 83 | 18.0 |
| Every 2 h | 37 | 8.0 |
| Every 3 h or less | 60 | 13.0 |
| Total | 461 | 100 |

3.2. Correlation Analysis

In the item correlation matrix of block 2, we observed variables that correlate moderately, with the rest of the variables exhibiting low correlations. However, the determinant value of the correlation matrix is close to 0, which indicates that the matrix variables are linearly related, which, in turn, supports the continuity of the analysis in the main components. See Table 7 for these results.

**Table 7.** Correlation matrix for the 16 items in the questionnaire.

| Items | Q-1 | Q-2 | Q-3 | Q-4 | Q-5 | Q-6 | Q-7 | Q-8 | Q-9 | Q-10 | Q-11 | Q-12 | Q-13 | Q-14 | Q-15 | Q-16 |
|---|---|---|---|---|---|---|---|---|---|---|---|---|---|---|---|---|
| Q-1  | 1.000 | 0.600 | 0.482 | 0.408 | 0.271 | 0.273 | 0.190 | 0.292 | 0.229 | 0.276 | 0.213 | 0.234 | 0.244 | 0.268 | 0.261 | 0.367 |
| Q-2  | 0.600 | 1.000 | 0.507 | 0.457 | 0.313 | 0.258 | 0.236 | 0.402 | 0.406 | 0.400 | 0.247 | 0.252 | 0.302 | 0.343 | 0.435 | 0.480 |
| Q-3  | 0.482 | 0.507 | 1.000 | 0.450 | 0.336 | 0.239 | 0.196 | 0.365 | 0.450 | 0.404 | 0.206 | 0.162 | 0.179 | 0.307 | 0.419 | 0.406 |
| Q-4  | 0.408 | 0.457 | 0.450 | 1.000 | 0.374 | 0.390 | 0.261 | 0.306 | 0.273 | 0.369 | 0.281 | 0.356 | 0.356 | 0.316 | 0.313 | 0.445 |
| Q-5  | 0.271 | 0.313 | 0.336 | 0.374 | 1.000 | 0.475 | 0.350 | 0.351 | 0.286 | 0.427 | 0.320 | 0.324 | 0.334 | 0.378 | 0.335 | 0.345 |
| Q-6  | 0.273 | 0.258 | 0.239 | 0.390 | 0.475 | 1.000 | 0.316 | 0.292 | 0.181 | 0.334 | 0.302 | 0.366 | 0.320 | 0.275 | 0.219 | 0.283 |
| Q-7  | 0.190 | 0.236 | 0.196 | 0.261 | 0.350 | 0.316 | 1.000 | 0.332 | 0.241 | 0.255 | 0.193 | 0.277 | 0.288 | 0.328 | 0.274 | 0.313 |
| Q-8  | 0.292 | 0.402 | 0.365 | 0.306 | 0.351 | 0.292 | 0.332 | 1.000 | 0.396 | 0.457 | 0.211 | 0.262 | 0.254 | 0.452 | 0.437 | 0.415 |
| Q-9  | 0.229 | 0.406 | 0.450 | 0.273 | 0.286 | 0.181 | 0.241 | 0.396 | 1.000 | 0.533 | 0.211 | 0.169 | 0.262 | 0.417 | 0.606 | 0.506 |
| Q-10 | 0.276 | 0.400 | 0.404 | 0.369 | 0.427 | 0.334 | 0.255 | 0.457 | 0.533 | 1.000 | 0.198 | 0.341 | 0.295 | 0.472 | 0.495 | 0.479 |
| Q-11 | 0.213 | 0.247 | 0.206 | 0.281 | 0.320 | 0.302 | 0.193 | 0.211 | 0.211 | 0.198 | 1.000 | 0.269 | 0.394 | 0.172 | 252   | 263   |
| Q-12 | 0.234 | 0.252 | 0.162 | 0.356 | 0.324 | 0.366 | 0.277 | 0.262 | 0.169 | 0.341 | 0.269 | 1.000 | 0.426 | 0.371 | 0.234 | 0.369 |
| Q-13 | 0.244 | 0.302 | 0.179 | 0.356 | 0.334 | 0.320 | 0.288 | 0.254 | 0.262 | 0.295 | 0.394 | 0.426 | 1.000 | 0.314 | 0.313 | 0.321 |
| Q-14 | 0.268 | 0.343 | 0.307 | 0.316 | 0.378 | 0.275 | 0.328 | 0.452 | 0.417 | 0.472 | 0.172 | 0.371 | 0.314 | 1.000 | 0.469 | 0.529 |
| Q-15 | 0.261 | 0.435 | 0.419 | 0.313 | 0.335 | 0.219 | 0.274 | 0.437 | 0.606 | 0.495 | 0.252 | 0.234 | 0.313 | 0.469 | 1.000 | 0.601 |
| Q-16 | 0.367 | 0.480 | 0.406 | 0.445 | 0.345 | 0.283 | 0.313 | 0.415 | 0.506 | 0.479 | 0.263 | 0.369 | 0.321 | 0.529 | 0.601 | 1.000 |

## 3.3. Kaiser–Meyer–Olkin (KMO) Measurement

This indicates the percentage of variance that the analyzed variables have in common; 0.6 and above is considered a good sample adaptation for a factor analysis [37,38]:

$$KMO = \frac{\sum_{i \neq j} r_{ij}^2}{\sum_{i \neq j} r_{ij}^2 + \sum_{i \neq j} r_{ij,m}^2}, \tag{3}$$

where:
$r_{ij}$: Represents the simple correlation coefficient between the variables $i$ and $j$.
$r_{ij,m}$: Represents the partial correlation coefficient between the variables $i$ and $j$, eliminating the effect of the remaining m variables.

In Table 8, we see that the Kaiser–Meyer–Olkin (KMO) that was obtained, take the value = 0.913 > 0.6; hence, it indicates that the data reduction process is good.

Table 8. Kaiser–Meyer–Olkin and Bartlett Test.

| Kaiser–Meyer–Olkin sampling adequacy measurement | | 0.913 |
|---|---|---|
| Barlett's sphericity test | Approx. Chi squared | 2748.056 |
| | df | 120 |
| | Sig. | 0.000 |

## 3.4. Bartlett's Sphericity Test

The Bartlett sphericity test result that contrasts its null hypothesis that the correlation matrix is an identity matrix (there is no correlation between the variables) has been obtained as shown in Table 8 ($p$-value = 0.000 < 0.05); hence, the Bartlett null hypothesis is rejected. Thus, the results of these tests indicate that the factor analysis can be considered to be appropriate [39–41].

## 3.5. Factor Analysis

In Table 9, which shows explained variance; three factors explain 55.166% of the variance. These factors are extracted via the analysis of main components, and the criteria that support its application are the Kaiser–Meyer–Olkin measurement test result, which takes a value of 0.913, and the Bartlett sphericity test, in which the $p$-value < 0.05; hence, it makes sense to perform the factor analysis.

Table 9. Total explained variance. Extraction method: Principal component analysis.

| Component | Initial Eigenvalues | | | Extraction Sums of Squared Loadings | | | Rotation Sums of Squared Loadings | | |
|---|---|---|---|---|---|---|---|---|---|
| | Total | % Variance | % Gathered | Total | % Variance | % Gathered | Total | % Variance | % Gathered |
| 1 | 6.187 | 38.668 | 38.668 | 6.187 | 38.668 | 38.668 | 3.517 | 21.984 | 21.984 |
| 2 | 1.453 | 9.084 | 47.752 | 1.453 | 9.085 | 47.752 | 2.917 | 18.231 | 40.214 |
| 3 | 1.186 | 7.414 | 55.166 | 1.186 | 7.414 | 55.166 | 2.392 | 14.952 | 55.166 |

With regard to the component matrix, to be able to perform the interpretation of the factors, we used Table 10 on the rotated component matrix by rotating varimax [39–41] to discover hidden relationships within the components and the respective indicators, which facilitates the interpretability of the factors. The table highlights values above 0.45 to achieve better exposure of the initial variables obtained for each component or factor.

**Table 10.** Rotated component matrix and its associated indicators.

| Item | | Component | | |
|---|---|---|---|---|
| | | 1 | 2 | 3 |
| Q9 | I get angry or irritated when someone bothers me while I'm using my smartphone. | **0.784** | 0.039 | 0.186 |
| Q15 | I feel nervous if I do not receive messages, calls, and notifications from social networks on my smartphone. | **0.783** | 0.146 | 0.201 |
| Q10 | If my smartphone is with me, I can't stop using it. | **0.678** | 0.264 | 0.206 |
| Q16 | If I didn't have my smartphone with me, I would feel bad because I wouldn't be able to check social networks. | **0.666** | 0.271 | 0.302 |
| Q14 | Right now, I would grab my smartphone and send a message, make a call, or check social networks. | **0.658** | 0.339 | 0.074 |
| Q8 | I need to use my smartphone more often. | **0.585** | 0.243 | 0.212 |
| Q12 | As soon as I wake up in the morning, the first thing I do is see who called me or whether someone has sent me a message. | 0.198 | **0.689** | 0.057 |
| Q6 | I go to bed later or have slept less to use my smartphone. | 0.090 | **0.684** | 0.215 |
| Q13 | When I feel lonely, I use my smartphone to make calls, send messages, etc. | 0.191 | **0.667** | 0.100 |
| Q5 | I spend more time than I should talking on my smartphone, sending messages, and using other apps. | 0.295 | **0.581** | 0.197 |
| Q11 | Ever since I have had smartphone, I have increased sent messages. | 0.059 | **0.560** | 0.207 |
| Q7 | I use my smartphone (for calls, reading, or sending messages and using WhatsApp, among other things), in situations that may not be dangerous but are not appropriate for smartphone use (such as while others are talking to me, etc.). | 0.326 | **0.495** | 0.007 |
| Q1 | If my smartphone wasn't working for a long time and it would take a long time to fix it, I would feel very bad | 0.104 | 0.219 | **0.809** |
| Q2 | If I don't have my smartphone, I feel bad. | 0.373 | 0.176 | **0.731** |
| Q3 | I don't think I could handle a week without my smartphone. | 0.393 | 0.049 | **0.692** |
| Q4 | If I couldn't check my smartphone for a while, I would want to check it. | 0.166 | 0.461 | **0.570** |

Extraction method: analysis of main components. Rotation method: Varimax with Kaiser standardization.
a: The rotation converged in six iterations.

The matrix shows three components, where each component has 16 items, and on the basis of Table 10, we can interpret each of them:

**Component 1:** This component includes the set of attributes of the nomophobia questionnaire that describe the students' sense of need to be with their smartphones. This component will consist of the following items: Q9, Q15, Q10, Q16, Q14 and Q8. They will be the factor that we call the "Anxiety Sensation" factor, which explains 38.668% of the total variability. The sense of anxiety of UNI students is related to the unfounded need for smartphones. This factor is basically caused by "not being able to communicate"; it refers to the feelings of losing instant communication with people and not being able to use the services that allow instant communication.

**Component 2:** This component contains six variables that are considered to be within those that do not find alternative resources to entertain themselves. This component will consist of the following items: Q12, Q6, Q13, Q5, Q11 and Q7. They will be the factor that we call "Compulsive Smartphone Use" factor, which explains 9.084% of the total variability, and which is reflected in the students compulsive need to interact with their smartphones. This factor is basically caused by "abuse and interference with other activities"; it refers to the excessive use of mobile devices even in situations where such use is dangerous or inconvenient.

**Component 3:** This includes the characteristics of low emotion. This component will consist of the following items: Q1, Q2, Q3 and Q4. They will be the factor that we call "Anxiety and Panic Sensation" factor, which explains 7.414% of the total variability. This factor reflects the mood of UNI students if they feel that they have been away from their smartphones for a long period of time. It is basically caused by "abstinence"; it refers to the withdrawal symptoms that appear if an addicted person cannot use the mobile.

The symptomatic nomophobia factors obtained in our research with engineering, sciences, and architecture students in Peru are very similar to those obtained in other studies cited by literature nomophobia with other students. For example, we mentioned some studies:

First, in [28], they found the following factors: problematic internet use, social appearance anxiety, and social media use. Second, in [16], they found the following factors: giving up convenience, fear due to running out of battery, nervousness due to disconnection from online identity, being uncomfortable when unable to stay up-to-date with social media, and anxious when unable to check e-mails. Third, in [23], they found the following factors: losing connectedness and giving up convenience. Then, in [14], they found the following factors: not being able to communicate, losing connectedness, not being able to access information, and giving up convenience. After that, in [42], they found the following factors: anxiety and depression. Finally, in [30], they found the following factors: abstinence, abuse and interference with other activities, tolerance, and lack of control.

This indicates that characteristic personality problems are common, regardless of the studies that are carried out and the region of the world where it occurs, because they are characteristic of human addiction. In university students of engineering, sciences, and architecture, the use of new technologies favors the academic training, the smartphone being one of them. The smartphone can be used as a self-learning tool; its benefits lead to excessive use resulting in nomophobia. This is a cause of concern for university teachers around the world.

In addition to the research cited in the literature, we find that none of them uses the focus group technique. This tool facilitated the ability for all the test questions evaluated to be answered completely by the students.

In Figure 2, we show in greater detail the structural model and testing results.

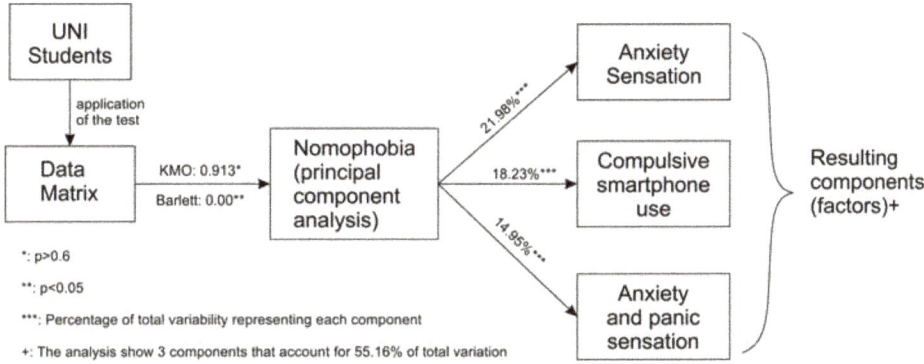

**Figure 2.** Structural model and results of applied analysis.

## 4. Conclusions

As a result of the process performed, following a research methodology adopted and validating the study, we obtain the following conclusions.

From the factor analysis, we concluded that there are three symptomatic factors of nomophobia in students at the National University of Engineering that describe the sensation that students experience when they feel the need to be with their smartphones and these are: sensation of anxiety, compulsive smartphone use, and sensation of anxiety and panic. These conclusions support our proposition that there is indeed enough evidence to state that there are symptomatic factors presented by UNI students due to indiscriminate use of smartphones. Based on the factors obtained in our study, we recommend implementing a program of prevention of levels of nomophobia that should be carried out by a medical center with specialists in the subject.

The use of a focus group allowed improving the quality of the data collected for research, and it was an innovative strategy to detect qualitative findings which improved the queries described in our questionnaire.

As future work, we hope to conduct research that links the influence of the symptoms of nomophobia factors, and the academic evaluation of students of the other universities, where the results obtained in our work would serve as a baseline for these research. Finally, we wish to expand the research to other social interest groups that will be necessary to have an instrument for the identification of symptomatic factors of nomophobia.

**Author Contributions:** J.A.R.-H. and J.L.C.-S. developed the ideas about the test adaptation, C.R.M.-A. designed the methodology, R.R.G.-L. implemented the questionnaire and validated the results obtained, E.E.A.-V. built the database and processed them. All of the authors were involved in preparing the manuscript.

**Funding:** The study was funded by the Vice-Rector for Research of the National University of Engineering.

**Conflicts of Interest:** The authors declare no conflict of interest.

## Abbreviations

The following abbreviations are used in this manuscript:

MDPI   Multidisciplinary Digital Publishing Institute
DOAJ   Directory of open access journals
TLA    Three letter acronym
LD     linear dichroism

## References

1. Oulasvirta, A.; Rattenbury, T.; Ma, L.; Raita, E. Habits make smartphone use more pervasive. *Pers. Ubiquitous Comput.* **2012**, *16*, 105–114. [CrossRef]
2. Calvete, E.; Londres, U. Adaptación al español del cuestionario Nomophobia Questionnaire (NMP-Q) en una muestra de adolescentes. *Actas Esp Psiquiatr* **2017**, *45*, 137–144.
3. Pavithra, M.; Madhukumar, S.; Mahadeva, M. A study on nomophobia-mobile phone dependence, among students of a medical college in Bangalore. *Natl. J. Community Med.* **2015**, *6*, 340–344.
4. Osiptel. Suscripciones de Internet Movil. Available online: https://www.osiptel.gob.pe/repositorioaps/data/1/1/1/par/62-suscripciones-de-internet-movil-segun-modalid/IntMovil_C6.2_Terminal.pdf (accessed on 24 December 2018).
5. Argumosa-Villar, L.; Boada-Grau, J.; Vigil-Colet, A. Exploratory investigation of theoretical predictors of nomophobia using the Mobile Phone Involvement Questionnaire (MPIQ). *J. Adolesc.* **2017**, *56*, 127–135. [CrossRef]
6. Dongre, A.S.; Inamdar, I.F.; Gattani, P.L. Nomophobia: A Study to Evaluate Mobile Phone Dependence and Impact of Cell Phone on Health. *Natl. J. Community Med.* **2017**, *8*, 688–693.
7. Akun, A.; Andreani, W. Powerfully tecnologized, powerlessly connected: The psychosemiotics of nomophobia. In Proceedings of the 2017 10th International Conference on Human System Interactions (HSI), Ulsan, Korea, 17–19 July 2017; pp. 306–310.
8. Walsh, S.P.; White, K.M.; Young, R.M. Needing to connect: The effect of self and others on young people's involvement with their mobile phones. *Aust. J. Psychol.* **2010**, *62*, 194–203. [CrossRef]
9. King, A.L.S.; Valença, A.M.; Nardi, A.E. Nomophobia: The mobile phone in panic disorder with agoraphobia: Reducing phobias or worsening of dependence? *Cognit. Behav. Neurol.* **2010**, *23*, 52–54. [CrossRef]
10. Krajewska-Kulak, E.; Kulak, W.; Stryzhak, A.; Szpakow, A.; Prokopowicz, W.; Marcinkowski, J. Problematic mobile phone using among the Polish and Belarusian University students, a comparative study. *Prog. Health Sci.* **2012**, *2*, 45–51.
11. King, A.L.S.; Valença, A.M.; Silva, A.C.; Sancassiani, F.; Machado, S.; Nardi, A.E. "Nomophobia": Impact of cell phone use interfering with symptoms and emotions of individuals with panic disorder compared with a control group. *Clin. Pract. Epidemiol. Ment. Health* **2014**, *10*, 28. [CrossRef]

12. Castilla Toribio, M.Y.; Páez Viciana, A. *Adicciones Sin Sustancias: Los JÓvenes Y EL MÓVIL*; Central Board of Secondary Education: Delhi, India, 2017.
13. Billieux, J.; Maurage, P.; Lopez-Fernandez, O.; Kuss, D.J.; Griffiths, M.D. Can disordered mobile phone use be considered a behavioral addiction? An update on current evidence and a comprehensive model for future research. *Curr. Addict. Rep.* **2015**, *2*, 156–162. [CrossRef]
14. Yildirim, C.; Correia, A.P. Exploring the dimensions of nomophobia: Development and validation of a self-reported questionnaire. *Comput. Hum. Behav.* **2015**, *49*, 130–137. [CrossRef]
15. Arpaci, I. Culture and nomophobia: The role of vertical versus horizontal collectivism in predicting nomophobia. *Inf. Dev.* **2019**, *35*, 96–106. [CrossRef]
16. Dasgupta, P.; Bhattacherjee, S.; Dasgupta, S.; Roy, J.K.; Mukherjee, A.; Biswas, R. Author's reply for article "nomophobic behaviors among smartphone using medical and engineering students in two colleges of West Bengal". *Indian J. Public Health* **2018**, *62*, 70.
17. Aguilera-Manrique, G.; Márquez-Hernández, V.V.; Alcaraz-Córdoba, T.; Granados-Gámez, G.; Gutiérrez-Puertas, V.; Gutiérrez-Puertas, L. The relationship between nomophobia and the distraction associated with smartphone use among nursing students in their clinical practicum. *PLoS ONE* **2018**, *13*, e0202953. [CrossRef]
18. Froese, A.D.; Carpenter, C.N.; Inman, D.A.; Schooley, J.R.; Barnes, R.B.; Brecht, P.W.; Chacon, J.D. Effects of classroom cell phone use on expected and actual learning. *Coll. Stud. J.* **2012**, *46*, 323–332.
19. End, C.M.; Worthman, S.; Mathews, M.B.; Wetterau, K. Costly cell phones: The impact of cell phone rings on academic performance. *Teach. Psychol.* **2009**, *37*, 55–57. [CrossRef]
20. Shelton, J.T.; Elliott, E.M.; Eaves, S.D.; Exner, A.L. The distracting effects of a ringing cell phone: An investigation of the laboratory and the classroom setting. *J. Environ. Psychol.* **2009**, *29*, 513–521. [CrossRef] [PubMed]
21. Prasad, M.; Patthi, B.; Singla, A.; Gupta, R.; Saha, S.; Kumar, J.K.; Malhi, R.; Pandita, V. Nomophobia: A cross-sectional study to assess mobile phone usage among dental students. *J. Clin. Diagn. Res.* **2017**, *11*, ZC34. [CrossRef] [PubMed]
22. Arpaci, I.; Baloğlu, M.; Kozan, H.İ.Ö.; Kesici, Ş. Individual differences in the relationship between attachment and nomophobia among college students: The mediating role of mindfulness. *J. Med. Internet Res.* **2017**, *19*, e404. [CrossRef]
23. Mendoza, J.S.; Pody, B.C.; Lee, S.; Kim, M.; McDonough, I.M. The effect of cellphones on attention and learning: The influences of time, distraction, and nomophobia. *Comput. Hum. Behav.* **2018**, *86*, 52–60. [CrossRef]
24. Bychkov, D.; Young, S.D. Facing Up to Nomophobia: A Systematic Review of Mobile Phone Apps that Reduce Smartphone Usage. In *Big Data in Engineering Applications*; Springer: Berlin, Germany, 2018; pp. 161–171.
25. Lee, S.; Kim, M.; Mendoza, J.S.; McDonough, I.M. Addicted to cellphones: exploring the psychometric properties between the nomophobia questionnaire and obsessiveness in college students. *Heliyon* **2018**, *4*, e00895. [CrossRef]
26. Al-Balhan, E.M.; Khabbache, H.; Watfa, A.; Re, T.S.; Zerbetto, R.; Bragazzi, N.L. Psychometric evaluation of the arabic version of the nomophobia questionnaire: confirmatory and exploratory factor analysis—Implications from a pilot study in Kuwait among university students. *Psychol. Res. Behav. Manag.* **2018**, *11*, 471. [CrossRef]
27. Ahmed, S.; Pokhrel, N.; Roy, S.; Samuel, A.J. Impact of nomophobia: A nondrug addiction among students of physiotherapy course using an online cross-sectional survey. *Indian J. Psychiatry* **2019**, *61*, 77.
28. Ayar, D.; Gerçeker, G.Ö.; Özdemir, E.Z.; Bektas, M. The Effect of Problematic Internet Use, Social Appearance Anxiety, and Social Media Use on Nursing Students' Nomophobia Levels. *Comput. Inform. Nurs.* **2018**, *36*, 589–595. [CrossRef]
29. Gutiérrez-Puertas, L.; Márquez-Hernández, V.V.; São-Romão-Preto, L.; Granados-Gámez, G.; Gutiérrez-Puertas, V.; Aguilera-Manrique, G. Comparative study of nomophobia among Spanish and Portuguese nursing students. *Nurse Educ. Pract.* **2019**, *34*, 79–84. [CrossRef]
30. Chóliz, M.; Pinto, L.; Phansalkar, S.S.; Corr, E.; Mujjahid, A.; Flores, C.; Barrientos, P.E. Development of a Brief Multicultural Version of the Test of Mobile Phone Dependence Questionnaire. *Front. Psychol.* **2016**, *7*, 650. [CrossRef] [PubMed]

31. Vacaru, M.; Shepherd, R.; Sheridan, J. New Zealand youth and their relationships with mobile phone technology. *Int. J. Ment. Health Addict.* **2014**, *12*, 572–584. [CrossRef]
32. Balakrishnan, J.; Griffiths, M.D. An Exploratory Study of "Selfitis" and the Development of the Selfitis Behavior Scale. *Int. J. Ment. Health Addict.* **2018**, *16*, 722–736. [CrossRef] [PubMed]
33. Cronbach, L.J. Coefficient alpha and the internal structure of tests. *Psychometrika* **1951**, *16*, 297–334. [CrossRef]
34. Celina Oviedo, H.; Campo Arias, A. Aproximación al uso del coeficiente alfa de Cronbach. *Rev. Colomb. Psiquiatr.* **2005**, *34*, 572–580.
35. Malhotra, N.K. *Investigación de Mercados: Un Enfoque Aplicado*; Pearson Educación: London, UK, 2004.
36. Pértigas, S.; Pita, S. Determinación del tamaño de la muestra para calcular la significación del coeficiente de correlación lineal. In *Unidad de Epidemiología Clínica y Bioestadística*; INIBIC: La Coruña, Spain, 2002.
37. Cerny, B.A.; Kaiser, H.F. A study of a measure of sampling adequacy for factor-analytic correlation matrices. *Multivar. Behav. Res.* **1977**, *12*, 43–47. [CrossRef] [PubMed]
38. Kaiser, H.F. An index of factorial simplicity. *Psychometrika* **1974**, *39*, 31–36. [CrossRef]
39. Peña, D. *Análisis de Datos Multivariantes*; McGraw-Hill España: Madrid, Spain, 2013.
40. Chatfield, C. *Introduction to Multivariate Analysis*; Routledge: Abingdon, UK, 2018.
41. Tatsuoka, M.M.; Lohnes, P.R. *Multivariate Analysis: Techniques for Educational and Psychological Research*; Macmillan Publishing Co., Inc.: London, UK, 1988.
42. Estévez, A.; Urbiola, I.; Iruarrizaga, I.; Onaindia, J.; Jauregui, P. Dependencia emocional y consecuencias psicológicas del abuso de internet y móvil en jóvenes. *Ann. Psychol.* **2017**, *33*, 260–268. [CrossRef]

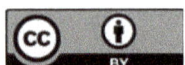

© 2019 by the authors. Licensee MDPI, Basel, Switzerland. This article is an open access article distributed under the terms and conditions of the Creative Commons Attribution (CC BY) license (http://creativecommons.org/licenses/by/4.0/).

*Article*

# Estimating Airway Resistance from Forced Expiration in Spirometry

**Nilakash Das [1], Kenneth Verstraete [1], Marko Topalovic [1], Jean-Marie Aerts [2] and Wim Janssens [1,\*]**

1 Laboratory for Respiratory Diseases, Department of Chronic Diseases, Metabolism and Ageing (CHROMETA), KU Leuven, 3000 Leuven, Belgium
2 Measure, Model & Manage Bioresponses (M3-BIORES), Division Animal and Human Health Engineering, Department of Biosystems, KU Leuven, 3000 Leuven, Belgium
\* Correspondence: wim.janssens@uzleuven.be

Received: 6 June 2019; Accepted: 11 July 2019; Published: 16 July 2019

**Featured Application:** Authors are encouraged to provide a concise description of the specific application or a potential application of the work. This section is not mandatory.

**Abstract:** Spirometry is the gold standard to detect airflow limitation, but it does not measure airway resistance, which is one of the physiological factors behind airflow limitation. In this study, we describe the dynamics of forced expiration in spirometry using a deflating balloon and using this model. We propose a methodology to estimate $\zeta$ (zeta), a dimensionless and effort-independent parameter quantifying airway resistance. In N = 462 (65 ± 8 years), we showed that $\zeta$ is significantly ($p < 0.0001$) greater in COPD (2.59 ± 0.99) than healthy smokers (1.64 ± 0.18), it increased significantly ($p < 0.0001$) with the severity of airflow limitation and it correlated significantly ($p < 0.0001$) with airway resistance (r = 0.55) and specific conductance (r = −0.60) obtained from body-plethysmography. $\zeta$ also showed significant associations ($p < 0.001$) with diffusion capacity (r = −0.64), air-trapping (r = 0.68), and CT densitometry of emphysema (r = 0.40 against % below −950 HU and r = −0.34 against 15th percentile HU). Moreover, simulation studies demonstrated that an increase in $\zeta$ resulted in lower airflows from baseline. Therefore, we conclude that $\zeta$ quantifies airway resistance from forced expiration in spirometry—a method that is more abundantly available in primary care than traditional but expensive methods of measuring airway resistance such as body-plethysmography and forced oscillation technique.

**Keywords:** spirometry; airflow limitation; airway resistance; specific airway conductance; COPD; body-plethysmography; forced expiration; alveolar pressure; emphysema; computed tomography; air-trapping

## 1. Introduction

Airflow limitation or obstruction is the characteristic feature of obstructive lung diseases such as chronic obstructive pulmonary disease (COPD) and asthma. In COPD, it arises out of the dual effects of permanent parenchymal destruction (emphysema) and small airway dysfunction due to prolonged exposure of the lungs to cigarette smoke [1]. While in asthma, it arises due to narrowing of airways from excessive inflammation and mucus production as a result of bronchial hyper- responsiveness to allergens [2].

In clinical practice, spirometry is the gold standard to measure airflow limitation [3]. During a spirometry test, a subject performs a forced expiration using a spirometer that measures the flow and volume of exhaled air. Several indices of diagnostic importance, such as forced expiratory volume in 1 second (FEV1), forced vital capacity (FVC), and Tiffeneau's index (FEV1/FVC) are obtained from spirometry [4]. Two widely accepted criteria for the presence of airflow limitation are a FEV1/FVC ratio below a fixed cutoff of 0.7 [3] or below the lower limits of normal (LLN, defined as the 5th percentile of a normally distributed set of values of FEV1/FVC for a population of non-smoking, normal individuals) [5]. The plot of expiratory flow against volume measurements is termed as maximal expiratory flow-volume curve (MEFVC), and it is also known to be associated with different pathological states [6].

Although spirometry is used to indicate airflow limitation, the latter itself is an end-result of many factors. One of these factors is an increased airway resistance, and therefore, measuring it may directly provide additional insight into the occurrence of airflow limitation. Traditionally, body-plethysmography has been used to determine airway resistance (Raw) as a ratio of driving alveolar pressure to airflow. Other methods of measuring airway resistance include forced oscillation technique (FOT), which estimates respiratory system resistance ($R_{RS}$) and reactance ($X_{RS}$), and the interrupter technique which measures interrupter resistance ($R_{int}$) at a single moment of tidal breathing [7].

All of the above-mentioned techniques measure airway resistance during tidal breathing. Nevertheless, factors affecting airway resistance during a forced expiration such as loss of lung elasticity [8] and dynamic airway collapse cannot be underestimated [9], and often compose the main reason for airflow limitation and clinical symptoms [10]. Measures of airway resistance obtained during forced expiration will provide better insight into these mechanisms, which are potentially amendable for intervention. Currently, there exists no method in the literature to calculate dynamic airway resistance from the forced expiratory manoeuvre. The consensus is that spirometry cannot be used to estimate airway resistance since it does not measure alveolar pressure [7,11,12]. In the past, researchers have proposed parameters reflective of airway resistance [13] that only describes the shape of MEFVC, without any physiological basis.

In this study, we describe the dynamics of forced expiration using a model of a deflating balloon, and thereby propose a method to estimate a parameter representative of airway resistance from spirometry. We hypothesized that this resistance parameter would be significantly higher in COPD compared to healthy smokers, increase with the severity of airflow limitation in COPD patients [14] and show a significant correlation with Raw and its flow standardized inverse, specific airway conductance (sGaw). We investigated the relationship of this parameter with other pulmonary function tests (PFT) parameters such as diffusion capacity for carbon monoxide (DLCO) [15] and the ratio of residual volume (RV) to total lung capacity (TLC), an index that quantifies air-trapping in COPD subjects [16]. We also associated this parameter with computed tomography (CT)-based densitometric quantification of emphysema, a condition of severe airflow limitation in COPD when lung parenchyma is permanently destroyed [17]. Finally, we studied how changes in the resistance parameters affect the shape of the MEFVC.

## 2. Materials and Methods

### 2.1. Study Population

We used data of 462 COPD individuals and healthy smokers from the Leuven COPD cohort. All subjects were Caucasian with an age range between 50 and 90 years, and with a smoking history of at least 15 pack-years. Individuals with a suspicion or diagnosis of asthma, with exacerbations due to COPD within the last 6 weeks of enrolment or with a diagnosis of other respiratory diseases were excluded. These individuals performed complete PFT including post-bronchodilator spirometry, body-plethysmography, and diffusion capacity at the time of enrolment, while a CT scan was carried out within one year of enrolment. COPD was defined based on a post-bronchodilator ratio of FEV1/FVC < 70 % [3], while the severity airflow limitation was based on FEV1 expressed as a percentage of healthy reference value (FEV1 %pred) as described in the Global Initiative of Chronic

Obstructive Lung Diseases (GOLD) [14]. The study design of the Leuven COPD cohort can be found at www.clinicaltrials.gov (NCT00858520).

*2.2. Pulmonary Function Tests*

2.2.1. Spirometry

Subjects performed spirometry using a MasterScreen Pneumo spirometer (available from Vyaire Medical Inc., Illinois, USA). Post-bronchodilator spirometry manoeuvres, the ones with the highest sum of FEV1 and FVC among three acceptable and repeatable manoeuvres, were used for the study [4].

2.2.2. Whole-body Plethysmography

Whole-body plethysmography was carried out using MasterScreen Body (available from Vyaire Medical Inc., Illinois, USA). Airway resistance (Raw), defined as a ratio of the difference of alveolar pressure and mouth pressure (or total driving pressure) to flow rate, was determined by a surrogate ratio of specific resistance (sRaw, the slope of shift volume to flow rate) to functional residual capacity (FRC) under tidal breathing conditions. Specific conductance (sGaw) was determined as a ratio of inverse of Raw to FRC. Finally, lung volumes including residual volume (RV) and total lung capacity (TLC) were also measured, and their ratio was defined as an index for air-trapping [1].

2.2.3. Diffusion Capacity

Diffusing capacity (DLCO) was measured by the single-breath carbon monoxide gas transfer method and corrected for alveolar ventilation but not hemoglobin concentration [18].

*2.3. Computed Tomography Densiometry*

CT scans were obtained in a routine setting using different multi-detector row scanners with different acquisition parameters. Patients were examined in supine position and the scans were conducted at end-inspiration. The severity of emphysema was calculated using the percentage of total voxels with an X-ray attenuation value below -950 HU, and using the attenuation value of the 15th percentile along a histogram of voxels [17].

*2.4. Airway Resistance from Spirometry*

2.4.1. Deflating Balloon Model of Forced Expiration

During forced expiration, a person empties his lungs forcefully from total lung capacity (TLC) until a residual volume (RV) is reached [4]. As such, one can draw an analogy with an elastic balloon that deflates from a volume of TLC until RV (Figure 1) or from a volume of FVC until 0 (since FVC is the difference between TLC and RV), under the influence of a driving pressure. At a given time t, we denote the volume of the balloon as x, and the velocity of deflation as $\dot{x}$. If we ignore the effect of intra-thoracic gas compression [19], then the volume of air coming out of the balloon is FVC- x and the magnitude of airflow is $\dot{x}$, which we assume to be laminar. Furthermore, we considered a coordinate system such that all vectors in the direction of deflation are negative.

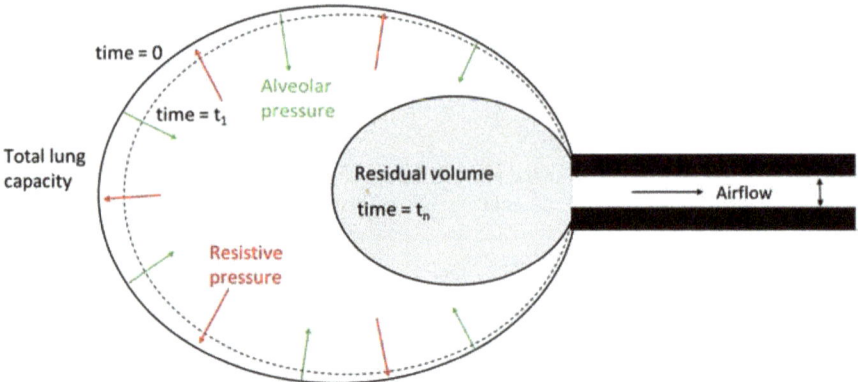

**Figure 1.** Model of a balloon that deflates from total lung capacity (or a volume of FVC) at time time (t) = 0 until residual volume (or a volume of 0) at t = $t_n$ with a peak airflow resulting at t = $t_1$. The deflation process is driven by alveolar pressure, which arises due to a combination of expiratory muscle effort and elastic recoil of the lungs; while it is opposed by a resistive pressure, which depends on the width of the outlet.

First, we write the equation of motion of the deflating balloon as:

$$I\ddot{x} = P_{alv} + P_{res} \qquad (1)$$

where $I\ddot{x}$ is the inertial pressure, $P_{alv}$ is the alveolar pressure, and $P_{res}$ is the resistive pressure. Equation (1) implies that the inertia of a deflating balloon is the result of $P_{alv}$, which is a driving pressure and $P_{res}$, which opposes deflation [9,20]. The initial conditions of Equation (1) at t = 0 are:

$$x(0) = FVC \text{ and } \dot{x}(0) = 0 \qquad (2)$$

and final conditions at t = $t_n$ (time at the end of forced expiration) are:

$$x(t_n) = 0 \text{ and } \dot{x}(t_n) = 0 \qquad (3)$$

At the beginning of the forced expiration, flow increases from zero to peak expiratory flow (PEF) within a very short interval $t_1$ (0 < $t_1$ << $t_n$). While the airflows in this phase are greatly influenced by expiratory muscle effort [21], the airflows during $t_1$ until $t_n$, generally after 50% of expired volume are known to be effort-independent [22]. To avoid effort-dependent biased estimates, we drop the former phase and consider only the later phase ($t_1 \leq t \leq t_n$) by modifying the initial conditions as:

$$x(t_1) = FVC - \Delta v \text{ and } \dot{x}(t_1) = -PEF \qquad (4)$$

where $\Delta v$ is the volume of air expired between 0 and $t_1$, and can be written in terms of measured airflow F(t) as:

$$\Delta = \int_0^{t_1} F(t) \, dt \qquad (5)$$

In Equation (1), the driving pressure $P_{alv}$ is a sum total of pleural pressure ($P_{pl}$), which arises purely out of expiratory muscle effort, and elastic recoil pressure ($P_{st}$), which is a restoring pressure generated by the inherent elasticity in the lungs [9]. According to the data produced by Agostani et al. [23], $P_{alv}$ decreases non-linearly with lung volume from a peak until zero during forced expiration. However, we make a simplifying assumption by representing $P_{alv}$ as a linear function of x with a coefficient k. Thus,

$$P_{alv} = -kx \tag{6}$$

The resistive pressure $P_{res}$ in Equation (1) is determined by the width of the outlet of the balloon (Figure 1a). $P_{res}$ decreases as the width of the outlet increases. We can represent it as a viscous damping pressure that dissipates the energy supplied to the system by $P_{alv}$, and denote it as a proportion of deflating velocity $\dot{x}$ with a damping coefficient c:

$$P_{res} = -c\dot{x}. \tag{7}$$

Putting Equations (6) and (7) in Equation (1) and rearranging the terms, we arrive at a familiar second-order linear differential equation describing free vibrations of a single-degree-of-freedom mass-spring-damper system:

$$\ddot{x} + 2\zeta\omega\dot{x} + \omega^2 x = 0. \tag{8}$$

here, $\zeta \left(= \frac{c}{2\sqrt{kI}}\right)$ is a dimensionless coefficient representative of resistance in the balloon while $\omega^2$ $\left(= \sqrt{\frac{k}{I}}\right)$ is a coefficient of driving pressure per unit inertance I. It is interesting to note that $\zeta$ turns out to be an effort-independent parameter unlike $\omega$. It quantifies the resistance of the small airways in the lungs. In the following section, we describe a method to estimate $\zeta$ and $\omega$.

2.4.2. Estimation of $\zeta$

Lung volumes decrease from TLC to RV during FE, unless noisy artifacts such as cough are present which we neglect in this study. So, we can consider the system in Equation (8) as an overdamped system, which implies $\zeta > 1$ [24]. In an overdamped system, the solution to Equation (8) is as follows:

$$x(t) = C_1 e^{s_1 (t - t_1)} + C_2 e^{s_2 (t - t_1)} \tag{9}$$

with

$$s_{1,2} = \left(-\zeta \pm \sqrt{\zeta^2 - 1}\right)\omega \tag{10}$$

There are four unknown terms, $C_1$, $C_2$, $\zeta$, and $\omega$ in solution 9, which can theoretically be determined using the two initial conditions (Equation (4)) and the two final conditions (Equation (3)). Applying the initial conditions (Equation (4)), we can rewrite $C_1$ and $C_2$ in terms of $\zeta$ and $\omega$ as follows (see Appendix A):

$$C_1 = \frac{\dot{x}(t_1) - s_2 x(t_1)}{s_3} \tag{11a}$$

$$C_2 = \frac{-\dot{x}(t_1) + s_1 x(t_1)}{s_3} \tag{11b}$$

with

$$s_3 = 2\omega\sqrt{\zeta^2 - 1} \tag{12}$$

We now use an optimization strategy to obtain the unknown parameters, $\zeta$ and $\omega$. There are two reasons for this step; the first is that final conditions (Equation (3)) could have anyway been solved numerically and the second, the estimate of the parameter $\zeta$ may not be robust if only a single data point at time $t_n$ is considered. Therefore, we consider the flow and volume of the entire manoeuver from $t_1$ until $t_n$ and express our cost function as follows:

$$J(\zeta, \omega) = \sum_{t=t_1}^{t_n} (V(t) - x(t))^2 + (F(t) - \dot{x}(t))^2 \tag{13}$$

where V(t) and F(t) are measured flow and volume of air during forced expiration. Then, we formulate the optimization as a minimization problem as follows:

$$\min_{\zeta,\omega} J(\zeta, \omega) \ s.t. \ \zeta > 1 \ and \ \omega > 0 \tag{14}$$

We can solve the above optimization problem for $\zeta$ and $\omega$ using any suitable method. In our study, we used differential evolution as implemented in Python by the original authors [25]. We defined a search space of [1,5] and (0, 5] for $\zeta$ and $\omega$, respectively. We wrote a Python script to automate the calculation of $\zeta$ and $\omega$ from flow-volume measurements of all subjects [26].

### 2.5. Statistical Analysis

We compared $\zeta$ between COPD and healthy smokers using a one-sided t-test. We studied $\zeta$ across different GOLD stages using one-way ANOVA followed by a post-hoc test using Tukey's honest significant difference test. We explored correlation of $\zeta$ against FEV1, FVC, FEV1/FVC, Raw, sGaw, DLCO, RV/TLC, and CT densitometry using Pearson's correlation coefficient. The significance level was set at 0.01 and all analyses were carried out in R Studio software [27]. Values were expressed as mean ± standard deviation (SD), unless specified otherwise. We used one-way ANOVA and logistic regression tests to assess group differences for continuous and categorical baseline variables.

## 3. Results

### 3.1. Baseline Characteristics

#### 3.1.1. Study Population

The baseline characteristics of the cohort are shown in Table 1. This cohort comprised of 63 GOLD I, 111 GOLD II, 92 GOLD III, 61 GOLD IV, and 135 healthy smokers. In this cohort, FEV1/FVC decreased with severity of airflow limitation from healthy (74 ± 4%) to GOLD I (64 ± 4%) until GOLD IV (30 ± 6%). In addition, Raw increased with severity of airflow limitation while other PFT parameters such as DLCO and air–trapping index (RV/TLC) also showed expected patterns. The extent of emphysema as quantified in CT by % below −950 HU and 15th percentile HU increased considerably with airflow limitation.

Table 1. Baseline characteristics of the Leuven COPD cohort with N = 462. Values are Mean (SD).

|  | Healthy | GOLD I | GOLD II | GOLD III | GOLD IV | p |
|---|---|---|---|---|---|---|
| N | 135 | 63 | 111 | 92 | 61 |  |
| Age (years) | 62 (6) | 63 (6) | 68 (8) | 69 (9) | 63 (7) | <0.001 |
| Sex (female %) | 21 | 24 | 23 | 20 | 26 | 0.9 |
| Smoking (pack-years) | 42 (21) | 50 (28) | 49 (23) | 49 (24) | 52 (25) | 0.06 |
| FEV1 (%pred) | 97 (13) | 93 (10) | 65 (9) | 40 (5) | 23 (5) | <0.001 |
| FVC (%pred) | 103 (14) | 115 (15) | 95 (16) | 82 (15) | 62 (14) | <0.001 |
| FEV1/FVC (%) | 74 (4) | 64 (4) | 55 (9) | 39 (8) | 30 (6) | <0.001 |
| Raw (kPa/L/s) | 0.32 (0.10) | 0.35 (0.12) | 0.44 (0.12) | 0.60 (0.16) | 0.82 (0.29) | <0.001 |
| sGaw (1/(kPa s)) | 0.9 (0.2) | 0.75 (0.21) | 0.55 (0.18) | 0.34 (0.11) | 0.22 (0.07) | 0.01 |
| RV/TLC (%) | 37 (6) | 38 (6) | 47 (7) | 57 (8) | 68 (8) | <0.001 |
| DLCO (mmol/min/kPa) | 7.7 (1.8) | 7.1 (2.2) | 5.5 (2.0) | 4.2 (1.4) | 2.9 (1) | <0.001 |
| 15th percentile (HU) | −935 (41) | −938 (34) | −943 (49) | −953 (39) | −968 (44) | <0.001 |
| % below -950 HU | 10 (12) | 11 (11) | 15 (16) | 19 (16) | 26 (17) | <0.001 |

### 3.1.2. Model Fit

The fit of the deflating balloon model was very good as evident by a low mean squared error (MSE) for both volume (0.01 ± 0.01) ($R^2$ = 0.99 ± 0.01)) and flow (0.02 ± 0.02) ($R^2$ = 0.98 ± 0.03). Figure 2 shows the fit of model flow-volume against actual measurements for a healthy and a COPD subject.

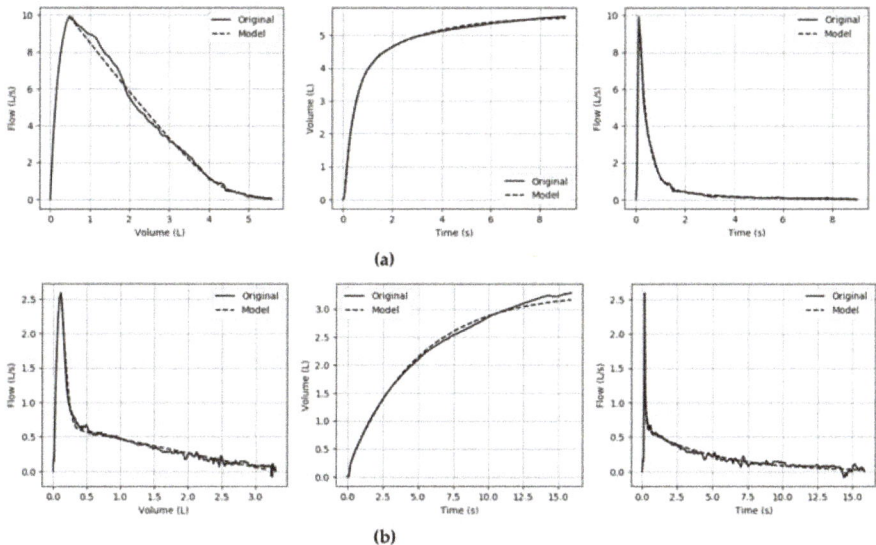

**Figure 2.** The fits of model flow-volume against original measurements in (**a**) a healthy individual with $\zeta$ = 1.52 ($R^2$ volume = 0.99 and $R^2$ flow = 0.99), and in (**b**) GOLD IV COPD with $\zeta$ = 4.93 ($R^2$ volume = 0.99 and $R^2$ flow = 0.98).

### 3.1.3. Model Parameters

While $\omega$ did not exhibit any discernible pattern, $\zeta$ confirmed our hypothesis. It was significantly greater ($p < 0.0001$) in COPD (2.59 ± 0.99) than healthy smokers (1.64 ± 0.18). Further, it increased with severity of airflow limitation (Table 2) from healthy until GOLD IV (3.96 ± 0.99) ($p < 0.0001$) with post-hoc tests confirming significant differences between each stage of airflow limitation. Further, $\zeta$ and $\omega$ were very weakly correlated among themselves ($r = 0.17, p < 0.01$).

**Table 2.** Mean (SD) of $\zeta$ and $\omega$ in different stages of airflow limitation. While $\zeta$ increases significantly ($p < 0.0001$) with severity of airflow limitation, $\omega$ does not show any discernible pattern.

|  | Healthy | GOLD I | GOLD II | GOLD III | GOLD IV | p |
|---|---|---|---|---|---|---|
| $\zeta$ | 1.64 (0.18) | 1.78 (0.23) | 2.10 (0.36) | 2.83 (0.77) | 3.96 (0.99) | <0.0001 |
| $\omega$ (rad/s)$^{0.5}$ | 1.58 (0.53) | 1.42 (0.61) | 1.43 (0.53) | 1.46 (0.49) | 1.75 (0.53) | <0.01 |

## 3.2. Association Studies of $\zeta$

### 3.2.1. Spirometry

Overall, $\zeta$ was strongly and negatively correlated ($r = -0.83, p < 0.0001$) with the FEV1/FVC, the primary index of airflow limitation (Table 2). It was also negatively correlated with FEV1 ($r = -0.72$, $p < 0.0001$) and with FVC ($r = -0.48, p < 0.0001$).

3.2.2. Raw and sGaw

$\zeta$ and Raw were positively correlated (r = 0.55, $p < 0.0001$), and both increased with severity of airflow limitation, thus confirming our hypothesis. Furthermore, it was negatively correlated with sGaw (r = −0.60, $p < 0.0001$), which was indeed a very logical observation as sGaw is inversely proportional to Raw. The trends of $\zeta$, Raw, and sGaw against severity of airflow limitation can be seen in Figure 3.

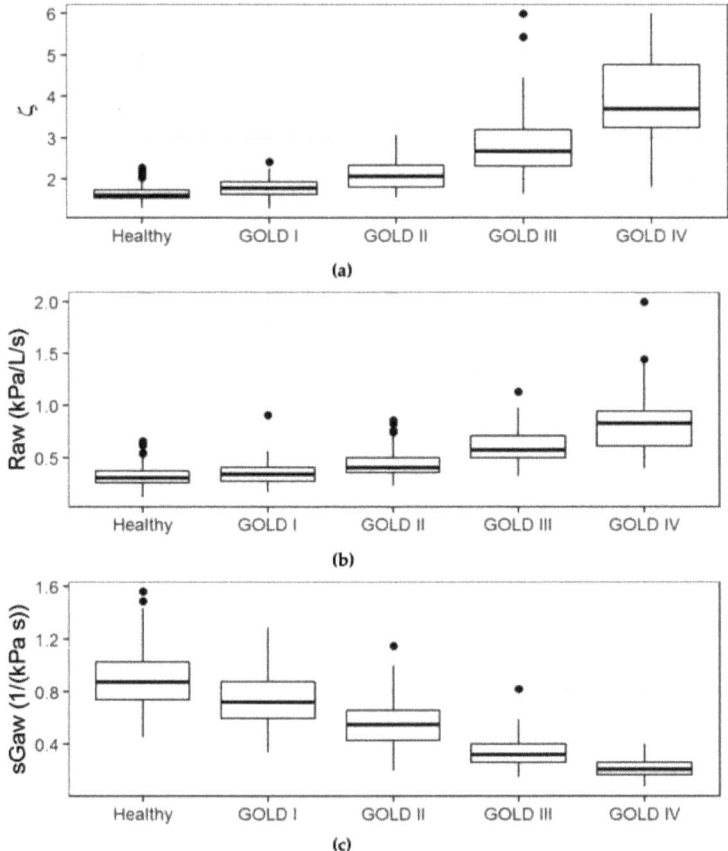

**Figure 3.** Boxplots (with median and inter-quartile range) of airway resistance parameters, $\zeta$ and Raw are positively correlated (r = 0.55, $p < 0.0001$) and they show an increasing trend with severity of airflow limitation in (**a**) and (**b**), respectively. Since sGaw is inversely proportional to Raw, it shows opposite trend in (**c**) with severity of airflow limitation.

3.2.3. DLCO and RV/TLC

As expected, $\zeta$ was negatively correlated with DLCO (r = −0.64, $p < 0.0001$) and positively correlated with RV/TLC (r = 0.68, $p < 0.0001$). We also observed that $\zeta$ was more strongly correlated with DLCO than known parameters quantifying airway resistance such Raw (r = −0.52, $p < 0.001$) and sGaw (r = 0.45, $p < 0.0001$). The correlations of Raw (r = −0.71, $p < 0.0001$) and sGaw (r = −0.77, $p < 0.0001$) with RV/TLC were higher than $\zeta$, which was expected as all these indexes were obtained from body-plethysmography.

### 3.2.4. CT Densitometry

We considered a cohort of COPD subjects only (N = 327), since emphysema is considered a trait of COPD only. We observed that $\zeta$ was significantly correlated with 15th percentile HU (r = −0.34, $p < 0.0001$) and with % below -950 HU (r = 0.40, $p < 0.0001$), although the magnitude of correlations was weak. Interestingly, the known parameters of airway resistance, Raw and sGaw, did not correlate with any of the densitometry indices ($p > 0.05$).

### 3.3. $\zeta$ simulation Studies

We studied how the shape of MEFVC changes when $\zeta$ changes from a baseline value. For a given manoeuver, we simulated MEFVCs by changing the baseline $\zeta$ by 20% while keeping $\omega$ as constant. Figure 4a,b shows the simulation of model flow and volume in the case of a healthy and a COPD individual for the baseline models shown in Figure 2a,b, respectively. As expected, an increase in $\zeta$ resulted in decreased airflows with a lower simulated FEV1 and FVC, while a decrease in $\zeta$ led to increased airflows with a higher simulated FEV1 and a slightly elevated FVC. The slight increase in FVC is seen as the model slightly underestimates the observed FVC. Furthermore, we also observed an increase in the concavity of the MEFVC as $\zeta$ increased in both the simulation studies.

## 4. Discussion

In this study, we described the dynamics of forced expiration in spirometry by using a model of a deflating balloon. With this model, we proposed a methodology to estimate a parameter $\zeta$ representative of airway resistance in the lungs. We proved our hypothesis by demonstrating that $\zeta$ was significantly ($p < 0.0001$) greater in COPD than in healthy smokers. It increased significantly with the severity of airflow limitation in COPD and it significantly correlated with Raw and sGaw, which are known indices of airway resistance. $\zeta$ also showed significant correlations with DLCO and air-trapping (RV/TLC), and with CT densitometric indices of emphysema in COPD patients. Moreover, simulation studies showed that an increase in $\zeta$ resulted in decreased airflows, and therefore a reduced FEV1 and FVC, which further validates our claim that $\zeta$ quantifies airway resistance.

The parameter $\zeta$ is not dependent on expiratory effort, but rather, it stems from the narrowing of the small airways (<2 mm diameter). Narrower airways result in increased airway resistance that is reflected by an elevated $\zeta$. In COPD, narrowing of the small airways during forced expiration is a result of a multitude of factors such as loss of elasticity in lung parenchyma leading to dynamic.

Airway collapse [9]; and airway abnormalities such as cellular inflammation [28], smooth muscle contraction [29], mucosal thickening [30], and fibrotic retraction [31]. Finally, a higher value of $\zeta$ also indicates the severity of airflow limitation, which itself is a functional consequence of a complex interaction between airway abnormalities and destruction of parenchyma elasticity.

Our method is the first to estimate airway resistance from forced expiration in spirometry. The use of a second-order linear differential equation in our method further validates the existence of second-order transfer functions to describe the dynamics of forced expiration [32]. Nevertheless, the application of second-order differential equations to describe respiratory mechanics is not a new concept [33]. In fact, the estimation of airway resistance during mechanical ventilation [34], body-plethysmography, and the interrupter technique is made possible by a simplification of these equations under tidal breathing conditions [7]. However, our method has an important distinction in that it does not require a measurement of alveolar pressure. Since spirometry does not measure alveolar pressure, we make a reasonable assumption on the variation of the latter (Equation (6)) that nonetheless, provides a good estimate of airway resistance. We believe that this is an important development in the field of respiratory mechanics because until now, the consensus has been that measuring alveolar pressure is indispensable for the calculation of airway resistance [7,35,36].

The clinical usefulness of $\zeta$ can be illustrated by the fact that it quantifies an important physiological phenomenon using spirometry alone, which is a simple but widely used pulmonary function test.

In fact, our results show that $\zeta$ is superior to its counterparts, Raw and sGaw, in their association with CT densitometry, which is considered as the most direct method for assessing the severity of emphysema [37]. It is also better correlated with DLCO, which is an index for alveolar destruction and loss of capillary bed in COPD [38]. Compared to the interrupter technique, which estimates airway resistance using measurements obtained at a single instant of time under tidal breathing [7], we achieve a more robust value of airway resistance as we consider the entire manoeuver of forced expiration. This motivates the application of our methodology, especially, in primary care where spirometers are more abundantly available than bulky and expensive equipment such as a body-box or FOT machine.

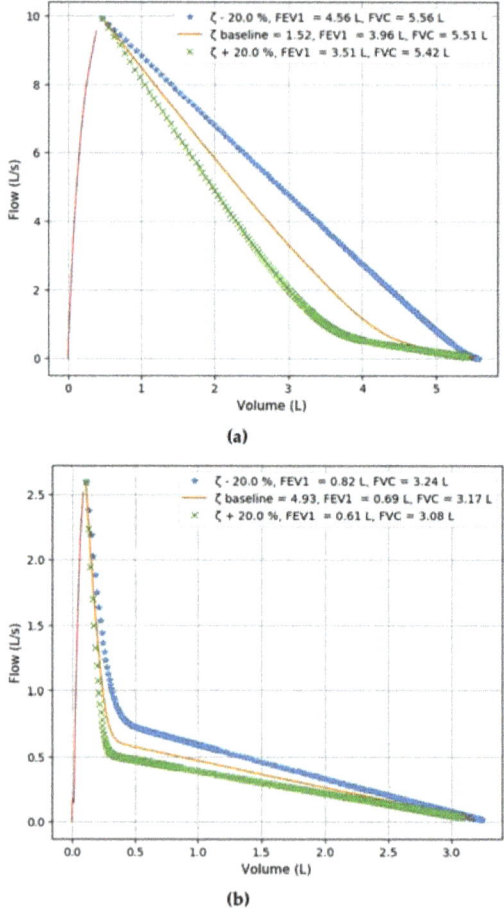

**Figure 4.** Simulation of model MEFVC when $\zeta$ is changed by 20% from baseline by keeping $\omega$ constant, shown in the case of (**a**) healthy and (**b**) COPD GOLD IV individuals. In both cases, an increase in $\zeta$ leads to lower airflows, and therefore, a lower FEV1 and FVC.

A major limitation of our methodology is that it does not shed any light on expiratory muscle effort and elastic recoil pressure, which are the components of alveolar pressure that drive forced expiration. The term $\omega$ proves to be of little use as it masks these underlying components. An interesting result would have been to estimate elastic recoil coefficient and then, to correlate it with elasticity loss in emphysema. However, such a step would have required pleural pressure measurements using an invasive and impractical esophageal balloon [39]. Another drawback is that $\zeta$ may not be sensitive to upper airway resistance. During forced expiration, the emptying of the upper airways occurs in the beginning, a phase that was neglected in our model (Equation (4)). It is also worth mentioning that validation of $\zeta$ by comparing it against Raw may not be completely appropriate. The latter quantifies total resistance during tidal breathing when resistance of the larger airways and viscoelastic properties of lung parenchyma account dominate over smaller airways resistance [40,41]. A better validation of $\zeta$ would have been to compare it against the difference of FOT resistance at 5 Hz and 20 Hz ($R_5$–$R_{20}$), metric that reflects small airway resistance [42]. Finally, our study was focused on airflow limitation associated with COPD only. A more inclusive study is required to evaluate the efficacy of $\zeta$ by considering other obstructive cohorts such as asthma, asthma-COPD overlap (ACO), and obstructive asthma.

## 5. Conclusions

In this study, we describe the dynamics of forced expiration in spirometry using a deflating balloon and using this model, we proposed a methodology to estimate $\zeta$, a dimensionless and effort-independent parameter quantifying airway resistance in the lungs. $\zeta$ correlated significantly with Raw and sGaw, which are traditional indices of airway resistance from body-plethysmography. It increases with the severity of airflow limitation as expected from an airway resistance, and in some cases, even showing better associations with DLCO and CT densitometry of emphysema than Raw and sGaw. Moreover, simulation studies showed that an increase in $\zeta$ resulted in decreased airflows, and therefore a reduced FEV1 and FVC. Thus, we conclude that $\zeta$ estimated from forced expiration in spirometry reflects airway resistance in the lungs. In primary care, $\zeta$ may be clinically useful, as spirometry is more widely available than traditional but expensive methods to measure airway resistance such as body-plethysmography or FOT. In the future, we aim to validate $\zeta$ in a more inclusive cohort of obstructive airway diseases with longitudinal follow-up, as well as study the association of $\zeta$ against airway resistance parameters obtained from the interrupter technique and FOT.

## 6. Patents

Based on the present study, we have filed a patent titled "Methods and apparatus for determining airflow limitation" (PCT/EP2019/059903) on 11 May 2019.

**Author Contributions:** N.D. performed conceptualization, methodology design, analysis, validation, software development and manuscript preparation. K.V. helped with validation and review editing. M.T. helped with data curation, review editing and supervision. J.M.A. helped with review editing and supervision. W.J. helped with conceptualization, methodology, review editing and supervision.

**Funding:** This research was funded by the Research Foundation-Flanders (FWO) strategic basic fellowship.

**Acknowledgments:** The authors would like to acknowledge the technical staff of the lung function unit at UZ Leuven for helping with the data collection.

**Conflicts of Interest:** M.T. and W.J. are the founders of a spin-off company ArtiQ at Leuven, Belgium. The funders had no role in the design of the study; in the collection, analyses, or interpretation of data; in the writing of the manuscript, or in the decision to publish the results.

## Appendix A

Applying initial conditions (Equation (4)), we get:

$$x(t_1) = C_1 + C_2 \quad (A1)$$

$$\dot{x}(t_1) = C_1 s_1 + C_2 s_2 \quad (A2)$$

multiplying (A1) by $s_2$ throughout, subtracting (A2) from it and rearranging for $C_1$, we get 11a

$$C_1 = \frac{\dot{x}(t_1) - s_2 x(1)}{s_3},$$

similarly, multiplying (A1) by $s_1$ throughout, subtracting (A1) from it and rearranging for $C_2$, we get 11b

$$C_2 = \frac{-\dot{x}(t_1) + s_1 x(t_1)}{s_3}$$

where

$$s_3 = s_1 - s_2 \tag{A3}$$

## References

1. O'Donnell, D.E.; Laveneziana, P. Physiology and consequences of lung hyperinflation in COPD. *Eur. Respir. Rev.* **2006**, *15*, 61–67. [CrossRef]
2. Bousquet, J.; Jeffery, P.K.; Busse, W.W.; Johnson, M.; Vignola, A.M. Asthma: From bronchoconstriction to airways inflammation and remodeling. *Am. J. Respir. Crit. Care Med.* **2000**, *161*, 1720–1745. [CrossRef]
3. Vestbo, J.; Hurd, S.S.; Agustí, A.G.; Jones, P.W.; Vogelmeier, C.; Anzueto, A.; Barnes, P.J.; Fabbri, L.M.; Martinez, F.J.; Nishimura, M.; et al. Global strategy for the diagnosis, management, and prevention of chronic obstructive pulmonary disease: GOLD executive summary (updated 2014). *Glob. Initiat. Chronic Obstr. Lung Dis.* **2014**, 21–26. [CrossRef]
4. Miller, M.R.; Hankinson, J.; Brusasco, V.; Burgos, F.; Casaburi, R.; Coates, A.; Crapo, R.; Enright, P.V.; Van Der Grinten, C.P.M.; Gustafsson, P.; et al. Standardisation of spirometry. *Eur. Respir. J.* **2005**, *26*, 319–338. [CrossRef]
5. Pellegrino, R.; Viegi, G.; Brusasco, V.; Crapo, R.O.; Burgos, F.; Casaburi, R.; Coates, A.; Van Der Grinten, C.P.M.; Gustafsson, P.; Hankinson, J.; et al. Interpretative strategies for lung function tests. *Eur. Respir. J.* **2005**, *26*, 948–968. [CrossRef]
6. Mead, J. Analysis of the configuration of maximum expiratory flow-volume curves. *J. Appl. Physiol.* **1978**, *44*, 156–165. [CrossRef]
7. Kaminsky, D.A. What Does Airway Resistance Tell Us about Lung Function? *Respir. Care* **2012**, *57*, 85–99. [CrossRef]
8. Petty, T.L.; Silvers, G.W.; Stanford, R.E. Radial Traction and Small Airways Disease in Excised Human Lungs. *Am. Rev. Respir. Dis.* **2015**, *133*, 132–135.
9. Zach, M.S. The physiology of forced expiration. *Paediatr. Respir. Rev.* **2000**, *1*, 36–39. [CrossRef]
10. Larsson, K. Aspects on pathophysiological mechanisms in COPD. *J. Intern. Med.* **2007**, *262*, 311–340. [CrossRef]
11. Criée, C.P.; Sorichter, S.; Smith, H.J.; Kardos, P.; Merget, R.; Heise, D.; Berdel, D.; Köhler, D.; Magnussen, H.; Marek, W.; et al. Body plethysmography—Its principles and clinical use. *Respir. Med.* **2011**, *105*, 959–971.
12. Stocks, J.; Godfrey, S.; Beardsmore, C.; Bar-Yishay, E.; Castile, R. Plethysmographic measurements of lung volume and airway resistance. *Eur. Respir. J.* **2001**, *17*, 302–312. [CrossRef]
13. Oh, A.; Morris, T.A.; Yoshii, I.T.; Morris, T.A. Flow Decay: A Novel Spirometric Index to Quantify Dynamic Airway Resistance. *Respir. Care* **2017**, *62*, 928–935. [CrossRef]
14. Vogelmeier, C.F.; Criner, G.J.; Martinez, F.J.; Anzueto, A.; Barnes, P.J.; Bourbeau, J.; Celli, B.R.; Chen, R.; Decramer, M.; Fabbri, L.M.; et al. Global Strategy for the Diagnosis, Management, and Prevention of Chronic Obstructive Lung Disease 2017 Report. GOLD Executive Summary. *Am. J. Respir. Crit. Care Med.* **2017**, *195*, 557–582. [CrossRef]
15. Jensen, R.L.; Crapo, R.O. Diffusing capacity: How to get it right. *Respir. Care* **2003**, *48*, 777–782.
16. O'Donnell, D.E.; Webb, K.A.; Neder, J.A. Lung hyperinflation in COPD: Applying physiology to clinical practice. *COPD Res. Pract.* **2015**, *1*, 4. [CrossRef]
17. Lynch, D.A.; Al-Qaisi, M.A. Quantitative computed tomography in chronic obstructive pulmonary disease. *J. Thorac. Imaging* **2013**, *28*, 284–290. [CrossRef]
18. Bencowitz, H.Z. Single breath diffusing capacity in a representative sample of the population of Michigan, a large industrial state. *Am. Rev. Respir. Dis.* **1983**, *127*, 270–277.
19. Krowka, M.J.; Enright, P.L.; Rodarte, J.R.; Hyatt, R.E. Effect of Effort on Measurement of Forced Expiratory Volume in One Second. *Am. Rev. Respir. Dis.* **1987**, *136*, 829–833. [CrossRef]
20. Hayes, D.; Kraman, S.S. The Physiologic Basis of Spirometry. *Respir. Care* **2009**, *54*, 1717–1726.

21. Quanjer, P.H.; Lebowitz, M.D.; Gregg, I.; Miller, M.R.; Pedersen, O.F. Peak expiratory flow: Conclusions and recommendations of a Working Party of the European Respiratory Society. *Eur. Respir. J. Suppl.* **1997**, *10*, 2s.
22. Fry, D.L.; Hyatt, R.E. Pulmonary mechanics. A unified analysis of the relationship between pressure, volume and gasflow in the lungs of normal and diseased human subjects. *Am. J. Med.* **1960**, *29*, 672–689. [CrossRef]
23. Agostoni, E.; Fenn, W.O. Velocity of Muscle Shortening As a Limiting Factor in Respiratory Air Flow. *J. Appl. Physiol.* **1960**, *15*, 349–353. [CrossRef]
24. Rao, S.S. *Mechanical Vibrations*; Addison-Wesley Longman: University of Michigan, MI, USA, 1990.
25. Storn, R.; Price, K. Differential Evolution—A Simple and Efficient Heuristic for Global Optimization over Continuous Spaces. *J. Glob. Optim.* **1997**, *11*, 341–359. [CrossRef]
26. Millman, K.J.; Aivazis, M. Python for scientists and engineers. *Comput. Sci. Eng.* **2011**, *13*, 9–12. [CrossRef]
27. RStudio Team. *RStudio: Integrated Development for R*; RStudio, Inc.: Boston, MA, USA, 2016; Available online: http//www.rstudio.com (accessed on 15 June 2019).
28. O'Donnell, R.; Breen, D.; Wilson, S.; Djukanovic, R. Inflammatory cells in the airways in COPD. *Thorax* **2006**, *61*, 448–454. [CrossRef]
29. Yan, F.; Gao, H.; Zhao, H.; Bhatia, M.; Zeng, Y. Roles of airway smooth muscle dysfunction in chronic obstructive pulmonary disease. *J. Transl. Med.* **2018**, *16*, 262. [CrossRef]
30. Ramos, F.L.; Krahnke, J.S.; Kim, V. Clinical issues of mucus accumulation in COPD. *Int. J. COPD* **2014**, *9*, 139.
31. Cottin, V.; Nunes, H.; Brillet, P.Y.; Delaval, P.; Devouassoux, G.; Tillie-Leblond, I.; Israel-Biet, D.; Valeyre, D.; Cordier, J.F. Combined pulmonary fibrosis and emphysema: A distinct underrecognised entity. *Eur. Respir. J.* **2005**, *26*, 586–593. [CrossRef]
32. Topalovic, M.; Exadaktylos, V.; Decramer, M.; Troosters, T.; Berckmans, D.; Janssens, W. Modelling the dynamics of expiratory airflow to describe chronic obstructive pulmonary disease. *Med. Biol. Eng. Comput.* **2014**, *52*, 997–1006. [CrossRef]
33. Mead, J. Mechanical properties of the lungs. *Acta Physiol. Pol.* **1961**, *41*, 281–330. [CrossRef]
34. Hess, D.R. Respiratory Mechanics in Mechanically Ventilated Patients. *Respir. Care* **2014**, *59*, 1773–1794. [CrossRef]
35. Grinnan, D.C.; Truwit, J.D. Clinical review: Respiratory mechanics in spontaneous and assisted ventilation. *Crit. Care* **2005**, *9*, 472. [CrossRef]
36. Dubois, A.B. Airway Resistance. *Am. J. Respir. Crit. Care Med.* **2000**, *162*, 345–346. [CrossRef]
37. Crossley, D.; Renton, M.; Khan, M.; Low, E.V.; Turner, A.M. CT densitometry in emphysema: A systematic review of its clinical utility. *Int. J. COPD* **2018**, *13*, 547. [CrossRef]
38. Bailey, K.L. The importance of the assessment of pulmonary function in COPD. *Med. Clin. N. Am.* **2012**, *96*, 745–752. [CrossRef]
39. Akoumianaki, E.; Maggiore, S.M.; Valenza, F.; Bellani, G.; Jubran, A.; Loring, S.H.; Pelosi, P.; Talmor, D.; Grasso, S.; Chiumello, D.; et al. The application of esophageal pressure measurement in patients with respiratory failure. *Am. J. Respir. Crit. Care Med.* **2014**, *189*, 520–531. [CrossRef]
40. Macklem, P.T.; Mead, J. Resistance of central and peripheral airways measured by a retrograde catheter. *J. Appl. Physiol.* **1967**, *22*, 395–401. [CrossRef]
41. Kaczka, D.W.; Ingenito, E.P.; Suki, B.; Lutchen, K.R. Partitioning airway and lung tissue resistances in humans: Effects of bronchoconstriction. *J. Appl. Physiol.* **1997**, *82*, 1531–1541. [CrossRef]
42. Brashier, B.; Salvi, S. Measuring lung function using sound waves: Role of the forced oscillation technique and impulse oscillometry system. *Breathe* **2015**, *11*, 57–65. [CrossRef]

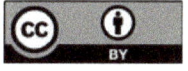

© 2019 by the authors. Licensee MDPI, Basel, Switzerland. This article is an open access article distributed under the terms and conditions of the Creative Commons Attribution (CC BY) license (http://creativecommons.org/licenses/by/4.0/).

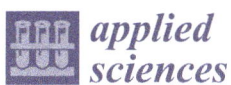 

*Article*

# Simulation Analysis of Knee Ligaments in the Landing Phase of Freestyle Skiing Aerial

Yanming Fu [1,2], Xin Wang [3,*] and Tianbiao Yu [1,*]

1. School of mechanical engineering and automation, Northeastern University, Shenyang 110819, China
2. Laboratory management center, Shenyang Sport University, Shenyang 110102, China
3. School of kinesiology, Shenyang Sport University, Shenyang 110102, China
* Correspondence: wangxin@syty.edu.cn (X.W.); tianbiaoyudyx@gmail.com (T.Y.)

Received: 22 July 2019; Accepted: 2 September 2019; Published: 6 September 2019

**Featured Application:** This paper focused on the knee joints of freestyle skiers in three landing conditions (neutral, backward, or forward landing). Aim to understanding the force inside the knee joints during the landing phase. The research results will be used in the design of athletes' protective gear.

**Abstract:** The risk of knee injuries in freestyle skiing athletes that perform aerials is high. The internal stresses in the knee joints of these athletes cannot easily be directly measured. In order to ascertain the mechanical response of knee joints during the landing phase, and to explore the mechanism of damage to the cartilage and ligaments, a finite element model of the knee joint was established. Three successful landing conditions (neutral, backward, or forward landing) from a triple kicker were analyzed. The results demonstrate that the risk of cruciate ligament damage during a neutral landing was lowest. A forward landing carried medium risk, while backward landing was of highest risk. Backward and forward landing carried risk of injury to the anterior cruciate ligament (ACL) and posterior cruciate ligament (PCL), respectively. The magnitude of stress on the meniscus and cartilage varied for all three landing scenarios. Stress was largest during neutral landing and least in backward landing, while forward landing resulted in a medium level of stress. The results also provide the basis for training that is scientifically robust so as to reduce the risk of injury and assist in the development of a professional knee joint protector.

**Keywords:** freestyle skiing aerials; knee joint; ligament; finite element simulation

## 1. Introduction

In the absence of trauma, the knee joint can operate effectively for decades while being subjected to high mechanical loads. The knees of athletes have a shorter life expectancy. After professional athletes retire, their knee joints often exhibit damage due to overwork. For example, the rate of knee joint injury in freestyle skiing aerialists in Chinese national team is close to 85% and higher in retired athletes. Studies have shown that instantaneous impact in the vertical direction will damage the cartilage of the knee joint, while long-term repeated impact will cause strain damage to the stress concentration region of the cartilage [1]. Other studies have shown that when the knee joint flexes at a certain angle, shear or torsion stress caused by instantaneous movement of the tibia may damage the cruciate ligaments [2,3], while instantaneous inversion or eversion of the knee may cause the medial or lateral collateral ligaments to be damaged [4,5]. In addition, the athletes' ankle joints are essentially locked in snowshoes, which do not provide sufficient cushioning at the moment of landing, resulting in greater impact force to be absorbed by the knee joints. For these reasons, freestyle skiing aerialists suffer a high rate of knee injuries.

In order to establish the internal force within the knee joint, a number of researchers have conducted in vitro experiments and with cadavers [6,7]. Other researchers have used the inverse dynamics technique to analyze knee movement [8,9]. Most researchers choose finite element analysis [10], which is possibly a more objective method of obtaining the specific movements of components within the knee joint. In this study, finite element simulation method had been adopted to analyze the knee joint at phase of landing, so as to obtain the stress of cartilage and ligament during landing buffering.

## 2. Methods

### 2.1. 3D Reconstruction

In the early stages of the study, CT (Computed Tomography) and MR (Magnetic Resonance) test data were obtained from a male athlete volunteer who had provided signed informed consent [11]. The height and weight of the volunteer was close to the mean value of male athletes. The CT and MR data were imported into Mimics software. After 3D reconstruction, the optimized model was imported into Abaqus software to complete finite element analysis.

Bone tissue 3D reconstruction was derived from CT data, while cartilage and ligament tissue models were derived from MR data [12–14]. Bone, cartilage, and ligament tissues were reconstructed independently using Mimics. The models were imported into Geomagic software in STL format. After image registration and model assembly, the bone, cartilage and ligament models were finally stored independently in IGES format.

### 2.2. Mechanical Models

From the motions observed during landing, a mechanical model of the landing phase was established in the X and Y directions, as shown in Figure 1. The angle between the femur and tibia was defined as $\alpha$. The angle between the tibia and the slope of the landing plane was defined as $\beta$. The angle between the trunk and the landing slope was defined as $\gamma$. $G$ and $G'$ represented force due to gravity and force on the tibial plateau, respectively. By combining theory with research [15,16] $G'$ was calculated as:

$$G' = 85.6\% \times G$$

The proportions of the force on the medial and lateral femoral condyles have been estimated to be 60% and 40%, respectively [17]. Therefore, if air resistance and wind direction are neglected, the impact force on the tibial plateau can be calculated from an analysis of the projectile motion of the human body.

### 2.3. Kinematic Analysis

Velocity of takeoff was obtained from a camera located at the kicker and the velocity of center of gravity, left and right knee joint movement angle, and duration of the balancing phase of landing at the point of impact were collected from cameras located on both sides of the landing site on the landing slope. Data relating to the kinematic parameters described above were obtained through SIMI Motion analysis. The maximum height of the trajectory above the landing site could be calculated from the takeoff velocity of a freestyle skiing aerialist completing a triple somersault having a prescribed action prior to landing (slope of 37.5°). This was approximately 17 m, as shown in Figure 1.

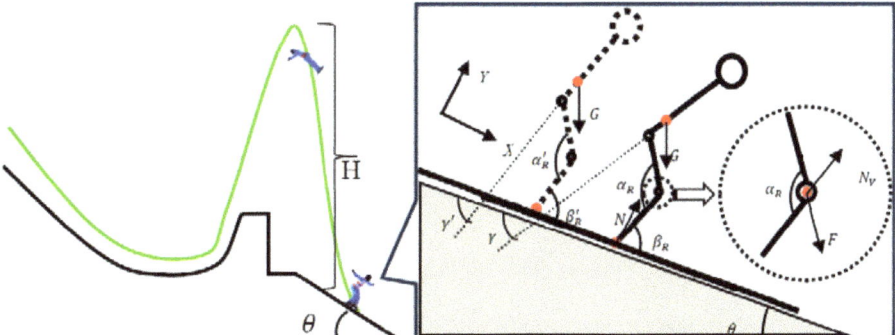

**Figure 1.** Freestyle skiing aerial motion curve and landing phase of the kinematic analysis diagram ($\alpha'_R$ and $\beta'_R$ represent the angles of the right knee and right ankle as landing begins, respectively, $\gamma'$ was the angle between the torso and the landing slope. $\alpha_R$ and $\beta_R$ represent the angles of the right knee and right ankle at the end of the balancing phase of landing, $\gamma$ represents the angle between the torso and the landing slope at the end of the balancing phase of landing. $H$ was the distance from the highest position of the trajectory to the landing position. $\theta$ was the landing slope angle. $G$ was the force experienced by the athlete due to gravity, $N$ was the reaction force from the landing slope, $N_v$ was the reaction force from the tibial plateau, $F$ was the impact force from the upper part of the knee joint in the direction of the femur).

In the process of image acquisition, 150 video files and 50 groups of images of the motion were collected in this study. After screening, 30 groups of images met the experimental requirements. After statistical analysis, no significant difference was detected between the experimental data and that of the mechanical model established in previous studies. The data collected were combined with the results calculated from the mechanical model and used as boundary conditions in the finite element calculation.

*2.4. Establishing the FEM (Finite Element Model)*

The 3D models obtained by 3D reconstruction were imported into Abaqus software in IGES format with the results of meshing (Figure 2a, using C3D10 meshing classification), attributes of materials and the assembled model displayed in Figure 2. The finite element calculations were completed using constraint conditions which were also configured in Abaqus, and then the density, elastic modulus and Poisson's ratio of bone, cartilage, and meniscus were set according to the data in Figure 2b [18–21]. An incompressible Neo-Hooke hyperelastic model was selected for the ligament model, expressed by C10 and D1 coefficients, as shown in Figure 2c [22]. The constraint conditions of the knee FEM were set according to the anatomical characteristics. All the contacts between ligaments and bones were "Tie" type constraint and tibia was set as "ENCASTRE".

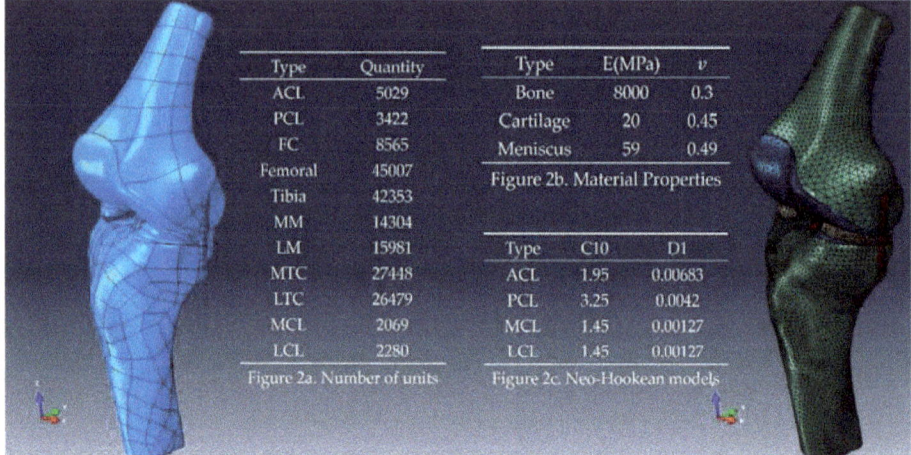

**Figure 2.** Mesh generation and material properties of knee models. The right figure represents assembled knee model. In the left figure, different colors define the different material properties. ACL: anterior cruciate ligament; PCL: posterior cruciate ligament; FC: femoral cartilage; MM: medial meniscus; LM: lateral meniscus; MTC: medial tibial cartilage; LTC: lateral tibial cartilage; MCL: medial collateral ligament; LCL: lateral collateral ligament.

## 3. Results

### 3.1. Results of Kinematic Analysis

Using SIMI Motion, 30 groups of motions were parsed. Mean velocity ($\bar{v}$) and standard deviation (SD) at takeoff were calculated as: $\bar{v} \pm SD = 16.62 \pm 2.51$ (m/s). In addition, the mean duration of the balancing phase ($\bar{t}$) and SD of landing were measured as: $\bar{t} \pm SD = 0.16 \pm 0.04$. The values of $\alpha_L$, $\alpha_R$, $\beta_L$, $\beta_R$, and $\gamma$ for the landing balancing phase are shown in Figure 3.

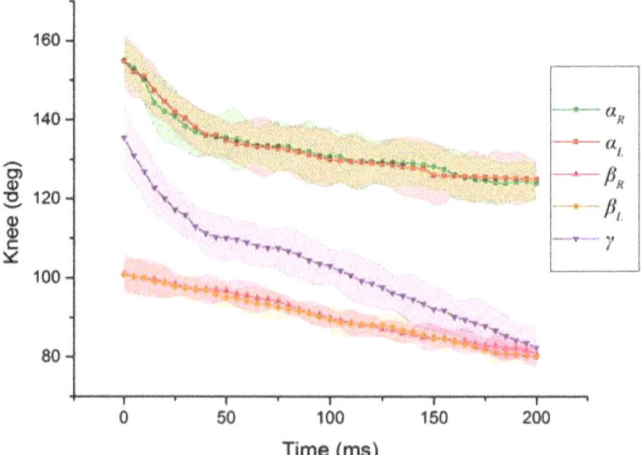

**Figure 3.** Variation trend of human body angle during the balancing stage, where $\alpha_L$ represents the angle of the left knee, $\alpha_R$ the angle of right knee, $\beta_L$ the angle of left ankle. $\beta_R$ the angle of right ankle. $\gamma$ represents the angle between the torso and landing slope.

From videos of successful landings, a successful landing can be approximately divided into three variations, as shown in Figure 4. The first can be denoted forward landing due to the front of the skis touching the snow first with the athlete's center of gravity being in a forward orientation. This requires an aerialist to adjust their center of gravity backward to ensure a successful landing. The second is denoted neutral landing, where the front and rear of the skis touch the snow simultaneously with the athlete's center of gravity mid-way of all the variations. This requires maintenance of knee joint stability and center of gravity to ensure a successful landing. The third is described as a backward landing, where the rear of the skis touch the snow first with the center of gravity of the athlete rearward. This requires an adjustment of the center of gravity forward to ensure a successful landing.

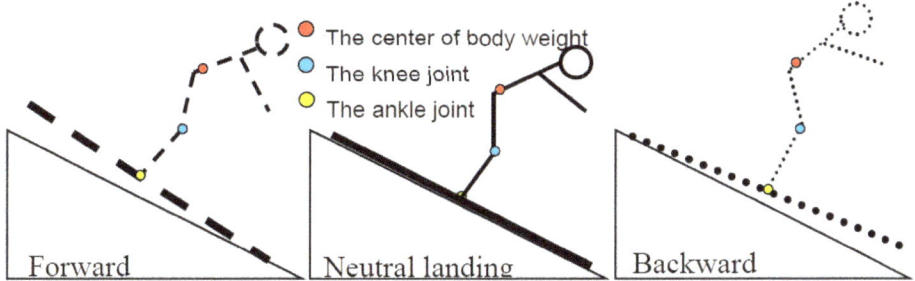

**Figure 4.** The three variations of successful landing.

More apparent differences can be observed if the three are combined into one image. An integrated image can be obtained when the center points of the knee and ankle joints from the three are overlain, as shown in Figure 5. Vertical lines from the center of body weight demonstrate the different positional features. In forward landing, this line is forward of the knee joint, essentially located within the boundaries of the knee joint in neutral landing and behind the knee joint in backward landing.

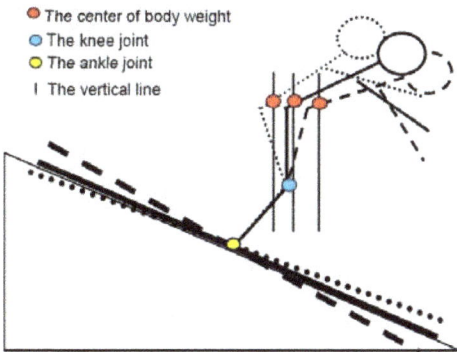

**Figure 5.** Overlay effect.

*3.2. Results of Mechanical Model Analysis*

$\alpha$, $\beta$, and $\gamma$ are the principal parameters for the mechanical model, with takeoff velocity ($v$) and landing balancing duration ($t$) critical variables for dynamic analysis. By adding results of tests using a force platform in the laboratory [23], vertical and shear force curves of the landing slope and tibial plateau were fitted by dynamic analysis, as shown in Figure 6. The balancing phase was 0–200 ms, maximum vertical force $F_\sigma$ and shear force $F_\tau$ on a single knee tibial plateau were approximately 2527 and 1699, respectively, with the range of knee angles from 155 to 120 degrees. Peak force was experienced at approximately 135°.

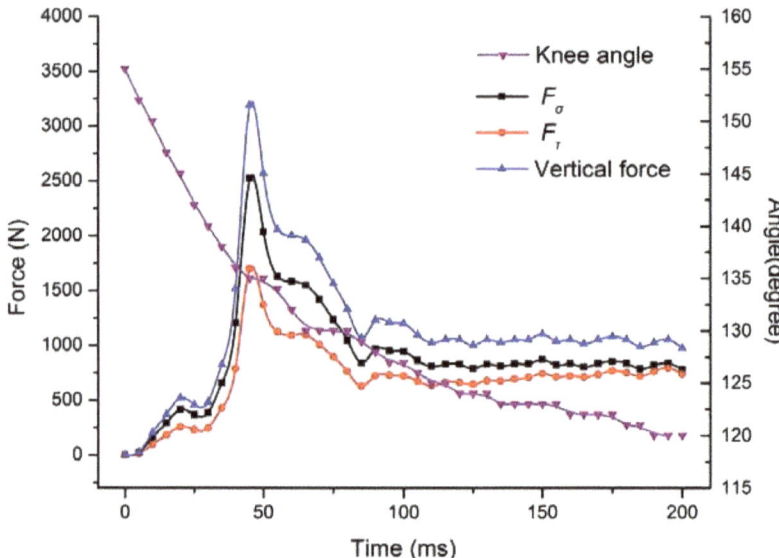

**Figure 6.** Force curve of a single knee joint in the balancing phase.

*3.3. Finite Element Simulation Results*

Combined with the three landing conditions described in Section 3.1, the external constraint conditions of the model were adjusted and finite element analysis performed on the ACL, PCL, MCL, and LCL. Time–stress curves were calculated according to the results of the analysis.

In forward landing (Figure 7), deformation of the front of the skis was minimal with elastic force in the balancing stage that could be ignored. According to the results of the analysis, due to the tendency of the tibia to move rearwards, the position of stress concentration was at the lower end of the posterior bundle of the ACL with a maximum stress value of 4.01 MPa. The position of stress concentration on the PCL was at the upper end of anterior bundle, with a maximum value of 6.81 MPa. The position of stress concentration on the LCL was in the middle, with a maximum stress value of 1.60 MPa. Maximum stress on the MCL was 1.96 MPa, with stress concentration in the middle and on the lower section. As the center of gravity was adjusted rearwards, the medial meniscus became squeezed, resulting in a region of stress concentration in the middle of the MCL.

In neutral landing (Figure 8), the skis were parallel to the landing slope and so elastic force in the balancing process was ignored. Although the impulse from the femur had a forward component at the tibial plateau, the tibial plateau also moved synchronously with flexion of the knee joint and so relative motion of the femur and tibial plateau were not apparent. According to the results of the finite element analysis, the position of stress concentration was at the lower end of posterior bundle of the ACL with a maximum stress of 3.16 MPa. Stress was concentrated in the upper part of the posterior bundle of the PCL to the lower end of anterior bundle with a maximum stress of 6.61 MPa. Maximum stress on the MCL was 2.49 MPa which was concentrated in the middle region. Stress concentration was in the middle of the LCL, to a maximum stress value of 1.67 MPa.

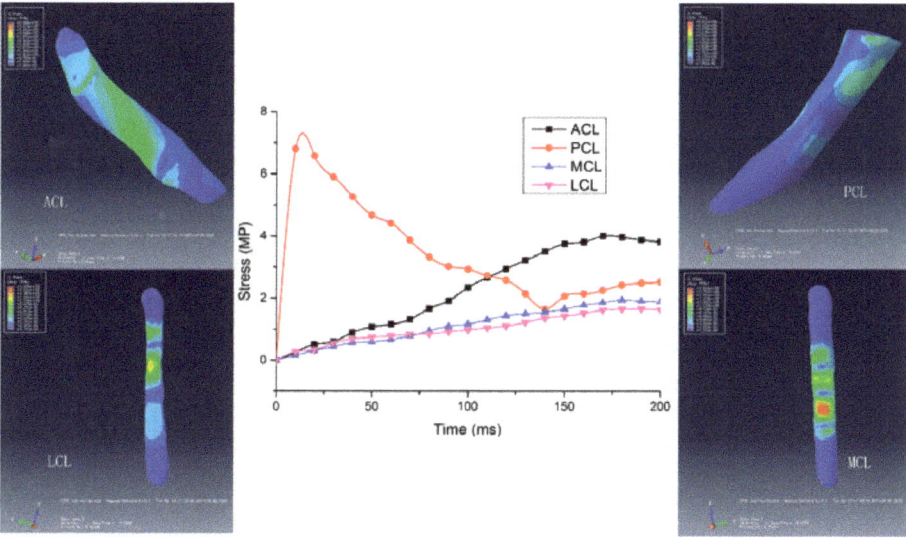

**Figure 7.** Stress distribution and stress-time curve of the ligaments in forward landing.

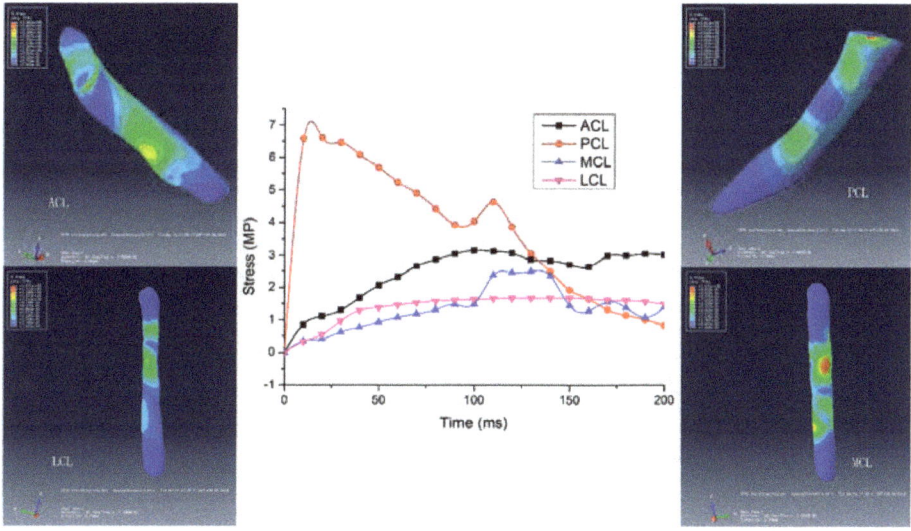

**Figure 8.** Stress distribution and stress–time curve of the ligaments in neutral landing.

During backward landing (Figure 9), elastic force from deformation of the tail of the skis provided an additional elastic force. Deformation of skis extended the duration of the balancing phase and reduced vertical impact force on the tibial plateau. According to the results of finite element analysis, maximum stress was experienced at the lower end of the posterior bundle of the ACL, at 4.52 MPa. On the PCL, stress was concentrated from the upper end of the posterior bundle to the lower end of anterior bundle, with a maximum value of 6.99 MPa. The middle of the MCL and LCL endured maximum stress, with values of 3.46 MPa and 1.39 MPa, respectively.

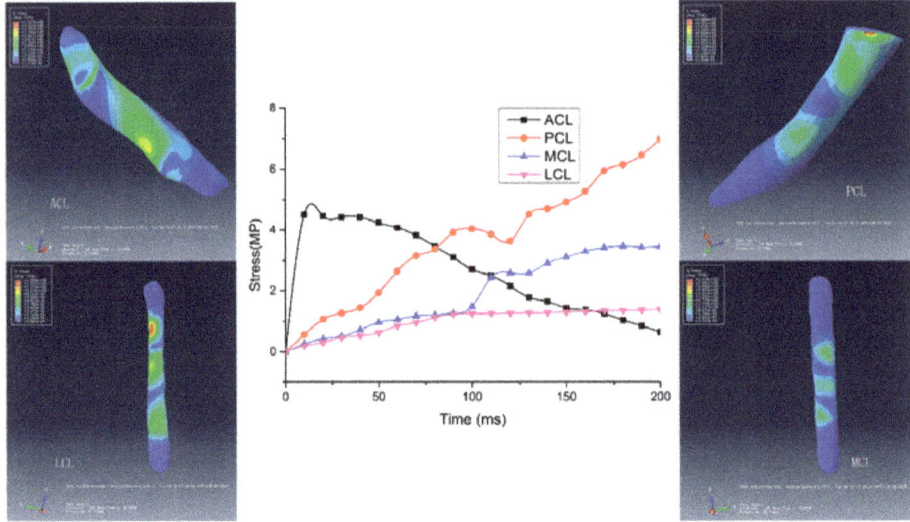

**Figure 9.** Distribution and stress–time curve of the ligaments in backward landing.

Simulation of stress at the tibial plateau are displayed in Figure 10, where the position of stress concentration was obvious. When the tibia moved rearwards relative to the femur, as in forward landing (Figure 10a), a region of stress concentration was observed at the front of the menisci and the middle of the medial meniscus. When the tibia is relatively immobile, such as during neutral landing (Figure 10b), the position of stress concentration was in the middle of the medial meniscus and the center of the lateral tibial cartilage. As the tibia moved forward relative to the femur such as in backward landing (Figure 10c), stress became concentrated in the middle of the medial meniscus and central position of the lateral tibial cartilage. Compared with neutral landing, the position and value of stress concentration in backward landing were relatively small and located towards the rear.

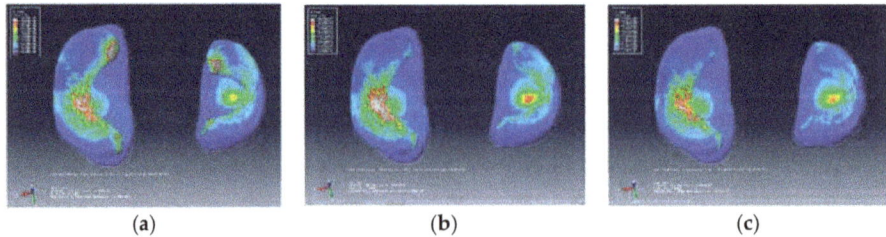

(a)　　　　　　　　　　(b)　　　　　　　　　　(c)

**Figure 10.** Stress distribution of tibial plateau and meniscus: (**a**) forward landing; (**b**) neutral landing; (**c**) backward landing.

## 4. Discussion and Implications

In the balancing phase of landing in freestyle skiing aerial sports, complex internal stresses are formed within the knee joint. In this study, only neutral, forward, and backward landing positions were considered. The principal differences between the three scenarios were position of center of gravity and the magnitude and direction of the reaction force.

In neutral landing, the reaction force provided by the landing slope was essentially perpendicular to the tibial plateau. Under the combined action of the impact force of falling and the frictional force of the snow, the analysis demonstrated that the tibia moved back and forth slightly within the knee joint. During knee flexion, the front and rear muscles of the thigh worked together to stabilize the knee joint.

According to the results of the simulation, peak stress on the tibial plateau and meniscus were greatest at this point in time for all three landing scenarios, but the relative displacement of the tibia was small. Stress on the cruciate ligaments in the balancing phase in neutral landing was the smallest of all three, and so was the safest form of landing.

In forward landing, slight backward motion of the tibia occurred within the knee joint and a vertical line through the center of gravity moved forward beyond the tibial plateau. As balancing progressed, the anterior thigh muscle was required to reposition the tibia [24]. According to the results of the simulation, peak stress in the tibial plateau and meniscus were smallest at this moment in all three conditions, with regions of stress concentrated in the anterior horn of the menisci. Because the medial meniscus was compressed by the femoral cartilage and resulted in lateral movement, stress in the middle of the MCL during the balancing phase of forward landing was the highest of all three landing scenarios.

In backward landing, elastic force of deformation of the skis and the impact force of falling resulted in the tibia exhibiting forward movement of the knee joint. As balancing progressed, the position of the tibia was adjusted towards the neutral position by action of the posterior thigh muscle [25] in a tangential direction, the tibia becoming pushed backwards. According to the results of the simulation, peak stress on the tibial plateau and meniscus was observed in forward and neutral landing, but of all three scenarios, stress on the ACL and PCL was largest in backward landing.

The results of the simulation in the three scenarios above demonstrate that the maximum value of stress (Table 1) in each ligament was less than the ultimate stress of the ligament. Even so, not all the ligaments are completely safe. Such as if athletes with the accumulated training, degenerative changes would occur within the region of stress concentration in the tibial cartilage and meniscus, in addition to fatigue and damage within the position of stress concentration in the cruciate ligament. If internal or external rotation of the knee joint occurred during landing, the risk of knee cartilage, meniscus or ligament injury would greatly increase. Over a controllable range, whether in forward or backward landing, aerialists require sufficiently strong anterior and posterior thigh muscles to maintain stability in the knee joint. If the strength of the anterior and posterior thigh muscles do not match, the risk of cruciate ligament injury is greatly increased.

Table 1. The stresses of the ligaments in three cases. (MPa).

| Type | Neutral Landing | Forward Landing | Backward Landing |
|------|-----------------|-----------------|------------------|
| ACL  | 3.16            | 4.01            | 4.52             |
| PCL  | 6.61            | 6.81            | 6.99             |
| MCL  | 2.49            | 1.96            | 3.46             |
| LCL  | 1.67            | 1.60            | 1.39             |

## 5. Conclusions

Although neutral landing had the greatest peak stress on the medial meniscus, stress on the ACL, PCL, MCL, and LCL were at their least of the three scenarios due to the slight relative displacement of the tibia, so neutral landing should be considered the safest and most successful technique of all three forms of landing.

During forward landing, a part of the femoral cartilage contacted with the front end of the meniscus, causing inward horizontal displacement of the meniscus. This allowed a greater likelihood that the medial meniscus would crush the MCL. The position of stress concentration in the medial meniscus was close to the anterior horn and middle edge, causing a high risk of meniscal damage. As the knee undergoes flexion, the tibia adjusted to a neutral position under action of the posterior thigh muscle. Therefore, athletes that have weakness in their posterior thigh muscle should avoid forward landing in order to reduce the possibility of PCL or MCL injury.

In backward landing, elastic deformation at the back of the skis created a cushion effect with deformation forces causing the tibia to move forward slightly. The tibia can be adjusted to a neutral position only using the power of an athlete's anterior thigh muscles. Therefore, those aerialists that have weak anterior thigh muscles should avoid backward landings to reduce the risk of ACL injury.

No matter which landing condition is adopted, due to the forward velocity and rotational inertia of the lower limbs, under the combined action of the reaction force of the landing slope and friction between the skis and surface of the snow, shear force is evident on the tibial plateau with a trend of forward and backward displacement. In this study, internal and external rotations of the tibia were not considered. If tibial rotation occurs on landing, risk of cruciate ligament injury is greatly increased [26].

Peak stress on the tibial plateau and meniscus is extremely large. The medial meniscus is particularly prominent. Therefore, the design of professional knee protection should consider a reduction in landing impact with increased joint stability. Professional knee protectors can be effective in reducing the occurrence of sports injury and prolonging the career of athletes. The results of this simulation for three landing conditions provide a theoretical basis for the design of knee protection for freestyle skiing aerialists.

**Author Contributions:** Conceptualization, T.Y.; methodology, X.W.; formal analysis, Y.F.; writing—original draft preparation, Y.F.; writing—review and editing, T.Y. and X.W.; visualization, Y.F.; supervision, T.Y. and X.W.

**Funding:** This research was funded by the Key Special Project of the National Key Research and Development Program "Technical Winter Olympics" (2018YFF0300502) and the Natural Science Foundation Guide Project of Liaoning Province (2019-ZD-0517).

**Conflicts of Interest:** The authors declare no conflict of interest.

### References

1. Meng, Q.; An, S.; Damion, R.A.; Jin, Z.; Wilcox, R.; Fisher, J.; Jones, A. The Effect of Collagen Fibril Orientation on the Biphasic Mechanics of Articular Cartilage. *J. Mech. Behav. Biomed. Mater.* **2017**, *65*, 439–453. [CrossRef]
2. Xie, F.; Yang, L.; Guo, L.; Wang, Z.J.; Dai, G. A study on construction three-dimensional nonlinear finite element model and stress distribution analysis of anterior cruciate ligament. *J. Biomech. Eng.* **2009**, *131*, 121007. [CrossRef]
3. Atarod, M.; Rosvold, J.M.; Kazemi, M. Inter-insertional distance is a poor correlate for ligament load: Analysis from in vivo gait kinetics data. *J. Biomech.* **2013**, *46*, 2264–2270. [CrossRef]
4. Gardiner, J.C.; Weiss, J.A. Subject-specific finite element analysis of the human medial collateral ligament during valgus knee loading. *J. Orthop. Res.* **2010**, *21*, 1098–1106. [CrossRef]
5. Luetkemeyer, C.M.; Marchi, B.C.; Ashton-Miller, J.A.; Arruda, E.M. Femoral entheseal shape and attachment angle as potential risk factors for anterior cruciate ligament injury. *J. Mech. Behav. Biomed. Mater.* **2018**, *88*, 313–321. [CrossRef]
6. Agneskirchner, J.D.; Hurschler, C.; Stukenborg-Colsman, C.; Imhoff, A.B.; Lobenhoffer, P. Effect of high tibial flexion osteotomy on cartilage pressure and joint kinematics: A biomechanical study in human cadaveric knees. *Arch. Orthop. Trauma Surg.* **2004**, *124*, 575–584. [CrossRef]
7. Ali, A.A.; Harris, M.D.; Shalhoub, S.; Maletsky, L.P.; Rullkoetter, P.J.; Shelburne, K.B. Combined measurement and modeling of specimen-specific knee mechanics for healthy and ACL-deficient conditions. *J. Biomech.* **2017**, *57*, 117–124. [CrossRef]
8. Adouni, M.; Shirazi-Adl, A.; Shirazi, R. Computational biodynamics of human knee joint in gait: From muscle forces to cartilage stresses. *J. Biomech.* **2012**, *45*, 2149–2156. [CrossRef]
9. Essinger, J.R.; Leyvraz, P.F.; Heegard, J.H.; Robertson, D.D. A mathematical model for the evaluation of the behaviour during flexion of condylar-type knee prostheses. *J. Biomech.* **1989**, *22*, 1229–1241. [CrossRef]
10. Trad, Z.; Barkaoui, A.; Chafra, M. A Three Dimensional Finite Element Analysis of Mechanical Stresses in the Human Knee Joint: Problem of Cartilage Destruction. *J. Biomim. Biomater. Biomed. Eng.* **2017**, *32*, 29–39. [CrossRef]
11. Fu, Y. Research of Injury Risk Assessment of Athlete Knee Joint Cartilage in Freestyle Skiing Aerial Skill in Stable Landing Moment. *J. Shenyang Sport Univ.* **2018**, *37*, 70–74.
12. Ali, A.A.; Shalhoub, S.S.; Cyr, A.J.; Fitzpatrick, C.K.; Maletsky, L.P.; Rullkoetter, P.J.; Shelburne, K.B. Validation of predicted patellofemoral mechanics in a finite element model of the healthy and cruciate-deficient knee. *J. Biomech.* **2016**, *49*, 302–309. [CrossRef]

13. Fu, Y.; Yu, T.; Wang, X.; Wang, W. Finite Element Analysis of Knee Joint Cartilage at Turning of Plough Type Ski. *J. Northeast. Univ. (Nat. Sci.)* **2017**, *38*, 1431–1435.
14. Jiang, Y.; Jason, S.; Michael, M.; Lerner, A.L. Stresses and strains in the medial meniscus of an ACL deficient knee under anterior loading: A finite element analysis with image-based experimental validation. *J. Biomech. Eng.* **2006**, *128*, 135.
15. Braune, W.; Fischer, O. *Determining the Position of the Centre of Gravity in the Living Body in Different Attitudes and with Different Loads*; Springer: Berlin/Heidelberg, Germany, 1985.
16. Landi, G. Properties of the center of gravity as an algorithm for position measurements: Two-dimensional geometry. *Nucl. Inst. Methods Phys. Res. A* **2003**, *497*, 511–534. [CrossRef]
17. Hao, Z. Biomechanics of the bone and the knee joint. *Chin. J. Solid Mech.* **2010**, *31*, 603–612.
18. Beillas, P.; Papaioannou, G.; Tashman, S.; Yang, K.H. A new method to investigate in vivo knee behavior using a finite element model of the lower limb. *J. Biomech.* **2004**, *37*, 1019–1030. [CrossRef]
19. Chao, W.; Zhixiu, H.; Shizhu, W. The Effect of the Variation in ACL Constitutive Model on Joint Kinematics and Biomechanics Under Different Loads: A Finite Element Study. *J. Biomech. Eng.* **2013**, *135*, 41002.
20. Donahue, T.L.H.; Hull, M.L.; Rashid, M.M.; Jacobs, C.R. How the stiffness of meniscal attachments and meniscal material properties affect tibio-femoral contact pressure computed using a validated finite element model of the human knee joint. *J. Biomech.* **2003**, *36*, 19–34. [CrossRef]
21. Peña, E.; Calvo, B.; Martínez, M.A.; Doblaré, M. A three-dimensional finite element analysis of the combined behavior of ligaments and menisci in the healthy human knee joint. *J. Biomech.* **2006**, *39*, 1686–1701. [CrossRef]
22. Zheng, K. The Effect of High Tibial Osteotomy Correction Angle on Cartilage and Meniscus Loading Using Finite Element Analysis. Master's Thesis, University of Sydney, Sydney, Australia, 2014.
23. Lou, Y. Biomechanical Characteristics of Lower Limbs in Freestyle Skiing Aerial Skill Athletes duringDifferent Landing Postures. *Chin. J. Sport. Med.* **2016**, *35*, 333–338.
24. Potthast, W.; Brueggemann, G.P.; Lundberg, A.; Arndt, A. Relative movements between the tibia and femur induced by external plantar shocks are controlled by muscle forces in vivo. *J. Biomech.* **2011**, *44*, 1144–1148. [CrossRef]
25. Ewing, K.A.; Fernandez, J.W.; Begg, R.K.; Galea, M.P.; Lee, P.V.S. Prophylactic knee bracing alters lower-limb muscle forces during a double-leg drop landing. *J. Biomech.* **2016**, *49*, 3347–3354. [CrossRef]
26. Zhao, X.; Gu, Y. Single leg landing movement differences between male and female badminton players after overhead stroke in the backhand-side court. *Hum. Mov. Sci.* **2019**, *66*, 142–148. [CrossRef]

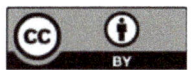 © 2019 by the authors. Licensee MDPI, Basel, Switzerland. This article is an open access article distributed under the terms and conditions of the Creative Commons Attribution (CC BY) license (http://creativecommons.org/licenses/by/4.0/).

*Article*

# Improvement of the Cardiac Oscillator Based Model for the Simulation of Bundle Branch Blocks

**Gian Carlo Cardarilli \*, Luca Di Nunzio \*, Rocco Fazzolari \*, Marco Re and Francesca Silvestri**

Department of Electronic Engineering, University of Rome Tor Vergata, 00133 Roma, Italy
\* Correspondence: g.cardarilli@uniroma2.it (G.C.C.); di.nunzio@ing.uniroma2.it (L.D.N.); fazzolari@ing.uniroma2.it (R.F.)

Received: 15 July 2019; Accepted: 27 August 2019; Published: 4 September 2019

**Abstract:** In this paper, we propose an improvement of the cardiac conduction system based on three modified Van der Pol oscillators. Each oscillator represents one of the components of the heart conduction system: Sino-Atrial node (*SA*), Atrio-Ventricular node (*AV*) and His–Purkinje system (*HP*). However, while *SA* and *AV* nodes can be modelled through a single oscillator, the modelling of *HP* by using a single oscillator is a rough simplification of the cardiac behaviour. In fact, the *HP* bundle is composed of Right (*RB*) and Left Bundle (*LB*) branches that serve, respectively, the right and left ventricles. In order to describe the behaviour of each bundle branch, we build a *phenomenological* model based on four oscillators: *SA*, *AV*, *RB* and *LB*. For the characterization of the atrial and ventricular muscles, we used the modified FitzHugh–Nagumo (*FHN*) equations. The numerical simulation of the model has been implemented in Simulink. The simulation results show that the new model is able to reproduce the heart dynamics generating, besides the physiological signal, also the pathological rhythm in case of Right Bundle Branch Block (RBBB) and Left Bundle Branch Block (LBBB). In particular, our model is able to describe the communication interruption of the conduction system, when one of the *HP* bundle branches is damaged.

**Keywords:** heart model; Van der Pol; FitzHugh–Nagumo; relaxation oscillator; electrocardiographic signal

---

## 1. Introduction

The human heart is a complex electro-pump that, through cycles of depolarization and repolarization, makes the propagation of the action potential, and consequently the contraction of the cardiac muscle tissue, possible. The electrical activity of the heart can be indirectly measured by the electrocardiogram (ECG), a non-invasive method based on 12 electrodes positioned on the body surface [1,2].

Considering the crucial role that the ECG signal plays in the clinical practice, different techniques were presented in the literature in order to model the dynamics of the heartbeat. The electrical and muscular activities of the heart were analyzed through both mathematical modeling and time series analysis [3]. By using mathematical modeling, it is possible to understand the electrical activation of the heart obtaining, by simulation, both normal and abnormal rhythms [4–6]. The generation of synthetic ECG signals with a wide range of waveform shapes and heart rates allows the modeling of the characteristics of each subpart composing the cardiac conduction system, and the understanding of its behaviour [7–11]. The nonlinearity and nonstationarity of the cardiovascular system make the use of nonlinear techniques for the modelling of heart activity useful [12–14]. Van der Pol (VdP) and Van der Mark described and modeled the behavior of heart using nonlinear relaxation oscillators [15].

FitzHugh [16] proposed an extended version of the Van der Pol equations for the generation of the action potential. In his work, he proposed a model for the emulation of the signal observed in an excitable cell of a living organism. The model is composed of two coupled, nonlinear ordinary differential equations. The first equation describes the evolution of the neuronal membrane voltage (fast action), while the second one the recovery action of the sodium and potassium channels (slow action) [17]. Grudzinski and Zebrowski modified the Van der Pol model to allow the reproduction of the time series of the action potential generated by a natural pacemaker [18,19]. In their model, the intrinsic frequency of the two pacemakers can be changed without the need to change the length of the refractory period. Although the model allows the manipulation of both the diastolic and the refractory period, the frequency obtained is too low if compared with the physiological values. Gois and Savi [20] proposed a mathematical model always based on the Van der Pol equations, but composed of three modified oscillators. This model is able to emulate the cardiac conduction system composed of a Sino-Atrial node (SA), Atrio-Ventricular node (AV) and His–Purkinje system (HS). The oscillators are connected to each other through time-delayed couplings. This model allows for generating the electrical response of the main cardiac pacemakers and obtaining the ECG wave as a composition of these signals. Although this model reproduces normal and pathological ECG signals, it does not model the activity of atrial and ventricular muscles. The characterization of muscle electrical responses proposed by Ryzhii [21] uses a quiescent excitable FitzHugh–Nagumo-type (FHN) oscillator. Successively, in [22,23], the authors improved this model by including the depolarization and repolarization waves of the atrial and ventricules generated by modified FHN systems for each ECG wave. The advanced model was able to generate normal ECG signals and several well-known rhythm disorders. In particular, it reproduces sinus tachycardia, sinus bradycardia, complete *SA–AV* block and complete *AV–HP* block [24].

In the models proposed in [20–22], the cardiac conduction system was treated as a network of three modified Van der Pol oscillators representing *SA*, *AV* nodes and the *HP* system. While *SA* and *AV* nodes can be modelled by using oscillators, the modeling of the *HP* system by using a single oscillator is a simplification of the cardiac activity as shown in [20–22] where the electrical behaviour of right and left bundle branches that composes the His–Purkinje system (Figure 1a) is modelled by using a single oscillator. By using this approach, it is not possible to characterize bundle branches of electrical conduction diseases. In the physiological condition, when the ventricular contraction occurs, the Purkinje fibers bring the impulse from the left and right bundle branches to the ventricles' myocardium. In this way, the contraction of ventricles muscle tissue and the ejection of blood outside the heart are allowed. However, the degradation of one of the bundle branches causes a defect called *Bundle Branch Block* (BBB) that implies an alteration of the pathways for the ventricular depolarization [25].

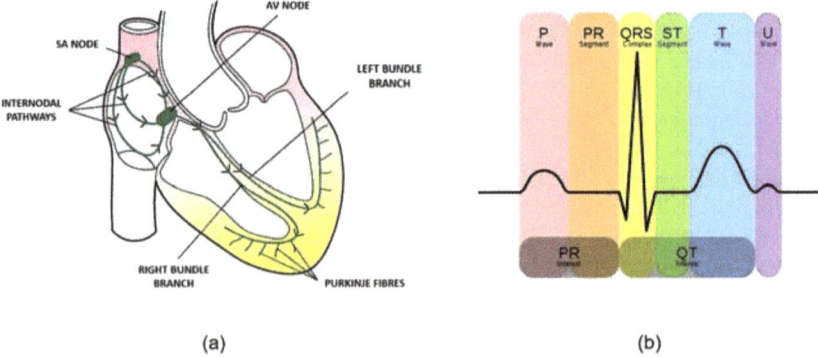

**Figure 1.** Electrophysiology of the heart (**a**) cardiac conduction system; (**b**) normal ECG waveform.

This work proposes a mathematical improvement of the Rizhii model [22] to better describe the heart rhythm by considering four coupled modified Van der Pol oscillators. Besides the use of two oscillators to describe *SA* and *AV* nodes, we use two additional oscillators to describe the right and left bundle branches of the His–Purkinje system. In this way, it is possible to reproduce different pathological conditions, such as the bundle branch blocks. Moreover, the FitzHugh–Nagumo (FHN) oscillators are used to describe the electrical process in the cardiac muscles. We underline that the proposed improved model corresponds to a phenomenological model [26]. The paper is organized as follows: in Section 2, the heart conduction system and mathematical models are shown. In Section 3, results of simulations are shown, and, finally, in Section 5, conclusions are drawn.

## 2. Heart Conduction System and Mathematical Models

Since the dynamic evolution of the heart action potential are close to the dynamical response of the Van der Pol oscillator (VdP) [15], this approach has been widely used in the modelling of the heart conduction system [18,20,21,27–31]. In our model, we modify the heterogeneous oscillator model used for the generation of the ECG signals as proposed by Ryzhii [21]. In addition to coupled VdP oscillators for the $SA$ and $AV$ nodes modeling, we use two additional oscillators to model the right and left bundle branches of the $HP$ system. Furthermore, we modify the excitable FitzHugo–Nagumo equations to take into account the two additional oscillators (right branch (RB) and left branch (LB)). Figure 2 shows the Ryzhii model and the proposed model. In order to better understand the improved model, in the first part of the following section, we provide a theoretical overview of the heart conduction system and a description of the Ryzhii model.

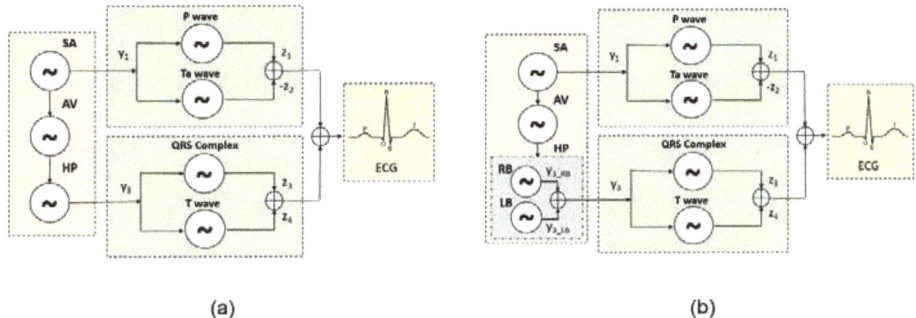

**Figure 2.** Heart mathematical models. (**a**) Ryzhii model [22], based on three oscillators; (**b**) modified model, based on four oscillators.

*2.1. Conduction System of the Heart*

The cardiac conduction system shown in Figure 1a is composed of a group of muscle cells characterized by their own electrical activity that generates the contraction of the cardiac muscles; the Sino-Atrial node ($SA$), the Atrio-Ventricular node ($AV$), branches of the right and left beam, and Purkinje fibers.

The $SA$ node is placed in the right atrium and it is the natural cardiac pacemaker. These cells are known as pacemakers because they manifest a spontaneous depolarization. They are able to reach the action potential threshold faster than every other cell. Thanks to this feature, they manage the heart rhythm [32]. The depolarization rises from the SA node, spreads in the whole right and left atria and finally reaches the $AV$ node.

Then, it proceeds along the bundle of his spreading to both left and right bundle branches depolarizing the left and right ventricles. The electrocardiogram (ECG) is a measure of how electrical activity changes during each cardiac cycle [33]. Figure 1b shows a typical ECG waveform.

The atrial depolarization phase is represented by the P wave, the ventricular depolarization by the QRS complex, and the ventricular repolarization by the T wave. In physiological conditions, the $SA$ node works at 60–100 bpm, faster than any other cell; the only conducting path from atria to ventricles is provided by the $AV$ node. If the $SA$ node has a disease and it fails to generate impulses, the cells of the *AV* node can stimulate the heart at a rate of about 40–60 bpm [32]. If this node also presents damaged cells, the atrial-ventricular conduction block occurs. Depending on the entity of the damage, the block can be complete or partial. In this case, not all the electrical signals generated by the *SA* node are transmitted to the *HP* system. If no excitation signal is delivered from *SA* or *AV* nodes, the *HP* cells can fire at a rate of about 20–40 bpm. However, if the right or left bundle branch of the *HP* system is corrupted, the respective ventricle is not contracted.

This condition is known as Bundle Branch Block (BBB) and it implies an alteration of the pathways for ventricular depolarization. When this condition occurs, the electrical impulse can move through muscle fibers both slowing the electrical activity and changing the propagation direction of the pulses [34].

### 2.2. Mathematical Model

Ryzhii in [22] describes the three natural pacemakers *SA*, *AV* and the *HP* bundle by a system of modified VdP equations:

$$\mathbf{SA} = \begin{cases} \dot{x}_1 = y_1, \\ \dot{y}_1 = -a_1 y_1 (x_1 - u_{11})(x_1 - u_{12}) - f_1 x_1 (x_1 + d_1)(x_1 + e_1), \end{cases} \quad (1)$$

$$\mathbf{AV} = \begin{cases} \dot{x}_2 = y_2, \\ \dot{y}_2 = -a_2 y_2 (x_2 - u_{21})(x_2 - u_{22}) - f_2 x_2 (x_2 + d_2)(x_2 + e_2) + K_{SA-AV}(y_1^{\tau_{SA-AV}} - y_2), \end{cases} \quad (2)$$

$$\mathbf{HP} = \begin{cases} \dot{x}_3 = y_3, \\ \dot{y}_3 = -a_3 y_3 (x_3 - u_{31})(x_3 - u_{32}) - f_3 x_3 (x_3 + d_3)(x_3 + e_3) + K_{AV-HP}(y_2^{\tau_{AV-HP}} - y_3), \end{cases} \quad (3)$$

where $x_i(t)$ and $y_i(t)$ correspond to the action potential and the transmembrane currents of the heart, $a_i(x_i - u_{ij})(x_i - u_{ik})$ are the damping factors, $f_i x_i (x_i - d_{ij})(x_i - e_{ik})$ are the harmonic force terms, $a_i > 0$, $u_{ij}$ represent the nonlinear damping force parameters, $f_i$ are the parameters related to the intrinsic frequency of the oscillator, the coupling coefficients $K_{SA-AV}$ and $K_{AV-HP}$ represent the unidirectional coupling between the SA, AV and HP pacemakers, $y_i^{\tau_n} \equiv y_i(t - \tau_n)$ are the velocity coupling components of the time-delay signal, and $\tau_n$ are the time delays [18,20]. The synchronism between the three oscillators depends on the coupling coefficients $K$ [35,36]. A lot of coupling methods can be found in the literature [37–39]. However, it is possible to avoid the use of delays $\tau_n$ in the coupling terms by choosing the appropriate coupling coefficients $K_{SA-AV}$ and $K_{AV-HP}$. In conclusion, the VdP Equations (1)–(3) become

$$\mathbf{SA} = \begin{cases} \dot{x}_1 = y_1, \\ \dot{y}_1 = -a_1 y_1 (x_1 - u_{11})(x_1 - u_{12}) - f_1 x_1 (x_1 + d_1)(x_1 + e_1), \end{cases} \quad (4)$$

$$\mathbf{AV} = \begin{cases} \dot{x}_2 = y_2, \\ \dot{y}_2 = -a_2 y_2 (x_2 - u_{21})(x_2 - u_{22}) - f_2 x_2 (x_2 + d_2)(x_2 + e_2) + K_{SA-AV}(x_1 - x_2), \end{cases} \quad (5)$$

$$\mathbf{HP} = \begin{cases} \dot{x}_3 = y_3, \\ \dot{y}_3 = -a_3 y_3 (x_3 - u_{31})(x_3 - u_{32}) - f_3 x_3 (x_3 + d_3)(x_3 + e_3) + K_{AV-HP}(x_2 - x_3). \end{cases} \quad (6)$$

Starting from this model, we propose improvements to describe the phenomenological behaviour of the right and left bundle branch. Leaving the *SA* and *AV* node equations (Equations (4) and (5)) unaltered, we describe the right bundle branch (*RB*) and the left bundle branch (*LB*) as

$$\text{SA} = \begin{cases} \dot{x}_1 = y_1, \\ \dot{y}_1 = -a_1 y_1 (x_1 - u_{11})(x_1 - u_{12}) - f_1 x_1 (x_1 + d_1)(x_1 + e_1), \end{cases} \quad (7)$$

$$\text{AV} = \begin{cases} \dot{x}_2 = y_2, \\ \dot{y}_2 = -a_2 y_2 (x_2 - u_{21})(x_2 - u_{22}) - f_2 x_2 (x_2 + d_2)(x_2 + e_2) + K_{SA-AV}(x_1 - x_2), \end{cases} \quad (8)$$

$$\text{RB} = \begin{cases} \dot{x}_{3_{RB}} = y_{3_{RB}}, \\ \dot{y}_{3_{RB}} = -a_3 y_{3_{RB}}(x_{3_{RB}} - u_{31})(x_{3_{RB}} - u_{32}) - f_3 x_{3_{RB}}(x_{3_{RB}} + d_3)(x_{3_{RB}} + e_3) + K_{AV-RB}(x_2 - x_{3_{RB}}), \end{cases} \quad (9)$$

$$\text{LB} = \begin{cases} \dot{x}_{3_{LB}} = y_{3_{LB}}, \\ \dot{y}_{3_{LB}} = -a_3 y_{3_{LB}}(x_{3_{LB}} - u_{31})(x_{3_{LB}} - u_{32}) - f_3 x_{3_{LB}}(x_{3_{LB}} + d_3)(x_{3_{LB}} + e_3) + K_{AV-LB}(x_2 - x_{3_{LB}}). \end{cases} \quad (10)$$

In the physiological condition, the right and left bundle branches are synchronized and the sum of their behaviour has to be the same as the *HP* oscillator:

$$y_{3_{HP}} = \alpha_1 y_{3_{RB}} + \alpha_2 y_{3_{LB}}, \quad (11)$$

where $\alpha_1$ and $\alpha_2$ are coefficients used to adjust the oscillation amplitudes. In order to obtain the physiological signal, we set $\alpha_1 = 0.5$ and $\alpha_2 = 0.5$. In this manner, each oscillator is weighted at 50% in the generation of the signal. This is because, in a normal rhythm, the contribution of the left and the right bundle branch is the same.

The parameters $a_i$, $u_{ij}$, $f_i$, $d_i$, $e_i$, are chosen to obtain intrinsic oscillation rates of 70 bpm, 50 bpm, 35 bpm and 35 bpm for uncoupled *SA*, *AV*, *RB* and *LB*, respectively (Figure 3) and with behaviour close to action potentials of real pacemakers: [40–42].

In particular, we use the following experimental parameters: $a_1 = 40$, $a_2 = 50$, $a_3 = 50$, $a_1 = 40$, $u_{11} = 0.83$, $u_{21} = 0.83$, $u_{31} = 0.83$, $u_{12} = -0.83$, $u_{22} = -0.83$, $u_{32} = -0.83$, $f_1 = 25$, $f_2 = 8.4$, $f_3 = 1.5$, $d_1 = 3$, $d_2 = 3$, $d_3 = 3$, $e_1 = 3.5$, $e_2 = 5$, $e_3 = 12$. The coupling coefficients are: $K_{SA-AV} = 100$, $K_{AV-RB} = 285$, $K_{AV-LB} = 285$.

We describe the depolarization and repolarization process for atrial (*AT*) and ventricular (*VN*) muscles starting from the modified FitzHugh–Nagumo model [16,43] proposed by Ryzhii in [22]:

$$\text{P wave} = \begin{cases} \dot{z}_1 = k_1(-c_1 z_1(z_1 - w_{11})(z_1 - w_{12}) - b_1 v_1 - d_1 v_1 z_1 + I_{AT_{De}}), \\ \dot{v}_1 = k_1 h_1(z_1 - g_1 v_1), \end{cases} \quad (12)$$

$$\text{Ta wave} = \begin{cases} \dot{z}_2 = k_2(-c_2 z_2(z_2 - w_{21})(z_2 - w_{22}) - b_2 v_2 - d_2 v_2 z_2 + I_{AT_{Re}}), \\ \dot{v}_2 = k_2 h_2(z_2 - g_2 v_2), \end{cases} \quad (13)$$

$$\text{QRS} = \begin{cases} \dot{z}_3 = k_3(-c_3 z_3(z_3 - w_{31})(z_3 - w_{32}) - b_3 v_3 - d_3 v_3 z_3 + I_{VN_{De}}), \\ \dot{v}_3 = k_3 h_3(z_3 - g_3 v_3), \end{cases} \quad (14)$$

$$\text{T wave} = \begin{cases} \dot{z}_4 = k_4(-c_4 z_4 (z_4 - w_{41})(z_4 - w_{42}) - b_4 v_4 - d_4 v_4 z_4 + I_{VN_{Re}}), \\ \dot{v}_4 = k_4 h_4 (z_4 - g_4 v_4), \end{cases} \quad (15)$$

where $k_i$ are the scaling coefficients. In our work, we used the experimental parameters: $k_1 = 2*10^3$, $k_2 = 4*10^4$, $k_3 = 10^4$, $k_4 = 2*10^3$, $c_1 = c_2 = 0.26$, $c_3 = 0.3$, $c_4 = 0.1$ $b_1 = b_2 = b_4 = 0$, $b_3 = 0.015$, $d_{m_1} = d_{m_2} = 0.4$, $d_{m_3} = 0.09$, $d_{m_4} = 0.1$, $h_1 = h_2 = 0.004$, $h_3 = h_4 = 0.008$, $g_1 = g_2 = g_3 = g_4 = 1$, $w_{11} = 0.13$, $w_{12} = 1.0$, $w_{22} = 1.0$, $w_{21} = 0.19$, $w_{31} = 0.12$, $w_{32} = 1.1$, $w_{41} = 0.22$, $w_{42} = 0.8$.

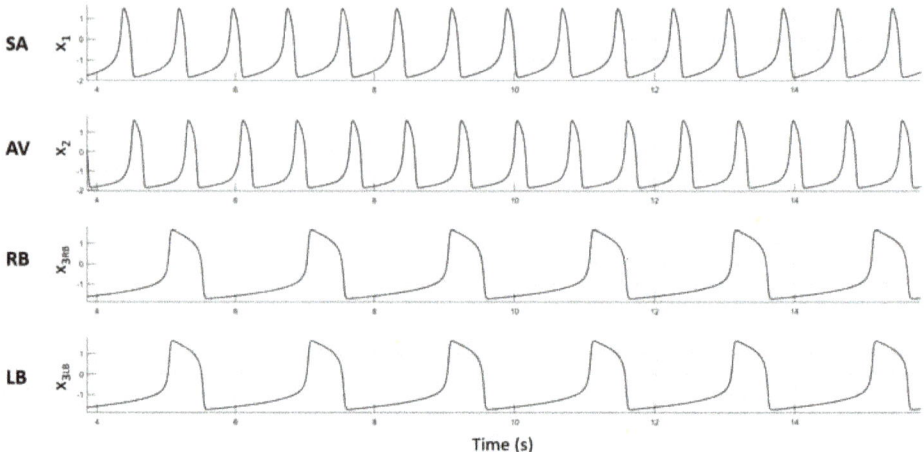

**Figure 3.** Action potentials of uncoupled oscillators. Intrinsic oscillation rates of 70 bpm, 50 bpm, 35 bpm and 35 bpm for uncoupled *SA, AV, RB* and *LB*, respectively.

The activation currents $I_i$ represent the coupling between the *SA* and the *AT* muscles and between the *RB*–*LB* pacemakers and the *VN* muscles. With respect to the Ryzhii model [22], we adjust the activation currents of the QRS complex and T wave in order to have the *HP* oscillator composed of the *RB* and *LB* oscillators:

$$I_{AT_{De}} = \begin{cases} 0, & \text{for } y_1 \leq 0, \\ K_{AT_{De}} y_1, & \text{for } y_1 > 0, \end{cases} \quad (16)$$

$$I_{AT_{Re}} = \begin{cases} -K_{AT_{Re}} y_1, & \text{for } y_1 \leq 0, \\ 0, & \text{for } y_1 > 0, \end{cases} \quad (17)$$

$$I_{VN_{De}} = \begin{cases} 0, & \text{for } y_{3_{HP}} \leq 0, \\ K_{VN_{De}} (y_{3_{RB}}^{tot} + y_{3_{LB}}^{tot}), & \text{for } y_{3_{HP}} > 0, \end{cases} \quad (18)$$

$$I_{VN_{Re}} = \begin{cases} -K_{VN_{Re}} (y_{3_{RB}}^{tot} + y_{3_{LB}}^{tot}), & \text{for } y_{3_{HP}} \leq 0, \\ 0, & \text{for } y_{3_{HP}} > 0. \end{cases} \quad (19)$$

In particular,

$$y_{3_{RB}}^{tot} = \alpha_1 y_{3_{RB}} + \alpha_3 y_{3_{LB}}^{TLB},$$

$$y_{3_{LB}}^{tot} = \alpha_2 y_{3_{LB}} + \alpha_3 y_{3_{RB}}^{TRB}, \tag{20}$$

where $y_{3_{HP}} = (y_{3_{RB}} + y_{3_{LB}})$, $K_{AT_{De}} = 9*10^{-5}$, $K_{AT_{Re}} = 1.5*10^{-5}$, $K_{VN_{De}} = 9*10^{-5}$, $K_{VN_{Re}} = 9*10^{-5}$, $\alpha_1 = 0.5$, $\alpha_2 = 0.5$ and $\alpha_3 = 0.001$.

In Equation (20), the terms $y_{3_{RB}}$ and $y_{3_{LB}}$ represent the impulses traveling through the right and left ventricles and through the bundle branches. The terms $y_{3_{RB}}^{TRB}$ and $y_{3_{LB}}^{TLB}$ represent the impulses traveling through the right and left ventricles through the myocardium cells. These secondary pathways are slower than the main path propagated through the bundle branches. In the physiological case, the contribution of these impulses is negligible with respect to the contribution of the main pathways [12]. On the other hand, in the pathological case, where one branch is damaged, the secondary pathways guarantee the contraction of the ventricle not served by the main pathway. To provide a complete model, we need to take into account the contribution of the secondary pathways. It can be described as an impulse that travels through the bundle branches delayed and attenuated by a multiplicative constant $\alpha_3$. We note that, in the actual case, these secondary impulses travel through the myocardium cells and the propagation of electrical activity should be described with a specific mathematical model. However, the scope of our work is to provide a phenomenological model. For this reason, we assumed that the impulses that travel through the myocardium cells can be modeled as an impulse attenuated and delayed in time.

In the model of the left bundle branch block (LBBB), the activation currents $I_{VN_{De}}$ and $I_{VN_{Re}}$ represent respectively the coupling between the $RB$ and $LB$ pacemakers with the $VN$ muscles; consequently, Equations (18) and (19) become

$$I_{VN_{De}}^{LBBB} = \begin{cases} 0, & \text{for } y_{3_{RB}} \leq 0, \\ K_{VN_{De}}(\alpha_1 y_{3_{RB}} + \alpha_3 y_{3_{RB}}^{TRB}), & \text{for } y_{3_{RB}} > 0, \end{cases} \tag{21}$$

$$I_{VN_{Re}}^{LBBB} = \begin{cases} -K_{VN_{Re}} \alpha_1 y_{3_{RB}}, & \text{for } y_{3_{RB}} \leq 0, \\ 0, & \text{for } y_{3_{RB}} > 0. \end{cases} \tag{22}$$

For LBBB simulation, we set the experimental parameters: $K_{SA-AV} = 100$, $K_{AV-BR} = 285$, $K_{AV-LB} = 0$, $K_{AT_{De}} = 9*10^{-5}$, $K_{AT_{Re}} = 3*10^{-5}$, $K_{VN_{De}} = 9*10^{-5}$, $K_{VN_{Re}} = -8*10^{-5}$, $\tau_{RB} = 0.78$, $\alpha_1 = 1$, $\alpha_3 = 1$ and $\alpha_2 = 0$.

In the model of right bundle branch block (RBBB) the activation currents, $I_{VN_{De}}$ and $I_{VN_{Re}}$ are

$$I_{VN_{De}}^{RBBB} = \begin{cases} K_{VN_{De}}(\alpha_2 y_{3_{LB}} + \alpha_3 y_{3_{LB}}^{TLB}), & \text{for } y_{3_{LB}} < 0, \\ K_{VN_{De}} \alpha_2 y_{3_{LB}}, & \text{for } y_{3_{LB}} > 0, \end{cases} \tag{23}$$

$$I_{VN_{Re}}^{RBBB} = \begin{cases} -K_{VN_{Re}} \alpha_2 y_{3_{LB}}, & \text{for } y_{3_{LB}} < 0, \\ 0, & \text{for } y_{3_{LB}} > 0. \end{cases} \tag{24}$$

For RBBB simulation, we set the experimental parameters: $K_{SA-AV} = 100$, $K_{AV-BR} = 0$, $K_{AV-LB} = 285$, $K_{AT_{De}} = 9*10^{-5}$, $K_{AT_{Re}} = 2*10^{-5}$, $K_{VN_{De}} = 5.5*10^{-5}$, $K_{VN_{Re}} = 7*10^{-5}$, $\tau_{RB} = 0.05$, $\alpha_1 = 0$, $\alpha_2 = 1$ and $\alpha_3 = 1$.

Finally, we obtain the synthetic ECG signal as a composition of the $AT$ and $VN$ waveforms

$$ECG = z_0 + z_1 - z_2 + k_R z_3 + z_4, \tag{25}$$

where $z_0 = 0.2$ provides the adjustment of the baseline and $k_R$ is a multiplicative coefficient to modulate the amplitude of the R peak.

## 3. Results

In order to validate our model, we performed different Simulink simulations reproducing either normal and pathological signals. Simulations are performed using a fixed step Runge–Kutta solver and a fixed step size of 0.0001 seconds. Figure 4 shows the normal condition where all pacemakers are dominated by the SA node. As a consequence, the heart rate follows the SA rate (70 bpm). In this case, both the right and left bundle branches are working, and they give the same contribution. The experimental parameters are the same used in the non-pathological as described in Section 2.

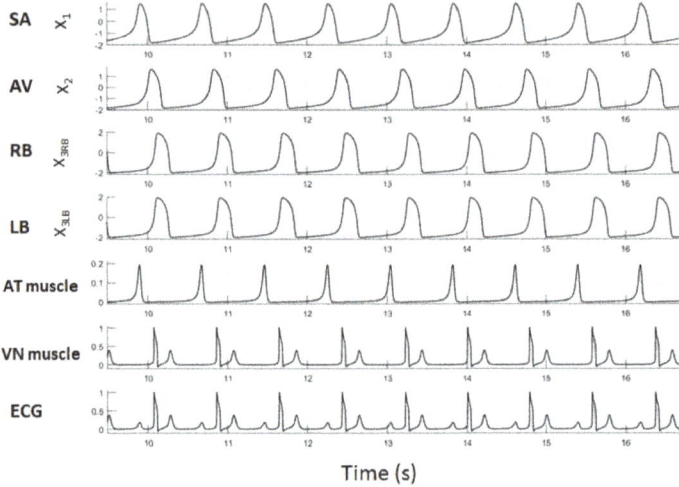

**Figure 4.** Action potentials, muscles response and ECG signal in non-pathological (70 bpm).

Then, we performed a simulation of a pathological condition of the His bundle. We obtain this condition by changing the physiological parameters with the pathological parameters in order to obtain both complete right bundle branch block (RBBB) and complete left bundle branch block (LBBB). The pathological parameters used are shown in Section 2.

**Left Bundle Branch Block** Figure 5 shows the left bundle branch block (LBBB). In this case, the left ventricle is not directly activated by the impulses travelling through the left bundle branch. The right ventricle is normally activated by the right bundle branch signal. These impulses are able to travel through the myocardium of the right ventricle to the left ventricle and depolarize it (yellow arrows in Figure 5). This activation extends the QRS duration to >120 ms [32,33]. The direction of the slow depolarization (from the right to the left) produces tall R-waves in the lateral leads (I, aVL, V5-6) of the electrocardiogram and deep S-waves in the right precordial leads (V1-3). Since the ventricles are activated sequentially (first right then left) rather than simultaneously, this produces a broad or notched ('M'-shaped) R-wave in the lateral leads (I, aVL, V5-6).

Figure 6a shows simulation results for the LBBB case. Experimental parameters: $K_{SA-AV} = 100$, $K_{AV-BR} = 285$, $K_{AV-LB} = 0$, $K_{AT_{De}} = 9*10^{-5}$, $K_{AT_{Re}} = 3*10^{-5}$, $K_{VN_{De}} = 9*10^{-5}$, $K_{VN_{Re}} = -8*10^{-5}$, $\tau_{RB} = 0.78$, $\alpha_1 = 1$, $\alpha_3 = 1$ and $\alpha_2 = 0$.

In this case, the term $y_{3_{LB}}$ in Equation (21) is not present because the contribution of the left bundle branch is zero. On the other hand, the impulse generated by the right bundle brunch $y_{3_{RB}}$ is able to both normally depolarize the right ventricle and to travel towards the left ventricle through the myocardium cells. As this second conduction way is slower than the main bundle of His–Purkinje fibres, the term $y_{3_{RB}}$ in Equation (21) (that represents the left ventricle depolarization) is delayed through the coefficient $\tau_{RB}$. This produces a broad or notched ('M'-shaped) R-wave in the ECG signal (Figure 6b). It is possible to compare simulation results with a real patient's ECG signal affected by LBBB shown in Figure 6c.

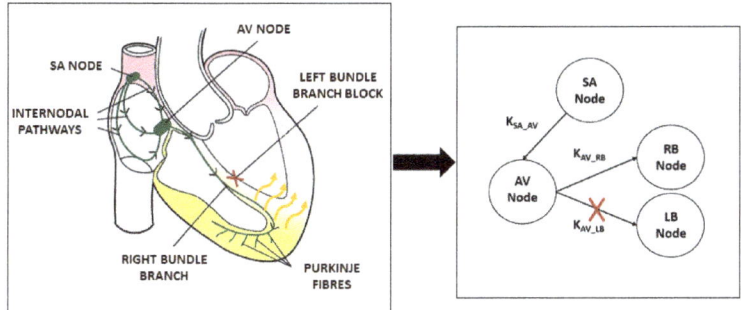

**Figure 5.** Left Bundle Branch Block (LBBB) and the four coupled oscillators model.

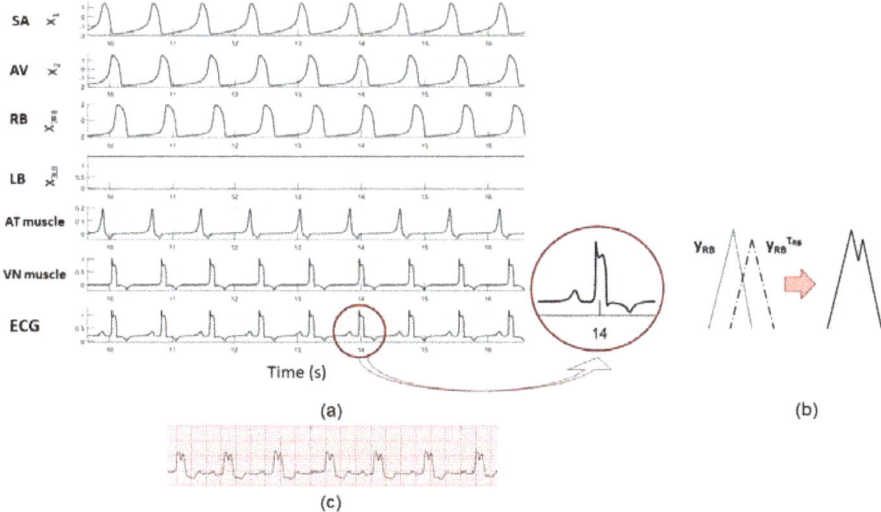

**Figure 6.** Simulation results for Left Bundle Branch Block (LBBB). (**a**) action potentials, muscles response and ECG signal in the LBBB case; (**b**) extra deflection of the QRS complex due to the rapid depolarization of the right ventricle followed by the slower depolarization of the left ventricle; (**c**) real ECG signal affected by LBBB [44].

**Right Bundle Branch Block** In the Right Bundle Branch Block (RBBB), the activation of the right ventricle is delayed because the depolarization has to spread from the left ventricle (yellow arrows in Figure 7). The left ventricle is activated normally and the early part of the QRS complex is unchanged. The delayed right ventricular activation produces a secondary R-wave (R') in the right precordial leads (V1-3) and a wide, slurred S-wave in the lateral leads [32,33] (Figure 7).

In this case, the term $y_{3_{RB}}$ in Equation (24) is not present because the contribution of the right bundle branch is zero. In this case, the impulse is generated by the left bundle brunch $y_{3_{LB}}$ that is able to both normally depolarize the left ventricle and to travel towards the right one through the myocardium cells. Figure 8a shows the simulation results for the RBBB case. For this simulation, we set the following experimental parameters: $K_{SA-AV} = 100$, $K_{AV-BR} = 0$, $K_{AV-LB} = 285$, $K_{AT_{De}} = 9*10^{-5}$, $K_{AT_{Re}} = 2*10^{-5}$, $K_{VN_{De}} = 5.5*10^{-5}$, $K_{VN_{Re}} = 7*10^{-5}$, $\tau_{LB} = 0.05$, $\alpha_1 = 0$, $\alpha_2 = 1$ and $\alpha_3 = 1$. In addition, in this case, it is possible to compare simulation results with a real patient's ECG signal affected by RBBB shown in Figure 8c.

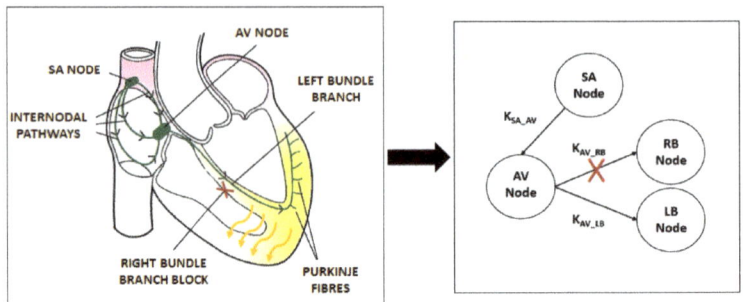

**Figure 7.** Right Bundle Branch Block (RBBB) and relative four coupled oscillators model.

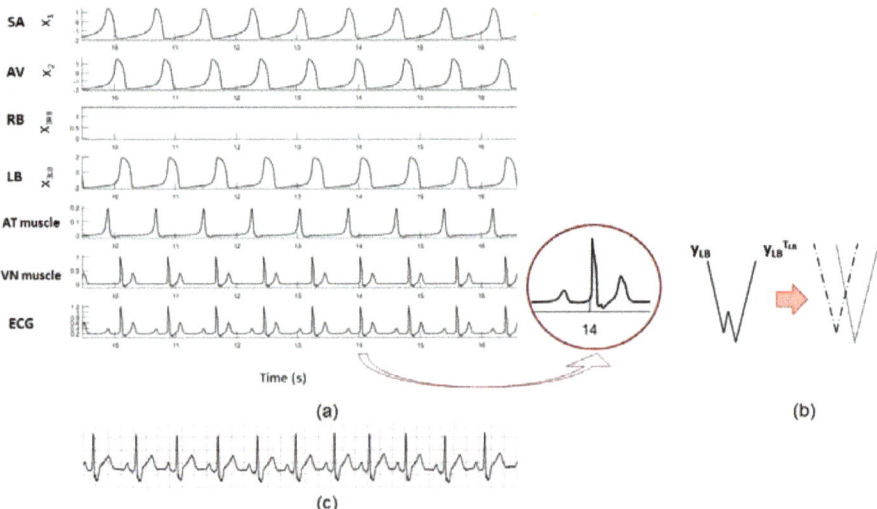

**Figure 8.** Simulation results for Right Bundle Branch block (RBBB). (**a**) action potentials, muscles response and ECG signal in the RBBB case; (**b**) slurred S-wave due to the rapid depolarization of the left ventricle followed by the slower depolarization of the right ventricle; (**c**) real ECG signal affected by RBBB [45].

## 4. Discussion

The model discussed in this paper is an extension of the one proposed in [22]. Both the models (the original proposed by Ryzhii and the one proposed in this paper) are able to generate realistic ECG signals in order to simulate normal and pathological rhythms. The analysis of the synthetic ECG signal generated by the two models can be performed like a real signal of the patient, which is conducted by observing the morphology of different waves and their behavior in time, with specific interest on the QRS complex. This means that, for RBBB and LBBB, as for the other pathologies discussed in this paper and in [22], the anomalies are identified analyzing the shape of the signal and identifying the interest points in which the waves change their morphology. For example, if we want to reproduce the LBBB, we need to modify the shape of the QRS complex, as well as the polarity of the T wave [46]. As shown in Figure 6, selecting proper parameters, our model is able to reproduce the main typical characteristics of the signal related to this pathology.

However, it is important to note that the synthetic signal may not be exactly the same as the patient's actual ECG signal. To generate a synthetic signal closer, but not equal, to the real one, it is possible to modify, inside a specific operating range, the model parameters to obtain different nuances of the same pathological behaviour. This difference is due to the uniqueness of the signal generated by the cardiac activity of each person. It means that it is possible to compare two signals belonging to two different people by observing the waveforms in time and searching the features of interest, but not comparing the shape of the tracks point by point. In addition to personal traits, there are several factors that make any real signal different from any other—for example, the noise due to the acquisition method, the constitution of patient that influenced the transmission of the electrical signal from heart to body surface, the coexistence of different pathologies, and so on. For this reason, nowadays, the interpretation of an ECG signal is mainly performed by physicians by observing the specific characteristics of tracks.

## 5. Conclusions

In the paper, we improve the mathematical model of the heart by using four modified Van der Pol oscillators to describe the electrical activity and we modify the FitzHugh–Nagumo equations to reproduce the behaviour of the cardiac muscle cells. Each oscillator represents one of the main natural pacemakers: Sino-Atrial node (*SA*), Atrio-Ventricular node (*AV*), Right Bundle Branch (*RBB*) and Left Bundle Branch (*LBB*).

Numerical simulations show that the proposed model, based on four oscillators, is able to reproduce the heart behavior by generating the physiological signal like the model proposed by Ryzhii in [22] (based on three oscillators). The main improvement of the proposed model is the description of the His–Purkinje system with two additional oscillators, in order to better describe the behavior of each bundle branch. The model is able to reproduce the communication interruption in the heart electrical conduction system when one of the His bundle branches does not work. In this case, the model reproduces both normal ventricle contraction due to healthy bundle branch and the propagation of action potential through myocardial cells to the ventricle where the bundle branch is pathologically altered.

The waveforms obtained by simulation are comparable with the real ECG signals of patients affected by the LBBB and RBBB pathologies. In other words, the clinical phenotypes observed in the patient's signals are similar to waveform features obtained with our model. In conclusion, the proposed model makes the study of interactions between the main components of the heart possible. It allows simulation and evaluation of heart activity and dynamics under different types of pacemaker coupling. These aspects are widely useful in clinical practice.

**Author Contributions:** Conceptualization, F.S.; methodology, G.C.C. and M.R.; software, F.S, L.D.N and R.F.; validation, F.S, L.D.N and R.F.; formal analysis, F.S.; data curation, F.S, L.D.N and R.F.; writing–original draft preparation, F.S; writing–review and editing, L.D.N and R.F.; supervision, G.C.C. and M.R.

**Conflicts of Interest:** The authors declare no conflict of interest.

## References

1. Kusumoto, F.M. *ECG Interpretation: From Pathophysiology to Clinical Application*; Springer: New York, NY, USA, 2009.
2. Silvestri, F.; Acciarito, S.; Cardarilli, G.C.; Khanal, G.M.; Nunzio, G.M.L.D.; Fazzolari, R.; Re, M. *FPGA Implementation of a Low-Power QRS Extractor*; Lecture Notes in Electrical Engineering; Springer: New York, NY, USA, 2009; pp. 9–15.

3. Silvestri, F.; Cardarilli, G.C.; Nunzio, L.D.; Fazzolari, R.; Re, M. Comparison of Low-Complexity Algorithms for Real-Time QRS Detection using Standard ECG Database. *Int. J. Adv. Sci. Eng. Inf. Technol.* **2018**, *8*, 307–314.
4. Breitenstein, D.S. Cardiovascular Modeling: The Mathematical Exspression of Blood Circulation. Master's Thesis, University of Pittsburgh, Pittsburgh, PA, USA, 1993.
5. Denis, N. Modelling the heart: Insights, failures and progress. *BioEssays* **2002**, *24*, 1155–1163.
6. Cloherty, S.L.; Dokos, S.; Lovell, N.H. *Electrical Activity in Cardiac Tissue, Modeling of American Cancer Society*; John Wiley and Sons: Hoboken, NJ, USA, 2006.
7. McSherry, P.E.; Clifford, G.; Tarassenko, L.; Smith, L.A. A dynamical model for generating synthetic electrocardiogram signals. *IEEE Trans. Biomed. Eng.* **2003**, *50*, 289–294. [CrossRef] [PubMed]
8. McSherry, P.E.; Clifford, G. Open-source software for generating electrocardiogram signals. In Proceedings of the 3rd IASTED International Conference on Biomedical Engineering, Innsbruck, Austria, 16–18 February 2005; pp. 410–414.
9. Pullan, A.J.; Buist, M.L.; Cheg, L.K. *Mathematical Modeling the Electrical Activity of Heart: From Cell to Body Surface and Back Again*; World Scientific: Singapore, 2005.
10. Tusscher, K.H.T.; Panfilov, A.V. Modelling of the ventricular conduction system. *Progr. Biophys. Mol. Biol.* **2008**, *96*, 152–170. [CrossRef] [PubMed]
11. Gidea, M.; Gidea, C.; Byrd, W. Deterministic models for simulating electrocardiographic signals. *Commun. Nonlin. Sci. Numer. Simul.* **2011**, *16*, 3871–3880. [CrossRef]
12. Acharya, U.R. *Advances in Cardiac Signal Processing*; Springer: Berlin, Germany, 2007; p. 33.
13. Thanom, W.; Loh, R.N.K. Nonlinear control of heartbeat models. *Syst. Cybern. Inform.* **2011**, *9*, 21–27.
14. Acharya, U.R.; Faust, O.; Sree, V.; Swapna, G.; Martis, R.J.; Kadri, N.A.; Suri, J.S. Linear and nonlinear analysis of normal and CAD affected heart rate signals. *Comput. Methods Prog. Biomed.* **2014**, *6*, 55–68. [CrossRef]
15. Van der Pol, B.; Van der Mark, J. The heartbeat considered as a relaxation oscillator and an electrical model of the heart. *Phys. A* **1928**, *6*, 763–775.
16. FitzHugh, R. Impulses and physiological states in theoretical models of nerve membrane. *Biophys. J.* **1961**, *1*, 445–446. [CrossRef]
17. Sherwood, W.E. *FitzHugh–Nagumo Model, Encyclopedia of Computational Neuroscience*; Springer: Berlin, Germany, 2014.
18. Grudzinski, K.; Zebrowski, J.J. Modeling cardiac pacemakers with relaxation oscillators. *Phys. A* **2004**, *336*, 153–162. [CrossRef]
19. Zebrowski, J.J.; Grudzinski, K.; Buchner, T.; Kuklik, P.; Gac, J.; Gielark, G.; Sanders, P.; Baranowski, R. Nonlinear oscillator model reproducing various phenomena in the dynamics of the conduction system of the heart. *Chaos* **2007**, *17*, 1–10. [CrossRef] [PubMed]
20. Gois, S.R.S.M.; Savi, M.A. An analysis of heart rhythm dynamics using three-coupled oscillator model. *Chaos Solitons Fractals* **2009**, *41*, 2553–2565. [CrossRef]
21. Ryzhii, E.; Ryzhii, M. Modeling of heartbeat dynamics with a system of coupled nonlinear oscillators. *Commun. Comput. Inf. Sci.* **2014**, *404*, 67–75.
22. Ryzhii, E.; Ryzhii, M. A heterogeneous coupled oscillator model for simulation of ECG signals. *Comput. Methods Programs Biomed.* **2014**, *117*, 40–49. [CrossRef] [PubMed]
23. Ryzhii, E.; Ryzhii, M. Simulink heart model for simulation of the effect of external signals. In Proceedings of the 2016 IEEE Conference on Computational Intelligence in Bioinformatics and Computational Biology (CIBCB), Chiang Mai, Thailand, 5–7 October 2016.
24. Ryzhii, E.; Ryzhii, M. Formation of second degree atrioventricular blocks in the cardiac heterogeneous oscillator model. In Proceedings of the 37th Annual International Conference of the IEEE Engineering in Medicine and Biology Society (EMBC), Milano, Italy, 25–29 August 2015.
25. Macfarlane, P.W.; van Oosterom, A.; Janse, M.; Kligfield, P.; Camm, J.; Pahlm, O. *Electrocardiology: Comprehensive Clinical ECG*; Springer: Berlin, Germany, 2012.
26. Wilholt, T. Explaining Models: Theoretical and Phenomenological Models and Their Role for the First, Explanation of the Hydrogen Spectrum. *Found Chem.* **2005**, *7*, 149–169. [CrossRef]
27. di Beranrdo, D.; Signorini, M.G.; Cerutti, S. A model of two nonlinear coupled oscillators for the study of heartbeat dynamics. *Int. J. Bifurc. Chaos* **1998**, *8*, 1975–1985. [CrossRef]

28. Katholi, C.R.; Urthaler, F.; Macy, J., Jr.; James, T.N. A mathematical model of automaticity in the sinus node and AV junction based on weakly coupled relaxation oscillators. *Comput. Biomed. Res.* **1977**, *10*, 529–543. [CrossRef]
29. Postnov, D.; Kee, H.S.; Hyungtae, K. Synchronization of diffusively coupled oscillators near the homoclinic bifurcation. *Phys. Rev. E* **1999**, *60*, 2799–2807. [CrossRef]
30. Das, S.; Maharatna, K. Fractional dynamical model for the generation of ECG like signals from filtered coupled Van der pol oscillators. *Comput. Methods Prog. Biomed.* **2013**, *112*, 490–507. [CrossRef]
31. Suchorsky, M.; Rand, R. Three oscillator model of the heartbeat generator. *Commun. Nonlin. Sci. Numer. Simul.* **2009**, *14*, 2434–2449. [CrossRef]
32. Laske, T.G.; Iaizzo, P.A. *Handbook of Cardiac Anatomy, Physiology, and Devices, 9-The Cardiac Conduction System*; Springer: Berlin, Germany, 2005; pp. 123–136.
33. Dupre, A.; Vincent, S.; Iaizzo, P.A. *Handbook of Cardiac Anatomy, Physiology, and Devices, 15-Basic ECG Theory, Recordings and Interpretation*; Springer: Berlin, Germany, 2005; pp. 191–202.
34. Acharya, U.R. *Advances in Cardiac Signal Processing, 1-The Electrocardiogram*; Springer: Berlin, Germany, 2007.
35. Santos, A.M.D.; Lopes, S.R.; Viana, R.L. Rhythm syncronization land chaotic modulation of coupled van der Pol oscillators in a model for the heartbeat. *Phys. A* **2004**, *338*, 335–355. [CrossRef]
36. Ryzhii, E.; Ryzhii, M.; Savchenko, V. Effect of coupling on the pacemaker synchronization in coupled oscillator ECG model. In Proceedings of the Conference on Biomedical Engineering and Sciences: "Miri, Where Engineering in Medicine and Biology and Humanity Meet", Kuala Lumpur, Malaysia, 8–10 December 2014; pp. 281–286.
37. Yaneyama, M.; Kawahara, K. Coupled oscillator systems of cultured cardiac myocytes:fluctuation and scaling properties. *Phys. Rev. E* **2004**, *70*, 1–9.
38. Santos, A.M.D.; Lopes, S.R.; Viana, R.L. Syncronization regimes for two coupled noisy Lienard-type drive oscillators. *Chaos Solit. Fract.* **2008**, *36*, 901–910. [CrossRef]
39. Wirkus, S.; Rand, R. The dynamics of two coupled Van der Pol oscillators with delay coupling. *Nonlin. Dyn.* **2002**, *30*, 205–221. [CrossRef]
40. Boyett, M.R.; Honjo, H.; Kodama, I. The sinoatrial node, aheterogeneous pacemaker structure. *Cardiovasc. Res.* **2000**, *47*, 658–687. [CrossRef]
41. Meijler, F.L.; Janse, M.J. Morphology and electrophysiology ofthe mammalian atrioventricular node. *Physiol. Rev.* **1988**, *68*, 608–647. [CrossRef] [PubMed]
42. Boyden, P.A.; Hirose, M.; Dun, W. Cardiac Purkinje cells. *HeartRhythm* **2010**, *7*, 127–135. [CrossRef]
43. Rocşoreanu, C.; Georgescu, A.; Giurgiteanu, N. An active pulse trasmission line simulating nerve axon. *Proc. IRE* **1962**, *50*, 2061–2070.
44. Available online: https://en.ecgpedia.org (accessed on 27 March 2019).
45. Available online: https://www.physionet.org/physiobank/database/html/mitdbdir/mitdbdir.html (accessed on 21 March 2019).
46. Available online: http://courses.kcumb.edu/physio/blocks/index.htm (accessed on 12 March 2019).

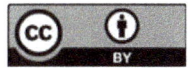

© 2019 by the authors. Licensee MDPI, Basel, Switzerland. This article is an open access article distributed under the terms and conditions of the Creative Commons Attribution (CC BY) license (http://creativecommons.org/licenses/by/4.0/).

*Article*

# PANDAS: Paediatric Attention-Deficit/Hyperactivity Disorder Application Software

### Hervé Mukenya Mwamba *[ID], Pieter Rousseau Fourie and Dawie van den Heever

Biomedical Engineering Research Group (BERG), Department of Mechanical & Mechatronic Engineering, University of Stellenbosch, Cape Town 7602, South Africa; pieter@innovation4life.com (P.R.F.); dawie@sun.ac.za (D.v.d.H.)
* Correspondence: hervemwamba279@gmail.com; Tel.: +27-60-821-1001

Received: 23 February 2019; Accepted: 28 March 2019; Published: 20 April 2019

**Abstract:** Attention-deficit/hyperactivity disorder (ADHD) is a common neuropsychiatric disorder that impairs social, academic and occupational functioning in children, adolescents and adults. In South Africa, youth prevalence of ADHD is estimated as 10%. It is therefore necessary to further investigate methods that objectively diagnose, treat and manage the disorder. The aim of the study was to develop a novel method that could be used as an aid to provide screening for ADHD. The study comprised of a beta-testing phase that included 30 children (19 non-ADHD and 11 ADHD) between the ages of 5 and 16 years old. The strategy was to use a tablet-based game that gathered real-time user data during game-play. This data was then used to train a linear binary support vector machine (SVM). The objective of the SVM was to differentiate between an ADHD individual versus a non-ADHD individual. A feature set was extracted from the gathered data and sequential forward selection (SFS) was performed to select the most significant features. The test set accuracy of 85.7% and leave-one-out cross-validation (LOOCV) accuracy of 83.5% were achieved. Overall, the classification accuracy of the trained SVM was 86.5%. Finally, the sensitivity of the model was 75% and this was seen as a moderate result. Since the sample size was fairly small, the results of the classifier were only seen as suggestive rather than conclusive. Therefore, the performance of the classifier was indicative that a quantitative tool could indeed be developed to perform screening for ADHD.

**Keywords:** ADHD; screening; machine learning; SVM; children; novel

## 1. Introduction

Attention-deficit/hyperactivity disorder (ADHD) is a brain disorder marked by an ongoing pattern of inattention and/or hyperactivity-impulsiveness that interferes with functioning or development [1]. Its exact origins are uncertain and complex [2] and its diagnosis relies almost exclusively on subjective assessments of perceived behaviour [3]. This presents some unresolved dilemmas. Firstly, there is a potential risk of over-diagnosis. Secondly, males are more likely to be diagnosed compared to females of the same age [4]. Finally, objective diagnostic methods are scarce. Furthermore, it is important to note the significant financial burden associated with the treatment and management of ADHD. It is estimated that for an adult with ADHD, the economic burden is approximately $3020 per annum [5].

Diagnosis of ADHD is based on clinical criteria defined by the Diagnostic and Statistical Manual of Mental Disorders (DSM 5), or the International Classification of Diseases (ICD 10) [2]. Proper diagnosis involves clinical interviews, patient history, psychometric testing and rating scales [6]. Since comorbidity may occur, diagnosis is patient-specific. It is observed that environmental factors such as peri/pre-natal, psychological and dietary, contribute to the development and severity of ADHD, but these factors may be consequential rather than causal [2]. Furthermore, the consensus is that ADHD is associated with dysfunction of the prefrontal cortex [7–9].

Various methods exist, where objective diagnosis was attempted, with some degree of success. The first category of method is computerized. The most popular and efficient computerized approach is continuous performance testing (CPT). The Conners CPT 3 test [10] is a commercially available test that evaluates attention disorders and neurological functioning. Its aim is to provide an objective evaluation of individuals aged eight years and older. During the 14-minute-long assessment, subjects are to click whenever any letter except 'X' appears on the screen. Using a normative sample of 1400 subjects, representative of an American population, it was found that the classification accuracy was 83.90%, the sensitivity 86% and the specificity 81%.

An example of a tool that integrates the Conners CPT 3 test in a more interactive manner is called MOXO. Instead of presenting the subject with the letter 'X', the subject must click whenever a specific face appears on the screen. Additional studies [11–13] have been done using MOXO to further validate the discriminatory ability of CPT testing. In these studies, comparisons were made between ADHD and non-ADHD groups with regards to the number of omission errors during the test. The difference between the studies was that different age groups were used, and different environmental distractors were used. It was found that when using MOXO, the sensitivity was between 81–91% (depending on the age group) and the specificity was between 85–89%. However, the studies did not focus on measuring the classification accuracy of MOXO and only used the sensitivity and specificity as the performance metrics.

In addition to MOXO, it was also found that objective diagnosis of ADHD could be attempted using inertial sensors that were mounted to subjects and that captured data for one hour through various scenarios [14]. Classification was then done with a linear support vector machine (SVM) model. The results found in the study were that the classification accuracy was 95.12%, the specificity 95.65% and the sensitivity 94.44%.

Additionally, there has been an FDA-approved device called NEBA that uses electroencephalogram signals to aid clinicians to make diagnoses. The most recent study [15] where NEBA was used was done in 2015. The aim of the study was to determine correlation between the diagnosis from NEBA and diagnosis from the consensus of a team of experts. It was found that the combination of NEBA and consensus diagnosis yielded 97% accuracy.

Finally, a study where neuroimaging was used to monitor activity in specific regions of the brain, namely, the pre-frontal cortex, is found in literature [8]. The major conclusions of this study were that a quantitative analysis of neuroanatomical abnormalities in ADHD was provided and that this could be used as the starting point of other studies.

Other challenges of ADHD are its treatment and management. For children between the ages of 6 and 18 years old, symptoms are typically identified in a classroom setting [2]. Specialists such as child psychologists will then interview the whole family and provide the parents and the teacher(s) with questionnaires called rating scales. Furthermore, the patient undergoes a series of psychometric tests. Based on the results of the rating scales as well as those of the psychometric tests, a thorough diagnosis is made, and a treatment plan is drawn up. The patient then goes for follow-up sessions, generally after every 6 months. This process represents the ideal case of identifying and diagnosing ADHD [2]. However, many schoolchildren are not identified as potential ADHD patients. This presents the need for a screening tool that may help identify the disorder from an early stage, such as in a classroom setting.

Since ADHD is defined by the Diagnostic and Statistical Manual for mental health, it can only be diagnosed clinically by a specialist (psychiatrist, psychologist, paediatrician etc.). Any other diagnosis cannot be given. Given this fact, the aim of the study was not to provide a diagnosis, but to provide screening. Ultimately, although there may be various methods and technologies that may claim to provide diagnosis, but clinically speaking, DSM 5 criteria must be met for an individual to be classified as having ADHD.

Thus, the aim of the study was to develop a novel method that provided rapid screening for the hyperactive subtype of ADHD. A concurrent study was done where the screening was done for the inattentive subtype. The output of the study was a diagnostic aid rather than a diagnostic tool. The final diagnosis was still to be given by a specialist. The study was broken down into the following different phases/objectives: (1) identification of measurable parameters for ADHD based on DSM-5 criteria and psychometric tests; (2) design and development of the tablet-based game; (3) performing beta-tests to gather data; (4) development of SVM classifier.

Since mobile tablets have become popular and very accessible to the general public, playing games on tablets has become a ubiquitous activity. The fact that tablet games are popular and enjoyable made it a good choice for the platform to use for the novel method developed in the study.

## 2. Software Design

The software that was used was in the form of a tablet-based game with an underlying layer of data processing. The main aspect of this two-layer approach was to use the game layer as input to the data-processing layer.

### 2.1. Game Design

A tablet-based game was developed using Unreal Engine v.4.18.0, one of the most popular and reliable platforms for game development for electronic devices. The device that was chosen was the NVIDIA K1 Shield Tablet. The theme that was chosen considered the age group of the subjects that were used for the research. Since the subjects were schoolchildren a jungle/tropical theme was a logical choice.

The objective of the task was to travel on a raft from one end of a river to the other end as quickly as possible. This had to be done while avoiding obstacles and collecting as many gems as possible. The speed of the raft increased as the game progressed, provided that no obstacles were hit. Three straight lanes were present, and the user was able to move to the left or right lane, while the middle lane was the default position. Figure 1 shows a screenshot of the game. The buttons can be seen at the bottom left and right corners of the screen. The buttons were used to navigate between the lanes, jump over incoming obstacles and throw objects at incoming obstacles in order to destroy them. The number of gems collected is displayed in the top left corner and the PANDA character is in the middle bottom section.

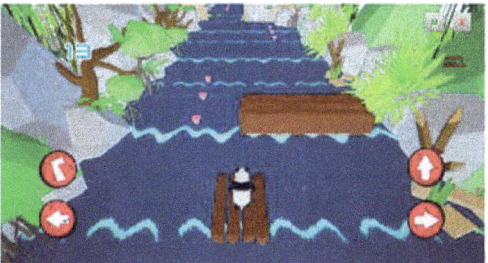

**Figure 1.** Screenshot of Game.

### 2.2. Data Processing

The data processing layer was broken down into three phases: data gathering, data storage and data extraction. This data processing was essential in building the SVM classifier. The raw data that was captured during game-play could be broken down into three categories: 1. personal user data; 2. game-play variables and; 3. accelerometer data. Personal user data was user-specific and included the following: age, gender, race, game enjoyment ("yes" or "no") and diagnosis (ADHD or non-ADHD). This data was captured manually by the test administrator at the end of a game session and recorded onto an Excel spreadsheet, where each user was given a unique identifier for traceability within the spreadsheet. The use of game-play variables and accelerometer variables was derived from translating the applicable DSM-V criteria into measurable parameters. Thus, the resulting parameters were the following: mistakes made, task completion time, task termination, distractibility, forgetfulness, sustained attention, sustained attention and device motion. The accelerometer data contained raw time-series data from the tri-axial accelerometer on the device. All this data was then stored on a cloud Firebase database. This is illustrated in Figure 2.

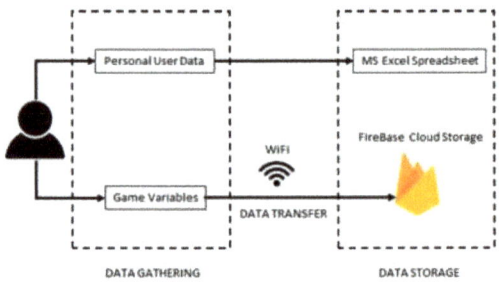

Figure 2. Data Gathering and Data Storage Flow.

Once the data was stored on the cloud, it could be downloaded from the Firebase database into .json files, where each .json file contained individual game session data. File processing was then done to extract the data from the .json files and store them into appropriate structures (matrices) for the SVM classifier. Figure 3 shows the file extraction process, which was implemented in MATLAB.

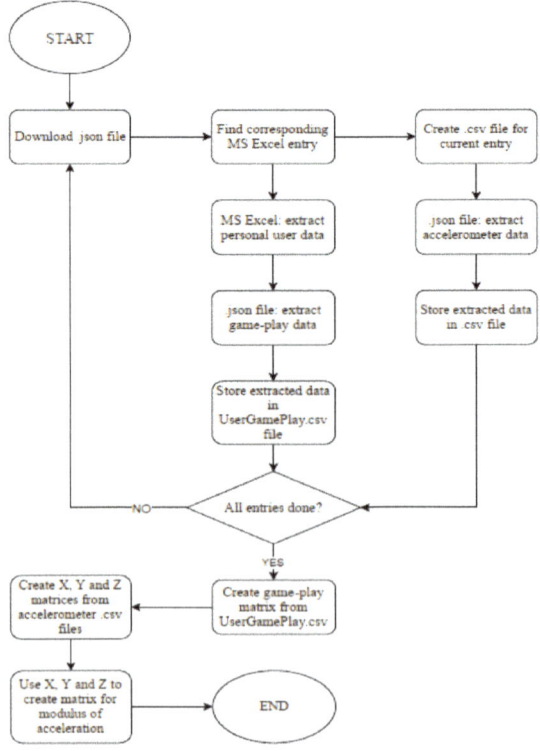

Figure 3. Data Extraction Process.

## 3. Methods

*3.1. Subjects*

The beta-test consisted of 30 subjects between the ages of 5 and 16 years of old. These subjects had been consulted by a specialist at a private paediatric practice at the Cape Gate Medi-Clinic. Subject participation was completely voluntary and parental consent was sought using information leaflets. The subjects also had to read and sign assent forms. The main inclusion criterion was age, since ADHD is most prevalent in minors. Furthermore, gender ratio was kept as closely as possible to 1:1. Children with a known history of severe mental illness were excluded. Additionally, children that suffered from photosensitive epilepsy were also excluded given the fact that the game images on the screen of the tablet could possibly trigger convulsions. Table 1 shows a breakdown of subject distribution.

**Table 1.** Subject Distribution; ADHD: Attention-deficit/hyperactivity disorder.

| Category | Value |
| --- | --- |
| Mean age | 10 y/o |
| Maximum age | 16 y/o |
| Minimum age | 5 y/o |
| Number of males | 16 |
| Number of females | 14 |
| Number of ADHD males | 6 |
| Number of ADHD females | 7 |
| Number of non-ADHD males | 10 |
| Number of non-ADHD females | 7 |
| **Total subjects** | **30** |

*3.2. Ethical Approval*

The ethical approval process was administered by the Health Research Ethics Committee (HREC) of Stellenbosch University. According to the HREC's definitions, the research was identified as a clinical trial because its purposes were to test effectiveness and efficacy of a diagnosis-aiding tool. The risk of the research was minimal since the testing only consisted of playing a game on a tablet. Ethical approval was obtained on the 14th July 2017 and is valid until the 13th July 2018. It was subsequently extended to July 2019.

*3.3. Power Analysis*

A power study was done in the initial stages of sample size estimation with consultation of a statistician. The McNemar test, as defined by [16], was used, as shown in Table 2 below.

**Table 2.** McNemar Test.

|  | Method 1 Positive | Method 2 Negative | Row Total |
| --- | --- | --- | --- |
| **Method 2 Positive** | A | b | a + b |
| **Method 2 Negative** | C | d | c + d |
| **Column Total** | a + c | b + d | N |

In this case, method 1 referred to the current diagnostic method and method 2 was the proposed method resulting from this study. The POWER analysis was performed using the Statistica software package and the following parameters were used as input:

- Delta: the difference in population proportion when Method 1 was positive and the population proportion when Method 2 was positive as described in McNemar's test;

- Nuisance parameter: the total proportion of times different events occur for the two methods. This was chosen as 0.4 based on the statistician's recommendation;
- Type-I error rate: This value is taken as 0.05 and means that one is willing to accept that there is a 5% chance that the null hypothesis is wrong. 0.05 is the standard accepted value.
- Power goal: 0.9

The POWER analysis was applied to various cases where the value of Delta was changed as shown in Table 3. Delta was kept less than 20%. The required sample size that was chosen was 156 subjects. This occurred with Delta = 0:16. In other words, the error in distinguishing between the gold standard method and the new method was 16% (84% accuracy). It was decided, however, that for the beta-testing, a sample size of only 30 subjects would be used to get preliminary results.

Table 3. POWER Analysis.

| $\delta$ | $\eta$ | $\alpha$ | Power Goal | Actual Power for Required N | Required Sample Size |
|---|---|---|---|---|---|
| 0.1 | 0.4 | 0.05 | 0.9 | 0.9004 | 412 |
| 0.15 | 0.4 | 0.05 | 0.9 | 0.9003 | 178 |
| 0.16 | 0.4 | 0.05 | 0.9 | 0.9016 | 156 |
| 0.17 | 0.4 | 0.05 | 0.9 | 0.9013 | 137 |
| 0.18 | 0.4 | 0.05 | 0.9 | 0.9009 | 121 |
| 0.2 | 0.4 | 0.05 | 0.9 | 0.9002 | 96 |

*3.4. Study Design*

The study consisted of two main phases: (1) design and development, (2) testing and data collection. The sequence of research activities is illustrated in Figure 4, where activities 5, 7 and 10 were the testing activities and where activities 3, 6, 8, 9, 11, 12 and 13 were the design and development activities.

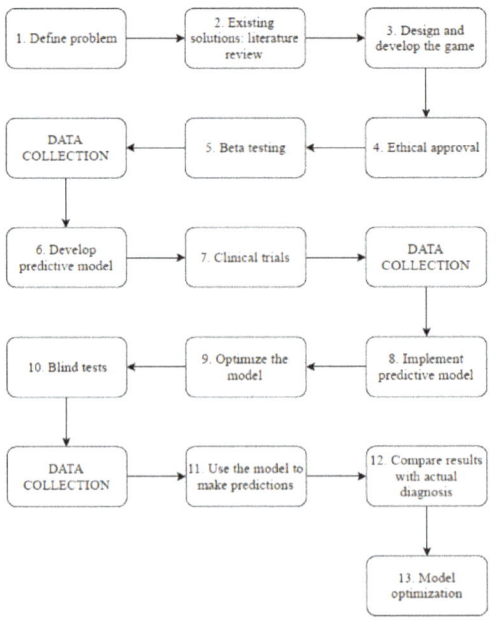

**Figure 4.** Sequence of Research Activities.

## 3.5. Standard Operating Procedure

Testing took place at Cape Gate Medi-Clinic. The subject was placed in a well-lit room and the tablet was presented to them on a table. The investigator then gave the subjects instructions before launching the game. The subject was given a maximum of 8 minutes to complete the task, unless he/she decided to quit. For each subject, the investigator recorded the name, age, diagnosis (for control group), race and additional comments/observations into an Excel spreadsheet. Data was recorded during game-play and sent to a secure FireBase database via a private WiFi connection.

## 3.6. Feature Extraction

Feature extraction is an important step in building a classifier, as it allows for raw data to be interpreted into meaningful information that can help the classifier distinguish one observation from another. Prior to calculating features to extract, outlier detection was performed. The method used took the interquartile range (IQR) into account where

$$IRQ = Q_3 - Q_1 \tag{1}$$

and $Q_3$ and $Q_1$ represent the middle values of the first and third half of the dataset respectively. A data-point $x_i$ was seen as an outlier if it satisfied one of the following two conditions:

$$x_i > Q_3 + 1.5 \times IRQ \tag{2}$$

$$x_i < Q_1 - 1.5 \times IRQ \tag{3}$$

If one of the conditions was met, then $x_i$ was replaced by the equation proposed by [17]:

$$x_i := \frac{x_{i-1} - x_{i+1}}{2} \tag{4}$$

Two feature sets were extracted from the datasets. The first one was referred to as the game feature set and the second one was the accelerometer feature set. The game feature set consisted of the following 16 features: number of left button presses, number of right button presses, number of jumps, number of throws, number of obstacles destroyed, number of obstacles hit, number of gems collected, game duration, game enjoyment (boolean: 1 = enjoyed, 2 = did not enjoy), throw efficiency, total button presses, directional button presses, frequency of button presses, age, race and gender. The accelerometer feature set consisted of the following 18 statistical features: mean, standard deviation, minimum, maximum, range, median, sum, variance, skewness, kurtosis, root mean square (RMS), percentiles (10th, 25th, 50th, 75th and 90th), interquartile range (IRQ) and crest factor. This resulted in a total of 72 features (18 × 4), where each of these features was calculated for the x, y, z axes and for the modulus which was calculated in the following way:

$$a_{total} = \sqrt{a_x^2 + a_y^2 + a_z^2} \tag{5}$$

The following 10 morphological features were extracted: exact Euclidean distance, autocorrelation coefficient, positive area, negative area, total area, absolute total area, total absolute area, number of zero crossings, latency time and peak-to- peak time-window. This resulted in a total of 39 features (10 × 4 − 1), where each of these features was calculated for the x, y, z axes and for the modulus, except for the exact Euclidean distance which was only calculated for the three possible axis pairings. Table 4 shows the breakdown of the feature set. The user specific features (race, age and gender) were important features in terms of correlating gender and age to the outcome of a diagnosis. Race was not necessarily significant for this sample size, but it was included more out of a speculative point of view. It was later seen that no conclusions could be made from this feature affecting the diagnosis. The game-play features were of significance because they gave insight into how subjects played the game (i.e., gaming behaviour). Statistical and morphological features were extracted from the multivariate accelerometer time series, as it has been proven to provide good results for this type of data.

Table 4. Breakdown of feature set.

| Feature Type | Number of Features |
|---|---|
| Statistical | 72 |
| Morphological | 39 |
| Game-play | 8 |
| Game-play-derived | 4 |
| User-specific | 3 |
| Total | 126 |

Once the features were extracted, feature normalization was then performed so that the mean of each feature in the set was equal to zero. This helped improve the efficiency of the classifier. Given a feature $f_i$, normalization performs the following:

$$f_i : \frac{f_i - \mu_i}{s_i} \quad (6)$$

where $\mu_i$ is the average of all the observations for that feature and $s_i$ is the range of the observations of that feature.

*3.7. Feature Selection*

Due to the small sample size, feature ranking could bias the classification accuracy and therefore was deemed unfit for this specific application. As a preliminary feature selection strategy, correlation matrices were used to visually inspect any strong correlations. One feature was removed using this method. Five combinations of feature sets were generated and evaluated. The first feature set was when all the features were used. The second feature set consisted of performing sequential forward selection (SFS) on the full feature set. The third feature set (combine set) was constructed from performing SFS both on the accelerometer features and, on the game, and user features and combining the resulting features. The last two feature sets were constructed from performing SFS on the game and user features and combining that with the morphological features for the one set and the statistical features for the other set. The feature selection sets are shown in Table 5. Ultimately, the feature set that yielded the lowest leave-one-out cross-validation (LOOCV) error was selected. LOOCV was used given the small sample size.

Table 5. Feature Selection Sets.

| Feature Set | Selection Method | Number of Features |
|---|---|---|
| $F_{all}$ | All features selected | 126 |
| $F_{SFS}$ | SFS | 10 |
| $F_{combined}$ | SFS | 21 |
| $F_{man1}$ | SFS and manual | 83 |
| $F_{man2}$ | SFS and manual | 55 |

## 4. Support Vector Machine Model

The approach that was taken in building the SVM classifier was based on the recommendation given by [18] in the following steps:

1. Transform extracted data into the format supported by the SVM package;
2. Perform simple scaling and normalization of the data;

3. Consider a linear kernel as an initial model;
4. Tune the parameter regularization parameter "C" using leave-one-out-cross-validation (LOOCV) method;
5. Use the tuned parameter C to train the whole training set;
6. Test the model on a test set.

The SVM model was implemented in Matlab using the "fitcsvm" function. The inputs to this function were the following:

1. A scaled and normalized dataset X;
2. Target values y, where y is part of [0,1];
3. Regularization parameter C. This parameter adds a penalty to features, thus reducing their overall effect. It is tuned to limit over-fitting;
4. The kernel type (linear);

The output of the "fitcsvm" function was an SVM model. Since five possible feature sets were evaluated, five models were created and the one with best performance was chosen. The process for creating and choosing the best feature set is shown below:

1. Choose an initial value for C: C = 10;
2. Perform LOOCV on each of the five feature sets;
3. Report LOOCV error for each of the five feature sets;
4. Repeat steps 1 to 3 for different values of C: C = 3, 1, 0.3;
5. Choose the feature set with the lowest LOOCV error;
6. Use the corresponding C value to build a final model;
7. Train the model using the whole training set (unlike for LOOCV that uses a subset of the training set);
8. Use the test set to make predictions with the new model

The results of this process are shown in Table 6 which simply shows that the smallest LOOCV error that was found was with a C value of 0.3. This corresponded to $F_{combined}$, where the LOOCV was at a minimum of 0.165. Once the classifier was trained, it was used on the test set to make predictions, using Matlab's "predict" function.

**Table 6.** Leave-one-out cross-validation (LOOCV) error on different feature sets and various C values.

| Feature Set | Features | C | | | |
|---|---|---|---|---|---|
| | | 10 | 3 | 1 | 0.3 |
| $F_{all}$ | 126 | 0.5 | 0.5 | 0.5 | 0.5 |
| $F_{SFS}$ | 10 | 0.25 | 0.1875 | 0.1875 | 0.1875 |
| $F_{combined}$ | 21 | 0.4375 | 0.4375 | 0.415 | **0.165** |
| $F_{man1}$ | 83 | 0.46 | 0.4375 | 0.437 | 0.437 |
| $F_{man2}$ | 55 | 0.43 | 0.4 | 0.4 | 0.4 |

## 5. Results

As mentioned previously, the small sample size that was used for the study induced certain limitations. Chief among them was the validity of the results. However, the results that will be discussed in this section are suggestive rather than conclusive. The main results of the performance of the classifier can be seen in the confusion matrix in Figure 5. The last column shows the percentages correctly classified examples (green) and incorrectly classified examples (red) for each class. The last row shows the same thing for each class. Respectively, the last column may be referred to as the recall, and the last row may be referred to as the false negative rate. These results came from the test set.

Since training accuracy is not a good indication of a classifier's performance, the training set confusion matrix was not calculated. Various performance metrics were derived from the confusion matrix and are explained next.

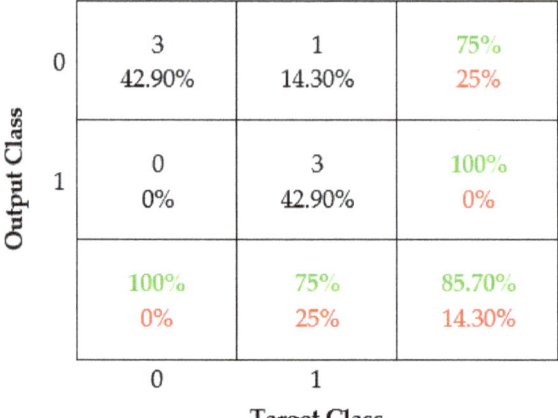

**Figure 5.** Confusion matrix of SVM classifier.

According to the confusion matrix, there were three true positives (TP), three true negatives (TN), one false negative (FN) and no false positives (FP). Table 7 shows the metrics that were used to evaluate the performance of the classifier. The LOOCV accuracy was calculated as 83.5%.

**Table 7.** Performance metrics of support vector machine (SVM).

| Metric | Equation | Value |
| --- | --- | --- |
| Test set accuracy (ACC) | $ACC = \frac{TP+TN}{TP+TN+FP+FN}$ | 0.857 |
| True positive rate (TPR) | $TPR = \frac{TP}{TP+FN}$ | 0.75 |
| True negative rate (TNR) | $TNR = \frac{TN}{TN+FP}$ | 1.00 |
| Positive predictive value (PPV) | $PPV = \frac{TP}{TP+FP}$ | 1.00 |
| Negative predictive value (NPV) | $NPV = \frac{TN}{TN+FN}$ | 0.75 |
| F1 score | $F_1 = 2\frac{PPV \times TPR}{PPV+TPR}$ | 0.857 |
| Type I error | $\alpha = 1 - TNR$ | 0 |
| Type II error | $\beta = 1 - TPR$ | 0.25 |

The reason for choosing 7 children was based on the train-test split when using machine learning, and more specifically SVM. It has been demonstrated that a good split is to use 75% of the full set for training, and 25% of the set for testing. For the sample size of N = 30, this resulted in a test set of 7 children, which is approximately 25%. The proportion of boys to girls is based on the fact that the training and test sets are chosen randomly, so long as the train-test split remains 75:25. The randomness insures that the designer is not biased to pick suitable subjects to yield maximum performance, but that the model will be robust enough to yield reliable results. As a result of the randomness, the proportion of boys to girl was 2:5. Should the study be repeated, a different proportion could be found in the test set, yet the conclusions of the results would still be the same.

## 6. Discussion and Conclusion

### 6.1. Discussion

As a concluding remark to the interpretation of the results, what was seen was that a classifier's performance does not solely rely on its test and cross-validation accuracies. Although cross-validation is a robust way to build classifiers and gives a general indication of how well the model will perform, models should be chosen based on their practical application as well. For example, the classifier built for this study was to be used for screening of ADHD. This means that other metrics become very relevant for assessing the model. Such metrics include sensitivity, specificity and recall.

According to the statistical analysis that was done to estimate a sample size, it was recommended that a total of 200 subjects be used in order to achieve a model accuracy of 84%. The main aim of the study was to conduct a clinical trial, given this sample size. The first step was to perform beta-tests on a smaller population (N = 30) in order to demonstrate the validity of the use of machine learning models. Although the beta-test results were seen as preliminary results, they were indicative enough to be used to demonstrate that the research question could be answered. Given the time constraints on the study, it was decided that clinical trials would form part of future work. The aim was to develop a screening tool for ADHD, and the beta-test was able to provide a solution for that.

The machine learning model that was implemented was SVM with a linear kernel. Due to the high dimensionality of the dataset, features were extracted through statistical and morphological analysis. Feature selection was then performed in order to have the most representative feature subset. Due to the small size of the dataset, leave-one-out cross-validation was chosen to determine the generalization error of the classifier, as well as to tune the regularization parameter. The feature set that was chosen consisted of 21 features that were selected using sequential forward selection. This feature selection method outperformed the other 3 methods that were used. The selected features included 11 of the game-play features and 10 of the features extracted from the accelerometer.

It can be seen that the test set accuracy and LOOCV accuracy are both high. This is expected given a small dataset. The sensitivity (TPR) relates to the classifier's ability to classify ADHD test subjects as having ADHD. Sensitivity was therefore an important characteristic of the classifier, especially for screening. Good classifier performance would require for the classifier to correctly identify subjects that are ADHD. Here the sensitivity is 0.75. This means that 75% of the time, the classifier will be able to detect the presence of ADHD. Although ADHD is sometimes difficult to detect, even with classical methods, a sensitivity of 75% is quite low. The specificity here of 1 shows that all non-ADHD test subjects were correctly classified.

Performance metrics of the classifier revealed that although the test and LOOCV accuracies were good (85.7% and 83.5% respectively) care had to be taken when selecting a classifier as being optimal. Important metrics, especially for diagnosing/screening conditions included specificity and sensitivity, which relate to how well a classifier correctly rules out negatives and correctly includes positives. From a screening point of view, the penalty is not as large as for diagnosis, but it is most desirable to have very high sensitivity and acceptable to high specificity. It was seen that the sensitivity was 75% while the specificity was 100%. The sensitivity was seen as low, while the specificity, although being high, was specific to this small dataset and would most likely decrease with a bigger dataset.

The positive predictive value (PPV) relates to the relevance of the outputs that were classified. A precision of 1 means that all the outputs that were classified were relevant. The negative predictive value (NPV) shows that 75% of relevant targets were selected.

The F1 score shows the balance between precision and recall. Values of F1 that are very high or very low, show that precision and recall are not well balanced. This appeared to be the case with this classifier. The high value of 85.7% suggests that the model may have high precision and low recall, or vice versa.

The type I error of 0 suggests that the null hypothesis was true, and accepted. Although this metric is not indicative given the dataset, it would have been approximately equal to 0.05 for a larger set. The type II error of 0.25 is quite large and suggests that there is 25% probability that the classifier may predict false positives.

In addition to the performance metrics that were discussed, a comparison of the test set distribution and target set distribution was made. The following observations were made: (1) the target values comprised of 4 ADHD subjects and 3 non-ADHD subjects; (2) the predicted values comprised of 3 ADHD subjects and 4 non-ADHD subjects; (3) the test set comprised of 2 boys, 1 of which was ADHD; (4) the test set comprised of 5 girls, 3 of which were ADHD; (6) all the boys with ADHD were classified correctly; (7) all the boys without ADHD were classified correctly; (8) Out of the 3 girls with ADHD in the test set, 2 were classified correctly; (9) all the girls without ADHD were classified correctly.

Although no major conclusions can be drawn from these few observations it is interesting to note that the classifier was able to correctly reject all the boys and girls that didn't have ADHD, as suggested by the 100% specificity. Contrary to the claim that boys are more misdiagnosed than girls, the test set shows that all boys were correctly classified. This observation does not resolve the claim, however, since the dataset was not representative enough of a wider ADHD population.

A comparison of this study's results with other studies and existing tools pertaining to the objective diagnosis of ADHD reveal that the results are close enough, especially considering the small size of the dataset. More specifically, the sensitivity of the proposed method was generally outperformed by the other methods by at least 5%. The specificity found for this method was 100% and this was seen as a biased result, that couldn't be used as representative of the method. The accuracy of the proposed method also performed moderately, although being lower than the other methods by at least 5–7%.

*6.2. Conclusion*

The biggest disadvantage of the method is the small sample size. The significance of this is that the results cannot be treated as conclusive but only indicative. The confidence in the classification is not great, as over-fitting is likely to occur with such a small sample size. However, it has been demonstrated by [2] that SVM can be used for ADHD diagnosis with a sample size of 42, which is the closest study in terms of sample size to date.

What is advantageous about this method is that the method has not yet been explored, in the sense that a game has not been used for screening purposes. Another advantage is the ability to provide screening, without the need of going to a specialist, as this tool could be used by parent's and teachers. The method could curb costs quite significantly, by doing early screening and possible detection, as well as limit over-diagnosis.

Due to the complexity of game development, a simple game with minimal features was implemented. Next, it is recommended that a more interactive and complex game be developed, where more features can be extracted, and more parameters can be monitored. A more complex implementation would give a feature set with higher quality and possibly better classifier performance. Furthermore, many studies have shown that the use of multivariate-time-series (MTS) can help accurately classify diseases such as cancer and even ADHD. Such MTS data is found in the signals of electroencephalograms (EEG), electrocardiograms (ECG) and electromyograms (EMG). These could be implemented into the game by placing sensors and electrodes on subjects. Additional physiological markers could be added, such as eye tracking and heart rate.

The study that was conducted was able to suggest an answer to the research question that was presented, that is: a person can be screened for ADHD using quantitative methods. It was seen that the classifier showed acceptable results, especially considering that those results were only preliminary. It was demonstrated that, given a data acquisition method, in this case being the game tablet, meaningful data could be extracted and used to build a predictive model. The methods that were used to build the model were based on an extensive literature review, where it was shown successfully how those methods were performed with reliability and repeatability. Therefore, the classifier developed for the study was not novel in itself, but it was the whole design process that was novel.

**Author Contributions:** Supervision, P.R.F. and D.v.d.H.; conceptualization, H.M.M. and P.R.F.; methodology, H.M.M. and P.R.F.; writing—review and editing, P.R.F. and D.v.d.H.

**Funding:** This research was privately funded by innovation4life.

**Acknowledgments:** The clinical assistance of Rose-Hannah Brown from the Cape Gate Therapy Centre is acknowledged. The development of the game software by Mark Atkinson is also acknowledged.

**Conflicts of Interest:** The authors declare no conflict of interest.

## References

1. nimh.nih.gov: NIMH: Attention Deficit Hyperactivity Disorder. 2016. Available online: http://www.nimh.nih.gov/health (accessed on 29 June 2016).
2. Schellack, N.; Meyer, H. The Management of Attention Deficit-Hyperactivity Disorder in Children: Evidence-Based Pharmacy Practice. *SA Pharm. J.* **2012**, *79*, 12–20.
3. Gualtieri, C.T.; Johnson, L.G. ADHD: Is Objective Diagnosis Possible? *Psychiatry* **2005**, *2*, 44.
4. Bruchmüller, K.; Margraf, J.; Schneider, S. Is ADHD Diagnosed in Accord with Diagnostic Criteria? Overdiagnosis and Influence of Client Gender on Diagnosis. *J. Consult. Clin. Psychol.* **2012**, *80*, 128. [CrossRef]
5. Schoeman, R.; Liebenberg, R. The South African Society of Psychiatrist/Psychiatry Management Group Management Guidelines for Adult Attention-Deficit/Hyperactivity Disorder. *S. Afr. J. Psychiatry* **2017**, *23*, 1–14. [CrossRef] [PubMed]
6. Dopheide, J.A.; Pliszka, S.R. Attention-Deficit-Hyperactivity Disorder: An Update. *Pharmacotherapy* **2009**, *29*, 656–679. [CrossRef] [PubMed]
7. Biederman, J. Attention-Deficit/Hyperactivity Disorder: A Selective Overview. *Biol. Psychiatry* **2005**, *57*, 1215–1220. [CrossRef] [PubMed]
8. Valera, E.M.; Faraone, S.V.; Murray, K.E.; Sideman, L.J. Meta-Analysis of Structural Imaging Findings in Attention-Deficit/Hyperactivity Disorder. *Biol. Psychiatry* **2007**, *61*, 1361–1369. [CrossRef] [PubMed]
9. Toplak, M.E.; Tannock, R. Time Perception: Modality and Duration Effects in Attention-Deficit/Hyperactivity Disorder (ADHD). *J. Abnorm. Child Psychol.* **2005**, *33*, 639–654. [CrossRef] [PubMed]
10. Multi Health Systems. 2019. Available online: https://www.mhs.com/MHS-Assessment?prodname=cpt3 (accessed on 26 March 2019).
11. Berger, I.; Cassuto, H. The Effect of Environmental Distractors Incorporation Into a CPT on Sustained Attention and ADHD Diagnosis Among Adolescents. *J. Neurosci. Methods* **2014**, *222*, 62–68. [CrossRef] [PubMed]
12. Berger, I.; Slobodan, O.; Cassuto, H. Usefulness and Validity of Continuous Performance Tests in the Diagnosis of Attention-Deficit Hyperactivity Disorder Children. *Arch. Clin. Neuropsychol.* **2017**, *32*, 81–93. [PubMed]
13. Cassuto, H.; Ben-Simon, A.; Berger, I. Using Environmental Distractors in the Diagnosis of ADHD. *Front. Hum. Neurosci.* **2013**, *7*, 805. [CrossRef] [PubMed]
14. O'Mahony, N.; Florentino-Liano, B.; Carballo, J.J.; Baca-Garcia, E.; Rodriguez, A.A. Objective Diagnosis of ADHD Using IMUs. *Med. Eng. Phys.* **2014**, *36*, 922–926. [CrossRef] [PubMed]
15. nebahealth.com: Neba Health. 2015. Available online: https://nebahealth.com/faq.html#1 (accessed on 20 September 2016).
16. McNemar, Q. Note on the sampling error of the difference between correlated proportions or percentages. *Psychometrika* **1947**, *12*, 153–157. [CrossRef] [PubMed]
17. Esmael, B.; Arnaout, A.; Fruhwirth, R.K.; Thonhauser, G. A Statistical Feature-based Approach for Operations Recognition in Drilling Time Series. *Int. J. Comput. Inf. Syst. Ind. Manag. Appl.* **2015**, *5*, 454–461.
18. Hsu, C.-W.; Chang, C.-C.; Lin, C.-J. A Practical Guide to Support Vector Classification. 2003. Available online: https://www.csie.ntu.edu.tw/~{}cjlin/papers/guide/guide.pdf (accessed on 10 August 2018).

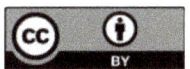

© 2019 by the authors. Licensee MDPI, Basel, Switzerland. This article is an open access article distributed under the terms and conditions of the Creative Commons Attribution (CC BY) license (http://creativecommons.org/licenses/by/4.0/).

Article

# Box-Jenkins Transfer Function Modelling for Reliable Determination of VO$_2$ Kinetics in Patients with COPD

Joren Buekers [1,2], Jan Theunis [1], Alberto Peña Fernández [2], Emiel F. M. Wouters [3,4], Martijn A. Spruit [3,4,5,6], Patrick De Boever [1,7] and Jean-Marie Aerts [2,*]

1. Health unit, Flemish Institute for Technological Research (VITO), 2400 Mol, Belgium; joren.buekers@vito.be (J.B.); jan.theunis@vito.be (J.T.); patrick.deboever@vito.be (P.D.B.)
2. Measure, Model & Manage Bioresponses (M3-BIORES), Department of Biosystems, KU Leuven, 3000 Leuven, Belgium; alberto.penafernandez@kuleuven.be
3. Department of Research and Education, Centre of Expertise for Chronic Organ Failure (CIRO), 6085 NM Horn, The Netherlands; e.wouters@mumc.nl (E.F.M.W.); martijnspruit@ciro-horn.nl (M.A.S.)
4. Department of Respiratory Medicine, Maastricht University Medical Centre, 6229 HX Maastricht, The Netherlands
5. REVAL—Rehabilitation Research Center, BIOMED—Biomedical Research Institute, Faculty of Rehabilitation Sciences, Hasselt University, 3500 Diepenbeek, Belgium
6. NUTRIM School of Nutrition and Translational Research in Metabolism, Maastricht University Medical Centre, 6211 LK Maastricht, The Netherlands
7. Centre for Environmental Sciences, Hasselt University, 3500 Diepenbeek, Belgium
* Correspondence: jean-marie.aerts@kuleuven.be

Received: 4 March 2019; Accepted: 29 April 2019; Published: 1 May 2019

**Abstract:** Oxygen uptake (VO$_2$) kinetics provide information about the ability to respond to the increased physical load during a constant work rate test (CWRT). Box-Jenkins transfer function (BJ-TF) models can extract kinetic features from the phase II VO$_2$ response during a CWRT, without being affected by unwanted noise contributions (e.g., phase I contribution or measurement noise). CWRT data of 18 COPD patients were used to compare model fits and kinetic feature values between BJ-TF models and three typically applied exponential modelling methods. Autocorrelation tests and normalised root-mean-squared error values (BJ-TF: 2.8 ± 1.3%; exponential methods A, B and C: 10.5 ± 5.8%, 11.3 ± 5.2% and 12.1 ± 7.0%; $p < 0.05$) showed that BJ-TF models, in contrast to exponential models, could account for the most important noise contributions. This led to more reliable kinetic feature values compared to methods A and B (e.g., mean response time (MRT), BJ-TF: 74 ± 20 s; methods A-B: 100 ± 56 s–88 ± 52 s; $p < 0.05$). Only exponential modelling method C provided kinetic feature values comparable to BJ-TF features values (e.g., MRT: 75 ± 20 s). Based on theoretical considerations, we recommend using BJ-TF models, rather than exponential models, for reliable determinations of VO$_2$ kinetics.

**Keywords:** chronic obstructive pulmonary disease; COPD; oxygen uptake; VO$_2$; kinetics; exercise testing

## 1. Introduction

Chronic obstructive pulmonary disease (COPD) is a common lung disease characterised by persistent airflow limitations due to a combination of airway and alveolar abnormalities. COPD is associated with high morbidity and mortality rates, posing a high economical and societal burden [1]. The most important symptom of COPD is dyspnoea during daily activities, but later also at rest. As a result, patients become physically less active, which is the start of a vicious circle of physical deconditioning [2]. Physical capacities can be assessed using standard exercise tests like a cardiopulmonary exercise test (CPET, incremental cycling load) or a constant work rate test (CWRT, constant cycling load) [3]. During a CPET, oxygen uptake ($VO_2$, ml.min$^{-1}$) increases linearly until the maximal or peak $VO_2$ value is reached. This maximal (or peak) $VO_2$ value, the maximal load reached during CPET and the endurance time during CWRT are the most frequently used metrics for evaluating physical capacities. However, there is additional information, besides these maximal values, that can be extracted from the breath-by-breath $VO_2$ time series that are generated during these tests.

During a CWRT, there is typically a 3-phase $VO_2$ response towards the step increase of cycling load (W). During phase I, the cardiodynamic phase, $VO_2$ shows an instant response driven by an increased cardiac output and pulmonary blood flow (Figure 1). In phase II, the primary component of the response, $VO_2$ increases exponentially, similar to the working muscle oxygen uptake. In phase III, $VO_2$ can reach a steady-state or can steadily keep increasing, i.e., $VO_2$ slow component (Figure 1), depending on the exercise intensity [4]. Kinetic analyses of the $VO_2$ response aim to quantify the speed and amplitude of the primary (phase II) response using a combination of features. Time delay (TD), time constant (TC) and mean response time (MRT = TD + TC) assess the speed of the response. Response amplitude (Amp) and steady state gain (SSG = Amp.$\Delta W^{-1}$) assess the magnitude of the response, with $\Delta W$ indicating the step increase of cycling load at the start of the exercise test (Figure 1). These features quantify the ability to respond to the increased physical load during a CWRT [4]. Generally, COPD patients exhibit a slower $VO_2$ response than healthy subjects [5,6], but supplemental oxygen [7], medication use [8,9] and exercise training [10], can speed up the $VO_2$ response to the step increase in cycling load.

Typically, exponential models are used to extract these kinetic features from the $VO_2$ time series. Three mono-exponential modelling methods have been described in COPD literature, which will be referred to as method A [6,8], B [10,11] and C [9,12]. Method A assumes there is no delay in the $VO_2$ response (TD = 0 s), whereas methods B and C estimate a TD value as one of the model parameters. Method B uses data starting from t = 0 s (load onset), while method C aims to exclude the contribution of the cardiodynamic phase by only using data starting from t = 20 s. Nevertheless, these exponential models are all still influenced by other unwanted noise contributions, such as measurement noise or cardiac output dynamics that are not related to the increased working muscle oxygen uptake.

In contrast to the generally applied exponential models, Box-Jenkins transfer function (BJ-TF) models can extract the same kinetic features [13] without being affected by these unwanted noise contributions. BJ-TF models are able to separate the unwanted contributions from the noise-free primary $VO_2$ response (i.e., phase II). Therefore, extraction of the kinetic features will not be influenced by the unwanted contribution of these additional components, and will only reflect the working muscle oxygen uptake. To the authors' knowledge, BJ-TF models have not yet been used to extract kinetic features from CWRT data. Therefore, the aim of this study was to compare model fits and kinetic feature values between BJ-TF models and the three different exponential modelling methods that were identified in COPD literature.

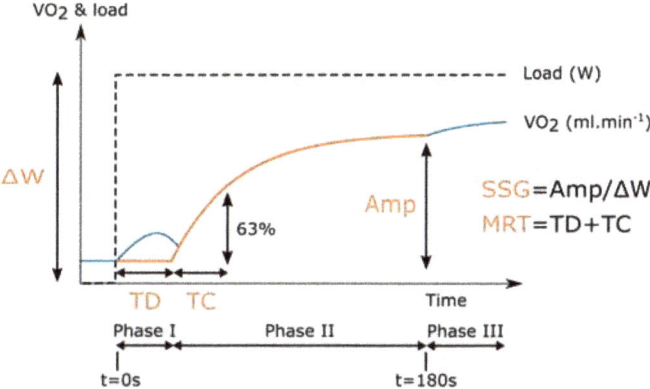

**Figure 1.** Graphical representation of the kinetic features that quantify the phase II response. The blue line represents the theoretical $VO_2$ response, the orange line shows the phase II contribution that should be modelled, the black dashed line visualises the load increase at t = 0 s. The blue and orange lines coincide during phase II. A slow component is visible in phase III. TD, Time delay; TC, time constant; MRT, mean response time; Amp, response amplitude; ΔW, the step increase in cycling load at t = 0 s; and SSG, steady state gain.

## 2. Materials and Methods

### 2.1. Study Design and Participants

Twenty COPD patients (GOLD II-IV) were recruited at CIRO (Horn, the Netherlands) during a standard baseline assessment prior to pulmonary rehabilitation [14]. Two patients were excluded from analyses because they failed to perform a CWRT during the baseline assessment. Demographics, partial pressure of oxygen and carbon dioxide, post-bronchodilator pulmonary function data (e.g., forced expiratory volume in 1 second, forced vital capacity and transfer factor for carbon monoxide) and modified Medical Research Council dyspnoea scores were collected during the standard baseline assessment at CIRO. The study was approved by the Medical Research Ethics Committees United (NL58079.100.16, MEC-U, the Netherlands) and all patients provided written informed consent.

### 2.2. Exercise Testing

Patients performed a CPET during the first day and a CWRT during the second day of the baseline assessment. The tests were performed on an electrically braked cycle ergometer and $VO_2$ data were collected breath-by-breath (Oxycon Pro, Carefusion, Houten, the Netherlands). Both tests started with 3 minutes of rest, followed by 3 minutes of unloaded cycling (W = 0). During CPET, the load then increased 1 Watt per 4, 6 or 12 seconds, depending on the relative fitness of the patient. During CWRT, the load remained constant at 75% of the maximal load obtained during the CPET. In both tests, patients were asked to keep their cycling speed constant between 60 and 70 rotations per minute and to cycle until limitation (exhaustion and/or severe dyspnoea). The tests ended with a 3-minute recovery period. CWRT time series data were used for the analyses described below.

### 2.3. Data Pre-Processing

Deviating breath values, identified as data samples deviating more than 3 standard deviations from the local mean (i.e., 31 s centred moving average), were deleted. An integrated random walk smoothing algorithm (CAPTAIN toolbox [15]) was used to converse the non-equidistant breath-by-breath $VO_2$ data into a smoothed 1 Hz time series, while still preserving the dynamics of the time series. Data after 180 s of loaded cycling were discarded to exclude any potential contribution of the $VO_2$ slow component.

## 2.4. Kinetic Analyses

The dynamic response of physiological variables towards an increase in physical load can be described by a number of features (Figure 1). These features were extracted using both exponential models and BJ-TF models. The following first order model was used as a basis for exponential modelling:

$$0 \leq t \leq TD: \quad \Delta VO_2(t) = 0,$$
$$TD < t \leq 180: \quad \Delta VO_2(t) = Amp \cdot \left(1 - e^{-\left(\frac{t-TD}{TC}\right)}\right), \tag{1}$$

where $\Delta VO_2(t)$ is the difference between the pre-processed $VO_2$ time series and the baseline $VO_2$ level ($VO_{2,baseline}$), i.e., $\Delta VO_2(t) = VO_2(t) - VO_{2,baseline}$. $VO_{2,baseline}$ is calculated as the mean $VO_2$ value of the last 30 s of unloaded cycling. The model parameters ($Amp$, $TD$ and $TC$) were estimated using non-linear least squares (Matlab 2015b, MathWorks Inc., Natick, Massachusetts, USA). Three mono-exponential modelling methods have been described in COPD literature. They will be referred to as method A [6,8], B [10,11] and C [9,12]. Method A assumes there is no $TD$ in the $VO_2$ response ($TD = 0$ s). Method B estimates the three model parameters using data from $t = 0$ s (load onset) until $t = 180$ s, whereas method C only uses data between $t = 20$ s and $t = 180$ s to exclude the contribution of the cardiodynamic phase (phase I).

Time evolutions and autocorrelation tests of the model residuals were checked to assess whether the model residuals retained any meaningful structure. Remaining structure in the model residuals indicates that the residuals contain information that is not captured by the model. The relative amplitude of these residuals was assessed by the normalised root-mean-squared error (NRMSE), defined as the root-mean-squared error divided by the amplitude of the $VO_2$ response:

$$NRMSE = \sqrt{\frac{\sum_{t=1}^{n} residuals(t)^2}{n}} \cdot Amp^{-1}. \tag{2}$$

A discrete-time, single-input, single-output BJ-TF model with time-invariant parameters can generally be written as follows:

$$y(t) = \frac{B(z^{-1})}{A(z^{-1})} u(t - TD) + \frac{C(z^{-1})}{D(z^{-1})} e(t), \tag{3}$$

where $y(t)$ is the model output at time t, $u(t)$ is the model input at time t, $z^{-1}$ is the backwards shift operator (i.e. $z^{-s} y(t) = y(t-s)$), $e(t)$ is zero mean white noise and $A(z^{-1})$, $B(z^{-1})$, $C(z^{-1})$ and $D(z^{-1})$ are polynomials containing the model parameters:

$$A(z^{-1}) = 1 + a_1 z^{-1} + \cdots + a_m z^{-m},$$
$$B(z^{-1}) = b_0 + b_1 z^{-1} + \cdots + b_n z^{-n},$$
$$C(z^{-1}) = 1 + c_1 z^{-1} + \cdots + c_p z^{-p},$$
$$D(z^{-1}) = 1 + d_1 z^{-1} + \cdots + d_q z^{-q}. \tag{4}$$

Thus, the full BJ-TF model (3) is a combination of a 'noise-free' system model (first term) and a noise model (second term). As phase II is known to follow a first-order exponential response, the system model was defined as a first order model with one gain parameter. This transformed the full model (3) as follows:

$$\Delta VO_2(t) = \frac{b_0}{1 + a_1 z^{-1}} W(t - TD) + \frac{C(z^{-1})}{D(z^{-1})} e(t), \quad (5)$$

where the input variable $W(t)$ was defined as:

$$t \leq 0 : \quad W = 0 \text{ Watt,}$$
$$t > 0 : \quad W = 75\% \text{ of the maximal load reached during CPET.}$$

The order of the noise model, given by the order of polynomial $D(z^{-1})$, was unknown and was therefore identified by comparing the performances of models with noise models up to order three in $C(z^{-1})$ and/or $D(z^{-1})$. Full model fits were inspected visually and the residuals were checked using autocorrelation tests and NRMSE values. In addition, the full models with different noise structures were compared by their Young Identification Criterion (YIC) value [16]. YIC combines goodness of fit and reliability of the parameter estimations, while penalising for over-parameterisation. A more negative YIC value indicates a better model performance. The noise model structure will be referred to as [p q], where p and q are the orders of polynomials $D(z^{-1})$ and $Z(z^{-1})$, respectively.

The parameters of the full model were estimated using the refined instrumental variable approach of the CAPTAIN toolbox in Matlab [16,17]. From the system model parameters $a_1$ and $b_0$, TC and SSG were calculated as follows:

$$TC = \frac{-\Delta t}{\log(-a_1)}, \quad (6)$$

$$SSG = \frac{b_0}{1 + a_1}. \quad (7)$$

where $\Delta t$ is the sampling time (= 1 s). MRT was calculated as the sum of TD and TC, Amp was calculated by multiplying SSG with the load increase ($\Delta W$).

## 2.5. Statistical Analysis

Patient characteristics were summarised for all patients as mean and standard deviation (SD). NRMSE and kinetic feature values were summarised as median and interquartile range (IQR). Wilcoxon signed-rank tests were used to look for differences in NRMSE and kinetic feature values as calculated with the different exponential modelling methods and BJ-TF modelling. A $p$-value lower than 0.05 was considered to provide statistical significance. All analyses were performed using Matlab 2015b (MathWorks Inc., Natick, Massachusetts, USA).

## 3. Results

Eighteen patients (14 male and four female) performed a CWRT. Table 1 summarises the clinical characteristics of the participants. On average, the elderly patients had a moderate-to-severe degree of airflow limitation, an impaired diffusing capacity and a slightly overweight body mass index. None of the patients were on long-term oxygen therapy. A median of 1.5 (± 2) deviating breath values were deleted per patient.

Table 1. Patient characteristics.

| | Value Mean (SD) |
|---|---|
| Age (years) | 63 (7) |
| Body mass index (kg/m$^2$) | 26 (5) |
| Forced expiratory volume in 1 second (FEV1) % predicted | 48 (14) |
| Forced vital capacity (FVC) % predicted | 105 (18) |
| FEV1/FVC (%) | 37 (13) |
| Transfer factor for carbon monoxide % predicted | 55 (15) |
| Partial pressure of oxygen (kPa) | 8.8 (1.8) |
| Partial pressure of carbon dioxide (kPa) | 5.3 (0.7) |
| Modified Medical Research Council dyspnoea scores (scores 1-2-3) | 2-14-2 |
| CPET maximal cycling load % predicted [18] | 50 (23) |
| CPET maximal oxygen uptake (ml/min) | 1133 (231) |
| CPET maximal oxygen uptake % predicted [18] | 55 (21) |
| CWRT cycling load (W) | 57 (16) |
| CWRT endurance time (s) | 243 (81) |

CPET, cardiopulmonary exercise test; CWRT, constant work rate test.

*3.1. Exponential Modelling*

Figure 2 shows an example of the three exponential modelling methods fitted to data of the same patient. NRMSE values differed between the three methods (method A: 10.5 ± 5.8; method B: 11.3 ± 5.2; method C: 12.1 ± 7.0; $p < 0.05$ for all pairwise comparisons). As shown in Figure 2, method C is the only method that can completely surpass the cardiodynamic phase.

The exponential model residuals contained remaining structure, as can be seen by plotting the relative residual values in function of time and the autocorrelation coefficients from lag 1 to 10 (example shown in Figure 3a). The same behaviour was obtained for all patients for all three methods.

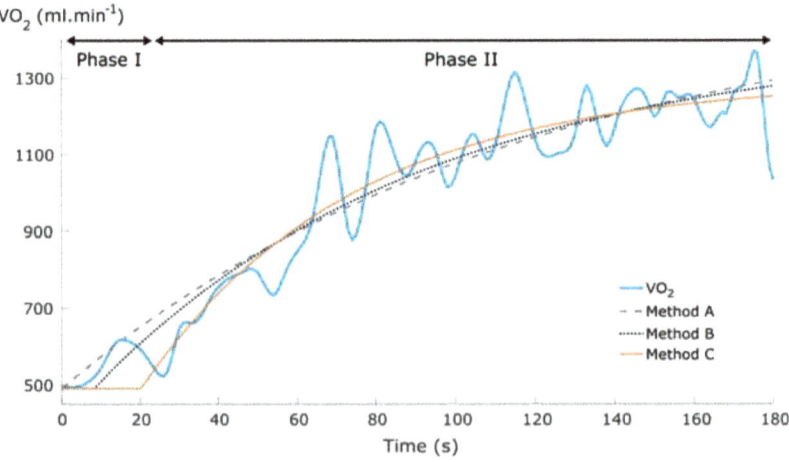

**Figure 2.** Example plot of VO$_2$ data and the three different exponential modelling methods. The estimated time delay (TD) values for methods B and C were 8.3 s and 20.3 s, respectively.

*3.2. Box-Jenkins Transfer Function Modelling*

Based on the full model fits, YIC values and NRMSE values (see below and Discussion), a first order system model with a [2 0] noise model order was selected and used for comparing kinetic feature values between exponential and BJ-TF models in the next section. An example of applying this BJ-TF model is shown in Figure 4.

BJ-TF models with first order noise models (i.e., first order in $D(z^{-1})$) resulted in visually inappropriate model fits. Noise models of order [1 0] and [1 1] led to the full model (i.e., system + noise model) lagging behind the measured $VO_2$ data. This lag was solved in the noise models of order [1 2] and [1 3]. However, for both these noise model structures the full model fits were completely off for some patients. Similarly, noise model orders [2 3] and [3 3] led to bad fits for some patients. YIC and NRMSE values of the remaining noise model orders are summarised in Table 2. Second order noise models had more negative (i.e., better) YIC values, but slightly higher residual values compared to third order models. Example residual and autocorrelation plots for [2 0] and [3 2] noise models are shown in Figure 3b,c, respectively. These noise model orders were chosen as examples because they had the lowest YIC value of all second and third order noise models, respectively. All second order noise models exhibited similar residual and autocorrelation plots, whereas some third order noise models still had a significant autocorrelation coefficient at lag 1, opposite to the example in Figure 3c.

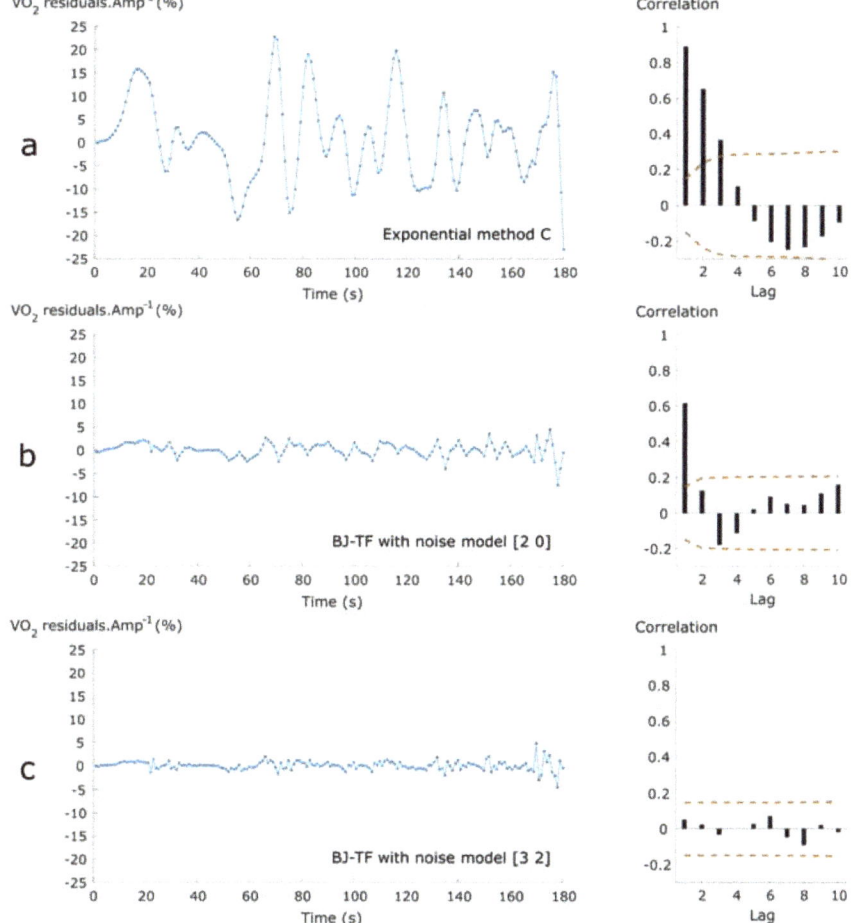

**Figure 3.** Residual analyses of the residuals from (**a**) exponential method C (representative for methods A and B) and Box-Jenkins transfer function (BJ-TF) models with noise model orders (**b**) [2 0] and (**c**) [3 2]. Left: residual values divided by the model parameter Amp, plotted in function of time. Right: autocorrelation coefficients up to lag 10.

**Table 2.** Model performance characteristics for identification of the noise model order. Dark squares show noise model orders that resulted in visually inappropriate full model fits. Upper values for every noise model structure are Young Identification Criterion (YIC) values, and lower values are normalised root-mean-squared error values (NRMSE) (%).

|  |  | Order $D(z^{-1})$ | | |
|---|---|---|---|---|
|  |  | 1 | 2 | 3 |
| Order $C(z^{-1})$ | 0 |  | −6.94 (2.31) 2.8 (1.3) | −5.69 (2.12) 2.1 (1.1) |
|  | 1 |  | −6.82 (2.91) 2.5 (1.7) | −6.20 (2.11) 2.0 (2.6) |
|  | 2 |  | −6.75 (2.63) 2.1 (1.6) | −6.21 (2.69) 2.0 (1.6) |
|  | 3 |  |  |  |

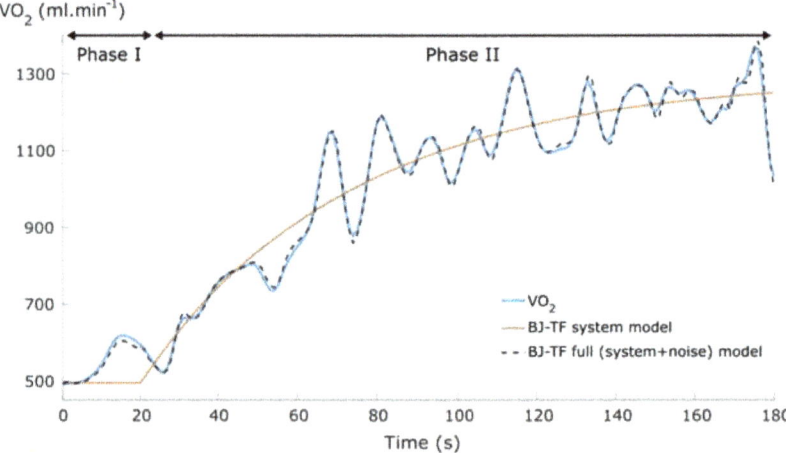

**Figure 4.** Example plot of $VO_2$ data and the BJ-TF system and full (system + noise) model. The estimated TD value was 20 s.

### 3.3. Kinetic Features

Figure 5 provides an overview of the $VO_2$ kinetic feature values as calculated with the different exponential (methods A, B and C) and full BJ-TF models. Methods A and B resulted in a smaller TD and a higher TC, MRT, Amp and SSG compared to method C and the BJ-TF full model (Figure 5). On a group level, method C and BJ-TF did not show significant differences between the kinetic feature values of the included patients (Figure 5). On an individual level, the median (± IQR) of the absolute differences between the feature values as calculated with method C and BJ-TF were 4 ± 13 s, 11 ± 17 s, 7 ± 8 s, 27 ± 43 ml·min$^{-1}$ and 0.5 ± 0.7 ml·min$^{-1}$·W$^{-1}$ for TD, TC, MRT, Amp and SSG, respectively. These absolute differences were respectively 24%, 20%, 9%, 4% and 4% of the respective median feature values as extracted from BJ-TF models. MRT values varied less than TC values between the different methods (Figure 5).

Two patients had extremely large kinetic feature values in all applied models (e.g., TC > 200 s and/or SSG > 20 ml·min$^{-1}$·W$^{-1}$). One of these patients cycled at a very low load during CWRT (22 W), the other patient showed a $VO_2$ response that increased almost linearly. When applying method A, one additional patient had extremely large kinetic feature values.

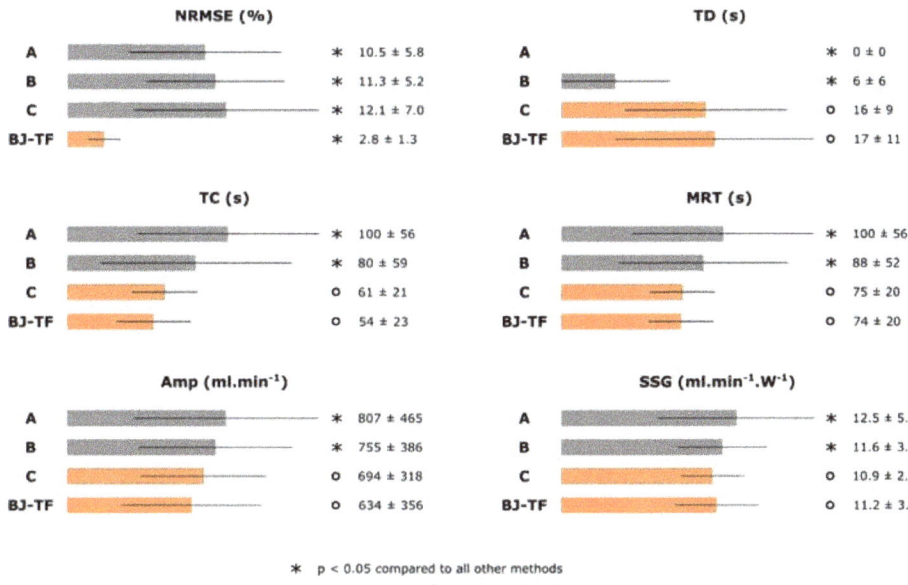

**Figure 5.** NRMSE and kinetic feature values summarised as median (bar) and interquartile range (line) for exponential modelling methods A, B, C and the BJ-TF model with noise model order [2 0].

## 4. Discussion

This is the first study to apply BJ-TF models to determine $VO_2$ kinetics during a CWRT. BJ-TF models provided better fits than the typically applied exponential models and were able to account for unwanted contributions (e.g., phase I contribution or measurement noise). When applying exponential models, method C succeeded best at surpassing the phase I contribution and most closely resembled the "noise-free" system model of BJ-TF models.

Exponential models are most commonly used to examine $VO_2$ kinetics [4]. However, none of the applied exponential modelling methods were able to account for the noise components in the $VO_2$ time series, as could be seen in the $VO_2$ time series, residual and autocorrelation plots (Figures 2 and 3). NRMSE values showed that the residuals acted on a magnitude of 10–12% of the total response amplitude, indicating that these noise components should not be neglected. Methods B and C had higher NRMSE values because they tried to surpass the contribution of the cardiodynamic phase (phase I), leading to higher residual values at the start of the test when the cardiodynamic phase plays an important role (Figures 2 and 3). However, method A is mechanistically unrealistic, as it does not assume any transit delays between muscle oxygen uptake and oxygen uptake at the mouth [19]. Only method C was able to fully discard the phase I contribution by removing the first 20 s of data. The ability to (partly) surpass the cardiodynamic phase was mainly reflected in the TD values, which in turn greatly affected all other feature values (Figure 5). This shows that for COPD patients, similar to healthy subjects [19,20], the applied exponential modelling method had a significant effect on the kinetic feature values.

Another strategy to exclude the phase I contribution might be applying a second-order exponential model, which aims to separately model the phase I and phase II contributions [4,20]. However, a second-order exponential model is based on the unproven assumption that the phase I response is exponential of nature [20]. Furthermore, the phase I contribution was not the only unwanted noise component in the data, as can be seen in Figure 3a. These other noise contributions acted at a similar level as phase I, making it difficult to distinguish phase I from other noise contributions (Figure 3a). The relatively small phase I contributions, compared to the other noise contributions, might be a result of the patients suffering from COPD [5] or because the test was preceded by unloaded cycling [19]. Averaging the $VO_2$ response of several repetitions of the same exercise can cancel out the noise contributions that are not related to the phase I contribution [21,22], but this requires unnecessarily strenuous exercise sessions. Therefore, BJ-TF models were preferred because of their ability to account for all unwanted components at once.

A [2 0] noise model structure was considered the most suitable for BJ-TF modelling. When considering all second order noise models, NRMSE values were all at the same magnitude, and a [2 0] structure had the best YIC values. This indicates that increasing the order of $C(z^{-1})$ above zero induced unnecessary complexity. Some structure remained in the residuals when applying a second order noise model, but at a very low magnitude (Figure 3b and Table 2). When increasing the noise model dynamics to order three, this low-magnitude structure in the residuals disappeared in most patients (Figure 3c) and NRMSE values became slightly lower, but were still at a similar magnitude as second order models (Table 2). The improvements of increasing the noise model order were thus minimal compared to the cost of the increased complexity (i.e., more difficult to interpret, greater risk of overfitting and more computationally expensive), resulting in higher YIC values for third order noise models (Table 2). A [2 0] noise model showed the best balance between model fit and model complexity.

BJ-TF models provided better fits than the exponential modelling methods. Whereas exponential models only provided an estimate of the general trend of the $VO_2$ response (Figure 2), BJ-TF models were able to account for the unwanted noise contributions around the general trend (Figure 5), without having to average $VO_2$ responses over several repetitions [21,22]. These noise contributions are especially important for COPD patients, as the reduced $VO_2$ responses, due to the lower workloads that are feasible for COPD patients [3], increase the relative magnitude of the noise contributions (i.e., lower signal to noise ratio). Residual and autocorrelation plots confirmed that the noise models accounted for the most important noise contributions (Figure 3), and the remaining residuals were four times smaller than residuals from exponential models (Figure 5). Whereas exponential modelling models A and B failed to provide satisfying estimates of TD, BJ-TF models with a [2 0] noise model always provided satisfactory results without having to manipulate the data manually (cf. method C).

The ability of BJ-TF models to separate the phase II contribution from other unwanted noise contributions ensured that these noise contributions could not influence the extracted kinetic feature values, which is a key advantage compared to exponential modelling. The influence of the unwanted contributions, mostly phase I, led to lower TD and higher TC, MRT, Amp and SSG values when applying methods A and B. Only method C produced similar feature values as BJ-TF models on a group level, pointing out that this method should be preferred over methods A and B when exponential models are applied on CWRT data from COPD patients. Nevertheless, median absolute differences between the feature values of individual patients, as calculated with method C and BJ-TF models, were up to 24%, showing that different feature values were obtained for individual patients when the two different methods were applied. Unfortunately, due to the unwanted noise components in $VO_2$ responses, the true $VO_2$ kinetic feature values are never exactly known. As a result, no quantitative evidence could be provided that indicates which model (method C or BJ-TF) was mainly responsible for these differences in feature values on an individual level. Nevertheless, some theoretical considerations favour BJ-TF models over exponential models, as discussed below.

Unwanted noise contributions influencing $VO_2$ kinetic features values are a general concern when applying exponential models [22–24]. In contrast, BJ-TF models explicitly account for the unwanted contributions and the extracted feature values will thus be less influenced by these contributions. Furthermore, parameters in the exponential models were estimated using the generally applied method of least squares, which can be influenced by unwanted noise contributions in the data, in contrast to the more robust refined instrumental variable approach that was used to estimate the model parameters in BJ-TF models [16,25]. In addition, BJ-TF models do not require data manipulation by removing the first 20 s of data after the load onset. Although this method has been proven robust for changes in the amount of removed data under specific conditions, e.g., using the averaged data of four repetitions of the test and a sampling time of 10 s [26], the effect of changing the amount of removed data under less strict conditions, e.g., when only a single test is available, is still unclear and could thus influence the extracted feature values. Based on these elements, BJ-TF models are believed to be more reliable than exponential method C for the determination of kinetic feature values.

MRT varied less than TC over the different modelling methods for quantifying the speed of the primary $VO_2$ response (Figure 5). This confirms the findings from test–retest reliability studies that determine $VO_2$ kinetics from healthy subjects using a treadmill [27] or step test [28]. Inaccurate TD estimates will directly affect TC estimates in the opposite direction. These opposing effects are balanced in the calculation of MRT, making MRT more robust towards inaccurate TD estimations. This study also confirms earlier findings that not all CWRT datasets of COPD patients are well-suited for kinetic analyses [29]. One patient showed no meaningful $VO_2$ response due to a very low cycling load (22 W). More interestingly, another patient had an almost linear primary $VO_2$ response that was not due to a low cycling load. The airway and alveolar abnormalities in COPD patients, which can limit the oxygen delivery to the working muscles [4], might have led to this alteration of the $VO_2$ response. Analyses of larger COPD populations will be required to confirm this hypothesis.

In addition to the more reliable determination of kinetic feature values compared to exponential methods, A and B, BJ-TF models can also be applied more broadly than exponential models. Exponential models do not explicitly include an input variable in their model, limiting their use to experiments with a single input transition (e.g., non-active to active or unloaded to loaded cycling). BJ-TF, however, are able to estimate kinetic feature values with multiple input transitions, e.g., for time-domain analyses of pseudo-random binary sequences of the cycling load [30], or during unsupervised physical activities. As physical activity and $VO_2$ can nowadays be measured with wearable devices [31,32], combining these measurements with BJ-TF modelling can produce frequent estimates of kinetic feature values during standard unsupervised training sessions, without the need for elaborate testing procedures. Similar models have already been successfully used to model heart rate responses during road cycling [33].

Although this study showed the advantages of applying BJ-TF models, some considerations should be taken into account. We only examined a specific population, which exhibits a reduced signal to noise ratio (due to the reduced $VO_2$ response amplitudes [3]) and phase I contribution [5]. It would thus be interesting to test the performance of BJ-TF models in other population types (e.g., athletes or other disease states). Furthermore, other exercise modalities (e.g., treadmill walking) and exercise intensities should be examined to test the general applicability of BJ-TF models for analysing $VO_2$ kinetics.

In conclusion, low residual values showed that BJ-TF models accurately model the $VO_2$ response of COPD patients during a CWRT. These models, in contrast to the typically used exponential models, were able to account for unwanted noise contributions (e.g., the phase I contribution), leading to more reliable determinations of kinetic feature values compared to methods A and B. Only exponential modelling method C, which excludes the data during the cardiodynamic phase, led to comparable kinetic feature values as extracted from BJ-TF models. Based on theoretical considerations, we recommend using BJ-TF, rather than exponential models, for reliable determinations of $VO_2$ kinetics.

**Author Contributions:** Conceptualization, J.B., J.T., M.A.S., P.D.B. and J.-M.A.; methodology, J.B., A.P.F. and J.-M.A.; formal analysis, J.B.; writing—original draft preparation, J.B.; writing—review and editing, J.T., A.P.F., E.F.M.W., M.A.S., P.D.B. and J.-M.A.; visualization, J.B.; supervision, J.T., M.A.S., P.D.B. and J.-M.A.

**Funding:** This research received no external funding.

**Acknowledgments:** This research is part of a PhD research funded by Flemish Institute for Technological Research (VITO), Mol, Belgium.

**Conflicts of Interest:** The authors declare no conflict of interest.

## References

1. Global Initiative for Chronic Obstructive Lung Disease (GOLD). Global strategy for the diagnosis, management, and prevention of Chronic Obstructive Pulmonary Disease—2019 Report 2019. Available online: https://goldcopd.org/wp-content/uploads/2018/11/GOLD-2019-v1.7-FINAL-14Nov2018-WMS.pdf (accessed on 30 January 2019).
2. Watz, H.; Pitta, F.; Rochester, C.L.; Garcia-Aymerich, J.; ZuWallack, R.; Troosters, T.; Vaes, A.W.; Puhan, M.A.; Jehn, M.; Polkey, M.I.; et al. An official European respiratory society statement on physical activity in COPD. *Eur. Respir. J.* **2014**, *44*, 1521–1537. [CrossRef] [PubMed]
3. American Thoracic Society (ATS); American College of Chest Physicians (ACCP). ATS/ACCP Statement on cardiopulmonary exercise testing. *Am. J. Respir. Crit. Care Med.* **2003**, *167*, 211–277. [CrossRef] [PubMed]
4. Poole, D.C.; Jones, A.M. Towards an understanding of the mechanistic bases of $VO_2$ kinetics. *Compr. Physiol.* **2012**, *2*, 933–996.
5. Nery, L.E.; Wasserman, K.; Andrews, J.D.; Huntsman, D.J.; Hansen, J.E.; Whipp, B.J. Ventilatory and gas exchange kinetics during exercise in chronic airways obstruction. *J. Appl. Physiol.* **1982**, *53*, 1594–1602. [CrossRef] [PubMed]
6. Somfay, A.; Porszasz, J.; Lee, S.-M.; Casaburi, R. Effect of hyperoxia on gas exchange and lactate kinetics following exercise onset in nonhypoxemic COPD patients. *Chest* **2002**, *121*, 393–400. [CrossRef] [PubMed]
7. Palange, P.; Galassetti, P.; Mannix, E.T.; Farber, M.O.; Manfredi, F.; Serra, P.; Carlone, S. Oxygen effect on $O_2$ deficit and $VO_2$ kinetics during exercise in obstructive pulmonary disease. *J. Appl. Physiol.* **1995**, *78*, 2228–2234. [CrossRef] [PubMed]
8. Laveneziana, P.; Palange, P.; Ora, J.; Martolini, D.; O'Donnell, D.E. Bronchodilator effect on ventilatory, pulmonary gas exchange, and heart rate kinetics during high-intensity exercise in COPD. *Eur. J. Appl. Physiol.* **2009**, *107*, 633–643. [CrossRef]
9. Berton, D.C.; Barbosa, P.B.; Takara, L.S.; Chiappa, G.R.; Siqueira, A.C.B.; Bravo, D.M.; Ferreira, L.F.; Neder, J.A. Bronchodilators accelerate the dynamics of muscle $O_2$ delivery and utilisation during exercise in COPD. *Thorax* **2010**, *65*, 588–593. [CrossRef] [PubMed]
10. Puente-Maestu, L.; Sánz, M.L.; Sánz, P.; De Oña, J.M.R.; Rodríguez-Hermosa, J.L.; Whipp, B.J. Effects of two types of training on pulmonary and cardiac responses to moderate exercise in patients with COPD. *Eur. Respir. J.* **2000**, *15*, 1026–1032. [CrossRef]
11. Faisal, A.; Zoumot, Z.; Shah, P.L.; Neder, J.A.; Polkey, M.I.; Hopkinson, N.S. Effective bronchoscopic lung volume reduction accelerates exercise oxygen uptake kinetics in emphysema. *Chest* **2016**, *149*, 435–446. [CrossRef] [PubMed]
12. Chiappa, G.R.; Borghi-Silva, A.; Ferreira, L.F.; Carrascosa, C.; Oliveira, C.C.; Maia, J.; Gimenes, A.C.; Queiroga, F.; Berton, D.; Ferreira, E.M.V.; et al. Kinetics of muscle deoxygenation are accelerated at the onset of heavy-intensity exercise in patients with COPD: Relationship to central cardiovascular dynamics. *J. Appl. Physiol.* **2008**, *104*, 1341–1350. [CrossRef]
13. Box, G.E.; Jenkins, G.M.; Reinsel, G.C.; Ljung, G.M. *Time Series Analysis*, 4th ed.; Quigley, S., Van Horn, L., Eds.; John Wiley & Sons, Inc.: New York, NY, USA, 2008; ISBN 9780470272848.
14. Spruit, M.A.; Vanderhoven-Augustin, I.; Janssen, P.P.; Wouters, E.F. Integration of pulmonary rehabilitation in COPD. *Lancet* **2008**, *371*, 12–13. [CrossRef]
15. Pedregal, D.J.; Taylor, C.J.; Young, P.C. *System Identification, Time Series Analysis and Forecasting: The Captain Toolbox handbook*; Lancaster University: Lancaster, UK, 2007.
16. Young, P.C. *Recursive Estimation and Time-Series Analysis: An Introduction for the Student and Practitioner*, 2nd ed.; Springer: Berlin/Heidelberg, Germany; New York, NY, USA, 2011; ISBN 978-3-642-21980-1.
17. Taylor, C.J.; Pedregal, D.J.; Young, P.C.; Tych, W. Environmental time series analysis and forecasting with the Captain toolbox. *Environ. Model. Softw.* **2007**, *22*, 797–814. [CrossRef]
18. Jones, N.L.; Makrides, L.; Hitchcock, C.; Chypchar, T.; McCartney, N. Normal Standards for an Incremental Progressive Cycle Ergometer Test. *Am. Thorac. Soc. J.* **1985**, *131*, 700–708.
19. Whipp, B.J.; Ward, S.A.; Lamarra, N.; Davis, J.A.; Wasserman, K. Parameters of ventilatory dynamics during exercise. *J. Appl. Physiol. Respir. Environ. Exerc. Physiol.* **1982**, *52*, 1506–1513.

20. Bell, C.; Paterson, D.H.; Kowalchuk, J.M.; Padilla, J.; Cunningham, D.A. A comparison of modelling techniques used to characterise oxygen uptake kinetics during the on-transient of exercise. *Exp. Physiol.* **2001**, *86*, 667–676. [CrossRef] [PubMed]
21. Spencer, M.D.; Murias, J.M.; Lamb, H.P.; Kowalchuk, J.M.; Paterson, D.H. Are the parameters of VO2, heart rate and muscle deoxygenation kinetics affected by serial moderate-intensity exercise transitions in a single day? *Eur. J. Appl. Physiol.* **2011**, *111*, 591–600. [CrossRef]
22. Lamarra, N.; Whipp, B.J.; Ward, A.; Wasserman, K. Effect of interbreath fluctuations on characterizing exercise gas exchange kinetics. *J. Appl. Physiol.* **1987**, *62*, 2003–2012. [CrossRef]
23. Puente-Maestu, L.; Buendía Abad, M.J.; Godoy, R.; Pérez-Parra, J.M.; Cubillo, J.M.; Whipp, B.J. Breath-by-breath fluctuations of pulmonary gas exchange and ventilation in COPD patients. *Eur. J. Appl. Physiol.* **2002**, *87*, 535–541. [CrossRef] [PubMed]
24. Markovitz, G.H.; Sayre, J.W.; Storer, T.W.; Cooper, C.B. On issues of confidence in determining the time constant for oxygen uptake kinetics. *Br. J. Sports Med.* **2004**, *38*, 553–560. [CrossRef]
25. Söderström, T. *Errors-in-Variables Methods in System Identification*; Springer International Publishing: Cham, Switzerland, 2018; ISBN 978-3-319-75000-2.
26. Murias, J.M.; Spencer, M.D.; Kowalchuk, J.M.; Paterson, D.H. Influence of phase I duration on phase II VO$_2$ kinetics parameter estimates in older and young adults. *Am. J. Physiol. Regul. Integr. Comp. Physiol* **2011**, *301*, 218–224. [CrossRef] [PubMed]
27. Kilding, A.E.; Challis, N.V.; Winter, E.M.; Fysh, M. Characterisation, asymmetry and reproducibility of on-and off-transient pulmonary oxygen uptake kinetics in endurance-trained runners. *Eur. J. Appl. Physiol.* **2005**, *93*, 588–597. [CrossRef]
28. De Müller, P.T.; Christofoletti, G.; Zagatto, A.M.; Paulin, F.V.; Neder, J.A. Reliability of peak O$_2$ uptake and O$_2$ uptake kinetics in step exercise tests in healthy subjects. *Respir. Physiol. Neurobiol.* **2015**, *207*, 7–13. [CrossRef]
29. Puente-Maestu, L.; Sánz, M.L.; Sánz, P.; Nuñez, A.; González, F.; Whipp, B.J. Reproducibility of the parameters of the on-transient cardiopulmonary responses during moderate exercise in patients with chronic obstructive pulmonary disease. *Eur. J. Appl. Physiol.* **2001**, *85*, 434–441. [CrossRef] [PubMed]
30. Edwards, A.M.; Claxton, D.B.; Fysh, M.L. A comparison of two time-domain analysis procedures in the determination of VO$_2$ kinetics by pseudorandom binary sequence exercise testing. *Eur. J. Appl. Physiol.* **2003**, *88*, 411–416. [CrossRef] [PubMed]
31. Macfarlane, D.J. Open-circuit respirometry: A historical review of portable gas analysis systems. *Eur. J. Appl. Physiol.* **2017**, *117*, 2369–2386. [CrossRef]
32. Van Remoortel, H.; Raste, Y.; Louvaris, Z.; Giavedoni, S.; Burtin, C.; Langer, D.; Wilson, F.; Rabinovich, R.; Vogiatzis, I.; Hopkinson, N.S.; et al. Validity of Six Activity Monitors in Chronic Obstructive Pulmonary Disease: A Comparison with Indirect Calorimetry. *PLoS ONE* **2012**, *7*, e39198. [CrossRef]
33. Lefever, J.; Berckmans, D.; Aerts, J.-M. Time-variant modelling of heart rate responses to exercise intensity during road cycling. *Eur. J. Sport Sci.* **2014**, *14*, S406–S412. [CrossRef] [PubMed]

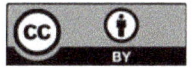

© 2019 by the authors. Licensee MDPI, Basel, Switzerland. This article is an open access article distributed under the terms and conditions of the Creative Commons Attribution (CC BY) license (http://creativecommons.org/licenses/by/4.0/).

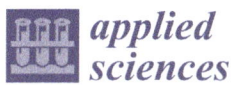 

*Article*

# Reverse Engineering of Thermoregulatory Cold-Induced Vasoconstriction/Vasodilation during Localized Cooling

**Ali Youssef [1], Anne Verachtert [1], Guido De Bruyne [2] and Jean-Marie Aerts [1,*]**

[1] Department of Biosystems, Animal and Human Health Engineering Division, M3-BIORES: Measure, Model & Manage of Bioresponses Laboratory, KU Leuven, Kasteelpark Arenberg 30, 3001 Heverlee, Belgium
[2] Department of Product Development, University of Antwerp, 2000 Antwerp, Belgium
* Correspondence: jean-marie.aerts@kuleuven.be

Received: 10 July 2019; Accepted: 8 August 2019; Published: 16 August 2019

**Abstract:** Biological systems, in general, represent a special type of control system. The physiological processes of homeostasis, which serve to maintain the organism's internal equilibrium against external influences, are clear forms of biological control system. An example of the homeostasis is the control of the organism thermal state or the thermoregulation. The thermoregulatory control of human skin blood flow, via vasoconstriction and vasodilation, is vital to maintaining normal body temperatures during challenges to thermal homeostasis such as localised cooling. The main objective of this paper is to reverse engineer the localised thermoregulatory cold-induced vasoconstriction/vasodilation (CIVC/CIVD) reactions using a data-based mechanistic approach. Two types of localised cooling were applied to the fingers of 33 healthy participants, namely, continuous and intermittent cooling. Modelling of the thermoregulatory cold-induced vasoconstriction/vasodilation reactions suggested two underlying processes, with one process being 10 times faster. A new term is suggested in this paper, namely, the latent heat of CIVD, which represents the amount of dissipated heat required to trigger the CIVD. Moreover, a new model for the thermoregulatory localised CIVC/CIVD reactions is proposed. The suggested new model states that, with an initial vasodilation state, the initial localised CIVC is triggered based on a certain threshold in the rate of heat dissipation from the skin to the surrounding environment.

**Keywords:** thermoregulation; homeostasis; cold-induced-vasodilation; cold-induced-vasoconstriction; control system; dynamic modelling

## 1. Introduction

Biological systems represent a special type of control system. In all of these, control is exercised over the flows of matter and energy to maintain a range of stationarity of their existence [1]. Hence, all living organisms are equipped with numerous interconnected control systems, which serve to maintain the organism's internal equilibrium regardless of outside influences. This condition is known as *homeostasis*. In the 19th century, Claude Bernard discovered the "amazing constancy" of the internal environment of the organism [2], and in 1927, Cannon named it the *homeostasis* [3].

An example of homeostasis is the control of an organism's thermal state (thermoregulation system). Heat in biological systems is generated in the course of metabolic conversion and scattered by conduction, convection, radiation and evaporation [4–6].

The hands and feet form powerful thermoregulatory regulators in the body, serving as heat radiators (exchanger) and evaporators in hot environments and as thermal insulators in the cold [7]. Taylor et al. [8] estimated that each hand and foot can dissipate 150–220 W·m$^{-2}$ through radiation and convection at rest in an ambient temperature of 27 °C, with even greater heat dissipation through sweating. Additionally, the extremities can serve as thermal sensor acting in feedback and feedforward fashion to the thermoregulation system of the body [7].

Arteriovenous anastomoses (AVAs) are direct connections between small arteries and small veins (Figure 1), with no capillary section between them. Since there is no capillary transportation, the only transport function they could possibly have is the transport of heat from the body core to surface areas containing AVAs [9].

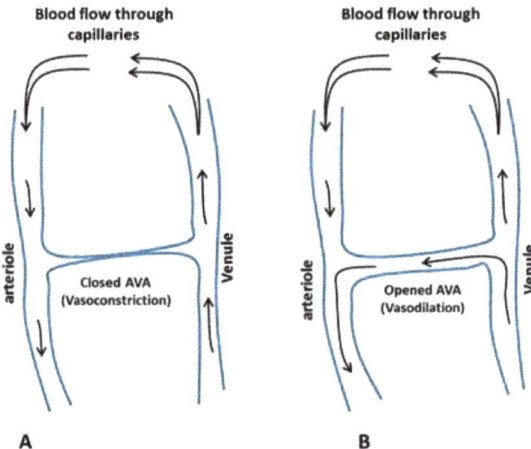

**Figure 1.** Schematic diagram showing the effect of a closed (**A**) and an open (**B**) arteriovenous anastomoses on the blood flow during cold-induced vasoconstriction and cold-induced vasodilation, respectively.

Grant and Blond [10] investigated the role of AVA in thermoregulation. They found a relation between the number of AVAs in a body part and the change in local skin temperature due to local cold [11]. When the extremities of the hand and feet are exposed locally to a cold environment, their AVAs respond with sympathetically mediated vasoconstriction, which is termed cold-induced vasoconstriction (CIVC). CIVC reduces the blood flow to the peripheries in favour of a central pooling of blood in the torso and deep body core [7,12,13]. Due to this vasoconstriction and the high surface area-to-volume ratio, the skin temperature of the extremities tends and exponentially decreases to a level approaching that of the ambient environment. After a brief period of lowered skin blood flow and temperature, due to the CIVC, a temporary increase in blood flow and rewarming occurs. During these episodes, skin temperature can rise by as much as 10 °C, and this fall and rise can occur repeatedly in a cyclic fashion [7]. This pattern of periodic warming was first reported by Lewis [14], who labelled it the "hunting response", due to its apparent oscillatory pattern. This response is also termed the cold-induced vasodilation (CIVD) phenomenon [15]. There is a definite variation in the occurrence, magnitude, and duration of the CIVD [16].

It was found that the CIVD occurs in about 5 to 10 min after the exposure of the hand to cold [15,17], and is initiated by the dilation of the AVAs [7,13,15,18]. Because of the elevated extremity blood flow and temperature, CIVD has generally been presumed to provide a protective function by maintaining local tissue integrity and minimizing the risk of cold injuries. However, the mechanisms underlying CIVD are unclear, yet understanding the nature of CIVD is of important occupational and clinical relevance [7]. Additionally, the review studies of Cheung et al. [7,19] have shown that it is not easy to compare different research findings due to the inconsistent methodologies in the experimental protocols, and most of the studies on CIVD are largely descriptive, lacking sufficient quantification of CIVD responses.

The current study was originated based on the findings of previous study by Youssef et. al. [20], in which the authors tried to take advantage of the CIVC reaction to prevent nail toxicity during chemotherapy. During their study [20], Youssef et al. aimed to model the CIVC responses to localized cooling for the purpose of developing a model-based controller of the finger skin temperature. However, the developed controller exhibited unpredictable disturbances, represented by abrupt increases in the skin temperature due to the CIVD reaction.

The main goal of this study it to try to understand and quantify the mechanism of CIVC and CIVD by reverse engineering the dynamic responses of the hands' skin temperature to localised cooling using a databased mechanistic (DBM) modelling approach.

## 2. Materials and Methods

### 2.1. Controllable Active Cooling Device and Measurements (iGlove-1)

An in-house (University of Antwerp, Antwerp, Belgium) developed active localised cooling device (*iGlove-1*, Figure 2) was developed to investigate the possibility of localised active cooling of hand fingers [21]. The *iGlove-1* device was developed in such way as to provide a stable localised low temperature (cooling) to the five fingers of the subject's left hand. The *iGlove-1* was equipped with 20 *Peltier* elements (two elements positioned on both sides of each finger) to apply localised cooling of the fingers. Each element had a size about 12 × 12 × 5 mm.

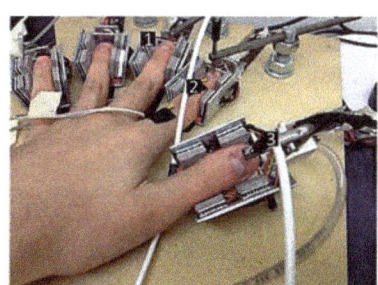

**Figure 2.** The *iGlove-1*-controlled cooling device for the left hand. (1) Peltier cooling elements; (2) NTC temperature sensor to measure the finger skin temperature; (3) one probe of the blood flow Laser Doppler meter.

The *iGlove-1* device consisted of a wooden construction on which the subject's left hand can rest. The construction was equipped with five mechanically adjustable holders to ensure a good contact between the Peltier elements and the fingers of different hand sizes. The two Peltier elements located on each side of the finger (two on the fingertip and another below the first phalanx, Figure 2) were always electrically connected in series.

The *iGlove-1* device was equipped with five NTC sensors (with an accuracy of ±0.1 °C) to continuously measure the temperatures of the left-hand fingers. Another 20 NTC sensors measured the temperature of the Peltier elements (one sensor for each element). A Laser Doppler blood flow meter (MoorVMS-LDF2® by Moor Instruments) was used to measure the changes in the blood flow underneath the nail bed. The blood flow measurements were performed on only two fingers, the index finger and the thumb, of the subject's left hand as a representation of the changes in the blood flow to the five fingers.

The temperature sensors were positioned on the underside of each fingertip, while the probes of the Laser-Doppler blood flow meter were placed on the middle of the nails of the thumb and index fingers. The skin temperatures of the five fingers and that of the ambient air (in degrees Celsius, °C) were recorded, as well as the blood flow (in Perfusion Units, PU) of the thumb and the index finger, every second (for more information see [20–22]).

## 2.2. Experiments

Data from two sets of experiments were used during the course of this work. The first set (Exp.1) was conducted during a previous study [20] with the objective of designing a model-based control system for localised cooling of hand termites to avoid nail toxicity during chemotherapy. The second set (Exp.2) of experiments was conducted during the course of this study to test the effect of intermittent cooling on the CIVD phenomena.

### 2.2.1. Test Subjects

Data from two different sets of experiments (Table 1) was obtained from 33 participants (test subjects). During the first set of experiments (Exp.1), a homogeneous group of 11 healthy women between the ages of 35 and 55 years performed the tests. This age range was chosen for the sake of the objective of the previous study [21], since a high incidence rate of breast cancer is recorded within this age range. The second set of experiments was performed using 12 test subjects, of which six were males and six were females with an age range between 18 and 24 years old.

**Table 1.** The number of test subjects participating in each of the conducted sets of experiments, showing the average-age and gender.

| Experiment | Number of Participants | Age | Gender | |
|---|---|---|---|---|
| | | | M | F |
| Exp.1 | 11 | 44.9 (±5.84) | 0 | 11 |
| Exp.2 | 12 | 20.4 (±2.60) | 6 | 6 |

During the course of both sets (Exp.1 and Exp.2), all the test subjects were in healthy condition, non-smokers, having no hand injuries and with no evidence of the *Perniosis* or *Raynaud* phenomena. The absence of (excessive) alcohol consumption was ensured in all of the test subjects, starting from the evening (6–8 pm) before the test, with a normal (7–9) h of sleep during the night. During the two sets of experiments, all participants were asked to keep only light clothing (no jackets or pullovers) consisting of shirts (or sweaters) and pants (or skirts).

### 2.2.2. Experimental Protocol

*Acclimatisation stage*: for both sets of experiments (Exp.1 and Exp.2), each test subject was seated at the start of the measurements in the test room for ±30 min to acclimatise them to the continuously measured ambient air temperature (22.4 ± 0.6 °C) within the test room.

*Step experiment stage*: after placing the subject's left hand fingers in their appropriate positions on the *iGlove-1* device (Figure 2), for the first set of experiments, the set-point temperature on the controller of the Peltier elements was set to 20 °C for 15 min. For the next 30 min, a step-down decrease in the temperature of the Peltier element was applied by setting the controller set-point to 2 °C. These applied set-points were chosen in such way as to ensure that both the CIVC and CIVD phenomenon were triggered [20,21].

During the first set of experiments (Exp.1), for each test subject, the previous test protocol was repeated three times in three consecutive days at the same time of day, giving a total of 33 full experimental trials. The second set of experiments (Exp.2) consisted of two different phases (Figure 3).

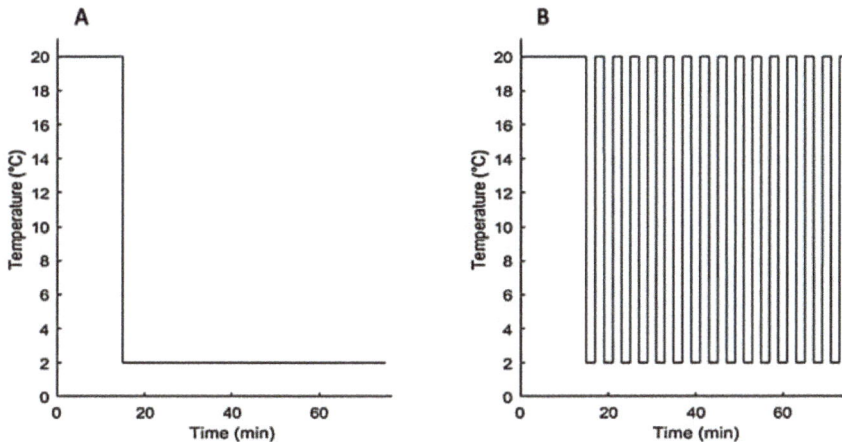

**Figure 3.** The different set temperature of the Peltier elements for (**A**) experimental phase (I) and (**B**) phase (II) of the second set of experiments.

During the first experimental phase (I), the set-point temperature of the controller of the Peltier elements was set to 20 °C for 15 min. For the next 60 min, a step-down decrease in the temperature of the Peltier element was applied by setting the controller set-point to 2 °C. During the second phase (II), a pulse train (a rectangular pulse wave) of set temperatures to the Peltier elements was applied for 60 min. More specifically, we set a pulse time of 2 min, a minimum and maximum set temperatures of 2 °C and 20 °C, respectively (see Figure 3B).

### 2.3. System Identification and Modelling of CIVC/CIVD

Although the system under study (the finger/blood circulation) is inherently a non-linear system, the essential perturbation behaviour can often be approximated well by simple linearized Transfer Function (TF) models [20,23–29].

For the purposes of the present paper, the following linear, single-input, single-output (SISO) discrete-time transfer function (DTF) is considered [20],

$$y(k) = \frac{b_1 z^{-1} + \ldots + b_m z^{-m}}{1 + a_1 z^{-1} + \ldots + a_n z^{-n}} u(k - \delta) + (k) = \frac{B(z^{-1})}{A(z^{-1})} u(k) + (k)$$
$$y(k) = \frac{b_1 z^{-1} + \ldots + b_m z^{-m}}{1 + a_1 z^{-1} + \ldots + a_n z^{-n}} u(k - \delta) + \xi(k) = \frac{B(z^{-1})}{A(z^{-1})} u(k) + \xi(k) \quad (1)$$

where $y(k)$ is the finger skin temperature (°C) and $u(k)$ is the temperature of the Peltier elements (°C), while $A(z^{-1})$ and $B(z^{-1})$ are appropriately defined polynomials in the backshift operator $z^{-1}$, i.e., $z^{-i} y(k) = y(k-i)$ and $\xi(k)$ is additive noise, a serially uncorrelated sequence of random variables with variance $\sigma^2$ that accounts for measurement noise, modelling errors and effects of unmeasured inputs to the process (assumed to be a zero mean). For convenience, any pure time delay of $\delta > 1$ samples can be accounted for by setting the $\delta - 1$ leading parameters of the $B(z^{-1})$ polynomial to zero, i.e., $b_1, \ldots \ldots, b_{\delta-1} = 0$.

A step-input was applied, as explained earlier, by suddenly decreasing the temperature of the Peltier elements from 20 to 2 °C. In practice, the transition of the input to the new steady state is taking some time (transition time). However, for convenience, in this paper the step-input was idealised and normalised by assuming that it starts from zero and changes instantaneously at a time equal to zero,

$$u(t) = \begin{cases} 0 \text{ for } t < 0 \\ 1 \text{ for } t \geq 0 \end{cases} \quad (2)$$

The *Simplified Refined Instrumental Variable* (SRIV) algorithm was utilised in the identification and estimation of the models (model parameters and model structure) [30,31].

Firstly, the appropriate model structure was identified, i.e., the most appropriate values for the triad [$n, m, \delta$] (see Equation (1)), where $n$ and $m$ are the number of poles and zeros, respectively. Two main statistical measures were employed to determine the most appropriate values of this triad. Namely, the coefficient of determination $R_2^T$, based on the response error; and YIC (Young's Information Criterion), which provides a combined measure of model fit and parametric efficiency, with large negative values indicating a model that explains the output data well and yet avoids over-parameterisation [31,32].

## 3. Results and Discussion

### 3.1. System Identification

#### 3.1.1. Data-Based Mechanistic Modelling of CIVC

The measured blood flow, conducted during the first set of experiments (Exp.1), showed a decreasing pattern (average drop of 400 ± 53 PU) coupled with decreased finger skin temperatures in response to the applied localized cooling (for more information see [20]).

In agreement with previous study [20], the SRIV algorithm combined with YIC and $R_2^T$ suggested that a second-order (with number of poles $n$ = 2 and zeros $m$ = 2) discrete-time TF described the dynamic responses of finger skin temperature to step-decreases in the input (Peltier element's temperature) most accurately (i.e., $R_2^T$ = 0.91 ± 0.04 and YIC = −11.23 ± 2.33) for all 33 test subjects. More specifically, the SRIV algorithm identified the following general discrete-time DTF model structure,

$$y(k) = \frac{b_1 z^{-1} + b_2 z^{-2}}{1 + a_1 z^{-1} + a_2 z^{-2}} u(k - \delta) + \xi(k) \qquad (3)$$

where the pure time delay ($\delta$) was different from test subject to another (interpersonal variation) with an average ($\bar{\delta}$ = 2.3 min) and standard deviation (SD = 1). The variations in the time delay of the model reflects the different individual biological responses to colder environment. Figure 4 shows a simulation example of the resulting model (3), showing the simulated dynamic responses of the finger skin temperature to step decrease (cooling) in the Peltier element temperature.

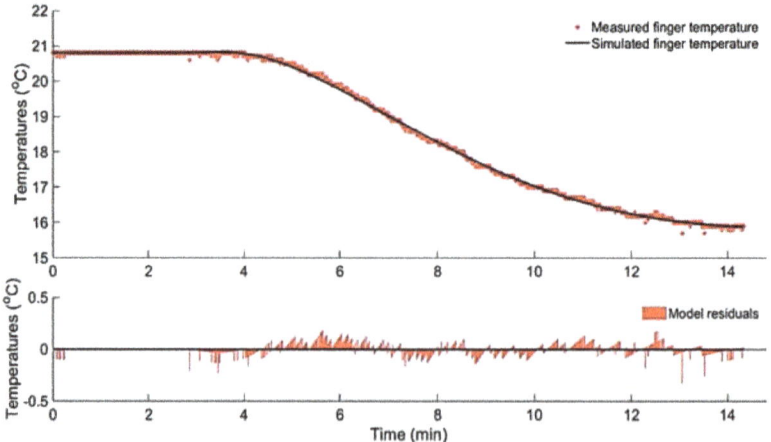

**Figure 4.** A simulation example of the second-order DTF (3) that represents the finger's temperature response (CIVC reaction) to the step decrease in Peltier element temperature (cooling).

To understand the underlying mechanism of the resulting second-order system (3), describing the CIVC process, it was decomposed into two simpler first-order transfer functions (TF). These two first-order TFs can be interconnected in three well-known configurations, namely, series, parallel and feedback configurations. The results showed that the parallel configuration (Figure 5) was mathematically most suitable (average $R_2^T$ = 0.91 ± 0.01) for describing the dynamic response of the CIVC process in all test subjects. As depicted in Figure 5, the second-order system (3), representing the CIVC process, was decomposed into two first-order TFs, defined as follows:

$$TF_1 = \frac{b_1}{1 + a_1 z^{-1}}$$

$$TF_2 = \frac{b_2}{1 + a_2 z^{-1}}$$

$$y(k) = [TF_1 + TF_2] \cdot u(k - \delta) \tag{4}$$

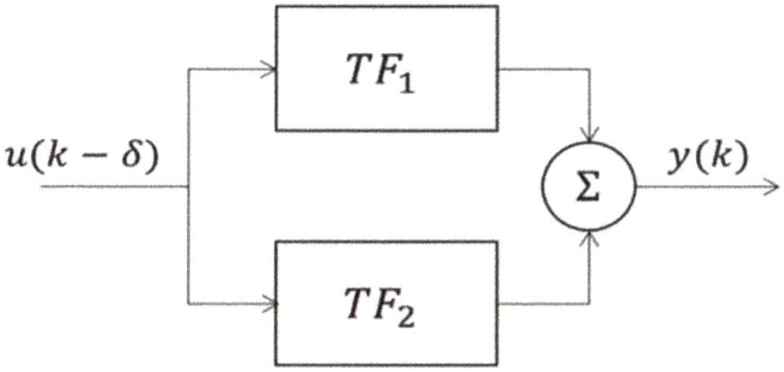

**Figure 5.** The parallel configuration of the interconnection between the two first-order TFs resulting from the decomposition of the second-order system (Equation (3)).

The time constants $\tau_1$ and $\tau_2$ of $TF_1$ and $TF_2$, respectively, were calculated and compared for all test subjects, where $\tau = 1/\ln(-a)$. Table 2 shows the mean and standard deviation of the calculated time constants obtained from all test-subjects during the two sets of experiments (Exp.1 and Exp.2, Phase I).

**Table 2.** Mean and standard deviation of the calculated time constants, of the decomposed two first-order TF, obtained from all test subjects (33) during the two sets of experiments (Exp.1 and Exp.2, Phase I).

|  | $\tau_1$ (min) | $\tau_2$ (min) |
| --- | --- | --- |
| Mean | 7.34 | 0.73 |
| Standard deviation | 3.2 | 0.56 |

The aforementioned results suggested two parallel underlying processes taking place during the CIVC action. However, by comparing the calculated time constants, it became clear that the process represented by $TF_2$ was, on average, 10 times faster ($\tau_2 \approx 0.73$ min) than the one represented by $TF_1$ ($\tau_1 \approx 7.34$ min).

Physical and physiological insights into the resulting mathematical model were investigated using first principles (e.g., Fourier's law and Newton's law of cooling) and other mechanistic models (e.g., [12]).

The heat flow through any object, including the finger, can be described conventionally by lumped quantities such as thermal resistance (or conductance) and thermal capacitance [27]. The heat balance equation representing the heat flow (W) between the finger and the colder Peltier's element can be given by:

$$\frac{dT_{skin}}{dt} = \frac{h_{vein}A_{vein}}{C_{skin}}(T_{bld} - T_{skin}) + \left\{\frac{h_{cap}A_{cap}}{C_{skin}}(T_{bld} - T_{skin}) - \frac{K_{skin}A_{skin}}{C_{skin}}(T_{skin} - T_\infty)\right\} \quad (5)$$

where $C_{skin}$ (J.°C$^{-1}$) is the skin thermal capacitance, $T_{skin}$ is the finger skin temperature, $h_{vein}$ (W m$^{-2}$ °C$^{-1}$) is the convective heat transfer coefficient of flowing blood in the superficial vein, $A_{vein}$ is the cross-section area of the superficial vein, $T_{bld}$ is the blood temperature, $h_{cap}$ (W m$^{-2}$ °C$^{-1}$) is the convective heat transfer coefficient of the blood in the superficial capillaries network, $K_{skin}$ (W m$^{-2}$ °C$^{-1}$) is the skin conductance.

Under normal temperature (normothermia), before applying the step cooling using the Peltier's element, there is a baseline level of vasoconstrictive tone [33], where the blood velocity fluctuates, between a high level and a very low level, with about 2–3 vasoconstrictions per minute [17]. The high level corresponds to a state when the AVAs were open. However, when the local environmental temperature (Peltier's element temperature) drops, the AVAs close, causing the direct blood flow from the artery to the superficial vein to stop quite abruptly. Hence, the convective heat transfer ($\dot{Q}_{vein} = h_{vein}A_{vein}(T_{bld} - T_{skin})$) from the blood in the superficial veins (Figure 6) decreases dramatically, causing a fast reduction in the skin temperature, which can be represented by the transfer function $TF_2$. On the other hand, the convective heat transfer from capillaries ($\dot{Q}_{cap} = h_{cap}A_{cap}(T_{blood} - T_{skin})$) together with the conductive heat exchange ($\dot{Q}_{skin} = K_{skin}A_{skin}(T_{skin} - T_\infty)$) between the skin and colder Peltier's element are dissipating the heat much slower. This is mainly due to the effect of skin thermal capacitance and the high resistance of the capillaries to blood flow. Hence, TF1, with the slow time constant, is suitable for describing the dynamic response of both the convective heat transfer from capillaries and conductive heat exchange between the skin and the Peltier's element.

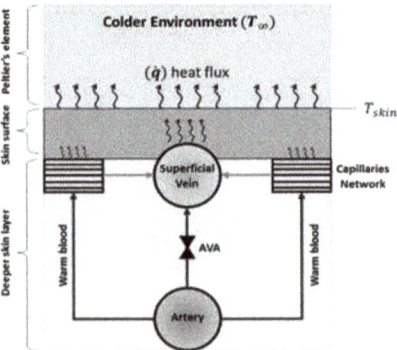

**Figure 6.** Schematic representation of the heat transfer between the finger and the Peltier element through three different layers, namely, deep skin layer, surface skin layer and the Peltier's element. The AVA controls the direct flow between the artery and the surface vein.

### 3.1.2. Data-Based Mechanistic Modelling of CIVD

Among the 33 test subjects, 27 showed the hunting reaction with cycles of CIVC and CIVD. Figure 7 shows an example of the resulting hunting reaction to continuous localised cooling using Peltier's element temperature at 2 °C.

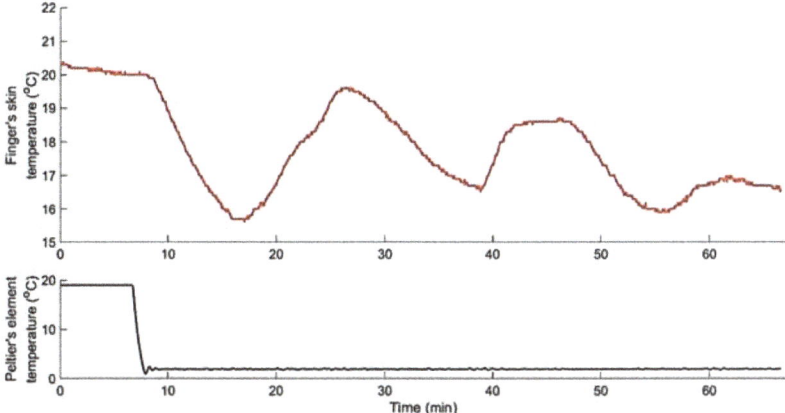

**Figure 7.** Dynamic response of finger skin temperature to step decrease in Peltier's element temperature from 20 °C to 2 °C, showing an example of the hunting reaction in a test subject.

Within the cooling period of 60 min, all test subjects exhibiting hunting reactions showed three consecutive cycles of CIVC/CIVD (an example is shown in Figure 7).

A second-order DTF with two poles ($n = 2$) and two zeroes ($m = 2$) was the best model structure (with average $R_T^2 = 0.92 \pm 0.04$ and $YIC = -10.61 \pm 3.45$) to describe the CIVD response to localised cooling for all test subjects with the hunting reaction:

$$y(k) = \frac{b_1 z^{-1} + b_2 z^{-2}}{1 + a_1 z^{-1} + a_2 z^{-2}} u(k - \delta) + \xi(k) \tag{6}$$

The structure of the identified model, represented by the triad $[n = 2, m = 2, \delta]$, showed an average time delay $\delta$ of 10.23 min ($\pm$3.50 min). In other words, for all test subjects that showing the hunting reaction, the first episode of CIVD started, on average, after 10.23 $\pm$ 3.50 min from the start of applying the localised cooling. Table 3 shows the estimation results of the identified model (6) for all test subjects showing the hunting reaction.

**Table 3.** Average and standard deviation of parameter estimates, $R_T^2$ and $YIC$ of the second-order DTF model describing the CIVD reaction to continuous localised cooling experiments obtained from the test-subjects that shown hunting reaction (i.e., cycles of CIVC/CIVD episodes).

| $A(z^{-1})$ | | $B(z^{-1})$ | | | $\delta$ (min) | $R_T^2$ | YIC |
|---|---|---|---|---|---|---|---|
| $a_1$ | $a_2$ | $b_0$ | $b_1$ | $b_2$ | | | |
| −1.989 | 0.980 | 0.0 | −0.0047 | 0.0045 | 10.23 | 0.92 | −10.61 |
| ±0.005 | ±0.002 | ±0.0 | ±0.0010 | ±0.0010 | ±3.50 | ±0.04 | ±3.45 |

This relatively long time delay, compared to the CIVC case, was somehow misleading in terms of system causality, since during this lag of time between the cause (step cooling) and the modelled effect (CIVD), there was another effect, namely the CIVC. Therefore, the model input, represented by the step decrease in the Peltier's element temperature, cannot fully explain the CIVD effect. However, the rate of heat dissipation ($\dot{Q}_{dis}$, Watt), from the finger to the Peltier's elements, shows more dynamics in relation to both CIVC and CIVD. The heat dissipation rate ($\dot{Q}_{dis}$) is calculated based on Newton's law of cooling as follows [34]:

$$\dot{Q}_{dis} = -h_P A_P (T_{sk} - T_\infty) \tag{7}$$

where $h_P$ is the heat transfer coefficient between the finger's skin and Peltier's element (=15 W m$^{-2}$ °C$^{-1}$, from the datasheet of the Peltier's element) and $A_P$ is the total surface area of the Peltier's elements in contact with the skin (=5.76 × 10$^{-4}$ m$^2$).

An example of the simulated finger skin temperature during the CIVD reaction using the identified second-order DTF (6) is shown in Figure 8. Additionally, Figure 8 shows the calculated dissipated heat rate ($\dot{Q}_{dis}$) using Equation (7), while the area-under-the-curve represents the amount of the dissipated heat ($Q_{dis}$, Joules) from the finger to the Peltier's elements.

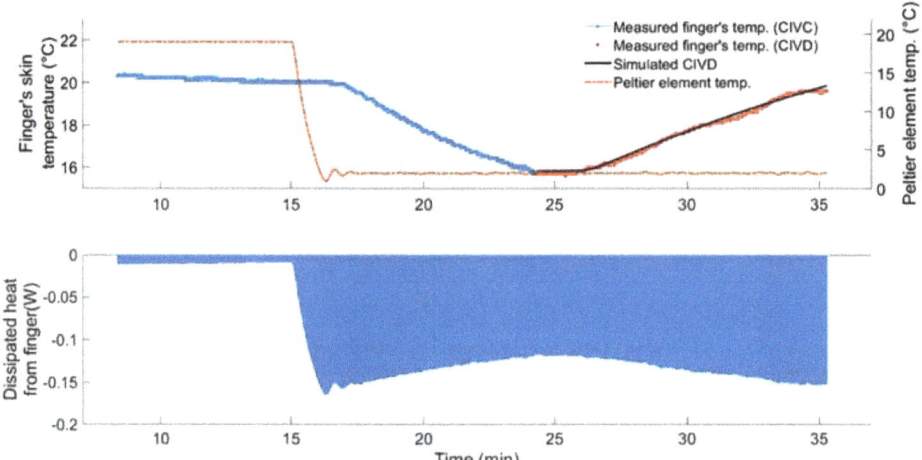

**Figure 8.** Measured and simulated finger skin temperature during the CIVD (upper graph), the dissipated heat rate from the finger and the area-under-the-curve represents the amount of dissipated heat in joules (lower graph).

The results showed that the average amount of dissipated heat from the skin of the finger before the CIVD kick-off (termed here as *latent heat for CIVD* or *LH-CIVD*) is 102.10 (±22.36) joules. We found that there was a significant difference between the test subjects (interpersonal) that exhibited the hunting effect with respect to their latent heat for CIVD (LH-CIVD), and this at a significance level of 1%. In other words, the LH-CIVD can be considered an individual-dependent characteristic. The proposed LH-CIVD term combined three main factors that are believed to affect the thermostatic responses, namely, the rate of cooling [35], the temperature to which the skin is cooled [36], and the duration of exposure [37].

The second-order TF (6) describing the CIVD reaction was decomposed into two first-order TFs with a parallel configuration (the same as described in Figure 5) as the most mathematically suitable configuration (average $R_2^T$ = 0.93 ± 0.01). The resulting time constants $\tau_1$ and $\tau_2$ of $TF_1$ and $TF_2$, respectively, were calculated and compared for all test subjects exhibiting the CIVD reaction, as shown in Table 4.

**Table 4.** Mean and standard deviation of the calculated time constants, of the decomposed two first-order TF, obtained from all test subjects with CIVD reaction during the two sets of experiments (Exp.1 and Exp.2, Phase I).

|  | $\tau_1$ (min) | $\tau_2$ (min) |
|---|---|---|
| Mean | 7.96 | 0.81 |
| Standard deviation | 4.35 | 0.65 |

In the same fashion as with the CIVC reaction, the calculated time constants suggested two parallel responses with clear and different dynamics. The first response, represented by the first-order model $TF_1$, was slow ($\tau_1 \approx 7.96$ min) in comparison to that represented by the first-order $TF_2$ ($\tau_1 \approx 0.81$ min). The fast response can be attributed to the gradual opening of the AVAs during the CIVD.

The time constants, $\tau_1$ and $\tau_2$, for the CIVC and CIVD responses were compared by the Kruskal-Wallis test. It was found that there was no significant difference, at a significance level of 1%, in the first time constant ($\tau_1$) for both CIVC and CIVD. The same results were noticed for the second time constant ($\tau_2$).

### 3.1.3. Modelling of Localized Intermittent Cooling Effect

During the localised intermittent cooling (Exp.2, Phase II), none of the test subjects that showed the hunting reaction (CIVC/CIVD cycles) during the continuous cooling (Phase I) showed any episodes of CIVD. On the other hand, intermittent cooling induced an episode of CIVC, causing the finger's temperature to drop to the same level reached during continuous cooling (on average, 16.2 ± 0.7 °C) and continued until the end of the experiment. Figure 9 shows an example of the finger's temperature response to intermittent cooling. Additionally, a second-order (with number of poles $n = 2$ and zeros $m = 2$) discrete-time TF described the dynamic responses of finger skin temperature (CIVC) to a series of cooling pulses (intermittent cooling) in the input (Peltier element's temperature) most accurately (i.e., $R_2^T = 0.92 \pm 0.02$ and $YIC = -11.67 \pm 3.55$) with same structure as the TF represented by (3). Table 5 shows the resulting average parameter estimates and delays from the identified DTF model describing the CIVC reaction to intermittent cooling.

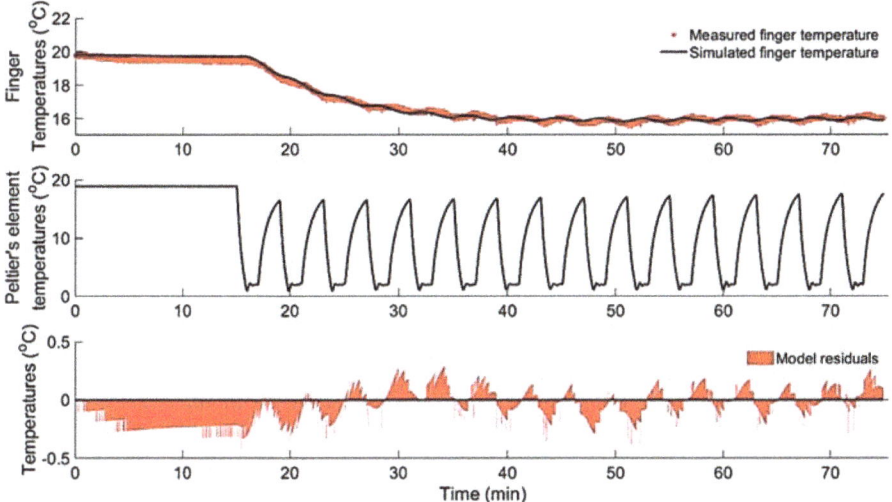

**Figure 9.** The dynamic response (upper graph) of the finger's temperature (CIVC) to a series of pulses in Peltier's element temperature (middle graph). Showing the measured and simulated finger's temperature (upper graph) using a second-order DTF and the model residuals (lower graph).

**Table 5.** Average and standard deviation of parameter estimates, $R_T^2$ and YIC of the identified second-order DTF model describing the CIVC reaction to the localised intermittent cooling experiment (Exp.2, Phase II).

| $A(z^{-1})$ | | $B(z^{-1})$ | | | $\delta$ (min) | $R_T^2$ | YIC |
|---|---|---|---|---|---|---|---|
| $a_1$ | $a_2$ | $b_0$ | $b_1$ | $b_2$ | | | |
| −1.987 | 0.987 | 0.0 | −0.0016 | 0.0018 | 2.34 | 0.92 | −11.67 |
| ±0.006 | ±0.001 | ±0.0 | ±0.0010 | ±0.0010 | ±1.21 | ±0.02 | ±3.55 |

Although the finger skin temperature, under intermittent cooling, reached the same level (on average, 16.2 ± 0.7 °C) as that under continuous cooling, the intermittent cooling did not induce reheating of the fingers (i.e., CIVD). This indicates that the temperature to which the skin was cooled is not the only triggering factor for the CIVD. Additionally, it was clear that the vasodilation here (CIVD) is typically transient, which may interrupt the original vasoconstriction. The current work suggests that the rate at which the skin was cooled (rate of dissipated heat from the skin) is one of the main triggering factors, aside from the skin temperature and the duration of cooling [7,15,19,38]. The results showed that all test subjects exhibited the hunting reaction (i.e., episodes of CIVD occurred) during continuous cooling (Exp.2, phase I), when the rate of change in the dissipated heat from skin ($\frac{dQ_{dis}}{dt}$) was quasi zero (an example from one test subject is shown in Figure 10). On the other hand, for the same test subjects, under intermittent cooling (Exp.2, Phase II) the rate of change ($\frac{dQ_{dis}}{dt}$) oscillated around zero (±0.0016), and no evidence of vasodilation was noticed (an example from one test subject is shown in Figure 11).

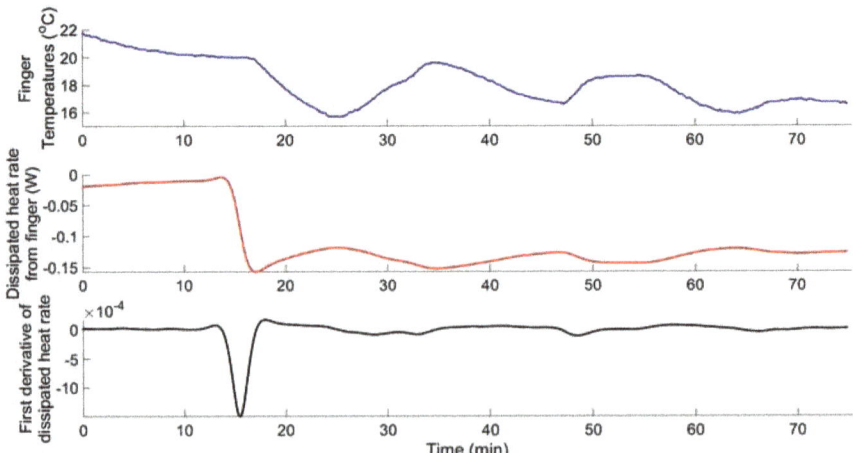

**Figure 10.** Dynamic response of finger skin temperature (upper graph), dissipated heat rate ($\dot{Q}_{dis}$, middle graph), and first derivative of the dissipated heat rate ($\frac{dQ_{dis}}{dt}$, lower graph) to localised continuous cooling obtained from test subject (s5) during the experiment (Exp.2, Phase I).

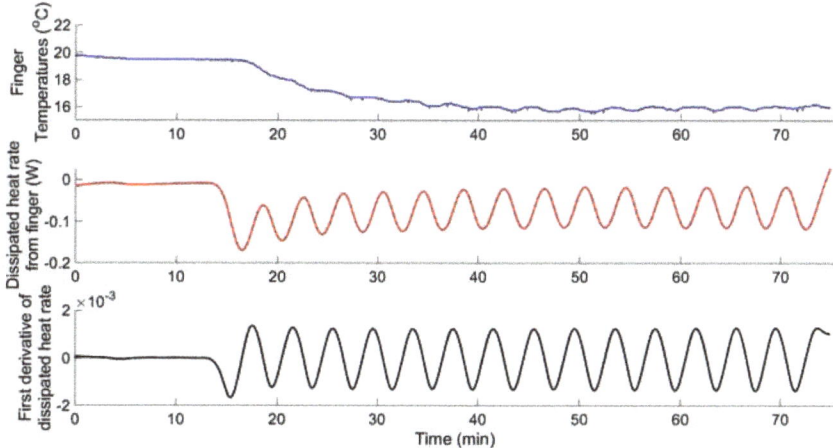

**Figure 11.** Dynamic response of finger skin temperature (upper graph), dissipated heat rate ($\dot{Q}_{dis}$, middle graph), and first derivative of the dissipated heat rate ($\frac{dQ_{dis}}{dt}$, lower graph) to localised intermittent cooling obtained from test subject (s5) during the experiment (Exp.2, Phase II).

The following section of this paper explores the different theories and mechanisms explaining the thermoregulatory CIVC/CIVD reactions.

*3.2. Physiological/Mechanistic Interpretation of Thermoregulatory CIVC/CIVD Reactions*

3.2.1. Mechanisms of CIVC/CIVD Reactions during Localised Cooling

The initial response to cold exposure is a sympathetically mediated peripheral vasoconstriction, resulting in reduced local tissue temperature [11,15,39,40]. With continued cold exposure, this vasoconstriction may be interrupted, resulting in periods of vasodilation, which correspond to an increase in tissue temperature [41]. The local cooling vasoconstrictor response is dependent on intact noradrenergic cutaneous active vasoconstrictor nerves [36,39,42]. Johnson et al. [36] concluded in their work that local cooling of skin occurs in two phases (biphasic): an initial phase, which lasts for few minutes (in accordance to the aforementioned results) and a prolonged phase. The initial phase is mediated by activation of cold-sensitive afferent neurons that affect the release of norepinephrine from sympathetic cutaneous vasoconstrictor nerves. Norepinephrine then vasoconstricts skin vessels (mainly the AVAs, in this case) through post-junctional α-receptors. On the other hand, the mechanisms for the prolonged phase, which follows an initial CIVD (hunting reaction), are suggested to be non-neurogenic [36], because no manipulations altered the prolonged cutaneous vasoconstriction during prolonged local cooling. However, these mechanisms have not been defined further [36]. Additionally, prolonged local cooling also mediates an initial "non-neurogenic" vasodilation (CIVD) that competes with the initial noradrenergically mediated vasoconstriction. Several hypotheses have been postulated on the mechanism of CIVD [15]. The main hypotheses to explain the initial CIVD and prolonged CIVC are depicted in Figure 12. In the case of prolonged localised cooling, and after an initial episode of CIVC (Figure 12A), an initial CIVD might occur. Based on previous research work (e.g., [15,18,43,44]), three different mechanisms are suggested to explain this initial CIVD (Figure 12). The first hypothesized mechanism (*pathway* 1) states that the smooth muscles in the blood-vessel walls become paralysed, for example, by a decreased concentration of $Ca^{2+}$ ions. Consequently, the paralysed smooth muscles will not be able to maintain vasoconstriction, and then vasodilation occurs. The second hypothesized mechanism (*pathway* 2) states that the smooth muscles become less sensitive to norepinephrine, for example, due to the resorption of the receptors from the cell membrane. The more resorption, the less norepinephrine can interact, the less the increase in intracellular $Ca^{2+}$ ion concentration, and the less the constriction. The third and final hypothesized mechanism (*pathway* 3) states that the adrenergic vasoconstrictor nerves release less norepinephrine. Thereby, the concentration of epinephrine in the synaptic cleft decreases. The bound epinephrine will detach from the receptors due to the concentration difference (diffusion), resulting in vasodilation.

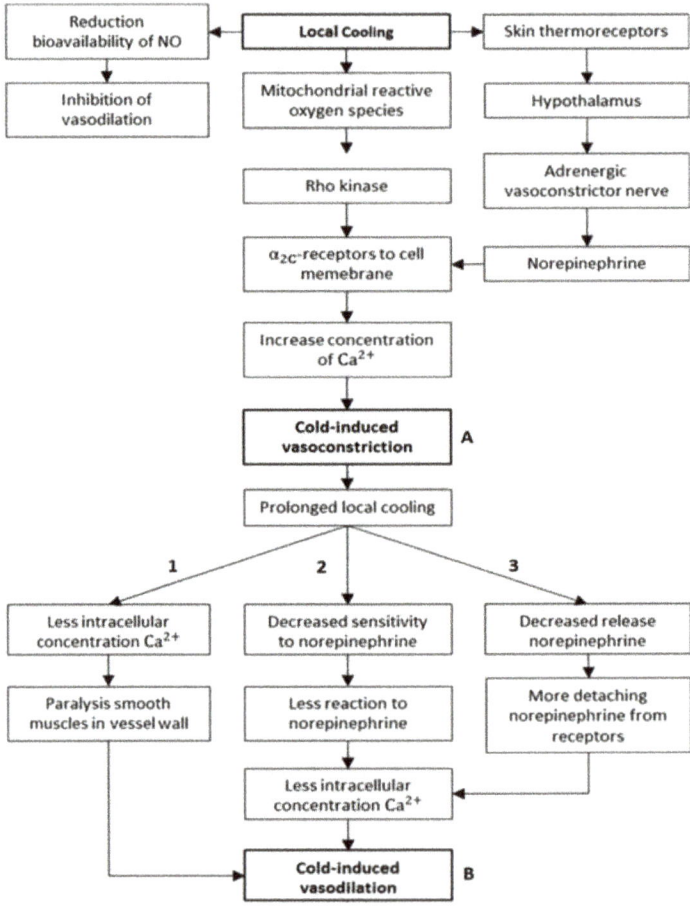

**Figure 12.** Main hypotheses explaining the hunting reaction (with *pathways* 1,2 and 3 representing the three proposed hypotheses from literature to explain the initial CIVD).

The findings of the current study do not support the first hypothesis (*pathway* 1), since it is clear from the case of intermittent localised cooling that the skin was cooled to the same temperature as in case of continuous cooling and yet no vasodilation evidence is recorded.

In agreement with the work of Yamazaki et al. [35], the present study suggests that the triggering of local cooling induced-vasodilation in the finger's skin is dependent on the heat dissipation rate ($\dot{Q}_{dis}$) or the rate of cooling as termed in [35,38].

Although the aforementioned hypotheses suggest non-neurogenic CIVD mechanisms, it is undisputed that CIVD magnitude and onset time are strongly dependent on central factors and sympathetic activity [45–48]. Mekjavic et al. [49] showed that after 13 days of immersing one hand, for 30 min daily, in 8 °C water, both the acclimated and contralateral (non-acclimated) hand decreased

CIVD frequency and finger temperatures. Such observations resulted in an additional central model explaining CIVD, wherein the release of peripheral vasoconstriction serves to release excess heat from the body assuming sufficient body heat content in the core.

3.2.2. A New Model for Thermoregulatory Localised CIVC/CIVD Reactions

In the present paper, we suggest a new model for thermoregulatory localised CIVC/CIVD reactions. Figure 13 depicts the main workflow of the suggested CIVC/CIVD thermoregulatory model. The proposed model is based on the suggestion that there have to be rate-sensitive receptors, which are able to detect the changes in the heat dissipation rate ($\dot{Q}_{dis}$). This rate-sensitive mechanism, which is not yet clear, is also suggested by Yamazaki et al. [35]. It is clear from the current work and the presented results by Youssef et al. [20] that the CIVC, indicated by drop in blood flow rate (320 ± 92 PU), starts earlier (1.55 ± 21 min), before the drop in the skin temperature. This suggests that the initial CIVC is triggered not based on skin temperature threshold, but rather on a certain threshold in the rate of heat dissipation from the skin to the surrounding environment. Under normal temperature (normothermia), the blood vessels are dilated (initial state = vasodilation), with a baseline level of vasoconstrcitive tone [33]. Due to the temperature difference ($\Delta T = T_{sk} - T_{\infty}$) between skin and the environment, which is the driving force for heat flow, there is always a certain level of negative heat flux (dissipation) from the skin to the surrounding environment. Once the step-localised cooling is applied, this results in a sudden increase in the temperature difference ($\Delta T = 18 \pm 0.6$ °C in the first two minutes), and consequently, a sudden increase in the heat dissipation rate ($\dot{Q}_{dis} = -0.15 \pm 0.2$ W in the first two minutes). If this change in the heat dissipation rate is above a certain threshold, the CIVC mechanisms are activated and vasoconstriction prevailed. Then, if the heat dissipation rate reaches a constant threshold level ($\frac{d\dot{Q}_{dis}}{dt} = 0$), the vasoconstriction mechanism will be interrupted and revert to vasodilation. Otherwise, the vasoconstriction state is prolonged.

It should be stated here that this proposed model leaves a number of questions open for further investigation. One very important question, here, is about the nature of the rate-sensitive receptors and their working mechanism. In their work on the coding of cutaneous temperature and thermal receptors [50], Ran et. al. observed that the responses of cold-responding neurons peaked during the transient cooling phase and rapidly adapted to steady cold stimuli, suggesting that these neurons report temperature changes. In other word, cold-responding neurons report the relative drop in skin temperature (i.e., rate of temperature change $\frac{dT_{sk}}{dt}$), rather than the absolute value [51].

Additionally, many questions are still open regarding the nature of thermal sensation and thermal-sensory system in relation to thermoregulation [52]. It is possible in our case to use many of the control-system terms to describe autonomic thermoregulation reactions (CIVC/CIVD), such as the regulated (controlled) variable (finger skin temperature), sensors (skin and preoptic area of the hypothalamus), integrator/controller, and effectors or actuators (blood vessels). However, a concept such as the set point in thermoregulation, and in homeostatic regulation in general, has eluded precise identification. Determination of where such a set point is precisely located, how it is consulted, and even more fundamentally, how the precise set-point value is established has been elusive [53]. Therefore, the "balance point" term [54] is suggested to be more suitable in our case, whereby the multiple pathways act independently [55]; integration (or balancing) of the independent pathways, each of which might have different thresholds of activation and inactivation, allows for a relatively well-maintained internal temperature [33,56]. The balance-point framework aids in explaining the physiology while still allowing for a negative feedback approach [53] in describing and reverse engineering the thermoregulatory reactions.

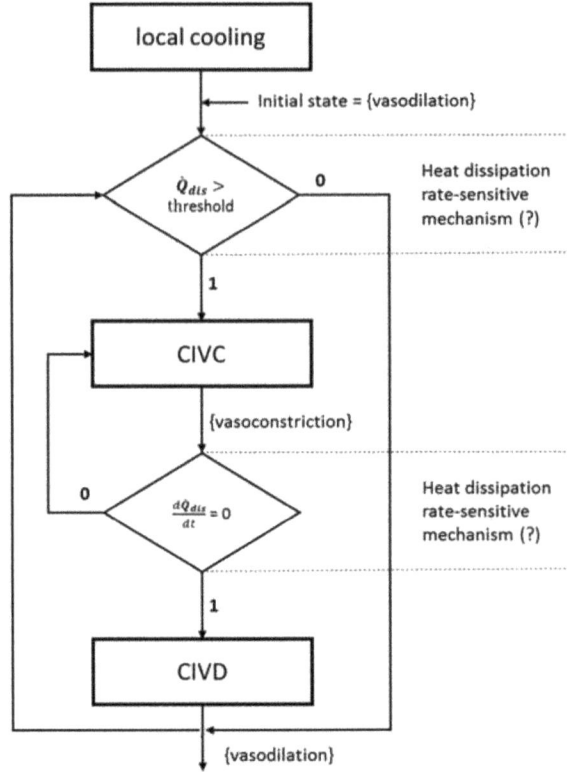

**Figure 13.** Flow chart explaining the suggested model of thermoregulatory localised CIVC/CIVD reactions.

## 4. Conclusions

The main goal of this study was to gain more physiological and mechanistic insights into the underlying processes of thermoregulatory localised CIVC/CIVD reactions using a data-based mechanistic modelling (DBM) approach. Two types of localised cooling were applied on the fingers of 33 healthy participants (test subjects), namely, continuous and intermittent cooling, during the course of the conducted experiments. During the first set of experiments. The results showed that 27 participants out of 33 showed clear evidence of the hunting reaction (i.e., cycles of CIVC/CIVD episodes) during continuous localised cooling. Two different, yet connected, thermoregulatory reactions representing the hunting reaction, namely, CIVC and CIVD were mathematically modelled and described as two separate processes or dynamic systems using the DBM approach. A second-order discrete-time transfer function (two poles and two zeros) was the best ($R_2^T$ = 0.91 ± 0.06 and $YIC$ = −11.43 ± 2.65) for mathematically representing the dynamic responses of the finger skin temperature to step localised cooling and for describing both CIVC and CIVD reactions. For both reactions, it was possible to decompose the obtained second-order system into two first-order TF systems in parallel configurations. The calculated time constants from the two first-order systems suggested two underlying processes for both CIVC and CIVD reactions, one of which is almost 10 times faster. Mechanistic and physiological insights into the suggested underlying processes suggested that the slower (with average $\tau$ = 7.36 min) process represents slow convective heat transfer from the capillaries and the conductive heat exchange between the skin and Peltier's elements. On the other hand, the faster process represents the closing/opening of the AVAs during the CIVC/CIVD reactions, which causes a fast change in the convective heat transfer from the superficial veins. During the intermittent localised cooling, no test subjects of Exp.2 (in total 12) showed any episodes of CIVD, although the skin temperature reached the same level (16.2 ± 0.7 °C) as that under continuous cooling. A new term is suggested in this paper, namely, the latent heat of CIVD (LH-CIVD), which represents the amount of dissipated heat required to trigger the CIVD. It should be stated here that the identified models are limited to the presented methodology of localized cooling. Additionally, in future investigations, interpersonal variations (e.g., physiological and anthropometric variations) should be considered and studied. Moreover, the present work suggested a new model for the thermoregulatory localised CIVC/CIVD reactions. The new model suggested states that, with an initial vasodilation state, the initial localised CIVC is triggered not based on skin temperature threshold, but rather on a certain threshold in the rate of heat dissipation from the skin to the surrounding environment.

**Author Contributions:** Conceptualisation, A.Y. and J.-M.A.; methodology, A.Y. and A.V.; software, A.Y. and A.V.; validation, A.Y.; formal analysis, A.Y. and A.V.; investigation, A.Y. and A.V.; resources, G.D.B and J-N.A.; data curation, A.Y. and A.V.; writing—original draft preparation, A.Y. and A.V.; writing—review and editing, A.Y. and J.-M.A.; visualisation, A.Y.; supervision, J.-M.A. and A.Y.; project administration, J.-M.A.; funding acquisition, J.-M.A.

**Funding:** This research received no external funding.

**Conflicts of Interest:** The authors declare no conflict of interest.

## References

1. Novosel'tsev, V.N. Homeostasis and health: Analysis from a standpoint of the control theory. *Autom. Remote Control* **2012**, *73*, 841–851. [CrossRef]
2. Bernard, C. *De la Physiologie Générale*; Librairie Hachette Et: Paris, France, 1872.
3. Cannon, W.B. *The Wisdom of the Body*; W.W. Norton: New York, NY, USA, 1939.
4. Ivanov, K.P. The development of the concepts of homeothermy and thermoregulation. *J. Therm. Biol.* **2006**, *31*, 24–29. [CrossRef]
5. Ivanov, K. Restoration of vital activity of cooled animals without rewarming the body. *Eur. J. Appl. Physiol.* **2009**, *105*, 5–12. [CrossRef] [PubMed]
6. Turner, J.S. On the thermal capacity of a bird's egg warmed by a brood patch. *Physiol. Zool.* **1997**, *70*, 470–480. [CrossRef] [PubMed]
7. Cheung, S.S. Responses of the hands and feet to cold exposure. *Temperature* **2015**, *2*, 105–120. [CrossRef] [PubMed]
8. Taylor, N.A.S.; Machado-Moreira, C.A.; van den Heuvel, A.M.J.; Caldwell, J.N. Hands and feet: Physiological insulators, radiators and evaporators. *Eur. J. Appl. Physiol.* **2014**, *114*, 2037–2060. [CrossRef] [PubMed]
9. Walløe, L. Arterio-venous anastomoses in the human skin and their role in temperature control. *Temp. (Austin. Tex.)* **2016**, *3*, 92–103. [CrossRef] [PubMed]
10. Grant, R.T.; Bland, E. Observations on arterio venous anastomoses in human skin and in the bird's foot with special reference to the reaction to cold. *Heart* **1931**, *15*, 385–411.
11. Heus, R.; Daanen, H.A.M.; Havenith, G. Physiological criteria for functioning of hands in the cold. *Appl. Ergon.* **1995**, *26*, 5–13. [CrossRef]
12. Karaki, W.; Ghaddar, N.; Ghali, K.; Kuklane, K.; Holmér, I.; Vanggaard, L. Human thermal response with improved AVA modeling of the digits. *Int. J. Therm. Sci.* **2013**, *67*, 41–52. [CrossRef]
13. Rida, M.; Karaki, W.; Ghaddar, N.; Ghali, K.; Hoballah, J. A new mathematical model to simulate AVA cold-induced vasodilation reaction to local cooling. *Int. J. Biometeorol.* **2014**, *58*, 1905–1918. [CrossRef] [PubMed]
14. Lewis, T. Observations upon the reactions of the vessels of the human skin to cold. *Heart* **1930**, *15*, 177–208.
15. Daanen, H.A.M. Finger cold-induced vasodilation: A review. *Eur. J. Appl. Physiol.* **2003**, *89*, 411–426. [CrossRef] [PubMed]
16. Teichner, W.H. Individual Thermal and Behavioral Factors in Cold-Induced Vasodilation. *Psychophysiology* **1966**, *2*, 295–304. [CrossRef]

17. Bergersen, T.K.; Hisdal, J.; Walløe, L. Perfusion of the human finger during cold-induced vasodilatation. *Am. J. Physiol.* **1999**, *276*, R731–R737. [CrossRef] [PubMed]
18. Lee, J.Y.; Bakri, I.; Matsuo, A.; Tochihara, Y. Cold-induced vasodilation and vasoconstriction in the finger of tropical and temperate indigenes. *J. Therm. Biol.* **2013**, *38*, 70–78. [CrossRef]
19. Cheung, S.S.; Daanen, H.A.M. Dynamic Adaptation of the Peripheral Circulation to Cold Exposure. *Microcirculation* **2012**, *19*, 65–77. [CrossRef]
20. Youssef, A.; D'Haene, M.; Vleugels, J.; de Bruyne, G.; Aerts, J.-M. Localised Model-Based Active Controlling of Blood Flow During Chemotherapy to Prevent Nail Toxicity and Onycholysis. *J. Med. Biol. Eng.* **2018**, *39*, 139–150. [CrossRef]
21. Bladt, L.; De Clercq, J.; Janssens, T.; Van Hulle, J.; Vleugels, J.; Aerts, J.M.; De Bruyne, G. Cold-induced vasoconstriction for preventing onycholysis during cancer treatment. *Extrem. Physiol. Med.* **2015**, *4*, A60. [CrossRef]
22. Steckel, J.; Goethijn, F.; de Bruyne, G. A research platform using active local cooling directed at minimizing the blood flow in human fingers. In Proceedings of the 7th International Conference on Pervasive Computing Technologies for Healthcare and Workshops, Venice, Italy, 5–8 May 2013; pp. 81–84.
23. Aerts, J.M.; Berckmans, D.; Saevels, P.; Decuypere, E.; Buyse, J. Modelling the static and dynamic responses of total heat production of broiler chickens to step changes in air temperature and light intensity. *Br. Poult. Sci.* **2000**, *41*, 651–659. [CrossRef]
24. Young, P.C. *Control and Dynamic Systems: Advances in Theory and Applications*; Leondes, C.T., Ed.; New Academic Press Inc Elsevier Science: New York, NY, USA, 1989.
25. Young, P.C. Data-based mechanistic modelling of environmental, ecological, economic and engineering systems. *Environ. Model. Softw.* **1998**, *13*, 105–122. [CrossRef]
26. Youssef, A.; Dekock, J.; Ozcan, S.E.; Berckmans, D. Data-Based Approach to Model the Dynamic Behaviour of Greenhouse Temperature. *Acta Hortic.* **2011**, *893*, 931–938. [CrossRef]
27. Youssef, A.; Exadaktylos, V.; Berckmans, D. Modelling and quantification of the thermoregulatory responses of the developing avian embryo: Electrical analogies of a physiological system. *J. Therm. Biol.* **2014**, *44*, 14–19. [CrossRef] [PubMed]
28. Youssef, A.; Exadaktylos, V.; Ozcan, S.E.; Berckmans, D. Proportional-Integral-Plus (PIP) Control System for Individual Thermal Zones in a Small Ventilated Space. *ASHRAE Trans.* **2011**, *117*, 48–56.
29. Youssef, A.; Yen, H.; Özcan, S.E.; Berckmans, D. Data-based mechanistic modelling of indoor temperature distributions based on energy input. *Energy Build.* **2011**, *43*, 2965–2972. [CrossRef]
30. Young, P.C.; Jakeman, A. Refined instrumental variable methods of recursive time-series analysis Part III. Extensions. *Int. J. Control* **1980**, *31*, 741–764. [CrossRef]
31. Young, P.C. *Recursive Estimation and Time-Series Analysis: An Introduction for the Student and Practitioner*; Springer: Heidelberg, Berlin, 2011.
32. Young, P.C.; Chotai, A.; Tych, W. *Identification, Estimation and Control of Continuous-Time Systems Described by Delta Operator Models*; Kluwer Academic Publishers: Dordrecht, the Netherlands, 1991.
33. Tansey, E.A.; Johnson, C.D. Recent advances in thermoregulation. *Adv. Physiol. Educ.* **2015**, *39*, 139–148. [CrossRef]
34. Lienhard, J.H. *A Heat Transfer Textbook*; Phlogiston Press: Cambridge, MA, USA, 2001.
35. Yamazaki, F.; Sone, R.; Zhao, K.; Alvarez, G.E.; Kosiba, W.A.; Johnson, J.M. Rate dependency and role of nitric oxide in the vascular response to direct cooling in human skin. *J. Appl. Physiol.* **2006**, *100*, 42–50. [CrossRef]
36. Johnson, J.M.; Yen, T.C.; Zhao, K.; Kosiba, W.A. Sympathetic, sensory, and nonneuronal contributions to the cutaneous vasoconstrictor response to local cooling. *Am. J. Physiol. Circ. Physiol.* **2005**, *288*, H1573–H1579. [CrossRef]
37. Nuzzaci, G.; Evangelisti, A.; Righi, D.; Giannico, G.; Nuzzaci, I. Is There Any Relationship between Cold-Induced Vasodilatation and Vasomotion? *Microvasc. Res.* **1999**, *57*, 1–7. [CrossRef]
38. Sheppard, L.W.; Vuksanović, V.; McClintock, P.V.E.; Stefanovska, A. Oscillatory dynamics of vasoconstriction and vasodilation identified by time-localized phase coherence. *Phys. Med. Biol.* **2011**, *56*, 3583–3601. [CrossRef] [PubMed]
39. Kellogg, D.L. In vivo mechanisms of cutaneous vasodilation and vasoconstriction in humans during thermoregulatory challenges. *J. Appl. Physiol.* **2006**, *100*, 1709–1718. [CrossRef] [PubMed]

40. Johnson, J.M.; Minson, C.T.; Kellogg, D.L. Cutaneous vasodilator and vasoconstrictor mechanisms in temperature regulation. *Compr. Physiol.* **2014**, *4*, 33–89. [PubMed]
41. Castellani, J.W.; O'Brien, C. Peripheral Vasodilation Responses to Prevent Local Cold Injuries. In *Prevention of Cold Injuries*; RTO: Neuilly-sur-Seine, France, 2005; pp. KN2-1–K2-14.
42. Pérgola, P.E.; Kellogg, D.L.; Johnson, J.M.; Kosiba, W.A.; Solomon, D.E. Role of sympathetic nerves in the vascular effects of local temperature in human forearm skin. *Am. J. Physiol.* **1993**, *265*, H785–H792. [CrossRef] [PubMed]
43. Sendowski, I.; Sarourey, G.; Besnard, Y.; Bittel, J. Cold induced vasodilatation and cardiovascular responses in humans during cold water immersion of various upper limb areas. *Eur. J. Appl. Physiol. Occup. Physiol.* **1997**, *75*, 471–477. [CrossRef]
44. Keramidas, M.E.; Musizza, B.; Kounalakis, S.N.; Mekjavic, I.B. Enhancement of the finger cold-induced vasodilation response with exercise training. *Eur. J. Appl. Physiol.* **2010**, *109*, 133–140. [CrossRef]
45. Flouris, A.D.; Westwood, D.A.; Mekjavic, I.B.; Cheung, S.S. Effect of body temperature on cold induced vasodilation. *Eur. J. Appl. Physiol.* **2008**, *104*, 491–499. [CrossRef]
46. Flouris, A.D.; Cheung, S.S. Thermal Basis of Finger Blood Flow Adaptations During Abrupt Perturbations in Thermal Homeostasis. *Microcirculation* **2011**, *18*, 56–62. [CrossRef]
47. Flouris, A.D.; Cheung, S.S. Influence of thermal balance on cold-induced vasodilation. *J. Appl. Physiol.* **2009**, *106*, 1264–1271. [CrossRef]
48. Daanen, H.A.; Ducharme, M.B. Finger cold-induced vasodilation during mild hypothermia, hyperthermia and at thermoneutrality. *Aviat. Space Environ. Med.* **1999**, *70*, 1206–1210.
49. Mekjavic, I.B.; Dobnikar, U.; Kounalakis, S.N.; Musizza, B.; Cheung, S.S. The trainability and contralateral response of cold-induced vasodilatation in the fingers following repeated cold exposure. *Eur. J. Appl. Physiol.* **2008**, *104*, 193–199. [CrossRef] [PubMed]
50. Ran, C.; Hoon, M.A.; Chen, X. The coding of cutaneous temperature in the spinal cord. *Nat. Neurosci.* **2016**, *19*, 1201–1209. [CrossRef] [PubMed]
51. Vandewauw, I.; Voets, T. Heat is absolute, cold is relative. *Nat. Neurosci.* **2016**, *19*, 1188–1189. [CrossRef] [PubMed]
52. Kobayashi, S. Temperature receptors in cutaneous nerve endings are thermostat molecules that induce thermoregulatory behaviors against thermal load. *Temp. (Austin. Tex.)* **2015**, *2*, 346–351. [CrossRef] [PubMed]
53. Tan, C.L.; Cooke, E.K.; Leib, D.E.; Lin, Y.C.; Daly, G.E.; Zimmerman, C.A.; Knight, Z.A. Warm-Sensitive Neurons that Control Body Temperature. *Cell* **2016**, *167*, 47–59. [CrossRef] [PubMed]
54. Romanovsky, A.A. Thermoregulation: Some concepts have changed. Functional architecture of the thermoregulatory system. *Am. J. Physiol. Integr. Comp. Physiol.* **2007**, *292*, R37–R46. [CrossRef]
55. McAllen, R.M.; Tanaka, M.; Ootsuka, Y.; McKinley, M.J. Multiple thermoregulatory effectors with independent central controls. *Eur. J. Appl. Physiol.* **2010**, *109*, 27–33. [CrossRef] [PubMed]
56. Fealey, R.D. Interoception and autonomic nervous system reflexes thermoregulation. *Handb. Clin. Neurol.* **2013**, *117*, 79–88.

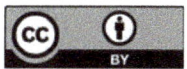

© 2019 by the authors. Licensee MDPI, Basel, Switzerland. This article is an open access article distributed under the terms and conditions of the Creative Commons Attribution (CC BY) license (http://creativecommons.org/licenses/by/4.0/).

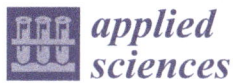 

*Review*

# Overview of Federated Facility to Harmonize, Analyze and Management of Missing Data in Cohorts

**Hema Sekhar Reddy Rajula [1,2,*], Veronika Odintsova [3,4], Mirko Manchia [5,6] and Vassilios Fanos [1]**

1. Neonatal Intensive Care Unit, Department of Surgical Sciences, AOU and University of Cagliari, 09042 Cagliari, Italy; vafanos@tin.it
2. Ph.D. student Marie Sklodowska-Curie CAPICE Project, Department of Surgical Sciences, University of Cagliari, 09042 Cagliari, Italy
3. Biological Psychology Department, Vrije Universiteit Amsterdam, 1081 BT Amsterdam, The Netherlands; v.v.odintsova@vu.nl
4. VI Kulakov National Medical Research Center for Obstetrics, Gynecology and Perinatology, Moscow 117198, Russia
5. Section of Psychiatry, Department of Medical Science and Public Health, University of Cagliari, 09125 Cagliari, Italy; mirkomanchia@unica.it
6. Department of Pharmacology, Dalhousie University, Halifax, NS B3H 4R2, Canada
* Correspondence: reddy@unica.it

Received: 10 July 2019; Accepted: 27 September 2019; Published: 1 October 2019

**Abstract:** Cohorts are instrumental for epidemiologically oriented observational studies. Cohort studies usually observe large groups of individuals for a specific period of time to identify the contributing factors to a specific outcome (for instance an illness) and create associations between risk factors and the outcome under study. In collaborative projects, federated data facilities are meta-database systems that are distributed across multiple locations that permit to analyze, combine, or harmonize data from different sources making them suitable for mega- and meta-analyses. The harmonization of data can increase the statistical power of studies through maximization of sample size, allowing for additional refined statistical analyses, which ultimately lead to answer research questions that could not be addressed while using a single study. Indeed, harmonized data can be analyzed through mega-analysis of raw data or fixed effects meta-analysis. Other types of data might be analyzed by e.g., random-effects meta-analyses or Bayesian evidence synthesis. In this article, we describe some methodological aspects related to the construction of a federated facility to optimize analyses of multiple datasets, the impact of missing data, and some methods for handling missing data in cohort studies.

**Keywords:** harmonization; meta-analysis; missing data; multiple imputations; information technology; remoteness; cohort studies

## 1. Introduction

Cohort studies are widely used in epidemiology to measure how the exposure to certain factors influences the risk of a specific disease. The role of large cohort studies is increasing with the development of multi-omics approaches and with the search of methods for the translation of omics findings, especially those that are derived from genome-wide association studies (GWAS) in clinical settings [1]. Many research efforts have been made to link vast amounts of phenotypic data across diverse centers. This procedure concerns molecular information, as well as data regarding environmental factors, such as those recorded in and obtained from health-care databases and epidemiological registers [2]. Cohort studies can be prospective (forward-looking) or retrospective (backward-looking).

Large-scale initiatives of cohort studies have been initiated worldwide, such as the NIG Roadmap Epigenomics Project [3] and the 500 Functional Genomics cohort [4] due to the increasing need of integration of data for genomic analysis. An example of the former is the Nurses' Health Study, a large prospective cohort study that revealed several significant associations between lifestyle choices and health by following up hundreds of thousands of women in North America [5]. Similarly, the National Health and Nutrition Examination Survey (http://www.cdc.gov/nchs/nhanes.htm) discovered the association between cholesterol levels and heart disease. Furthermore, another large prospective cohort study, the Framingham Heart Study (https://www.framinghamheartstudy.org), demonstrated the cardiovascular health risks of tobacco smoking. However, the integration of data from multiple cohort studies faces a variety of challenges [6].

Database federation is a method for data integration that offers constant access to a number of various data sources in which middleware can operate, including interactive database management systems [6]. Individual-level data indicate information about participants, being either contributed by the participants themselves in surveys etc., or collected from registers. In fact, individual-level data assembling of large population-based studies across centers in international collaborations faces several difficulties [7]. On the one hand, merging cohort datasets extends the capability of these studies by allowing research questions of mutual interest to be addressed, by enabling the harmonization of standard measures, and by authorizing the investigation of a range of psychosocial, physical, and contextual factors over time. However, on the other hand, data are often collected in different locations and systems, and they are rarely aggregated into larger datasets, an aspect that limits their utility. Additionally, it is essential to accurately address privacy, legal, and ethical issues that are associated with data usage [8].

Meta-analysis is a common approach to pool results from multiple cohorts and it is consistently used, for example, in GWAS [9] epidemiological studies [10], case-control studies [11] and randomized controlled trials [12]. Several studies are pooled to increase the sample size to increase the statistical power to detect true association signals (decreasing type 1 error). Due to the restrictions of participants confidentiality and the refusal by authors to provide anonymized dataset, individual-level data often cannot be pooled among studies, so meta-analytical approaches are typically used to combine summary statistics across studies, and they have been shown to be as powerful as the integration of individual datasets [9].

In cohort studies, retaining participants with several waves of follow-up is challenging. These waves of data collection give researchers an opportunity to get data regarding deviations in the measures of participants' exposure and outcome over time. The duration of follow-up waves of data can range from one to two years up to 20 to 30 years or even with longer post-baseline assessments. Missingness of the data can be related to study designs in which recurrent measures of exposure and outcome over time are needed. Specifically, the candidates might not available or might be too ill to participate, or they might refuse to respond to specific inquiries or could be deceased [13]. Thus, researchers often face missing data, which might introduce bias in the parameter estimations (for instance of risk calculation) as well as the loss of statistical power and accuracy [13]. Although further research is required to understand both the impact of missing data and the development of effective methodologies for their handling, there are approaches (discussed below) that may decrease the detrimental effect of missing information.

There are several ways of storing and integrating data, such as warehouses, federations, data hotels, etc. For example, the Dutch Techcentre for Life sciences (DTL) is an innovative solution for data hotels. DTL keenly supports FAIR (Findable, Accessible, Interoperable, and Reusable) data stewardship of life science data, within its partnership and in close collaboration with its international partners [14]. The principles of FAIR data serve as an international guideline for high quality data stewardship. A federated facility is a meta-database system that is distributed across multiple locations. It allows making the data from different sources comparable and useful for analyses [15]. Its main difference between federated facility and registries and warehouses is that data management is carried out via a remote distributed request from one federated server (or database manager) to multiple sources.

A federated facility allows for researchers to receive analytical insight from the pooled information of diverse datasets without having to move all the data to the main location, thus reducing the extent of data movement in the distribution of intermediate results, and maximizing the security of the local data in the distributed sources [16,17]. Most of the data are analyzed close to where they are produced in a federated analytical model. To enable collaboration at scale, federated analytics permits the integration of intermediate outcomes of data analytics while the raw data remains in its locked-down site. When the integrated results are pooled and explored, a substantial amount of knowledge is acquired, and researchers managing a single-center database have the ability to compare their results with the findings that were derived by the analyses of federated pooled data.

In this paper, we describe some methodological aspects that are related to the federated facility. Specifically, we review the methods of harmonization and analysis of multi-center datasets, focusing on the impact of missing data (as well as different approaches to deal with them) in cohorts. Thus, firstly, we aim to suggest a few examples of cohort studies and a data collection procedure for a cohort study, and, secondly, to offer approaches of harmonization and integrative data analysis over cohorts. To this end, we present different methods for handling missing data, such as complete case-analysis and multiple imputations. Finally, we offer a perspective on the future directions of this research area.

## 2. Examples of Cohort Studies and Integration of Cohorts

Cohort studies allow for one to answer different epidemiological questions regarding the association between an exposure factor and a disease, such as whether exposure to smoking is associated with the manifestation of lung cancer. The British Doctors Study, which started in 1951 (and continued until 2001), was a cohort study that comprised both smokers (the exposed group) and non-smokers (the unexposed group) [18]. The study delivered substantial evidence of the association of smoking with the prevalence of lung cancer by 1956. In a cohort study, the groups are selected in terms of many other variables (i.e., general health and economic status), such that the effect of the variable being evaluated, i.e., smoking (independent variable), is the only one that could be associated with lung cancer (dependent variable). In this study, a statistically significant increase in the prevalence of lung cancer in the smoking group when compared to the non-smoking group rejects the null hypothesis of the absence of a relationship between risk factor and outcome.

Another example is the Avon Longitudinal Study of Parents and Children (ALSPAC), a prospective observational study that examines the impacts on health and development across the life course [19]. ALSPAC is renowned for investigating how genetic and environmental factors affect health and growth in parents and children [20]. This study has examined multiple biological, (epi) genetic, psychological, social, and environmental factors that are associated with a series of health, social, and developmental outcomes. Enrollment sought to register pregnant women in the Bristol area in the UK during 1990–92. This was prolonged to comprise additional children that are eligible up to the age of 18 years. In 1990–92, the children from 14,541 pregnancies were enrolled, which increased the number of participants enrolled to include 15,247 pregnancies by the age of 18 years. The follow-up comprised 59 questionnaires (four weeks–18 years of age) and nine clinical assessment visits (7–17 years of age) [19]. Genetic (the DNA of 11,343 children, genome-wide data for 8365 children, complete genome sequencing for 2000 children) and epigenetic (methylation sampling of 1000 children) data were collected during this study [19].

The federated model is more often used in multi-center studies, large national biobanks, such as the UK Biobank [21], and meta-analyses projects combining data from different registries or databases. It requires new methods and systems to handle large data collection and storing.

One example is the Cross Study funded by the National Institutes of Health (NIH). In this project, data are combined from three current longitudinal studies of adolescent development with a specific emphasis on recognizing evolving pathways that are prominent in substance use and disorder [22].

All three studies oversampled offspring who had at least one biological parent affected by alcohol use disorder and comprised a matched sample of healthy control offspring of unaffected parents. The Michigan Longitudinal Study [23] is the first study that has collected a comprehensive dataset in a large sample of 2–5 year olds subjects who were evaluated via four waves of surveys up to early adulthood. The Adolescent and Family Developmental Project [24] is the second study that recruited families of adolescents aged 11–15, with the surveys being distributed well into adulthood. The Alcohol, Health, and Behavior Project [25] is the third study to include intensive assessments of college freshmen, who, up to their thirties, participated in more than six waves of surveys. Collectively, these three studies span the first four decades of life, mapping the phases when early risk factors for later substance outcomes first emerge (childhood), substance use initiation typically occurs (adolescence), top rates of substance use disorders are evident (young adulthood), and deceleration in substance involvement is evident (adulthood). One potential cause might be that conducting such analyses can be an extremely complex and challenging task. Key practical issues that are associated with data acquisition and data management are often exceed by a multitude of difficulties that arise from at times substantial study-to-study differences [22].

Similarly, the European Union-funded ongoing project Childhood and Adolescence Psychopathology: unraveling the complex etiology by a large Interdisciplinary Collaboration in Europe (CAPICE—https://www.capice-project.eu/) [26] is currently working to create a facility for federated analyses. This requires the databases to have a common structure. CAPICE brings together data from eight population-based birth and childhood (twin) cohorts to focus on the causes of individual differences in childhood and adolescent psychopathology and its course. However, different cohorts use a different measure to assess childhood and adolescent mental health. These different instruments assess the same dimensions of child psychopathology, but they phrase questions in different ways and use different response categories. Comparing and combining the results across cohorts is most efficient when a common unit of measurement is used.

Another project, the Biobank Standardisation and Harmonization for Research Excellence in the European Union (BioSHare) study, built the federated facility using the Mica-Opal federated framework aiming at building a cooperative group of researchers and developing tools for data harmonization, database integration, and federated data analyses [7]. New database management systems and web-based networking technologies are at the limelight of providing solutions to federated facility [7]. Furthermore, the GenomeEUtwin is a large-scale biobank-based research project that integrates massive amounts of genotypic and phenotypic data from distinct data sources that are located in specific European countries and Australia [2]. The federated system is a network called TwinNET used to exchange and pool analyses. The system pools data from over 600,000 twin pairs, and genotype information from a part of those with the goal to detect genetic variants related to common diseases. The network architecture of TwinNET consists of the Hub (the integration node) and Spokes (data-providing centers, such as twin registers). Data-providers initiate connections while using virtual private network tunnels that provide security. This approach also allows for the storage and combining of two databases: the genotypic and the phenotypic database, which are often stored in different locations [27]. The development of Genome EUtwin facility started from the integration of the limited number of variables that appear simple and non-controversial and it is intended to include more variables standard for the world twin community. Most of the European twin registries do not have genotypic or phenotypic information from non-twin individuals. But some do, and GenomEUtwin will want to take advantage of those samples. The advantage with this structure consists in the possibility to store completely new variables as soon as they emerge without changing the database structure. By applying the same variable names and value formats to variables in common to all databases, several advantages will be accomplished [27]. Here, we describe the process of building a federated facility, divided into separate steps (see Table 1).

Table 1. Main Steps of Federated Facility Process.

| Step | Description |
|---|---|
| Data collection in cohort studies | Study data is obtained from self-completed paper-based/online questionnaires, biosample analysis, clinical assessments, linkage to administrative records, etc. |
| Integration on cohorts | Remote access to aggregated data for statistical analysis is provided and data collected in multiple studies is integrated with the use of harmonization data tools (if needed) |
| Mega-analyses, meta-analyses or integrative data analyses | Statistical tools for analysis of combined data are applied |

## 3. Data Collection Procedure for a Cohort Study

Several sets of data might be collected in the context of a cohort study. These might include clinical, biological, and imaging data. Data from clinical assessments are comprised of physiological, cognitive, structured or semi-structured interviews measures and/or computer-based questionnaires. Genetic, transcriptomic, proteomic, metabolomic, epigenetic, biochemical, and environmental exposure data can be obtained from the analysis of biological samples [28]. Imaging data can be collected as a part of routine clinical assessment (including magnetic resonance imaging, computer tomography scans, dual-energy x-ray absorptiometry, retinal scan, peripheral quantitative computed tomography, and three-dimensional (3D) Face and body shape). Data are obtained through administrative records comprised of maternity and birth records, child health records, electronic health records, primary and secondary health care records, and social network channels. In the presence of applicable data formats, this information might be transferred while using innovative tools that are becoming increasingly available and that are now robust enough to allow for digital continuity. There will be meticulous management and stewardship of the valuable digital resources, to the benefit of the entire academic community [14].

## 4. Data Integration

Built-in security features of database management systems can limit access to the whole dataset of a federated facility, and security can be increased while using encryption. Some solutions can be applied, such as establishing a common variable format and standard, creating a unique identifier for all individuals in the cohorts, implementing security access to data and integrity constraints in the database management system, and making automated integration algorithms in the core module to synchronize or federate multiple heterogeneous data sources, to facilitate the integration of different datasets among various cohorts.

There are three steps in data integration: (1) extraction of data and harmonization into a common format at a data provider site; (2) transfer of harmonized data to a data-collecting center for checking; and, (3) data load into a common database [2].

Harmonization is a systematic approach, which allows the integration of data collected in multiple studies or multiple sources. Sample size can be increased by pooling data from different cohort studies. Conversely, individual datasets may be comprised of variables that measure the same hypothesis in different ways, which hinders the efficacy of pooled datasets [29]. Variable harmonization can help to handle this problem.

The federation facility might also be created without the need for harmonization (i.e., any cohorts that have some data (e.g., genotyping data) in one place and some data (e.g., phenotypic) in another or have a connection to national registries, etc.). For example, in the Genome of the Netherlands Project (http://www.nlgenome.nl/), nine large Dutch biobanks (~35,000 samples) were imputed with the population-specific reference panel, an approach that led to the identification of a variant within the ABCA6 gene that is associated with cholesterol levels [30].

The potential of harmonization can be evaluated with the studies' questionnaires, data dictionaries, and standard operating techniques. Harmonized datasets available on a server in every single research centers across Europe can be interlocked through a federated system to allow for integration and statistical analysis [7]. To co-analyze harmonized datasets, the Opal [31], Mica software [7], and the Data SHIELD package within the R environment are used to generate a federated infrastructure that allows for investigators to mutually analyze harmonized data while recollecting individual-level records within their corresponding host organizations [7]. The idea is to generate harmonized datasets on local servers in every single host organization that can be securely connected while using encrypted remote connections. Using a strong collaborative association among contributing centers, this approach can lead to effortless collateral analyses using globally harmonized research databases while permitting each study to maintain complete control over individual-level data [7].

Data harmonization is implemented in light of several factors, for instance, detailed or partial variable matching about the question asked/responded, the answer noted (value definition, value level, data type), the rate of measurement, the period of measurement, and missing values [29].

For instance, in the context of the CAPICE project, the important variables are those concerning demographics (i.e., sex, family structure, parental educational attainment, parental employment, socio-economic status (SES), individual's school achievements, mental health measures (both for psychopathology as well as for wellbeing and quality of life) by various raters (mother, father, self-report, teacher)), pregnancy/the perinatal period (i.e., alcohol and substance use during pregnancy, birth weight, parental mental health, breast feeding), general health (i.e., height, weight, physical conditions, medication, life events), family (i.e., divorce, family climate, parenting, parental mental health), and biomarkers (genomics, epigenetics, metabolomics, microbiome data, etc.). All of these pieces of data gathered in children and parents are harmonized while using various procedures.

Variable manipulation is not essential if the query asked/responded and the answer noted in both datasets is the same [29]. If the response verified is not the same, the response is re-categorized/re-organized to improve the comparability of records from both of the datasets. Missing values are generated for each subsequent unmatched variable and are switched by multiple imputations if the same pattern is calculated in both datasets, even if using different methods/scales. A scale that is applied in both datasets is recognized as a reference standard [29]. If the variables are calculated several times and/or in distinct periods, these are harmonized by gestation trimesters data. Lastly, the harmonized datasets are assembled into a single dataset.

## 5. Meta-analysis and mega-analysis

Researchers are currently analyzing large datasets to clarify the biological underpinnings of diseases that, particularly in complex disorders, remain obscure. However, due to privacy concerns and legal complexities, data hosted in different centers cannot always be directly shared. In practice, data sharing is also hindered by the administrative burden that is associated with the need to transfer huge volumes of data. This situation made researchers to look for an analytical solution within meta-analysis or federated learning paradigms. In the federated setting, a model is fitted without sharing individual data across centers, but only using model parameters. Meta-analysis instead performs statistical testing by combining results from several independent analyses, for instance, by sharing p-values, effect sizes, and/or standard errors across centers [32].

Lu and co-authors have recently proposed two additions to the splitting approach for meta-analysis: splitting in a cohort and splitting cohorts [9]. The first method implies that data for each cohort is divided, monitored by a choice of variables on one subset and calculation of p-values on the other subset, and by meta-analysis across all cohorts [9]. This is a typical addition of the data splitting approach that can be applied to numerous cohorts. The second method comprises splitting cohorts as an alternative. Cohorts are divided into two groups, one group is used for variable selection and the other is used for attaining p-values as well as meta-analysis. This is a more applicable method, since it simplifies the analysis burden for each study and decreases the possibility of errors [9].

As the focus of a meta-analysis is on the creation of summary statistics obtained from several studies, this method is most efficient when the original individual records used in prior analyses are not accessible or no longer collected [22]. The individual-level information can be pooled into a single harmonized dataset upon which mega-analyses are carried out [33]. The increased flexibility in handling confounders at the individual patient level and assessing the impact of missing data are substantial benefits of a mega-analytical method [34]. Mega-analyses have also been endorsed to evade the assumptions of within-study normality and recognize the within-study variances, which are particularly challenging with small samples. In spite of these benefits, mega-analysis requires homogeneous data sets and the creation of a shared centralized database [34].

Meta-analysis has several disadvantages, including the presence of high level of heterogeneity [35], unmeasured confounders [36], limitation by ecological fallacy [37]. In addition, most of the primary studies included in meta-analysis are conducted in developed or western countries [38]. However, there are numerous benefits to directly fitting models straight into the original raw data instead of creating the applicable summary statistics. Current technological developments (such as a superior capacity for data sharing and wide opportunities for electronic data storage and retrieval) have increased the feasibility of retrieving original individual records for secondary analysis. This gives new opportunities for the progress of different approaches to integrate results across studies by using original individual records to overcome some of the inevitable limitations of meta-analysis [22].

Here, we focus on approaches of integrative data analysis within the psychological sciences, as approaches to collecting current data can differ across disciplines.

## 6. Integrative Data Analysis

Integrative data analysis (IDA) is the statistical analysis of a dataset that contains two or more separate samples that have been combined into one [22]. The characteristics of a sample that allow for considering it as a separate entity can be defined on a case-by-case basis. In specific situations, there may be differences in the design of the studies from which samples were due to recruited participants. For instance, separate samples might be collected in a multi-site employing single-site strategy in which key design characteristics remain constant (e.g., recruitment, procedures, and measurement). However, in other situations, each study is designed in a distinct setting (e.g., distinct hospitals or regions of the country) or across distinct time periods (e.g., as recruitment moves across different birth cohorts or school years). These separate samples are combined for analysis or cohort differences [22].

However, though IDA may be applied to a variety of designs, the emphasis here is unambiguously on the later situation, and namely where numerous samples are drawn from independent current studies and assembled into a dataset for follow up analyses. This was exactly what the authors experienced in the project called Cross Study, in which their attention was on data collected from three independent studies where participants were different from one to another in both hypothetically and methodologically meaningful ways [22]. The investigators were confident that the greatest potential for upcoming applications of IDA in psychological research comes from the combination of data from two or more studies [22].

## 7. Different Approaches to Dealing with Missing Data in Cohorts

Different types of missing data in phenotypic and genotypic databases can appear in cohorts: these include, but are not limited to, the following: irrelevant non-response, responses of participants that were excluded from the study in the follow up, irrelevant missing structural data (when data are irrelevant in the context), responses of participants such as "do not know" responses, no answer to a specific item, and missing data due to error codes.

There are several approaches for dealing with missing data: complete-case analyses, last observational carried forward (LOCF) method, mean value substitution method, missing indicator method, and multiple imputations (MI).

The complete case-analysis only is comprised of applicants with full data in all waves of data collection, thus possibly decreasing the accuracy of the estimates of the exposure-outcome relations [13]. To be effective, complete case analyses should assume that applicants with missing data can be considered to be a random sample of those that were intended to be observed (generally referred as missing completely at random (MCAR)) [13], or at least that the probability of data being missing does not dependent on the observed value [39]. Further, LOCF is a method of imputing missing data in longitudinal studies with the non-missing value from the previously completed time-point for the same individual, since the imputed values are unrelated to a subject's other measurements. The mean value substitution replaces the missing value with the average value available from the other individual time-points of a longitudinal study [40]. The missing indicator method comprises an additional category for the analysis created for applicants with missing data [41].

Missing data can be handled by means of multiple imputation [42–45]. MI methods are used to address missing data and its assumptions are more flexible than those of complete case analysis [46]. The principle of MI is to substitute missing observations with plausible values multiple times and generate complete data sets [47]. Every single complete data set is individually analyzed and the effects of the analyses are then assembled. MI results are consistent when the missing mechanism satisfies the MCAR and the missing at random (MAR) assumptions [48,49]. Multiple imputation consists of three steps. The first step is (1) to determine which variables are used for imputation. The variables used for imputation should be selected on the basis of the presentation of their missing information as MAR [43], that is, whether or not a score that is missing depend on the missing value [42]. The variables that cause the missingness are unknown to the researcher unless missingness is, to some extent, expected. Practically, variables are selected in a way that expected to be good predictors containing missing values. One can choose the number of variables and which variables to use, but there is no alternate way to assess whether MAR is achieved, and MAR is an assumption. Binary or ordinal variables may be imputed under a normality assumption and then rounded off to discrete values. If a variable is right skewed, it might be modeled on a logarithmic scale and then transformed back to the original scale after imputation [42]. We should impute variables that are functions of other (incomplete) variables. Several data sets consist of transformed variables, sum scores, interaction variables, ratio's, and so on. It can be useful to integrate the transformed variables into the multiple imputation algorithms [50]. The second step is (2) to generate imputed data matrices. One of the tools that can be used is the R package Multiple Imputation by Chained Equations (MICE) [50], which uses an iterative procedure in which each variable is sequentially imputed and restricted on the real and imputed values of the other variables. The third step of the multiple imputation procedure is (3) to analyze each imputed data set as desired and pool the results [51].

## 8. Discussion and Future Perspective

The current narrative review focuses on the rationale of federated facility, as well as the challenges and solutions developed to when attempting to maximize the advantages that are obtained from the federated facility of cohort studies. Assembling individual-level data can be a useful, particularly when the results of interest are relevant. There are several benefits of federated facility and harmonizing cohorts: integrating harmonized data allows for an increase in sample sizes, improves the generalizability of results [1,7,52], ensures the validity of comparative research, creates opportunities to compare different population groups by filling the gaps in the distribution (different age groups, nationality, ethnicity etc.), facilitates extra proficient secondary use of data, and offers opportunities for collaborative and consortium research.

Data pooling of different cohort studies faces many hurdles, including interoperability, shared access, and ethical issues, when cohorts working under different national regulations are integrated.

It is essential that strong collaboration among different parties exists to effectively implement database federation and data harmonization [7]. A federated framework allows investigators to analyze data safely and remotely (i.e., produce summary statistics, contingency tables, logistic regressions) facilitating their accessibility and decreasing actual time restrictions without the burden of filing several data access requests at various research centers, thereby saving principal investigators and study managers time and resources [7].

An important aspect of our review is to provide insights into large samples that result from merging the datasets. Meta-analysis, or mega-analysis of studies, might lead to a more robust estimate of the magnitude of the associations ultimately increasingly the generalizability of findings [33]. As progressively thorough computations can be accomplished in a mega-analysis, some researchers reckon that mega-analysis of individual-participant data can be more efficient than meta-analysis of aggregated data [34]. The mega-analytical framework appears to be the more robust methodology due to the relatively high amount of variation detectable among cohorts in multi-center studies.

In cohort studies, several methods are used to deal with missing data in the exposure and outcome analyses. The most common method is to perform a complete case analysis, an approach that might generate biased consequences if the missing data are not followed by the assumptions of missing completely at random (MCAR). The complete-case analysis allows for consistent results only when the missing data probabilities do not depend on the disease and exposure status simultaneously. Nowadays, researchers are using advanced statistical modeling procedures (for example, *MI* and Bayesian) to handle missing data. Combining studies by Bayesian enable us to quantify the relative evidence with respect to multiple hypotheses using the information from multiple cohorts [44]. Missingness is a typical problem in cohort studies and it is likely to introduce substantial bias into the results. We highlighted how the unpredictable recording of missing data in cohort studies, if not dealt with properly, and the ongoing use of inappropriate approaches to handle missing data in the analysis can substantially affect the study findings leading to inaccurate estimates of associations [13]. Increasing the quality of the study design and phenotyping should be a priority to decrease the amount and impact of missing data. Robust and adequate study designs minimize the additional requests on participants and clinicians beyond routine clinical care, an aspect that encourages the implementation of pragmatic trial design [53].

An organization of databases can facilitate the use of innovative exploratory tools based on machine learning and data mining for data analyses due to data-harmonization techniques. In this narrative review, we proposed several approaches of data integration over cohorts, meta-analysis, mega-analysis in a framework for federated system, and various methods to handle missing data. Further developments of these studies will extend the proposed analysis, from multi-center facility to large-scale cohort data, such as in the context of the CAPICE project.

## 9. Conclusions

In our review, we highlighted the relevance of setting up reliable database management systems and innovative internet-based networking technologies to provide the resources to support collaborative, multi-center studies in a proficient and secure manner. Variable harmonization remains an essential feature for conducting research using several datasets and permits to increase the statistical power of a study capitalizing on sample size, allowing for more advanced statistical analyses, and answering research questions that might not be addressed by a single study. Future research in this area is needed to develop novel methods to handle missing data, which can substantially impact in very large scale analysis.

**Author Contributions:** Conceptualization, writing—original draft preparation, H.S.R.R.; added part of the content to the draft—review and editing, V.O.; review and editing, M.M.; supervision, V.F.

**Funding:** This research was funded by European Union's Horizon 2020 research and innovation program under the Marie Skłodowska-Curie Grant Agreement No. 721567, CAPICE project - Childhood and Adolescence Psychopathology: unravelling the complex etiology by a large Interdisciplinary Collaboration in Europe under Grant Agreement 721567. The APC was funded by the CAPICE project.

**Acknowledgments:** We acknowledge the support from the European Union's Horizon 2020 research and innovation program under the Marie Skłodowska-Curie Grant Agreement No. 721567, CAPICE project -

Childhood and Adolescence Psychopathology: unravelling the complex etiology by a large Interdisciplinary Collaboration in Europe under Grant Agreement 721567.

**Conflicts of Interest:** The authors declare no conflict of interest.

## References

1. Wijmenga, C.; Zhernakova, A. The importance of cohort studies in the post-GWAS era. *Nat. Genet.* **2018**, *50*, 322–328. [CrossRef] [PubMed]
2. Muilu, J.; Peltonen, L.; Litton, J.-E. The federated database – a basis for biobank-based post-genome studies, integrating phenome and genome data from 600 000 twin pairs in Europe. *Eur. J. Hum. Genet.* **2007**, *15*, 718–723. [CrossRef] [PubMed]
3. Bernstein, B.E.; Stamatoyannopoulos, J.A.; Costello, J.F.; Ren, B.; Milosavljevic, A.; Meissner, A.; Kellis, M.; Marra, M.A.; Beaudet, A.L.; Ecker, J.R.; et al. The NIH Roadmap Epigenomics Mapping Consortium. *Nat. Biotechnol.* **2010**, *28*, 1045–1048. [CrossRef] [PubMed]
4. Bakker, O.B.; Aguirre-Gamboa, R.; Sanna, S.; Oosting, M.; Smeekens, S.P.; Jaeger, M.; Zorro, M.; Võsa, U.; Withoff, S.; Netea-Maier, R.T.; et al. Integration of multi-omics data and deep phenotyping enables prediction of cytokine responses. *Nat. Immunol.* **2018**, *19*, 776–786. [CrossRef]
5. Colditz, G.A.; Philpott, S.E.; Hankinson, S.E. The Impact of the Nurses' Health Study on Population Health: Prevention, Translation, and Control. *Am. J. Public Health* **2016**, *106*, 1540–1545. [CrossRef]
6. Haas, L.M.; Lin, E.T.; Roth, M.A. Data integration through database federation. *IBM Syst. J.* **2010**, *41*, 578–596. [CrossRef]
7. Doiron, D.; Burton, P.; Marcon, Y.; Gaye, A.; Wolffenbuttel, B.H.R.; Perola, M.; Stolk, R.P.; Foco, L.; Minelli, C.; Waldenberger, M.; et al. Data harmonization and federated analysis of population-based studies: the BioSHaRE project. *Emerg. Themes Epidemiol.* **2013**, *10*, 12. [CrossRef]
8. Haynes, C.L.; Cook, G.A.; Jones, M.A. Legal and ethical considerations in processing patient-identifiable data without patient consent: lessons learnt from developing a disease register. *J. Med. Ethics* **2007**, *33*, 302–307. [CrossRef]
9. Lu, C.; O'Connor, G.T.; Dupuis, J.; Kolaczyk, E.D. Meta-analysis for penalized regression methods with multi-cohort Genome-wide Association Studies. *Hum. Hered.* **2016**, *81*, 142. [CrossRef]
10. Lim, G.Y.; Tam, W.W.; Lu, Y.; Ho, C.S.; Zhang, M.W.; Ho, R.C. Prevalence of Depression in the Community from 30 Countries between 1994 and 2014. *Sci. Rep.* **2018**, *8*. [CrossRef]
11. Ng, A.; Tam, W.W.; Zhang, M.W.; Ho, C.S.; Husain, S.F.; McIntyre, R.S.; Ho, R.C. IL-1β, IL-6, TNF- α and CRP in Elderly Patients with Depression or Alzheimer's disease: Systematic Review and Meta-Analysis. *Sci. Rep.* **2018**, *8*, 12050. [CrossRef] [PubMed]
12. Ng, J.H.; Ho, R.C.M.; Cheong, C.S.J.; Ng, A.; Yuen, H.W.; Ngo, R.Y.S. Intratympanic steroids as a salvage treatment for sudden sensorineural hearing loss? A meta-analysis. *Eur. Arch. Oto-Rhino-Laryngology* **2015**, *272*, 2777–2782. [CrossRef] [PubMed]
13. Karahalios, A.; Baglietto, L.; Carlin, J.B.; English, D.R.; Simpson, J.A. A review of the reporting and handling of missing data in cohort studies with repeated assessment of exposure measures. *BMC Med. Res. Methodol.* **2012**, *12*, 96. [CrossRef] [PubMed]
14. Wilkinson, M.D.; Dumontier, M.; Aalbersberg, I.J.; Appleton, G.; Axton, M.; Baak, A.; Blomberg, N.; Boiten, J.-W.; da Silva Santos, L.B.; Bourne, P.E.; et al. The FAIR Guiding Principles for scientific data management and stewardship. *Sci. Data* **2016**, *3*, 160018. [CrossRef] [PubMed]
15. Wade, T.D. Traits and types of health data repositories. *Heal. Inf. Sci. Syst.* **2014**, *2*, 4. [CrossRef] [PubMed]
16. Thomas, G.; Thompson, G.R.; Chung, C.-W.; Barkmeyer, E.; Carter, F.; Templeton, M.; Fox, S.; Hartman, B. Heterogeneous distributed database systems for production use. *ACM Comput. Surv.* **1990**, *22*, 237–266. [CrossRef]
17. Herscovitz, E. Secure virtual private networks: the future of data communications. *Int. J. Netw. Manag.* **1999**, *9*, 213–220. [CrossRef]
18. Di Cicco, M.E.; Ragazzo, V.; Jacinto, T. Mortality in relation to smoking: the British Doctors Study. *Breathe (Sheffield, England)* **2016**, *12*, 275–276. [CrossRef] [PubMed]

19. Boyd, A.; Golding, J.; Macleod, J.; Lawlor, D.A.; Fraser, A.; Henderson, J.; Molloy, L.; Ness, A.; Ring, S.; Davey Smith, G. Cohort Profile: the 'children of the 90s'–the index offspring of the Avon Longitudinal Study of Parents and Children. *Int. J. Epidemiol.* **2013**, *42*, 111–127. [CrossRef]
20. Fraser, A.; Macdonald-Wallis, C.; Tilling, K.; Boyd, A.; Golding, J.; Davey Smith, G.; Henderson, J.; Macleod, J.; Molloy, L.; Ness, A.; et al. Cohort Profile: the Avon Longitudinal Study of Parents and Children: ALSPAC mothers cohort. *Int. J. Epidemiol.* **2013**, *42*, 97–110. [CrossRef]
21. Manolio, T.A.; Weis, B.K.; Cowie, C.C.; Hoover, R.N.; Hudson, K.; Kramer, B.S.; Berg, C.; Collins, R.; Ewart, W.; Gaziano, J.M.; et al. New models for large prospective studies: is there a better way? *Am. J. Epidemiol.* **2012**, *175*, 859–866. [CrossRef]
22. Curran, P.J.; Hussong, A.M. Integrative data analysis: the simultaneous analysis of multiple data sets. *Psychol. Methods* **2009**, *14*, 81–100. [CrossRef] [PubMed]
23. Zucker, R.A.; Fitzgerald, H.E.; Refior, S.K.; Puttler, L.I.; Pallas, D.M.; Ellis, D.A.; Fitzgerald, H.E.; Refior, S.K.; Puttler, L.I.; Pallas, D.M.; et al. The Clinical and Social Ecology of Childhood for Children of Alcoholics: Description of a Study and Implications for a Differentiated Social Policy. In *Children of Addiction*; Routledge: Ann Arbor, MI, USA, 2002; pp. 125–158.
24. Chassin, L.; Rogosch, F.; Barrera, M. Substance use and symptomatology among adolescent children of alcoholics. *J. Abnorm. Psychol.* **1991**, *100*, 449–463. [CrossRef] [PubMed]
25. Sher, K.J.; Walitzer, K.S.; Wood, P.K.; Brent, E.E. Characteristics of children of alcoholics: putative risk factors, substance use and abuse, and psychopathology. *J. Abnorm. Psychol.* **1991**, *100*, 427–448. [CrossRef] [PubMed]
26. Revolution, T.H.E.; Microbiomics, O.F. Selected Abstracts of the 14 th International Workshop on Neonatology THE REVOLUTION OF MICROBIOMICS NUTRITION, BACTERIA AND PROBIOTICS IN PERINATAL AND PEDIATRIC HEALTH CAGLIARI (ITALY). *J Pediatr Neonat Individual Med.* **2018**, *7*, 1–66.
27. Litton, J.E.; Muilu, J.; Björklund, A.; Leinonen, A.; Pedersen, N.L. Data Modeling and Data Communication in GenomEUtwin. *Twin Res.* **2003**, *6*, 383–390. [CrossRef]
28. Rajula, H.S.R.; Mauri, M.; Fanos, V. Scale-free networks in metabolomics. *Bioinformation* **2018**, *14*, 140–144. [CrossRef]
29. Patel, A.; Patten, S.; Giesbrecht, G.; Williamson, T.; Tough, S.; Dahal, K.A.; Letourneau, N.; Premji, S. Harmonization of data from cohort studies– potential challenges and opportunities. *Int. J. Popul. Data Sci.* **2018**, *3*, 23889.
30. van Leeuwen, E.M.; Karssen, L.C.; Deelen, J.; Isaacs, A.; Medina-Gomez, C.; Mbarek, H.; Kanterakis, A.; Trompet, S.; Postmus, I.; Verweij, N.; et al. Genome of the Netherlands population-specific imputations identify an ABCA6 variant associated with cholesterol levels. *Nat. Commun.* **2015**, *6*, 6065. [CrossRef]
31. Open-source software for biobankers | BBMRI-ERIC: Making New Treatments Possible. Available online: http://www.bbmri-eric.eu/news-events/open-source-software-for-biobankers/ (accessed on 5 June 2019).
32. Silva, S.; Gutman, B.A.; Romero, E.; Thompson, P.M.; Altmann, A.; Lorenzi, M. Federated Learning in Distributed Medical Databases: Meta-Analysis of Large-Scale Subcortical Brain Data. *aeXiv* **2019**, arXiv:1810.08553.
33. Singh, A.; Babyak, M.A.; Brummett, B.H.; Kraus, W.E.; Siegler, I.C.; Hauser, E.R.; Williams, R.B. Developing a synthetic psychosocial stress measure and harmonizing CVD-risk data: a way forward to GxE meta- and mega-analyses. *BMC Res. Notes* **2018**, *11*, 504. [CrossRef]
34. Boedhoe, P.S.W.; Heymans, M.W.; Schmaal, L.; Abe, Y.; Alonso, P.; Ameis, S.H.; Anticevic, A.; Arnold, P.D.; Batistuzzo, M.C.; Benedetti, F.; et al. An Empirical Comparison of Meta- and Mega-Analysis With Data From the ENIGMA Obsessive-Compulsive Disorder Working Group. *Front. Neuroinform.* **2018**, *12*, 102. [CrossRef] [PubMed]
35. Abraham, N.; Buvanaswari, P.; Rathakrishnan, R.; Tran, B.X.; Thu, G.V.; Nguyen, L.H.; Ho, C.S.; Ho, R.C. A Meta-Analysis of the Rates of Suicide Ideation, Attempts and Deaths in People with Epilepsy. *Int. J. Environ. Res. Public Health* **2019**, *16*, 1451. [CrossRef] [PubMed]
36. Low, Z.X.; Yeo, K.A.; Sharma, V.K.; Leung, G.K.; McIntyre, R.S.; Guerrero, A.; Lu, B.; Sin Fai Lam, C.C.; Tran, B.X.; Nguyen, L.H.; et al. Prevalence of Burnout in Medical and Surgical Residents: A Meta-Analysis. *Int. J. Environ. Res. Public Health* **2019**, *16*, 1479. [CrossRef] [PubMed]
37. Foo, S.Q.; Tam, W.W.; Ho, C.S.; Tran, B.X.; Nguyen, L.H.; McIntyre, R.S.; Ho, R.C. Prevalence of Depression among Migrants: A Systematic Review and Meta-Analysis. *Int. J. Environ. Res. Public Health* **2018**, *15*, 1986. [CrossRef] [PubMed]

38. Ng, T.K.S.; Ho, C.S.H.; Tam, W.W.S.; Kua, E.H.; Ho, R.C.-M. Decreased Serum Brain-Derived Neurotrophic Factor (BDNF) Levels in Patients with Alzheimer's Disease (AD): A Systematic Review and Meta-Analysis. *Int. J. Mol. Sci.* **2019**, *20*, 257. [CrossRef] [PubMed]
39. White, I.R.; Carlin, J.B. Bias and efficiency of multiple imputation compared with complete-case analysis for missing covariate values. *Stat. Med.* **2010**, *29*, 2920–2931. [CrossRef] [PubMed]
40. Molenberghs, G. Analyzing incomplete longitudinal clinical trial data. *Biostatistics* **2004**, *5*, 445–464. [CrossRef] [PubMed]
41. Greenland, S.; Finkle, W.D. A Critical Look at Methods for Handling Missing Covariates in Epidemiologic Regression Analyses. *Am. J. Epidemiol.* **1995**, *142*, 1255–1264. [CrossRef]
42. Schafer, J.L.; Graham, J.W. Missing data: Our view of the state of the art. *Psychol. Methods* **2002**, *7*, 147–177. [CrossRef] [PubMed]
43. Demirtas, H. Flexible Imputation of Missing Data. *J. Stat. Softw.* **2018**, *85*. [CrossRef]
44. *Multiple Imputation for Nonresponse in Surveys*; Rubin, D.B. (Ed.) Wiley Series in Probability and Statistics; John Wiley & Sons, Inc.: Hoboken, NJ, USA, 1987; ISBN 9780470316696.
45. Sterne, J.A.C.; White, I.R.; Carlin, J.B.; Spratt, M.; Royston, P.; Kenward, M.G.; Wood, A.M.; Carpenter, J.R. Multiple imputation for missing data in epidemiological and clinical research: potential and pitfalls. *BMJ* **2009**, *338*, b2393. [CrossRef] [PubMed]
46. Montez-Rath, M.E.; Winkelmayer, W.C.; Desai, M. Addressing Missing Data in Clinical Studies of Kidney Diseases. *Clin. J. Am. Soc. Nephrol.* **2014**, *9*, 1328. [CrossRef] [PubMed]
47. Nooraee, N.; Molenberghs, G.; Ormel, J.; Van den Heuvel, E.R. Strategies for handling missing data in longitudinal studies with questionnaires. *J. Stat. Comput. Simul.* **2018**, *88*, 3415–3436. [CrossRef]
48. Ebrahim, G.J. Missing Data in Clinical Studies Molenberghs G. and Kenward M. G. *J. Trop. Pediatr.* **2007**, *53*, 294. [CrossRef]
49. Carpenter, J.R.; Kenward, M.G. *Multiple imputation and its application*; John Wiley & Sons: London, UK, 2013; ISBN 9780470740521.
50. van Buuren, S.; Groothuis-Oudshoorn, K. **mice**: Multivariate Imputation by Chained Equations in R. *J. Stat. Softw.* **2011**, *45*. [CrossRef]
51. Zondervan-Zwijnenburg, M.A.J.; Veldkamp, S.A.M. Parental age and offspring childhood mental health: a multi-cohort, population-based investigation. *Child Dev.*. (in Press)
52. Thompson, A. Thinking big: Large-scale collaborative research in observational epidemiology. *Eur. J. Epidemiol.* **2009**, *24*, 727–731. [CrossRef]
53. Ford, I.; Norrie, J. Pragmatic Trials. *N. Engl. J. Med.* **2016**, *375*, 454–463. [CrossRef] [PubMed]

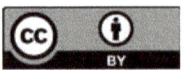

© 2019 by the authors. Licensee MDPI, Basel, Switzerland. This article is an open access article distributed under the terms and conditions of the Creative Commons Attribution (CC BY) license (http://creativecommons.org/licenses/by/4.0/).

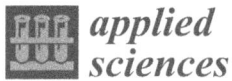 

Article

# Towards Model-Based Online Monitoring of Cyclist's Head Thermal Comfort: Smart Helmet Concept and Prototype

Ali Youssef [1], Jeroen Colon [1], Konstantinos Mantzios [2], Paraskevi Gkiata [2], Tiago S. Mayor [3], Andreas D. Flouris [2], Guido De Bruyne [4,5] and Jean-Marie Aerts [1,*]

1. Department of Biosystems, Animal and Human Health Engineering Division, M3-BIORES: Measure, Model & Manage of Bioresponses Laboratory, KU Leuven, Kasteelpark Arenberg 30, 3001 Heverlee, Belgium
2. FAME Laboratory, Department of Exercise Science, University of Thessaly, 410-00 Thessaly, Greece
3. SIMTECH Laboratory, Transport Phenomena Research Centre, Engineering Faculty of Porto University, Rua Dr. Roberto Frias, 4200-465 Porto, Portugal
4. Department of Product Development, University of Antwerp, 2018 Antwerp, Belgium
5. Lazer Sport NV, Lamorinierestraat 33-37, 2018 Antwerp, Belgium
* Correspondence: jean-marie.aerts@kuleuven.be

Received: 10 July 2019; Accepted: 1 August 2019; Published: 4 August 2019

**Featured Application: In this work, we introduce the basis for a personalised adaptive model to predict head thermal comfort using streaming data of easily measured variables, which can be used for real-time monitoring of a cyclist's thermal comfort and adaptive controlling of smart wearable applications.**

**Abstract:** Bicyclists can be subjected to crashes, which can cause injuries over the whole body, especially the head. Head injuries can be prevented by wearing bicycle helmets; however, bicycle helmets are frequently not worn due to a variety of reasons. One of the most common complaints about wearing bicycle helmets relates to thermal discomfort. So far, insufficient attention has been given to the thermal performance of helmets. This paper aimed to introduce and develop an adaptive model for the online monitoring of head thermal comfort based on easily measured variables, which can be measured continuously using impeded sensors in the helmet. During the course of this work, 22 participants in total were subjected to different levels of environmental conditions (air temperature, air velocity, mechanical work and helmet thermal resistance) to develop a general model to predict head thermal comfort. A reduced-order general linear regression model with three input variables, namely, temperature difference between ambient temperature and average under-helmet temperature, cyclist's heart rate and the interaction between ambient temperature and helmet thermal resistance, was the most suitable to predict the cyclist's head thermal comfort and showed maximum mean absolute percentage error (MAPE) of 8.4%. Based on the selected model variables, a smart helmet prototype (SmartHelmet) was developed using impeded sensing technology, which was used to validate the developed general model. Finally, we introduced a framework of calculation for an adaptive personalised model to predict head thermal comfort based on streaming data from the SmartHelmet prototype.

**Keywords:** thermal comfort; bicycle helmet; smart wearables; adaptive model; streaming data

## 1. Introduction

Bicycling, for recreational, transport and sport purposes, provides health benefits for the individual as well society [1]. However, due to different reasons, bicyclists can be subjected to crashes, which can cause injuries over the whole body. Of these, head injuries can lead to serious brain damage and, in extreme cases, death [2].

Head injuries can be prevented by wearing bicycle helmets, thereby increasing cycling safety [3]. However, while it is well known that bicycle helmets can be lifesaving in case of an accident, they are not worn frequently. A variety of barriers of social, psychological, cultural and biological origin have been reported [4].

One of the most common complaints associated with wearing bicycle helmets appears to be thermal comfort [5]. In a survey study by Finnoff et al. [5], it appeared that "uncomfortable" and "it's hot" were two of the most important barriers for wearing a bicycle helmet in all three age categories (children (7–10), adolescents (11–19) and adults (>19)). Furthermore, Bogerd et al. [6] concluded in their review study, which investigated the ergonomics of headgear, that unfavourable thermal sensation or thermal discomfort is frequently used as an argument for not wearing headgear. Wearing a bicycle helmet alters the local skin temperature and sweat rate, which can lead to thermal discomfort [6]. Moreover, under exertion, the human body dissipates a significant fraction of its excess heat through the head, which, during cycling, is placed in a strong air current. The helmet insulates the head, limiting the transfer of heat to the air and the evaporation of sweat [7]. Therefore, it is of utmost importance for bicycle helmets to be designed in a way that favours thermal comfort whilst meeting mechanical protection requirements. This dual goal of protection and comfort poses a great challenge because of the often-contradictory requirements of thermal comfort and impact protection [8].

Sensations concerning thermal comfort are the result of a cognitive process described by the American Society of Heating, Refrigerating and Air-Conditioning Engineers (ASHRAE) standard 55 [9] as "that condition of mind, which expresses satisfaction with the thermal environment" (ASHRAE standard 55–66). Comfort is a recognisable state of feeling which is the result of the entire environment, including psychological and physiological variables. It is usually associated with conditions that are pleasant and compatible with health and happiness, whereas discomfort is associated with pain, which is unpleasant [10].

Skin temperature and sweat rate are examples of the body's mechanisms to keep body temperature quasi-constant. These mechanisms are controlled by a region in the brain called the hypothalamus. This regulation centre monitors body temperature and controls it directly by physiological processes and/or indirectly by behaviour (i.e., behavioural thermoregulation). Although a person's reported state of thermal comfort is purely perceptive, the body's thermoregulatory actions influence thermal comfort by its outcomes (e.g., sweat rate, skin temperature, etc.) [10–12].

An often-used method to accurately assess thermal sensation (TS) and comfort ($T_C$) is to ask individuals directly about their thermal sensation perception [11,13]. Individuals express their opinion to rate their thermal sensation/comfort when they are exposed to given thermal conditions by using a scale from cold to hot that has a predefined number of points. Mathematical models of thermal sensation and comfort have been developed to overcome the difficulties of direct enquiry of subjects. The development of such models has mostly depended on statistical approaches that correlate experimental condition data (i.e., environmental and personal variables) with thermal sensation votes obtained from human subjects [11,14]. Thermal comfort models, such as predicted mean vote (PMV), predict the state of thermal comfort from thermoregulatory actions such as skin temperature and sweat secretion. These two types of models are therefore often combined to predict the thermal comfort of an average person under different environmental conditions [13,15]. Many advanced mechanistic thermoregulation models, such as the "Fiala thermal Physiology and Comfort" (FPC) model, were developed to predict the thermal comfort status of humans [16]. By implementing thermoregulation models in wearable devices connected to the body, thermal comfort can be monitored and, in a further stage, even controlled. However, for real-time applications, such models are too complex and have a high computational cost, thus making them less suitable for monitoring and control applications. Data-based models, on the other hand, are less complex and thus more adequate for real-time monitoring and control purposes. Youssef et. al. [17] demonstrated that such compact data-based mechanistic models are promising for modelling body temperature response using metabolic activity alone or metabolic activity and skin temperature as inputs by means of, respectively, a single-input single-output (SISO) or a multiple-input single-output (MISO) discrete-time transfer function model.

Recent developments in compact wireless sensors allow the implementation of sensors in wearable devices such as bicycle helmets. Considering this, bicycle helmet design should be optimised for thermal comfort, so that bicycle helmets not only allow monitoring an individual's thermal comfort but also support its active control.

In this reported research, we aimed at

(i) identifying a general model to estimate thermal comfort based on a few variables, the measurements of which can be integrated in helmets;
(ii) developing and testing a prototype of a smart helmet based on the identified general thermal comfort model; and
(iii) introducing the framework of calculation for an adaptive personalised reduced-order model to predict a cyclist's under-helmet thermal comfort using nonintrusive, easily measured variables.

## 2. Materials and Methods

The main goal of this paper is to introduce a framework for developing a personalised adaptive model for predicting a cyclist's head thermal comfort by utilising the smart helmet concept. Figure 1 presents the general framework introduced in the present paper.

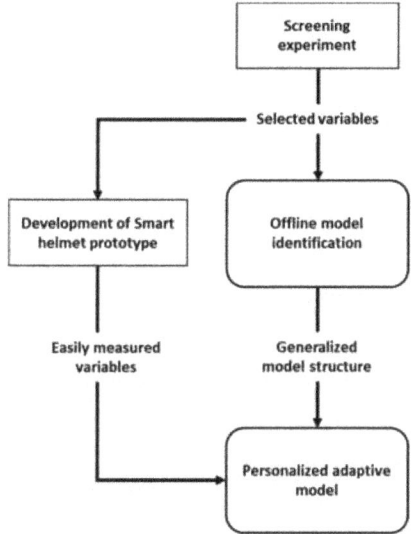

**Figure 1.** Schematic diagram showing the general framework of the development of a personalised adaptive model for the smart helmet prototype.

### 2.1. Development of General Thermal Comfort Predictive Model

2.1.1. Experimental Setup and Test Subjects

During the course of these experiments, 15 male test subjects with an average age ($\bar{\mu}_{age}$) of 22 (±1) years and an average weight ($\bar{\mu}_{mass}$) of 74.3 (±9.2) kg were used in this study. The experimental protocol was approved by the Social and Societal Ethics Committee (SMEC) of KU Leuven. The experiments were conducted using a professional bicycle trainer (Tacx Ironman Smart) with a fastened racing bicycle (BH L52C8 Speedrom) controlling the power delivery of the subject with a power brake.

The power brake itself was wirelessly controlled via the Tacx Trainer software. The bicycle trainer was placed in a customised wind tunnel to simulate the wind effect on the test subjects during the course of the experiment (Figure 2). The wind tunnel was 2.1 m high, 2.3 m long and 1.5 m wide. Four rows with three fans each (Fancom type 1435/L7-588 fans) were used as the actuators for wind speed. Each fan produced a maximum ventilation rate of 3000 m$^3 \cdot$h$^{-1}$. A 50 cm long honeycomb gauze structure, placed 25 cm from the fans, was used to obtain a quasi-laminar flow within the open-loop wind tunnel (for more information about the wind tunnel, see [18]). The air speed near the test subject's head was set to 2.5 m$\cdot$s$^{-1}$ to simulate recreational cycling for adults and children. The wind tunnel was placed inside a climate-controlled chamber (Figure 2), the inner dimensions of which were 4 × 11 × 5 m ($w \times l \times h$). The air temperature within the climate chamber was controllable within the range of 15–35 °C. Additionally, the ventilation rate within the climate chamber was controllable within the range of 0–2700 m$^3 \cdot$h$^{-1}$ (i.e., 0–11.25 volume refreshments per hour).

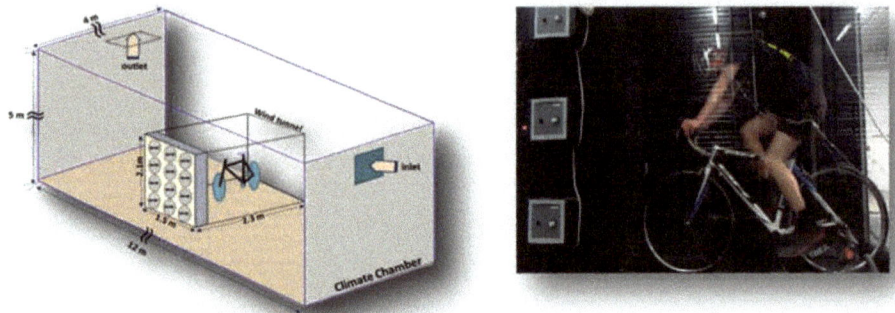

**Figure 2.** Schematic representation showing the used bicycle fixed inside a customised wind tunnel and placed within a climate chamber (**left**) and a photograph of a test subject riding the bike within the wind tunnel (**right**).

2.1.2. Pretest Experiments

The pretest was a modification of the widely used physiological test protocols described by the Australian Institute of Sport [19]. The aim of the pretest was to obtain a power ($P$) value that could be maintained by each of the 15 test subjects for a period of at least 20 min. The maximal lactate steady state ($MLSS$) and the corresponding workload steady state ($WLSS$) are presumed to be the maximum workload that can be maintained for endurance sports [20,21]. This lactate threshold is defined as the highest oxygen consumption rate that can be achieved during exercise without a systematic increase in blood lactate concentration [22]. A respiratory exchange ratio (RER) > 1.0 is an indication of the growing contribution of anaerobic metabolism, which causes muscle acidification and leads to muscle fatigue [23].

A bicycle incremental step test was designed in such way that the power increased 30 W every 5 min starting from 100 W. During the test, the subject's RER was measured with a spirometer (Metamax 3B) and the test was terminated when he exceeded an RER value of 1 for more than 20 s (the corresponding power, $P_{RER\,=\,1}$, was used further in the thermal comfort experiment). The tests were conducted at normal indoor climate conditions with 47% (±4%) relative humidity and an ambient temperature of 20 (±1) °C.

2.1.3. Thermal Comfort and Variable Screening Experimental Protocol

The main objective of this stage was to screen the most suitable variables to predict the cyclist's under-helmet thermal comfort which can also be easily measured so as to be combatable for smart helmet application. During the course of these experiments, each experimental trial lasted 80 min and was divided into four consecutive timeslots of 20 min each. At each timeslot, a combination of changes in the environmental variables, namely, relative air velocity imposed by the fan ($v$), ambient air temperature ($T_a$), thermal resistance of the scalp ($R_h$) and the delivered cycling power ($P$), was applied. The quantification of the scalp thermal resistance ($R_h$) was developed based on computational fluid dynamic (CFD) simulation for a bare head [24]. The thermal resistance was quantified (see Table 1) for the following cases: no-helmet wearing, where $R_h$ was 0; wearing helmet; and wearing helmet with helmet fast (aeroshell). The applied combinations of the different variables with their different levels (low, mid and high) are shown in Table 1.

Table 1. The applied values for each variable.

| | $T_a$ (°C) | $v$ (m·s$^{-1}$) | $P$ (W) | $R_h$ (m$^2$·°C·W$^{-1}$) |
|---|---|---|---|---|
| Low level | 20 | 0 | 50% (PRER = 1) | 0 (no helmet) |
| Midlevel | / | / | / | 0.045 (with helmet) |
| High level | 30 | 4 | 90% (PRER = 1) | 0.060 (helmet + aeroshell) |

During the course of each trial, the heart rate ($H_R$), in bpm, of the test subject was measured and logged with a validated heart rate belt sensor (Zephyr$^{TM}$ bioharness Bt) in combination with a built-in optical heart rate sensor (PPG, Lifebeam) in the bicycle helmet (Lazer Z1 and Lazer Z1 fast = Lazer Z1 + aeroshell). The temperatures of the subject's forehead, neck, inside of the ear and the air under the bicycle helmet (at front, back, right and left) were continuously measured using calibrated thermocouples (type-T) with a sampling frequency of 1 Hz.

During the experiment, all test subjects were verbally asked about their thermal comfort every 5 min from the start (minute 0) until the end (minute 80) based on the thermal comfort scale introduced by Gagge et al. [10]. For convenience, the cold thermal sensation votes were excluded, as shown in Table 2, as the present work only focused on discomfort perception due to high temperatures.

Table 2. Thermal comfort scale introduced by Gagge et al. [10], excluding the cold sensation votes.

| Scale | Thermal Comfort Perception |
|---|---|
| 1 | Comfortable |
| 2 | Slightly uncomfortable |
| 3 | Uncomfortable |
| 4 | Very uncomfortable |

The experimental design was done using JMP Pro software. A preliminary screening experiment was set up to investigate the contribution of the different variables that, potentially, have an effect on the thermal sensation and thermal comfort under the bicycle helmet. Therefore, each subject was subjected to a combination of different levels of environmental conditions during the experiment.

The experiment was designed to investigate the main effects of the defined environmental input variables, the two-variable interactions between these variables and, due to the particular interest in the effect of a bicycle helmet, the quadratic effect of $R_h$, which can be mathematically expressed as follows:

$$T_C = \beta_{T_a}T_a + \beta_{R_h}R_h + \beta_P P + \beta_v v + \beta_{Pv}Pv + \beta_{PT_a}PT_a + \beta_{PR_h}PR_h + \beta_{R_hT_a}R_hT_a + \beta_{R_h^2}R_h^2, \quad (1)$$

where $T_C$ is the thermal comfort and $\beta_i$ is the weighting factor for each variable or variable combination ($i$).

The inclusion of the quadratic effect, which is the interaction effect of the variable with itself, was necessary to generate an experiment that has multiple levels of $R_h$, so that analysis of a dynamic response due to the bicycle helmet was possible. With the help of the JMP Pro® software, different combinations (referred to as runs) of the input variables were generated. In general, each participant (test subject) was subjected to four runs (combinations) of the generated ones. Table 3 shows the experimental design for test subjects ($j$) 1 and 8 as an example, where each time slot corresponds to one run (a combination of the four input variables).

Table 3. Experimental design for test subjects 1 and 8, showing the four runs (combinations) of input variables with three different levels, namely, high (↑), mid (−) and low (↓).

| Participant (No. = $j$) | Variables | Timeslot (1) | Timeslot (2) | Timeslot (3) | Timeslot (4) |
|---|---|---|---|---|---|
| $j = 1$ | $T_a$ (°C) | ↓ | ↓ | ↓ | ↓ |
|  | $v$ (m·s$^{-1}$) | ↑ | ↓ | ↑ | ↓ |
|  | $P$ (% PPER = 1) | ↓ | ↓ | ↑ | ↑ |
|  | $R_h$ (m$^2$·°C·W$^{-1}$) | − | ↑ | − | ↓ |
| $j = 8$ | $T_a$ (°C) | ↑ | ↑ | ↑ | ↑ |
|  | $v$ (m·s$^{-1}$) | ↑ | ↑ | ↓ | ↓ |
|  | $P$ (% PPER = 1) | ↑ | ↓ | ↑ | ↑ |
|  | $R_h$ (m$^2$·°C·W$^{-1}$) | − | − | ↓ | ↑ |

2.1.4. General Linear Regression (LR) Model Identification and Offline Parameter Estimation

The main objective of this stage was to identify a general reduced-order and the most parametrically efficient (parsimonious) model structure with the minimum number of easily measured variables (based on the results of the previous stage) to predict the cyclist's under-helmet thermal comfort. For the sake of the main objective of the present work, the selected predictive model had to be suitable, concerning the computational cost, for wearable sensing technology. Due to the subjective nature of the thermal comfort data, it could not be performed in a continuous pattern, unlike the other input variables, which was a challenge for identifying the predictive model. Hence, in the present paper, we used a simple multivariate regression model with the following general form [25]:

$$T_{ci} = \alpha + \beta_1 u_{i1} + \beta_2 u_{i2} + \ldots + \beta_m u_{im} + \epsilon_i, \text{ for } i \in \{1, \ldots, n\},$$

where $T_{ci} \in \mathbb{R}$ is the response (thermal comfort) for the $i$th observation, $\alpha \in \mathbb{R}$ is the regression intercept, $\beta_j \in \mathbb{R}$ is the $j$th predictor's slope, $u_{ij} \in \mathbb{R}$ is the $j$th predictor for the $i$th observation and $\epsilon_i \sim N(0, \sigma^2)$ is an independent and identically distributed Gaussian error term. This can be formulated in matrix form as follows:

$$\mathbf{T_C} = \mathbf{X}\beta + \epsilon, \text{ subjected to}: \mathbf{T_C} \in \mathbb{R}^{n \times 1} \text{ and } \mathbf{X} \in \mathbb{R}^{n \times m}$$

where $n$ and $m$ are the number of samples and number of predictors (input variables), respectively. In the present paper, we used the ordinary least-squares (OLR) approach to find the regression coefficients estimates ($\hat{\beta}$) that minimised the sum of the squared errors as follows:

$$\hat{\beta} = \arg\min_{\beta}(\mathbf{T_C} - \mathbf{X}\beta)^T(\mathbf{T_C} - \mathbf{X}\beta) = (\mathbf{X}^T\mathbf{X})^{-1}\mathbf{X}^T\mathbf{T_C}.$$

2.2. Development of Smart Helmet Prototype

A standard cyclist helmet (312 g) was utilised for the development of the smart helmet prototype (Lazer Bullet 1.0, Lazer Sport, Antwerp, Belgium). The helmet was equipped with a Lifebeam heart rate sensor (Lazer Sport, Antwerp, Belgium; Figure 3) and a 3 × 3 mm digital humidity and temperature sensor (CJMCU-1080 HTC1080, Texas Instruments, Dallas, Texas; accuracy: ±2% for relative humidity and ±0.2 °C for temperature) to measure the surrounding air humidity and temperature. Additionally, four temperature sensors (Negative-Temperature-Coefficient "NTC" temperature sensors, 100 kΩ at 25 °C; Figure 4) were used at the front, back, right and left of the helmet inner body. The final weight of the equipped helmet was 358 g. All sensors were connected directly to a microcontroller (Adafruit Feather

32u4 Bluefruit, Adafruit Industries, New York, NY, USA) that transmitted all data from the helmet to a smartphone via Bluetooth. The Adafruit Bluefruit was chosen as it is the smallest "all-in-one" Arduino-compatible and Bluetooth Low Energy microcontroller with built-in USB and battery charging. The developed system was compatible with a 3.7 V Li-polymer rechargeable battery (LP-523450-1S-3) with the ability to power the system for up to 10 h. A circuit diagram of the used electronics and sensors is shown in Figure 4. The impeded electronics and sensor technology in the smart helmet increased the final original weight of the helmet (312 g) by only 14.7% and did not alter the geometric and aerodynamic characteristics of the original standard helmet. As such, the developed smart helmet is comparable to the original standard helmet (Lazer Bullet 1.0, Lazer Sport, Antwerp, Belgium).

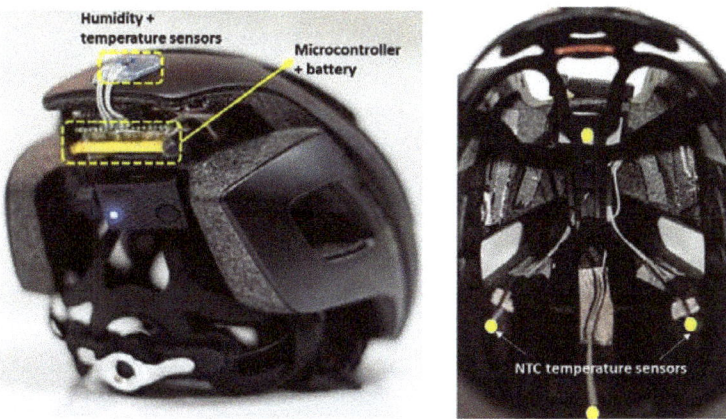

**Figure 3.** The developed smart helmet prototype showing the microcontroller and the humidity and temperature sensor on the back side of the helmet (**left picture**) and the four NTC temperature sensors placed in the inner body of the helmet (**right picture**).

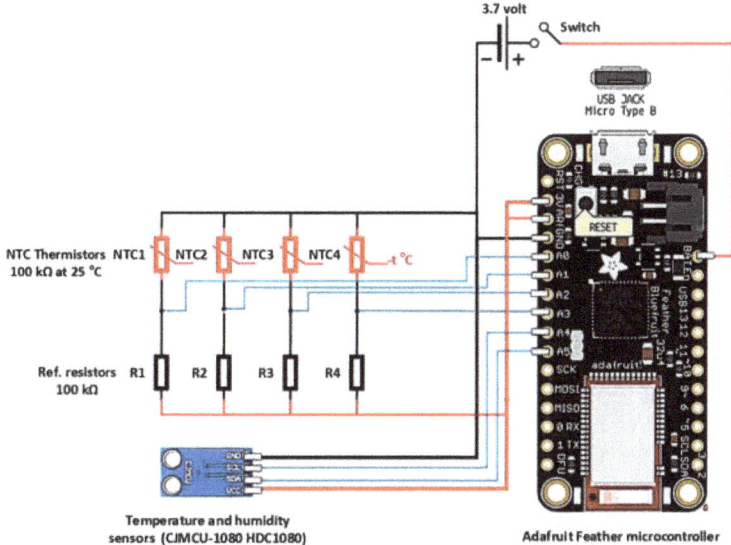

**Figure 4.** Circuit diagram of the stand-alone sensor system impeded in the smart helmet prototype.

An android-based application "SmartHelmet App" (Figure 5) was developed to simultaneously communicate with both the Adafruit Feather microcontroller and the Lifebeam heart rate monitor via a Bluetooth communication protocol. The SmartHelmet App was developed using the AppyBuilder online platform (App Inventor, Massachusetts Institute of Technology, Cambridge, Massachusetts, USA). The application was designed to receive, display in real-time and store all the data from the SmartHelmet at a 0.2 Hz sampling rate.

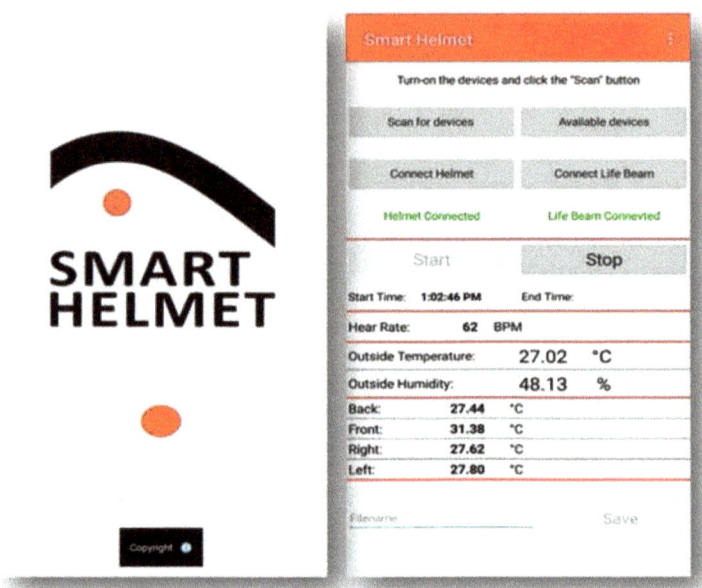

**Figure 5.** A screenshot of the designed SmartHelmet App.

*2.3. Testing the Developed Smart Helmet Prototype*

2.3.1. Test Subjects

In total, seven well-trained male cyclists were recruited for the course of this experiment. Their average physical characteristics were as follows: age—34.5 (±5) years; body mass—74.5 (±7.3) kg; body height—177.6 (±5.4) cm; body mass index (BMI)—23.6 (±1.8) kg·m$^{-2}$; and body surface area—1.9 (±0.1) m$^2$. Prior to the trial, a signed written consent form was obtained from all participants after a detailed description of the protocol, discomforts and benefits. The experimental protocol was approved by the ethical review board at the University of Thessaly, School of Exercise Science in accordance with the recommendations of the Declaration of Helsinki.

2.3.2. Experimental Design and Protocol

Participants were exposed to a hot (34 °C and 56% relative humidity) environment and completed a 30 km cycling time-trial (TT) inside an environmental chamber. In addition, exposure to 800 W of solar radiation was simulated using compact source iodide (CSI) lamps, while a constant wind speed of 5.1 m·s$^{-1}$ was provided with a large 80 cm diameter industrial fan positioned in front of the participant at a distance of 140 cm from the bicycle saddle. All participants were instructed to abstain from vigorous physical activity 24 h prior the experimental trial and consume at least 500 mL of water and a light meal 2 h before arrival at the laboratory.

Upon arrival at the laboratory, participants changed into their standardised cycling apparel and underwent basic anthropometric measurements. Body height was measured using a stadiometer (Seca

213; Seca GmbH & Co. KG; Hamburg, Germany), while body mass was determined with a digital weighing scale (Version 5.3 KERN & Sohn GmbH). BMI and body surface area were calculated from the measurements of body height and mass. After instrumentation, participants wore the SmartHelmet, entered the controlled environmental chamber and sat on the cycle for 10 min for a baseline period. Thereafter, they performed a 15 min warm-up followed by the 30 km TT. Participants were allowed to drink water ad libitum throughout the TT. No verbal encouragement was provided during the TT.

Cyclists performed the TT on an adjustable friction-braked cycle ergometer (CycleOps 400 Pro Serie Indoor Cycle, Fitchburg, MA, USA), which was combined with the commercially available software Rouvy (VirtualTraining, Vimperk, Czech Republic), allowing simulation of a route on a computer screen. During the 30 km TT, all cyclists were instructed to complete the race as fast as possible with free access to controlling power (W) and cadence (rpm). To simulate real cycling, participants could see their power, cadence and covered distance throughout the TT.

Ratings of perceived exertion (RPE) were reported with the 6–20 point Borg scale [26] before the baseline period, at the beginning of the warm-up period as well as at the start and end times of the TT. Thermal comfort ($T_C$) and thermal sensation ($T_S$) were measured at the same time points using 7- and 9-point scales, respectively [10].

The average power output, pedalling cadence and 30 km TT duration of all the participants (test subjects) are shown in Table 4.

**Table 4.** The mean average power output, pedalling cadence and 30 km time-trial (TT) obtained from all test subjects.

| Variable | Average (±Standard Deviation) |
|---|---|
| Power output (W) | 176.5 (±24.2) |
| Cadence (rpm) | 93.7 (±14.2) |
| 30 km TT duration (min) | 56.9 (±7.9) |

## 3. Results

### 3.1. Pretest Experiments

Figure 6 shows the resulting $P_{RER\,=\,1}$ value for each test subject and the corresponding low and high levels of power. The corresponding low ($P$ = 50% of $P_{RER\,=\,1}$) and high ($P$ = 90% of $P_{RER\,=\,1}$) levels for each test subject were used in the screening experiments.

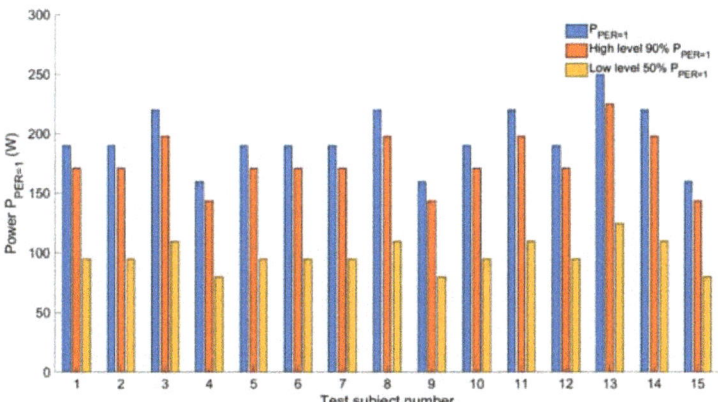

**Figure 6.** Obtained power values of the pretest. These power values correspond to the power value when they exceeded a respiratory exchange ratio (RER) of one.

## 3.2. Development of Offline (General) Thermal Comfort Model

Figure 7 shows the acquired measurements from test subject 1, including environment-related variables, namely, ambient temperature ($T_a$), air velocity ($v$), helmet thermal resistance and applied power level ($R_h$) and the applied mechanical work rate ($P$). Bioresponse-related variables, including heart rate ($H_R$), the temperature difference ($\Delta T$) between the average temperature beneath the helmet and the ambient air temperature, the temperature difference ($\Delta T_{ear}$) between the ear temperature and the ambient air temperature as well the thermal comfort ($T_C$), were considered.

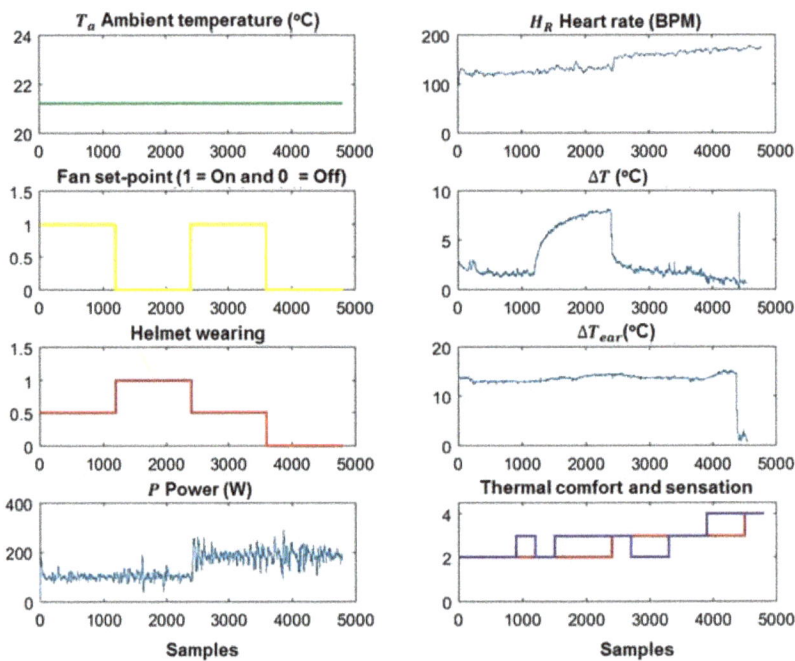

**Figure 7.** The recorded measurements of the different variables obtained from test subject 1.

The graphs show the environmental variables (left graphs), including the ambient air temperature ($T_a$, °C), fan set-points ($v$, 1 = 4 ms$^{-1}$), the helmet wearing level (0 = no helmet, 0.5 = helmet and 1 = helmet + aeroshell) and the applied mechanical work rate (power) level ($P$, W). The measured variables related to the bioresponses of the test subject (right graphs) were heart rate ($H_R$, bpm), the temperature difference ($\Delta T$, °C) between the average temperature beneath the helmet and the ambient air temperature, the temperature difference ($\Delta T_{ear}$, °C) between the ear temperature and the ambient air temperature and the thermal comfort (red line) and sensation (blue line) scores.

To investigate the effect of the different inputs on thermal comfort, different linear regression models (general models) were identified to estimate and predict the perceived under-helmet thermal comfort $T_C$ (output) using continuously measured variables (inputs), including the aforementioned environmental and bioresponse-related variables. The most suitable combination of input variables was selected by retaining only the input variables with a significant ($p < 0.05$) effect on thermal comfort. Additionally, the best model structure was selected based on two main selection criteria, namely, the goodness of fit ($R^2$) and Akaike information criterion (AIC). The results showed that the most suitable LR model structure, with the highest goodness of fit (average $R^2 = 0.87 \pm 0.05$) and lowest Akaike information criterion (average AIC = 138 ± 12), to predict the thermal comfort for all test subjects was as follows:

$$T_C = \alpha + \beta_1 T_a + \beta_2 v + \beta_3 P + \beta_4 [T_a R_h]. \tag{2}$$

The average parameter estimates, *t*-ratio and *p*-value of $P > |t|$ for each selected input variable are given in Table 5. The results showed that the main effect of the thermal resistance $R_h$ was not significant ($p > 0.05$); however, the variable interaction of $R_h$ with $T_a$ showed a significant ($p = 0.015$) effect on the prediction of the under-helmet thermal comfort.

Table 5. The estimation results of the selected linear regression model (3) to predict thermal comfort, showing the average model estimates for the 15 test subjects.

| Term | Parameter | Estimate | Std. Error | t-Ratio | P > \|t\| |
|---|---|---|---|---|---|
| intercept | $\alpha$ | 2.36 | 0.14 | 16.80 | <0.0001 * |
| $T_a$ | $\beta_1$ | −0.40 | 0.11 | −3.52 | 0.0025 * |
| $v$ | $\beta_2$ | −0.36 | 0.07 | −4.85 | <0.0001 * |
| $P$ | $\beta_3$ | 0.41 | 0.07 | 5.45 | <0.0001 * |
| $[T_a R_h]$ | $\beta_4$ | 0.25 | 0.01 | 2.52 | 0.015 * |

* significant ($p < 0.05$).

To understand the interaction effect of $R_h$ and $T_a$ on the prediction of thermal comfort, a prediction trace analysis of the model [27] was employed using prediction the JMP® profiler tool [28], as visualised in Figure 8. For convenience of this analysis, the values of each input variable were scaled (normalised) in such a way to lie in the closed interval [−1, +1], where -1 indicates the variable's low level and +1 indicates its high level (Figure 8). The scaling of each variable value $i(k)$ was done according to the following formula:

$$x_i(k) = \frac{i(k) - M_i}{\Delta_i}$$

where $x_i(k)$ is the scaled variable value at time instance $k$, $M_i$ is the midpoint ($M_i = \frac{L_i + U_i}{2}$) and $L_i$ and $U_i$ are the particular lower and upper limits of input variable $i$, respectively. The term $\Delta_i$ ($\frac{L_i - U_i}{2}$) is half of the range of the interval.

Table 6. The estimation results of the compact regression model (3) to predict thermal comfort, showing the average model estimates for the 15 test subjects.

| Term | Parameter | Estimate | Std. Error | t-Ratio | P > \|t\| |
|---|---|---|---|---|---|
| intercept | $\alpha$ | 1.86 | 0.21 | 13.61 | <0.0001 * |
| $\Delta T$ | $\beta_1$ | 1.30 | 0.19 | 5.22 | 0.0031 * |
| $H_R$ | $\beta_2$ | −0.62 | 0.13 | −5.67 | 0.0014 * |
| $[T_a R_h]$ | $\beta_3$ | 0.35 | 0.07 | 2.52 | 0.0140 * |

* significant ($p < 0.05$).

The prediction trace analysis [28] of the developed model (2) was based on computing the predicted response as one variable was changing while the others were held constant at certain values. The results showed that the effect of $R_h$ was dependent on the level of $T_a$. At a low level (−1) of ambient air temperature ($T_a = 20$ °C), for a change in thermal resistance $R_h$ from a low level (−1) (i.e., no-bicycle helmet) to a high level (1) (i.e., using the Lazer-Z1 Fast), the predicted thermal comfort scale (Table 2) decreased by 0.5 thermal comfort units but was perceived as comfortable. However, at a high level (1) of ambient air temperature ($T_a = 30$ °C), the comfort level increased by 0.5 thermal comfort units. This information is important for actively controlling under-helmet thermal comfort, which can be done by manipulating the helmet thermal resistance via, for instance, opening/closing some of the helmet's holes.

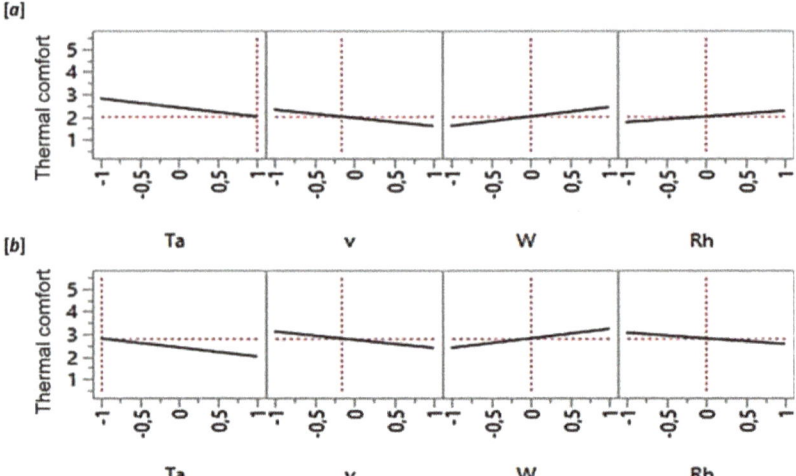

**Figure 8.** Visualisation of the model prediction traces showing the interaction effect of the thermal resistance ($R_h$) and ambient temperature ($T_a$) on the predicted thermal comfort. (**a**) When the temperature was low (20 °C), additional thermal resistance was perceived as comfortable. However, (**b**) when the temperature was high (30 °C), additional thermal resistance was perceived as uncomfortable. The values of the input variables were normalised in the range between -1 and 1, which correspond to low and high levels, respectively. Table 6 shows the average parameter estimates of the developed compact regression model (3) for the 15 test subjects.

As expected, the heart rate ($H_R$) of the test subjects was found to be highly correlated (Pearson's correlation coefficient, $r = 0.85$) with the power ($P$). Additionally, the heart rate was significantly correlated ($r = 0.68$) with the recorded thermal comfort for all 15 test subjects.

As expected, the temperature difference ($\Delta T$) between the average air temperature beneath the helmet ($\overline{T}_h$) and the ambient air temperature ($T_a$) was correlated with both relative air velocity ($v$) and helmet thermal resistance ($R_h$), with $r = 0.82$ and $0.78$, respectively.

By employing both heart rate ($H_R$) and the temperature difference ($\Delta T$) as input variables to the linear regression model, the best model structure that gave the highest average goodness of fit (with average $R^2 = 0.89 \pm 0.04$) and lowest Akaike information criterion (average AIC = $123 \pm 7$) was as follows:

$$T_C = \alpha + \beta_1 \Delta T + \beta_2 H_R + \beta_3 [T_a R_h], \qquad (3)$$

where $\Delta T = \overline{T}_h - T_a$ and $\overline{T}_h$ is the average air temperature under the helmet, which is calculated from the four temperature sensors located under the helmet. It can be noticed that the structure of model (3) is more compact, consisting of three input variables, compared with the structure of model (2), which consisted of five input variables. Model (3) showed better prediction performance for the thermal comfort level than model (2), which had maximum mean absolute percentage errors (MAPEs) of 8.4% and 11%, respectively. The MAPE is given by

$$MAPE = \frac{100\%}{N} \sum_{k=1}^{N} \left| \frac{\hat{T}_C(k) - T_C(k)}{T_C(k)} \right|$$

where $N$ is the number of data points and $\hat{T}_C$ is the predicted thermal comfort.

It can be noticed that both the mechanical work rate ($P$) and air velocity ($v$) disappeared from the compact model (3). The heart rate ($H_R$) variable included in the compact model (3) directly linked to the applied mechanical work rate ($P$), hence the effect of $P$, included in model (2), translated by the bioresponse represented by $H_R$ (e.g., [29]) included in model (3). According to Newton's law of cooling, temperature difference ($\Delta T$) is the driving force for the convective heat transfer ($Q_h$) between the cyclist's head and the ambient air. The heat flux ($q$) is proportional to $\Delta T$ and the convective heat transfer coefficient ($h_c$) links both variables as follows:

$$q = -h\Delta T \ [\text{W·m}^{-2}].$$

The heat transfer coefficient ($h_c$, W·m$^2$·°C) is a combination of the heat transfer coefficient of the air ($h_{air}$) and that of the helmet ($h_H = \frac{1}{R_h}$); hence,

$$\Delta T = -\left[\frac{1}{h_{air} + \frac{1}{R_h}}\right] q.$$

The heat transfer coefficients of the air ($h_{air}$) and the bicycle helmet ($\frac{1}{R_h}$) are dependent on air velocity ($v$). Hence, it is clear that the effect of $\Delta T$ is inherently connected to the effect of both $v$ and helmet thermal resistance ($R_h$).

It can be concluded from the presented results that the input variables included in model (3), namely, temperature difference ($\Delta T$), heart rate ($H_R$) of the cyclist and the interaction variable $[T_a R_h]$ between ambient temperature ($T_a$) and helmet thermal resistance ($R_h$), were suitable enough to estimate the cyclist's thermal comfort ($T_C$) under the bicycle helmet. These selected variables were the basis for developing a reduced-order personalised model for real-time monitoring of a cyclist's thermal comfort under the helmet. Additionally, from a practical point of view, these three variables were suitable to be measured using integrated sensors in the cyclist's helmet, as is shown in the following subsection.

*3.3. Testing the SmartHelmet Prototype and Validation of the Developed General Model*

In Figure 9, the average ratings of perceived exertion (RPE), thermal comfort ($T_C$) and thermal sensation ($T_S$) values at the start and end times of the TT are presented for all seven test subjects. The average values (±standard deviation) of all used subjective ratings showed a significant ($p < 0.05$) increase at the end of the TT (RPE = 17.6 ± 0.5, $T_C$ = 2.6 ± 0.5 and $T_S$ = 4.4 ± 0.6) compared with their values at the start of the trial.

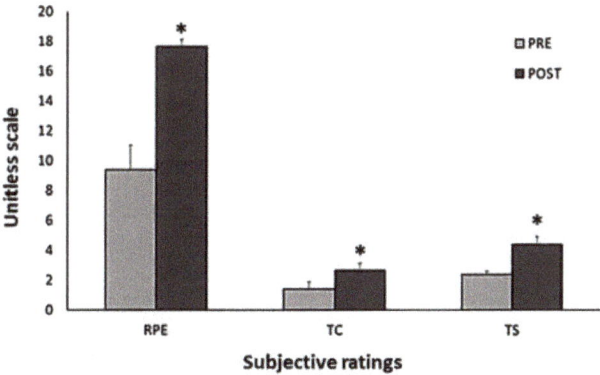

**Figure 9.** Average values of ratings of perceived exertion (RPE), thermal comfort ($T_C$) and thermal sensation ($T_S$) between the start (PRE) and end (POST) times of the TT (* indicates a significant difference of $p < 0.05$).

Figure 10 shows the real-time measured average temperatures ($\overline{T}_h$) under the helmet, average temperature difference ($\Delta T$) between the average temperature under the helmet and the ambient air temperature and the average heart rate ($H_R$) obtained during the TT from all seven test subjects using the developed prototype smart helmet.

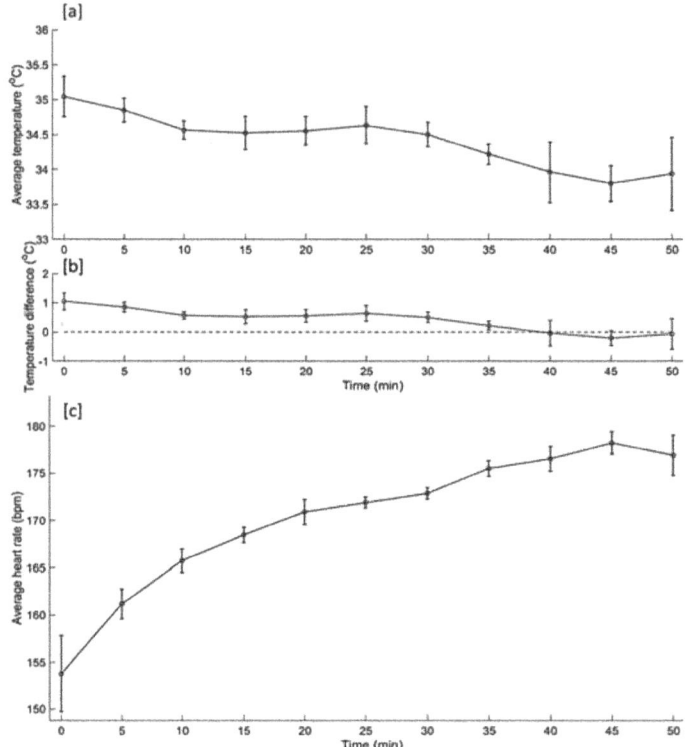

**Figure 10.** (**a**) Average temperature ($\overline{T}_h$) beneath the helmet, (**b**) average temperature difference ($\Delta T$) between the average temperature and the ambient air temperature and (**c**) average heart rate ($H_R$) obtained during the TT from all test subjects.

The developed offline liner regression model (3) was used to estimate the thermal comfort ($T_C$) of all seven test subjects based on the measurements acquired from the SmartHelmet prototype and for comparison with the thermal comfort subjective rating. The model was able to estimate the thermal comfort from all test subjects and revealed an average $R^2$ of 0.84 (±0.03). Model (3) was able to predict the cyclist's thermal comfort under the helmet and had a maximum MAPE of 10%. However, by retuning the model parameters using the data obtained from the TT experiment, the maximum MAPE was reduced to 7.8%.

The main advantage of the proposed model is that it is a conceptually simple yet very effective tool to explore linear relationships between a response variable (output) and a set of explanatory variables (input variables), which can be easily used for wearable technology such as the SmartHelmet. On the other hand, the disadvantage of such a model is the absence of the time component; in other words, the model is not able to explain the transient response of the output. Additionally, in practice, many factors can affect and change the relationship represented by the proposed model. These factors include helmet-related factors (e.g., helmet weight), other environmental conditions (e.g., wind direction) and personal-related factors, which were not included in the model (e.g., the surface area and contour of the cyclist's head). Hence, it is clear that such general models need to be adapted to new data (personal data) and different conditions for better performance. With the help of wearable sensing technologies

(SmartHelmet) and streaming modelling algorithms, an adaptive personalised model can be developed for real-time monitoring of a cyclist's head thermal comfort.

In the following subsection, we introduce the framework of online model adaptation and personalisation (streaming algorithm) based on the easily measured variables obtained from the wearable sensors impeded in the SmartHelmet.

### 3.4. Introduction of Online Personalisation and Adaptive Modelling Algorithm

Most of the available thermal sensation and comfort predictive models (e.g., [30–37]) are static models. That is, they predict the average vote of a large group of people based on, for example, the 7-point thermal sensation scale instead of individual thermal comfort, and they only describe the overall thermal sensation/comfort of multiple occupants in a shared thermal environment. To overcome the disadvantages of static models, adaptive thermal comfort models aim to provide insights and opportunities to personalise the thermal comfort prediction of individuals [38]. The idea behind adaptive models is that occupants and individuals are no longer regarded as passive recipients of the thermal environment, but rather, they play an active role in creating their own thermal preferences [39]. The suggested linear regression model, represented by (3), in the present paper is considered as a global model, also called an offline model [40,41], for an adaptive personalised model to assess and predict individual thermal comfort under a cyclist's helmet.

Figure 11 depicts the proposed steps for retuning and personalising the offline regression model (3). The suggested personalised adaptive tuning algorithm consists of the main components shown in Figure 11.

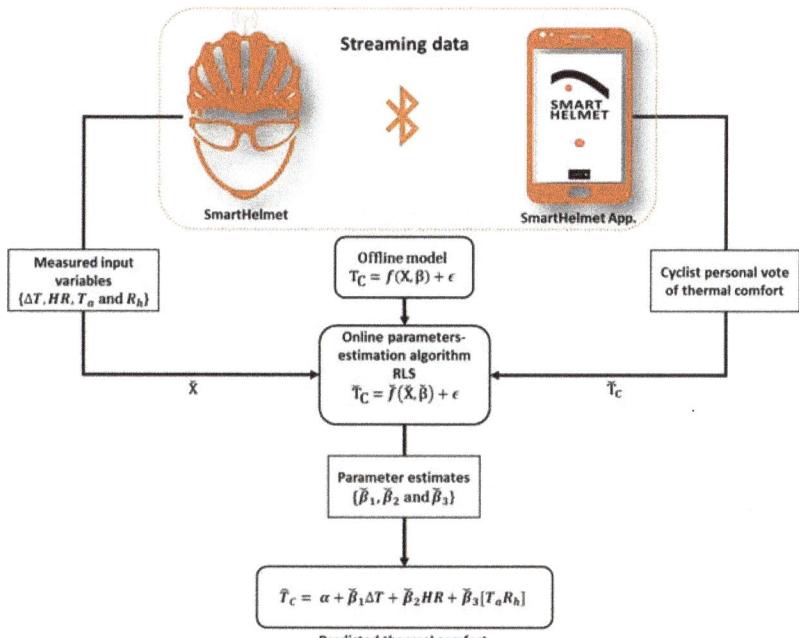

**Figure 11.** Schematic representation of the proposed online personalisation algorithm to predict thermal comfort under the helmet. The retuning and personalisation algorithm is based on data streaming obtained from the developed SmartHelmet prototype and the cyclist's personal vote of thermal comfort acquired from the developed SmartHelmet App. The streamed data is fed, together with the developed offline model, to an online parameter estimation algorithm based on a recursive least-squares (RLS) algorithm.

### 3.4.1. Offline Linear Regression Model

As mentioned earlier, the linear regression model (3), which was developed based on the data obtained from the 15 test subjects, is the offline base model for online prediction of personal under-helmet thermal comfort. The general form of the offline linear regression model (3) is as follows:

$$\mathbf{T_C} = \mathbf{X}\boldsymbol{\beta} + \boldsymbol{\epsilon} \tag{4}$$

and is subjected to $\mathbf{T_C} \in \mathbb{R}^{n \times 1}$ and $\mathbf{X} \in \mathbb{R}^{n \times 3}$, where $\mathbf{T_C}$ is the output vector ($n$ samples of thermal comfort votes); $\epsilon$ is the model residual vector, which consists of independent and Gaussian-distributed entries; and $\beta$ and $\mathbf{X}$ are the regression vector (of the size 3) and predictor matrix (of the size $n \times 3$), respectively, given by

$$\mathbf{X} = \begin{bmatrix} 1 & \Delta T_1 & H_{R1} & (T_a R_h)_1 \\ 1 & \Delta T_2 & H_{R2} & (T_a R_h)_2 \\ \vdots & \vdots & \vdots & \vdots \\ 1 & \Delta T_n & H_{Rn} & (T_a R_h)_n \end{bmatrix} \text{ and } \boldsymbol{\beta} = \begin{bmatrix} \alpha \\ \beta_1 \\ \beta_2 \\ \beta_3 \end{bmatrix}.$$

### 3.4.2. Streaming Data

The availability of real-time sensor data from the developed SmartHelmet prototype allows for streaming data, which is processed via an online algorithm (stream processing) to adapt the offline model [42]. The streaming data includes new $\check{n}$ samples of measured sensor data (new input matrix $\check{\mathbf{X}}$) acquired from the SmartHelmet sensors, and new personal thermal comfort votes (new output vector $\check{\mathbf{T}}_C$) acquired through an interactive query provided by the developed SmartHelmet App.

### 3.4.3. Online Parameter Estimation Algorithm

As explained earlier (Section 2.1.3), the general setting of regression analysis is to identify a relationship between a response variable ($Y$) and one or several explanatory variables (predictors) ($X$) by using a learning sample [43]. In a prediction framework, the main assumption for predicting $Y$ on a new sample of $X$ observations is that the regression model (with the general form $Y = f(X) + \epsilon$, where $\epsilon$ represents the model residuals) is still valid. Unfortunately, this assumption is not valid in the present case, where the thermal comfort of the individual cyclist is strongly dependent on many personal- and time-dependent factors [11]. Therefore, in this study, we adapted the original regression model (3) to a new sample (observations) by estimating a transformation [41,43] between the original regression function ($f(X)$) and the new one ($\check{f}(\check{X})$) while still using the same model variables and structure. Ordinary least squares (LS) is one of the most popular regression techniques, which was used here for parameter estimation of the developed offline model. However, for the online parameter estimation and in the presence of unknown parameter changes, its adaptive versions—the sliding or moving LS, recursive least squares (RLS) and recursive partial least squares (PLS)—are widely used [41,44,45].

In the present paper, the RLS algorithm is suggested for online personalisation and adaptive modelling of under-helmet thermal comfort. The suggested RLS algorithm has the advantage of being simple and computationally efficient for wearable and adaptive sensing, which was the case in the present work. In the RLS algorithm, the new regression vector $\check{\beta}$, as in Equation (4), can be estimated recursively as follows [25,46,47]:

$$\mathbf{P}_{n+1} = \mathbf{P}_n - \frac{\mathbf{P_n}(\mathbf{X}_{n+1})^T \mathbf{X}_{n+1} \mathbf{P}_n}{1 + \mathbf{X}_{n+1} \mathbf{P}_n (\mathbf{X}_{n+1})^T}, \tag{5}$$

$$\check{\beta}_{n+1} = \check{\beta}_n + \mathbf{P}_{n+1}(\mathbf{X}_{n+1})^T \left( \check{T}_{C_{n+1}} - \mathbf{X}_{n+1} \check{\beta}_n \right) \tag{6}$$

where $\mathbf{P}_n = \left(\mathbf{X}_n^T \mathbf{X}_n\right)^{-1}$. This recursive algorithm is efficient for cases where the regression vector $\check{\beta}$ is a function of time (time varying). However, in the case of adaptive modelling with streaming data, due to the arrival of new samples, the influence of new observations decreases gradually and the ability to track the changes in $\check{\beta}$ will be lost. Hence, to mitigate this, the widely used and popular forgetting factor approach [48] is proposed in this paper. The approach of forgetting here is based on gradually discarding older data in favour of more recent information. In the least-squares method, forgetting can be viewed as giving less weight to older data and more weight to recent data [48,49]. Hence, the forgetting factor, $\lambda$, was introduced to (5) as follows [41]:

$$\mathbf{P}_{n+1} = \frac{1}{\lambda}\left(\mathbf{P}_n - \frac{\mathbf{P}_n(\mathbf{X}_{n+1})^T \mathbf{X}_{n+1} \mathbf{P}_n}{\lambda + \mathbf{X}_{n+1} \mathbf{P}_n (\mathbf{X}_{n+1})^T}\right) \quad (7)$$

where $\lambda \in (0, 1]$. The forgettiing factor $\lambda$ operates as a weight, which diminishes for more remote data and expands for more recent data [48,49]. The main difference here between (5) and (7) is that in conventional RLS (5), the covariance vanishes to zero with time, losing its capability to keep track of changes in the regression vector $\check{\beta}$. In (7), however, the covariance matrix is divided by $0 \leq \lambda < 1$ at each update. This slows down the fading out of the covariance matrix [49].

## 4. Conclusions

In the present work, we aimed to develop a general model approach to predict a cyclist's head thermal comfort using nonintrusive and easily measured variables, which can be measured using impeded sensors in a bicycle helmet. During the first experimental stage, 15 participants were exposed to different levels of mechanical activity, ambient temperatures, helmet thermal resistance and wind velocities in order to develop a general model to predict a cyclist's head thermal comfort. The results showed that ambient temperature, average air temperature under the helmet, cyclist heart rate, cyclist mechanical work and helmet thermal resistance significantly influenced the cyclist's head thermal comfort. A reduced-order general linear regression model with three input variables, namely, temperature difference between ambient temperature and average under-helmet temperature, cyclist's heart rate and the interaction between ambient temperature and helmet thermal resistance, was the most suitable to predict the cyclist's head thermal comfort, showing a maximum MAPE of 8.4%. The developed general model structure was based on easily measured variables that can be measured continuously using impeded sensors in the bicycle helmet but is still of reduced order and low computational cost, which is suitable for streaming and adaptive modelling. Based on the selected model variables, a smart helmet prototype (SmartHelmet) was developed using impeded sensing technology as a proof of concept. The developed general model was validated using the developed SmartHelmet prototype. During the validation experimental phase, seven well-trained male cyclists were exposed to a hot (34 °C and 56% relative humidity) environment and completed a 30 km cycling TT inside an environmental chamber. The validation results showed that the developed general model was able to predict the thermal comfort of the seven participants and had a maximum MAPE of 10%. By retuning the model parameters, the maximum MAPE decreased to 7.8%. Finally, we introduced a calculation framework of an adaptive personalised model based on the developed general model to predict a cyclist's head thermal comfort based on streaming data from the SmartHelmet prototype.

**Author Contributions:** Conceptualisation, A.Y., J.-M.A. and G.D.B.; methodology, A.Y., J.C. and K.M.; software, A.Y., P.G. and K.M.; validation, A.Y., J.C. and K.M.; formal analysis, A.Y., J.C. and K.M.; investigation, A.Y., J.C. and K.M.; resources, P.G. and G.D.B and A.F.; data curation, A.Y., J.C. and K.M.; writing—original draft preparation, A.Y., J.C.; writing—review and editing, A.Y., J.-M.A., G.D.B, A.F. and T.M.; visualisation, A.Y. and J.C.; supervision, J.-M.A. and A.Y.; project administration, T.M. and J.-M.A.; funding acquisition, T.M. and J.-M.A.

**Funding:** Marie Skłodowska-Curie grant agreement no. 645770.

**Acknowledgments:** We acknowledge the support from the European Union's Horizon 2020 research and innovation programme under the Marie Skłodowska-Curie grant agreement no. 645770.

**Conflicts of Interest:** The authors declare no conflict of interest.

## References

1. Titze, S.; Bauman, A.; De Geus, B.; Krenn, P.; Kohlberger, T.; Reger-Nash, B.; Oja, P. Health benefits of cycling: A systematic review. *Scand. J. Med. Sci. Sports* **2011**, *21*, 496–509.
2. Zentner, J.; Franken, H.; Löbbecke, G. Head injuries from bicycle accidents. *Clin. Neurol. Neurosurg.* **1996**, *98*, 281–285. [CrossRef]
3. Elvik, R. Publication bias and time-trend bias in meta-analysis of bicycle helmet efficacy: A re-analysis of Attewell, Glase and McFadden, 2001. *Accid. Anal. Prev.* **2011**, *43*, 1245–1251. [CrossRef] [PubMed]
4. Action, A.C.; Hope, T.U. *Final Report of Working Group 2: Traffic Psychology*; COST Action TU1101/HOPE: Brussels, Belgium, 2015.
5. Finnoff, J.T.; Laskowski, E.R.; Altman, K.L.; Diehl, N.N. Barriers to Bicycle Helmet Use. *Pediatrics* **2001**, *108*, 2–10. [CrossRef] [PubMed]
6. Bogerd, C.P.; Aerts, J.M.; Annaheim, S.; Bröde, P.; De Bruyne, G.; Flouris, A.D.; Kuklane, K.; Mayor, T.S.; Rossi, R.M. A review on ergonomics of headgear: Thermal effects. *Int. J. Ind. Ergon.* **2015**, *45*, 1–12. [CrossRef]
7. Underwood, L.; Vircondelet, C.; Jermy, M. Thermal comfort and drag of a streamlined cycling helmet as a function of ventilation hole placement. *Proc. Inst. Mech. Eng. Part P J. Sports Eng. Technol.* **2018**, *232*, 15–21. [CrossRef]
8. Mayor, T.S.; Couto, S.; Psikuta, A.; Rossi, R.M. Advanced modelling of the transport phenomena across horizontal clothing microclimates with natural convection. *Int. J. Biometeorol.* **2015**, *59*, 1875–1889. [CrossRef] [PubMed]
9. ASHRAE. *ASHRAE Standard 55*; American Society of Heating, Refrigerating and Air-Conditioning Engineers, Inc.: Atlanta, GA, USA, 2017.
10. Gagge, A.P.; Stolwijk, J.A.J.; Hardy, J.D. Comfort and thermal sensations and associated physiological responses at various ambient temperatures. *Environ. Res.* **1967**, *1*, 1–20. [CrossRef]
11. Kenneth, C. *Human Thermal Environments: The Effects of Hot, Moderate, and Cold Environments on Human Health, Comfort, and Performance*, 3rd ed.; CRC Press: Boca Raton, FL, USA, 2014.
12. Fanger, P.O. *Thermal Comfort: Analysis and Applications in Environmental Engineering*, 1st ed.; Danish Technical Press: Lyngby, Denmark, 1970.
13. Enescu, D. Models and Indicators to Assess Thermal Sensation Under Steady-state and Transient Conditions. *Energies* **2019**, *12*, 841. [CrossRef]
14. Koelblen, B.; Psikuta, A.; Bogdan, A.; Annaheim, S.; Rossi, R.M. Thermal sensation models: A systematic comparison. *Indoor Air* **2017**, *27*, 680–689. [CrossRef]
15. Rugh, J.P.; Farrington, R.B.; Bharathan, D.; Vlahinos, A.; Burke, R.; Huizenga, C.; Zhang, H. Predicting human thermal comfort in a transient nonuniform thermal environment. *Eur. J. Appl. Physiol.* **2004**, *92*, 721–727. [CrossRef]
16. Havenith, G.; Fiala, D. Thermal Indices and Thermophysiological Modeling for Heat Stress. *Compr. Physiol.* **2015**, *6*, 255–302.
17. Youssef, A.; Truyen, P.; Brode, P.; Fiala, D.; Aerts, J.M. Towards Real-Time Model-Based Monitoring and Adoptive Controlling of Indoor Thermal Comfort. In Proceedings of the Ventilating Healthy Low-Energy Buildings, Nottingham, UK, 13–14 September 2017.
18. De Bruyne, G.; Aerts, J.M.; Sloten, J.V.; Goffin, J.; Verpoest, I.; Berckmans, D. Quantification of local ventilation efficiency under bicycle helmets. *Int. J. Ind. Ergon.* **2012**, *42*, 278–286. [CrossRef]
19. Gore, C.J. *Physiological Tests for Elite Athletes Australian Sports Commmission*; Human Kinetics: Champaign, IL, USA, 2000.
20. Biochemistry, B.B.; Science, S. The Concept of Maximal Lactate Steady State. *Sports Med.* **2003**, *33*, 407–426.

21. Beneke, R. Methodological aspects of maximal lactate steady state-implications for performance testing. *Eur. J. Appl. Physiol.* **2003**, *89*, 95–99. [CrossRef]
22. Sibernagl, S. *Atlas van de Fysiologie*; SESAM/HBuitgevers: Baarn, The Netherlands, 2008.
23. Fitts, R.H. Cellular mechanisms of muscle fatigue. *Physiol. Rev.* **1994**, *74*, 49–94. [CrossRef]
24. Mukunthan, S.; Vleugels, J.; Huysmans, T.; de Bruyne, G. Latent Heat Loss of a Virtual Thermal Manikin for Evaluating the Thermal Performance of Bicycle Helmets. In *Advances in Human Factors in Simulation and Modeling*; Springer: Cham, Switzerland, 2019; pp. 66–78.
25. Soong, T.T. *Fundamentals of Probability and Statistics for Engineers*; Wiley: Hoboken, NJ, USA, 2004.
26. Borg, G.A. Psychophysical bases of perceived exertion. *Med. Sci. Sports Exerc.* **1982**, *14*, 377–381. [CrossRef]
27. Box, G.E.P.; Draper, N.R. *Empirical Model-Building and Response Surfaces*; John Wiley & Sons: Oxford, UK, 1987.
28. JMP®14. *JMP®14 Profilers*; Institute Inc.: Cary, NC, USA, 2018.
29. Zinoubi, B.; Zbidi, S.; Vandewalle, H.; Chamari, K.; Driss, T. Relationships between rating of perceived exertion, heart rate and blood lactate during continuous and alternated-intensity cycling exercises. *Biol. Sport* **2018**, *35*, 29–37. [CrossRef]
30. Takada, S.; Matsumoto, S.; Matsushita, T. Prediction of whole-body thermal sensation in the non-steady state based on skin temperature. *Build. Environ.* **2013**, *68*, 123–133. [CrossRef]
31. Fiala, D. *Dynamic Simulation of Human Heat Transfer and Thermal Comfort*; De Montfort University: Leicester, UK, 1998.
32. Lomas, K.J.; Fiala, D.; Stohrer, M. First principles modeling of thermal sensation responses in steady-state and transient conditions. *ASHRAE Trans.* **2003**, *109*, 179–186.
33. Zhang, H. *Human Thermal Sensation and Comfort in Transient and Non-Uniform Thermal Environments*; University of California: Berkeley, CA, USA, 2003.
34. Guan, Y.D.; Hosni, M.H.; Jones, B.W.; Gielda, T.P. Investigation of Human Thermal Comfort Under Highly Transient Conditions for Automotive Applications-Part 2: Thermal Sensation Modeling. *ASHRAE Trans.* **2003**, *109*, 898–907.
35. Guan, Y.D.; Hosni, M.H.; Jones, B.W.; Gielda, T.P. Investigation of Human Thermal Comfort Under Highly Transient Conditions for Automotive Applications-Part 1: Experimental Design and Human Subject Testing Implementation. *ASHRAE Trans.* **2003**, *109*, 885–897.
36. Nilsson, H.O.; Holmer, I. Comfort climate evaluation with thermal manikin methods and computer simulation models. *Indoor Air* **2003**, *13*, 28–37. [CrossRef]
37. Kingma, B.R.M.; Schellen, L.; Frijns, A.J.H.; Lichtenbelt, W.D.V. Thermal sensation: A mathematical model based on neurophysiology. *Indoor Air* **2012**, *22*, 253–262. [CrossRef]
38. Lu, S.; Wang, W.; Wang, S.; Hameen, E.C. Thermal Comfort-Based Personalized Models with Non-Intrusive Sensing Technique in Office Buildings. *Appl. Sci.* **2019**, *9*, 1768. [CrossRef]
39. De Dear, R.; Brager, G.S. Developing an adaptive model of thermal comfort and preference. *ASHRAE Trans.* **1998**, *104*, 145–167.
40. Kadlec, P.; Grbić, R.; Gabrys, B. Review of adaptation mechanisms for data-driven soft sensors. *Comput. Chem. Eng.* **2011**, *35*, 1–24. [CrossRef]
41. Sharma, S.; Khare, S.; Huang, B. Robust online algorithm for adaptive linear regression parameter estimation and prediction. *J. Chemom.* **2016**, *30*, 308–323. [CrossRef]
42. Zimmer, A.M.; Kurze, M.; Seidl, T. Adaptive Model Tree for Streaming Data. In Proceedings of the 2013 IEEE 13th International Conference on Data Mining, Dallas, TX, USA, 7–10 December 2013; pp. 1319–1324.
43. Bouveyron, C.; Jacques, J. Adaptive linear models for regression: Improving prediction when population has changed. *Pattern Recognit. Lett.* **2010**, *31*, 2237–2247. [CrossRef]
44. Jiang, J.; Zhang, Y. A revisit to block and recursive least squares for parameter estimation. *Comput. Electr. Eng.* **2004**, *30*, 403–416. [CrossRef]
45. Young, P.C. *Recursive Estimation and Time-Series Analysis*; Springer: Berlin, Germany, 2011.
46. Benesty, J.; Paleologu, C.; Gänsler, T.; Ciochină, S. *Recursive Least-Squares Algorithms*; Springer: Berlin, Germany, 2011; pp. 63–69.
47. Plackett, R.L. Some Theorems in Least Squares. *Biometrika* **1950**, *37*, 149. [CrossRef]

48. Johnson, C.R. *Lectures on Adaptive Parameter Estimation*; Prentice-Hall: Upper Saddle River, NJ, USA, 1988.
49. Vahidi, A.; Stefanopoulou, A.; Peng, H. Recursive least squares with forgetting for online estimation of vehicle mass and road grade: Theory and experiments. *Veh. Syst. Dyn.* **2005**, *43*, 31–55. [CrossRef]

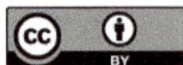
© 2019 by the authors. Licensee MDPI, Basel, Switzerland. This article is an open access article distributed under the terms and conditions of the Creative Commons Attribution (CC BY) license (http://creativecommons.org/licenses/by/4.0/).

*Article*

# Towards Online Personalized-Monitoring of Human Thermal Sensation Using Machine Learning Approach

Ali Youssef [1], Ahmed Youssef Ali Amer [1,2], Nicolás Caballero [1] and Jean-Marie Aerts [1,*]

[1] Department of Biosystems, Animal and Human Health Engineering Division, M3-BIORES: Measure, Model & Manage of Bioresponses Laboratory, KU Leuven, Kasteelpark Arenberg 30, 3001 Heverlee, Belgium

[2] Electrical Engineering (ESAT) TC, Group T Leuven Campus, Andreas Vesaliusstraat 13 - Box 2600, 3000 Leuven, Belgium

* Correspondence: jean-marie.aerts@kuleuven.be

Received: 20 July 2019; Accepted: 2 August 2019; Published: 12 August 2019

**Abstract:** Thermal comfort and sensation are important aspects of building design and indoor climate control, as modern man spends most of the day indoors. Conventional indoor climate design and control approaches are based on static thermal comfort/sensation models that view the building occupants as passive recipients of their thermal environment. To overcome the disadvantages of static models, adaptive thermal comfort models aim to provide opportunity for personalized climate control and thermal comfort enhancement. Recent advances in wearable technologies contributed to new possibilities in controlling and monitoring health conditions and human wellbeing in daily life. The generated streaming data generated from wearable sensors are providing a unique opportunity to develop a real-time monitor of an individual's thermal state. The main goal of this work is to introduce a personalized adaptive model to predict individual's thermal sensation based on non-intrusive and easily measured variables, which could be obtained from already available wearable sensors. In this paper, a personalized classification model for individual thermal sensation with a reduced-dimension input-space, including 12 features extracted from easily measured variables, which are obtained from wearable sensors, was developed using least-squares support vector machine algorithm. The developed classification model predicted the individual's thermal sensation with an overall average accuracy of 86%. Additionally, we introduced the main framework of streaming algorithm for personalized classification model to predict an individual's thermal sensation based on streaming data obtained from wearable sensors.

**Keywords:** thermal sensation; adaptive model; personalized model; machine leaning; support-vector-machine; adaptive control; streaming algorithm

## 1. Introduction

Thermal comfort (TC) is an ergonomic aspect determining satisfaction with the surrounding environment and is defined as 'that condition of mind which expresses satisfaction with the thermal environment and is assessed by subjective evaluation' [1]. The effect of thermal environments on occupants might also be assessed in terms of thermal sensation (TS), which can be defined as 'a conscious feeling commonly graded into the categories cold, cool, slightly cool, neutral, slightly warm, warm, and hot' [1]. Thermal sensation and thermal comfort are both subjective judgements, however, thermal sensation is related to the perception of one's thermal state, and thermal comfort is related to the evaluation of this perception [2]. In other words, TS expresses the perception of the occupants, while TC assesses this perception, taking into account physiological and psychological factors [3].

The assessment of thermal sensation has been regarded as more reliable and as such is often used to estimate thermal comfort [4].

Thermal sensation is the result of the body "psycho-physical reaction" to certain thermal stimuli related to indoor conditions [5]. Human thermal sensation mainly depends on the human body temperature (core body temperature), which is a function of sets of comfort factors [5,6]. These comfort factors include indoor environmental factors, such as mean air temperature around the body, relative air velocity around the body, humidity, and mean radiant temperature of the environment to the body [6]. Additionally, some personal (individual-related) factors, namely metabolic rate or internal heat production in the body, which vary with the activity level and clothing thermo-physical properties (such as clothing insulation and vapor clothing resistance), are included. It should be mentioned that the individual thermal perception is deepening, as well, on psychological factors, expectations and short/long-term experience, which directly affect individuals' perceptions, time of exposure, perceived control, and environmental stimulation [7]. The most considered way to have an accurate assessment of TS is to ask the individuals directly about their thermal sensation perception [5,6]. The thermal-sensation-vote (TSV) is one of the most used concepts to address the opinion of individuals concerning TS. That is, individuals express their vote to rate their TS when they are exposed to given thermal conditions, by using a scale from cold to hot, with a predefined number of points.

Thermal sensation mathematical models are developed in order to overcome the difficulties of direct enquiry of subjects. The development of such models is mostly dependent on statistical approaches by correlating experimental conditions (i.e., environmental and personal variables) data to thermal sensation votes obtained from human subjects [4,6]. The recent intensive review work of Enescu (2019), explored the most important contributions to model and predict thermal sensation (TS) under both steady-state and transient conditions. It is shown that the most used models to assess TS of the human body with respect to the environment have been developed starting from Fanger's predicted-mean-vote (PMV) empirical model [3] for steady-state conditions and from the Gagge model [8] for transient conditions. Since then, numurus models are developed to assess and predict TS (e.g., [9–16]). Most of the aforementioned models (e.g., PMV) are static in the sense that they predict the average vote of a large group of people based on the seven-point thermal sensation scale, instead of individual thermal comfort, they only describe the overall thermal sensation of multiple occupants in a shared thermal environment. To overcome the disadvantages of static models, adaptive thermal comfort models aim to provide insights in increasing opportunities for personal and responsive control, thermal comfort enhancement, energy consumption reduction and climatically responsive and environmentally responsible building design [17,18]. The idea behind adaptive models is that occupants and individuals are no longer regarded as passive recipients of the thermal environment but rather, play an active role in creating their own thermal preferences [18]. Many adaptive thermal comfort models are developed based on regression analysis (e.g., [18–20]).

Besides regression analysis, thermal sensation prediction can also be seen as a classification problem where various classification algorithms can be implemented [17]. In their work [21], Lee et al., proposed a method for learning personalized thermal preference profiles by formulating a combined classification and inference problem with 5-cluster models. Moreover, the thermal preference of a new user is inferred by a mixture of sub-models for each cluster, where clusters are used to group occupants with similar thermal preferences.

Recently, a number of research works (e.g., [22–26] have demonstrated the possibility of using machine learning techniques, such as support vector machine (SVM), to assess and predict human thermal sensation. It can be concluded, based on the published work (see the recent literature review [17] by Lu et al.), that classification-based models have performed as well as regression models.

Different related works investigated the problem of thermal sensation and comfort prediction via machine learning algorithms. Ghahramani et al. [27] applied the hidden Markov model (HMM) technique to the thermal comfort prediction problem with three levels of thermal comfort. There is a main issue in the used dataset in this study is the class imbalance, which is not tackled by the proposed methodology. In their study, Ghahramani et al. did not discuss the problem of streaming analytics and model personalisation.

In order to develop personalized models, Jiang et al. [28] applied support vector machines classifiers to the personal data of each subject to predict the thermal sensation level for the same subject. The obtained results are promising, however, their approach requires a sufficient number of data-points to obtain an acceptable performance, which is not applicable to our dataset (9 data-points per subject).

The very recent study of Lu et al. [17] proposed a personalized model, however, the study strictly investigated two subjects and developed a dedicated model for each subject.

In comparison with many relevant studies, our study is tackling several challenges at the same time. These issues are feature reduction, streaming, and online modeling compatibility and model personalization. The latter issue is tackled in a novel way by considering both personal and nonpersonal data relying on the similarity either inter or intra subjects. In general, it can be stated that it is a real modeling challenge to correlate the physiological variables with information concerning global and local sensation [5].

Recent advances in mobile technologies in healthcare, in particular, wearable technologies (m-health) and smart clothing, have positively contributed to new possibilities in controlling and monitoring health conditions and human wellbeing in daily life applications. The wearable sensing technologies and their generated streaming data are providing a unique opportunity to understand the user's behaviour and to predict future needs [29]. The generated streaming data is unique due to the personal nature of the wearable devices. However, the generated streaming data forms a challenge related to the need for personalized adaptive models that can handle newly arrived personal data.

The main goal of this work is to introduce a personalized adaptive modeling algorithm to predict an individual's thermal sensation based on non-intrusive and easily measured variables, which could be obtained from already available wearable sensors.

## 2. Methods

### 2.1. Data Processing and Classification

Thermal sensation prediction based on wearable sensors can be considered as a classification machine learning problem, the input of which is the set of extracted features from the measured variables and the output is the subjects' feedback with the standard thermal sensation labels. Several machine learning techniques can be used for such a problem. Support vector machines (SVMs) is one of the efficient classification techniques used in different relevant studies [21–23,25,26]. In this study, the least squares support vector machine (LS-SVM) is proposed to be used for general models as it is as powerful as standard SVMs, but, it has less computational cost [30]. Most, if not all, relevant studies of thermal sensation prediction rely on global general models. Global models are models that are trained using the whole available training dataset with a uniform weight (i.e., all training points are equally contributing to the training process). However, global models are not that efficient for online classification and streaming analytics applications in which a stream of new data is collected from subjects via wearable technology, especially when aiming at personalized models. Hence, for this purpose, we suggest a localized version of LS-SVM, namely K-Nearest Neighbours (KNN)-LS-SVM [31] to be compatible with the wearable sensors for online and streaming analytics.

The classification problem of thermal sensation is a multiclass classification problem, the input variables of this problem from which features are extracted are: aural temperature $T_{er}$, average skin temperature $\overline{T}_{sk} = \frac{1}{3}[T_{scap} + T_{ch} + T_{arm}]$, ambient temperature $T_a$, chest skin temperature $T_{ch}$, heart rate $H_r$, average heat flux from the skin $\overline{q}_{sk}$, temperature gradient between core and skin $\Delta T_{sk} = T_{er} - \overline{T}_{sk}$, age, gender, body mass index $BMI$, metabolic rate $M_r$. As some variables are time measurements of the different parameters, the process of feature extraction is applied to a specified time window from the recordings, namely the last five minutes preceding the sensation labeling by the test subjects. The extracted features from time-variant variables are: minimum (*min*), maximum (*max*), variance (*var*), energy, time-derivate ($\frac{d}{dt}$), root mean square (*rms*). Target labels are the seven classes of the standard thermal comfort sensation scores: *Cold* (-3), *Cool* (-2), *Slightly Cool* (-1), *Neutral* (0), *Slightly Warm* (1), *Warm* (2), and *Hot* (3).

### 2.1.1. Support Vector Machines (SVMs)

SVMs are originally presented as binary classifiers, that assign each data instance $X \in \mathbb{R}^d$ to one of two classes described by a class label $y \in \{-1, 1\}$ based on the decision boundary that maximizes the margin $2/\|\mathbf{w}\|_2$ between the two classes. Generally, a feature map $\phi : \mathbb{R}^d \Rightarrow \mathbb{R}^p$ is used to transform the geometric boundary between the two classes to a linear boundary $L : \mathbf{w}^T \varphi(x) + b = 0$ in feature space, for some weight vector $\mathbf{w} \in \mathbb{R}^{p \times 1}$ and $b \in \mathbb{R}$. The class of each instance can then be found by $y = sign(\mathbf{w}^T \varphi(x) + b)$, where *sign* refers to the sign function [30].

The estimation of the boundary $L$ is performed based on a set of training examples $x_i$ ($1 \le i \le N$) with corresponding class labels $y_i \in \{-1, 1\}$. An optimal boundary is found by maximizing the margin that is defined as the smallest distances between $L$ and any of the training instances. In particular, one is interested in constants $\mathbf{w}$ and $b$ that minimize a loss-function:

$$\min_{\mathbf{w},\, b;\, \xi} \frac{1}{2} \mathbf{w}^T \mathbf{w} + C \sum_{i=1}^{N} \xi_i \quad (1)$$

and are subject to:

$$y_i\left(\mathbf{w}^T \varphi(xi) + b\right) \ge 1 - \xi_i \text{ and } \xi_i \ge 0,\, i = 1, 2, \ldots, N. \quad (2)$$

The constant $C$ denotes the penalty term that is used to penalize misclassification through the slack variables $\xi_i$ in the optimization process.

The so-called kernel-trick avoids the explicit introduction of a feature map $\phi$ and implicitly allows for the use of feature spaces of infinite dimensionality. A commonly used kernel is given by the Gaussian kernel:

$$k(x_i, x_j) = exp\left(\frac{\|x_i - x_j\|^2}{2\sigma^2}\right) \quad (3)$$

where $\sigma$ denotes the kernel bandwidth. Both $\sigma$ and $C$ can be optimized as hyper-parameters in a cross-validation experiment.

### 2.1.2. Least Squares Support Vector Machine (LS-SVM)

LS-SVMs are obtained by using a least-squares error loss function [30]:

$$\min_{\mathbf{w},\, b;\, e} \frac{1}{2} \mathbf{w}^T \mathbf{w} + \gamma \sum_{i=1}^{N} e_i^2 \quad (4)$$

such that

$$y_i\left(\mathbf{w}^T \varphi(x_i) + b\right) \ge 1 - e_i \text{ and } e_i \ge 0,\, i = 1, 2, \ldots, N. \quad (5)$$

This optimization procedure introduces errors $e_i$ such that $1-e_i$ is proportional to the signed distance of $x_i$ from the decision boundary and $\gamma$ represents the regularization constant. In fact, the non-negative slack variable constraint is removed and the solution of the optimization problem can be obtained by a set of linear equations, reducing computational effort [30].

### 2.1.3. KNN-LS-SVM

While global SVMs consider the same weight for all training instances in the optimization process, local learning approaches allow for training samples near a test point to be more influential than others. Localized approaches of SVMs [31] are based on weighting functions $\lambda(x_s, x_i)$ that express the similarity between the features vectors of the $i^{th}$ data point $x_i$ and the test instance $x_s$. For an LS-SVM, this leads to the following cost function:

$$\min_{w, b; e} \frac{1}{2} w^T w + \gamma \sum_{i=1}^{N} \lambda(x_s, x_i) e_i^2 \qquad (6)$$

such that

$$y_i\left(w^T \varphi(x_i) + b\right) \geq 1 - e_i \text{ and } e_i \geq 0, \ i = 1, 2, \ldots, N. \qquad (7)$$

For KNN-LS-SVM a binary valued similarity criterion:

$$\lambda(x_s, x_i) = \begin{cases} 1 \text{ if } \|\varphi(x_s) - \varphi(x_i)\|^2 \leq r_s \\ 0 \text{ otherwise} \end{cases} \qquad (8)$$

where $r_s$ is the $K^{th}$ smallest distance among $\{\|\varphi(x_s) - \varphi(x_i)\|; 1 \leq j \leq N\}$. This formulation leads to the hybrid KNN-LS-SVM method [31]. In practice, implementing the hybrid classifier of KNN-LS-SVM, as shown in Figure 1, starts with receiving an unlabelled new test point $x_s$ and finding the nearest $K$ points from the training set in the feature space. Based on the nearest $K$ points, an LS-SVM model is trained only with the new subset, hence, for each test point a dedicated model is trained. The advantage of this localized approach is that it can enhance the classification performance in case of class imbalance, in addition to the computational and temporal efficiency especially for online modelling and streaming analytics. For more detail concerning localized learning, reference [31] includes a detailed explanation of the algorithms.

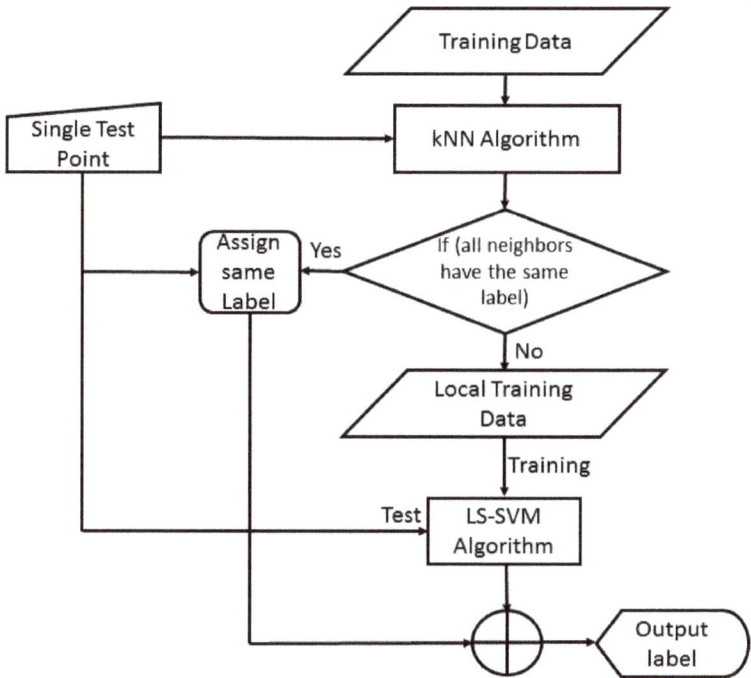

**Figure 1.** A flow chart illustrating the algorithm of K-Nearest Neighbours Least Squares Support Vector Machines (KNN-LS-SVM) classifier.

## 2.2. Experiments and Experimental Setup

### 2.2.1. Test Subjects

In total 25 healthy participants (6 females and 19 males), between the age of 25 and 35 (average age 26 ± 4.2) years, with average weight and height of 70.90 (± 12.70) kg and 1.74 (± 0.10) m, respectively, volunteered to perform the aforementioned experimental protocol. Detailed physical information about the test subjects is shown in Table 1.

Table 1. General physical information of the participants (test subjects).

| Subject | Gender | Height (cm) | Weight (kg) | Age (year) |
| --- | --- | --- | --- | --- |
| P1 | M | 1.69 | 59 | 23 |
| P2 | M | 1.77 | 75 | 20 |
| P3 | M | 1.82 | 73 | 29 |
| P4 | F | 1.61 | 53 | 31 |
| P5 | M | 1.86 | 88 | 21 |
| P6 | F | 1.57 | 50 | 22 |
| P7 | M | 1.73 | 86 | 33 |
| P8 | M | 1.81 | 67 | 21 |
| P9 | M | 1.86 | 92 | 36 |
| P10 | M | 1.65 | 62 | 31 |
| P11 | F | 1.7 | 61 | 23 |
| P12 | M | 1.86 | 80 | 23 |
| P13 | M | 1.82 | 86 | 27 |
| P14 | F | 1.6 | 51 | 22 |
| P15 | M | 1.7 | 58 | 29 |
| P16 | M | 1.75 | 74 | 26 |
| P17 | F | 1.68 | 76 | 26 |
| P18 | M | 1.8 | 74 | 29 |
| P19 | M | 1.78 | 79 | 29 |
| P20 | M | 1.83 | 81 | 22 |
| P21 | M | 1.78 | 78 | 28 |
| P22 | M | 1.81 | 69 | 22 |
| P23 | F | 1.57 | 49 | 26 |
| P24 | M | 1.75 | 68 | 24 |
| P25 | M | 1.78 | 83 | 28 |

### 2.2.2. Climate Chambers

During the course of this study, three (Rooms A, B and C) climate-controlled chambers designed and built to investigate the dynamic mental and physiological responses of humans to specific indoor climate conditions were used. Figure 2 shows a photographic picture of the three climate rooms, namely, A, B and C. The Body and Mind Rooms are experimental facilities at the M3-BIORES laboratory (Division of Animal and Human Health Engineering, KU Leuven). The three rooms are dimensionally identical; however, each room is designed to provide different ranges of climate conditions as shown in Table 2.

Table 2. Different temperature and relative humidity ranges that can be provided by the different Body and Mind (A, B and C).

| Room | Air Temperature Range (°C) | Relative Humidity Range (%) |
| --- | --- | --- |
| A | +23–+37 | 50–80 |
| B | +10–+25 | 50–80 |
| C | −5–+10 | 40–60 |

The three rooms are equipped with axial fans to simulate wind velocities between 2.5 and 50 km h$^{-1}$.

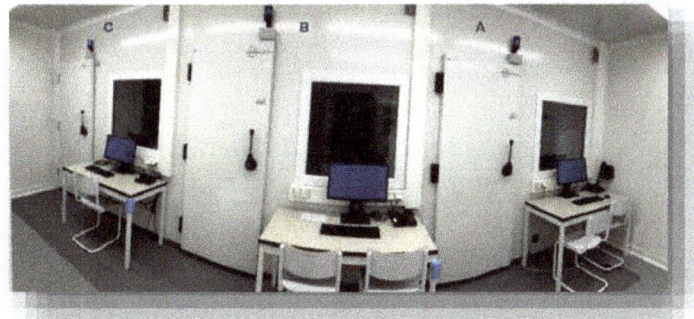

**Figure 2.** Photographic picture of the three climate-controlled rooms (from right to left, A–C).

2.2.3. Measurements and Gold Standards

During the course of the experiments, participants' heart rate $H_R$, metabolic rate $M_r$, average skin temperature $T_{sk}$, heat flux $q_{sk}$ between the skin and the ambient air, core body temperature $T_c$ represented by the aural temperature $T_{er}$ were measured continuously. The heart rate of each participants was monitored with a sampling rate of 128 Hz using the Polar H7 ECG strap that is placed under the chest. The metabolic rate as metabolic equivalent tasks (METs) of each participant was calculated based on indirect calorimetry using MetaMAX 3B spiroergometer sensor. The average skin temperature was calculated based on measurements from three body-places, namely, scapula $T_{scap}$, chest $T_{ch}$ and arm $T_{arm}$ (Figure 3). The skin temperature measurements were performed using one Shimmer temperature sensor and two gSKIN® bodyTEMP patches. Two heat flux gSKIN® patches were placed on both the chest and the left arm (Figure 3). The skin temperatures and heat flux measurements were acquired at sampling frequency of 1 Hz. Core body temperature was estimated based on aural temperature measure measurements, which was performed using in-ear wireless (Bluetooth) temperature sensors (Cosinuss One) with a sampling rate if 1 Hz. At the end of each applied temperature level during the course of both experimental phases, a thermal sensation questionnaire, based on ASHRAE 7-poins thermal scale, was performed for each test subject.

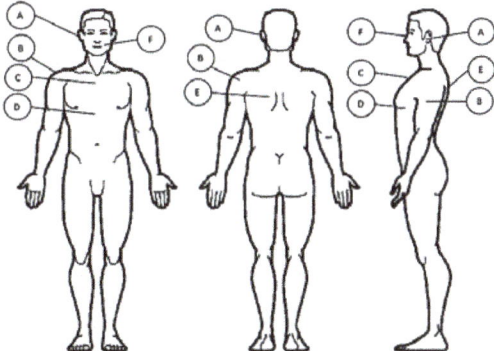

**Figure 3.** Sensor placement. (**A**) Ear channel for aural temperature measurement via the Cosinuss One, (**B**) upper arm where skin temperature and heat flux are measured with the gSKIN patch, (**C**) middle upper chest where skin temperature and heat flux are measured with the gSKIN patch, (**D**) lower chest where heart rate is measured with the Polar H7, (**E**) Scapula where skin temperature is measured with the shimmer, (**F**) mouth and nose where metabolic rate is measured via the MetaMAX-3B spiroergometer sensor.

### 2.2.4. Experimental Protocol

The experimental protocol used in the present study was designed in such way to investigate the subjects' thermal and physiological responses to three different temperature (*low, normal* and *high*) under two levels of physical activities (*low* and *high*).

The three predefined temperatures (*low* = 5 °C, *normal* = 24 °C and *high* = 37 °C) were chosen based on the *thermal-comfort-chart* of the ASHRAE-55 [32] and the effects on health according to the Wind Chill Chart for cold exposure (National Weather Service of the US) and for hot temperatures exposure according to [33]. The conducted experiments were consisted of two phases (Figure 4, upper graph), namely, low activity and high activity phases. During the first experimental phase, low activity phase, the test subjects (while being seated = low activity) were exposed, during 55 minutes, to three levels of temperatures in the following order: normal, low, high and normal again (Figure 4). During the high activity phase, the test subjects was exposed to a 15 minutes of light physical stress (80W of cycling on a fastened racing bicycle). During the course (75 minutes) of the active phase, each test subject was exposed to the predefined three temperature levels (Figure 4, lower graph). During each temperature level, starting from the normal level (24 °C), the test subjects are performed 15 minutes of cycling (with 80 W power) and followed 4 minutes of resting (seated). During the course of conducted experiments, the clothing insulation factor (*Col*) was kept constant at *Col* = 0.34, which accounted for a cotton short and t-shirt as a standard clothing for all test subjects. The experimental protocol was approved by the SMEC (Sociaal-Maatschappelijke Ethische Comissie), on the 16 January 2019 with number G-2018 12 1464.

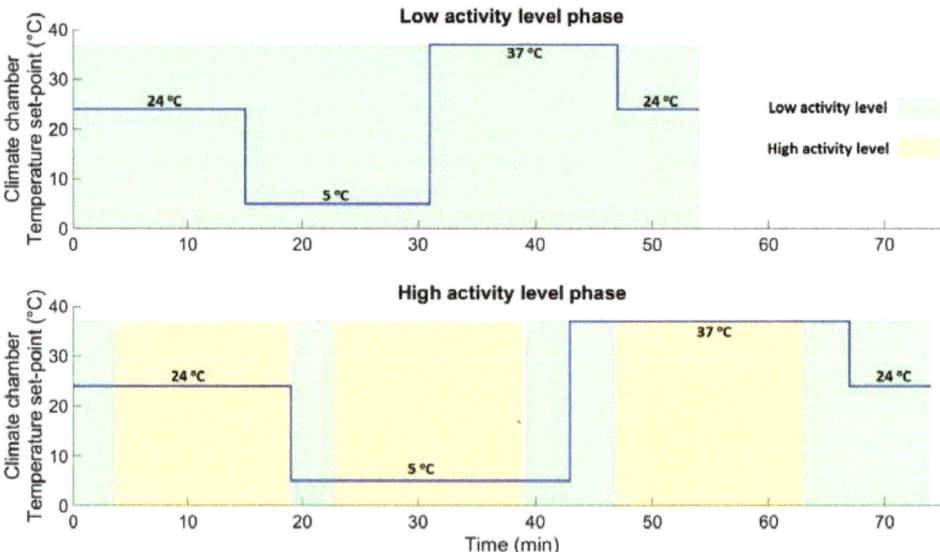

**Figure 4.** Plots showing the climate chambers' set-point temperatures programmed during the 55 min low activity phase (**upper graph**) and the 75 min high activity phase (**lower graph**).

## 3. Results and Discussions

### 3.1. General Classification Models

In this section, classification models are developed 'globally', in other words the classification models are trained using all available training dataset with the same weight (i.e., all training data-points are contributing equally to the training process). The whole dataset (*N*-subjects) are divided, based on leave-one-subject-out approach (LOSO), into $N - 1$ subjects for training and 1 subject for testing.

### 3.1.1. Developing General Model Using All Extracted Features for 7-Classes Problem (Model I)

Initially, in this stage of developing a general classification model to predict thermal sensation, in total 54 features have been used to form the input space of the classification model for the 7-classes classification problem. The extracted features are meant to be simple and basic features that are not computationally expensive and represent the basic characteristics of segmented time windows. A feature space includes the mean value of the measured input variables, namely, $T_{er}$, $H_R$, $\bar{q}_{sk}$, $\Delta \bar{T}$ and $M_r$. Additionally, other features are extracted by computing the variance, min, max, root mean squares (RMS), energy ($E = \frac{1}{N}\sum_{n=1}^{N} x^2(n)$, where $N$ is the number of samples of variable $x$) and first derivative ($\frac{dx}{dt}$) of the aforementioned measured variables as shown in Table 3. The age, gender, body-mass-index (BMI) and ambient temperature ($T_\infty$) are also included in the feature spaces.

The output confusion matrix is computed for each subject based on LOSO testing approach. The averaged normalized confusion matrix over all test subjects is shown in Table 4 where the value of each cell $(i, j)$ represents the number of times (as percentage '%') that class $j$ is classified as class $i$. Given that the optimal situation is 100% for $i = j$. From the resulted confusion matrix (Table 4) the overall accuracy of the developed classifier (Model I) is calculated to be 51%. In Table 4, there is the prediction result noted as 'Else', which represents the case that the classifier could not assign the test point to any of the presented classes. The error performance of the developed general model is depicted in Figure 5.

Table 3. Overview of the 54 extracted features (× = selected).

|  | Variance | Mean | Min | Max | RMS | E | $\frac{d}{dt}$ |
|---|---|---|---|---|---|---|---|
| $T_{er}$ | × | × | × | × | × | - | × |
| $H_R$ | × | × | × | × | × | - | × |
| $\bar{q}_{sk}$ | × | × | × | × | × | × | × |
| $\bar{T}_{sk}$ | × | × | × | × | × | - | × |
| $\Delta \bar{T}$ | × | × | × | × | × | - | × |
| $M_r$ | × | × | × | × | × | × | × |
| $T_{arm}$ | × | × | × | × | × | - | × |
| $T_{scap}$ | × | × | × | × | × | - | × |

Table 4. The normalized confusion matrix of Model I.

| | | Actual Label (j) | | | | | | |
|---|---|---|---|---|---|---|---|---|
| Prediction label (i) | | Cold % | Cool % | Slightly Cool % | Neutral % | Slightly Warm % | Warm % | Hot % |
| | Else | 0 | 0 | 3.30 | 2.80 | 4.20 | 8.00 | 6.70 |
| | Cold | 0 | 0 | 0 | 0 | 0 | 0 | 0 |
| | Cool | 33.3 | 52.3 | 23.4 | 1.40 | 0 | 0 | 0 |
| | Slightly cool | 66.7 | 42.9 | 40.0 | 12.7 | 2.10 | 0 | 0 |
| | Neutral | 0 | 4.80 | 33.3 | 60.6 | 27.1 | 0 | 0 |
| | Slightly Warm | 0 | 0 | 0 | 19.7 | 56.3 | 32.0 | 13.3 |
| | Warm | 0 | 0 | 0 | 1.40 | 10.4 | 44.0 | 40.0 |
| | Hot | 0 | 0 | 0 | 1.40 | 0 | 16.0 | 40.0 |

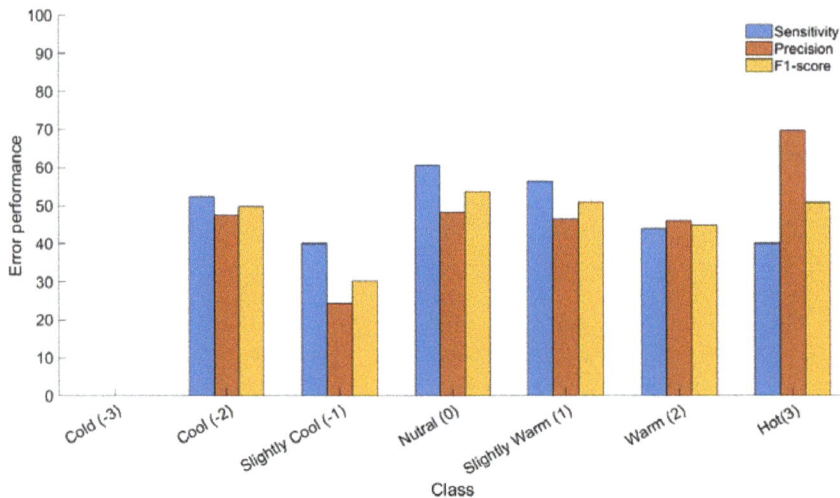

**Figure 5.** Error performance of the developed general classification model with 54 input features for 7-classes classification problem.

3.1.2. Developing a General Model for 7-Classes Classification Problem with Dimension Reduction (Model II)

As shown in Table 3, the input space of *Model I* included all extracted features (54 features) that were obtained from the measured variables. However, for the sake of the main objective of the present work, the computational cost of the developed algorithm should be low enough to be compatible with wearable technology and online modeling. Hence, a feature selection procedure was employed to obtain the most reduced-dimension input space for the classification model yet with the best error performance. Feature selection here is based on evaluating all possible feature combinations and selecting the combination with best error performance. The used feature selection procedure resulted in a reduced input space of only 12 features with optimal feature combination.

The selected features comprise: gender, age, $H_R$, $T_{er}$, $T_{sk}$, $\Delta \overline{T}$, $\overline{q}_{sk}$, rms ($H_r$, $T_c$, $T_{sk}$, $\dot{q}$), and $\frac{d\overline{q}_{sk}}{dt}$ (time-derivative of average heat flux). The feature selection step reduced the input space from 54 features to only 12, which effectively reduced the computational costs of the classification algorithm during online implementation.

The reduced dimension input space, including the selected 12 features, was used to develop a general classification model for the 7-classes classification problem to predict the thermal sensation of all test subjects. The resulted classification confusion matrix for the developed general model using the reduced-dimension input space is shown in Table 5. The results showed an overall accuracy of the developed classification model of 57% with an improvement of 6% compared to the results of model I. The overall error performance (sensitively, precision and F1-score) results are shown in Figure 6.

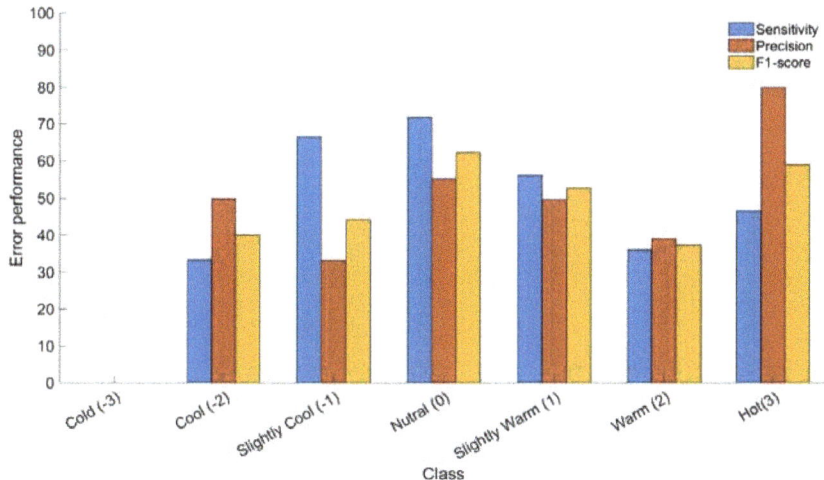

**Figure 6.** Error performance of the developed general classification model with the selected 12 input features (reduced dimension input space) for 7-classes classification problem.

**Table 5.** The normalized confusion matrix of Model II.

| | | Actual Label (*i*) | | | | | | |
|---|---|---|---|---|---|---|---|---|
| | | Cold % | Cool % | Slightly Cool % | Neutral % | Slightly Warm% | Warm % | Hot % |
| Prediction label (*j*) | Else | 0 | 4.79 | 6.65 | 0 | 10.40 | 16.03 | 0 |
| | Cold | 0 | 0 | 0 | 0 | 0 | 0 | 0 |
| | Cool | 33.20 | 33.33 | 0 | 0 | 0 | 0 | 0 |
| | Slightly cool | 66.80 | 57.08 | 66.69 | 8.45 | 2.10 | 0 | 0 |
| | Neutral | 0 | 4.79 | 26.66 | 71.81 | 22.90 | 4.03 | 0 |
| | Slightly Warm | 0 | 0 | 0 | 18.32 | 56.25 | 31.96 | 6.71 |
| | Warm | 0 | 0 | 0 | 1.42 | 8.35 | 35.99 | 46.65 |
| | Hot | 0 | 0 | 0 | 0 | 0 | 12.00 | 46.65 |

### 3.2. Class Reduction

From the confusion matrix in Table 5, it can be seen that the confusion is mostly observed between the adjacent classes. The main reason of such interclass confusion is that the features are not able to discriminate completely between these adjacent classes. For instance, the actual neutral class (0) is confused with 8.45% and 18.32% with slightly cool (−1) and slightly warm (1) classes, respectively. Hence, it is more convenient to reduce the seven thermal sensation classes into three classes representing thermal comfort (comfortable, uncomfortably cool, and uncomfortably warm). The class reduction is done based on three criteria, namely, maximum confusion, acceptable class imbalance, and avoiding overlap between classes. As mentioned earlier, the maximum confusion is observed between the adjacent classes (see Table 5). However, it is not possible to merge all adjacent confused classes due to the overlap. For example, the Slightly-Warm class is confused with the Neutral class by 22.9%, on the other hand, the Warm class is confused with the Slightly-warm by 31.96%. Hence, in order to merge the Slightly-warm class with the Neutral it should not be merged with Warm and vice versa. Therefore, merging must avoid any overlap between different classes. Another criterion is the class imbalance, as shown in Figure 7a and Table 5, where Cold is not recognized by the classifier due to the relatively very low number of instances labeled as Cold compared to the other classes. For an acceptable class imbalance, it is meant to consider the already existing class imbalance between the whole states that the frequency of a state occurrence is reducing by moving far from the Neutral state, as shown in Figure 7a.

Finally, it is necessary to avoid any overlap between the reduced classes by assigning each state to only one class. As there are different possibilities to obtain the new three classes, it is found that three configurations are the closest to the thermal comfort levels, considering the earlier mentioned criteria. Based on these criteria the seven classes were reduced into three classes with three different configurations as follows:

- **Configuration 1** Merging the states of Cold (−3) and Cool (−2) into 'Class 1' (27 instances), merging Slightly cool (−1), Neutral (0), and Slightly warm (1) into 'Class 2' (149 instances), and merging Warm (2) and Hot (3) into 'Class 3' (40 instances) (Figure 7b).
- **Configuration 2** Merging the states of Cold, Cool and Slightly-cool into 'Class 1' (57 instances), Neutral as 'Class 2' (71), and merging Slightly-warm, warm and Hot into 'Class 3' (88 instances) (Figure 7c).
- **Configuration 3** Merging the states of Cold, Cool and Slightly-cool into 'Class 1' (57 instances), merging Neutral, and Slightly-warm into 'Class 2' (119 instances), and merging warm and Hot into 'Class 3' (40 instances) (Figure 7d).

As shown in Figure 7, each configuration has a different class distribution (i.e., number of instances per class).

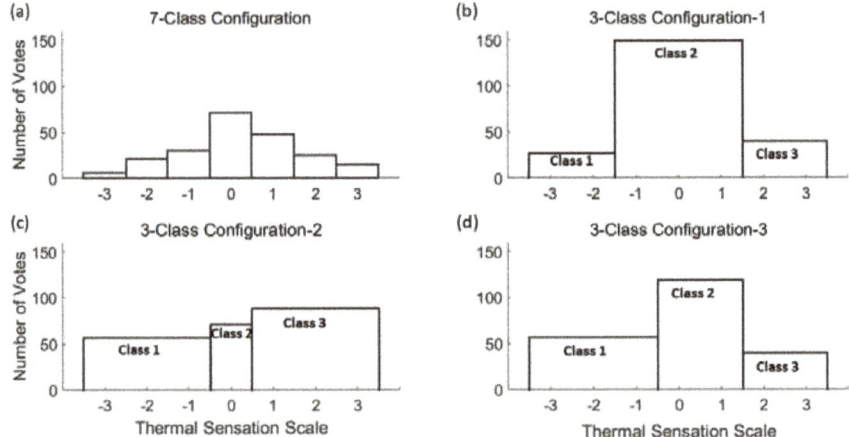

**Figure 7.** (**a**) A histogram of 7-class thermal sensation scale of ASHRAE system. (**b**) A histogram of 3-class thermal sensation of Configuration 1. (**c**) A histogram of 3-class thermal sensation of Configuration 2. (**d**) A histogram of 3-class of Configuration 3.

Developing General Models with the Selected Features for 3-Classes Problem with Different Class Configurations (Model III)

The error performance results of the developed classification model (Model III), based on the 12 selected features, for the three labelling configurations (Conf. 1, Conf. 2 and Conf. 3) are shown in Table 6. Comparing the three configurations is not consistent, as for each configuration, the number of data-pointdata-points change, which influences the performance especially for such small size dataset.

**Table 6.** The error performance (precision, sensitivity, F1-score, and accuracy) of general Least Squares Support Vector Machine (LS-SVM) model for the three different 3-class configurations.

| Configurations | Classes | Precision | Sensitivity | F1-Score | Accuracy |
|---|---|---|---|---|---|
| Conf. 1 | Class 1 | 0.53 | 0.37 | 0.44 | 0.81 |
|  | Class 2 | 0.83 | 0.89 | 0.86 |  |
|  | Class 3 | 0.79 | 0.75 | 0.77 |  |
| Conf. 2 | Class 1 | 0.88 | 0.88 | 0.88 | 0.81 |
|  | Class 2 | 0.75 | 0.66 | 0.70 |  |
|  | Class 3 | 0.82 | 0.89 | 0.86 |  |
| Conf. 3 | Class 1 | 0.88 | 0.88 | 0.88 | 0.85 |
|  | Class 2 | 0.88 | 0.91 | 0.89 |  |
|  | Class 3 | 0.88 | 0.78 | 0.83 |  |

*3.3. Personalized Classification Models*

In order to develop online-personalized models, it is necessary to consider two main challenges, first the developed model should be able to handle the new, personal, data in the training set. Additionally, the developed model should be adapted to the new personal data without any bias to the majority of the old (non-personal) data. Different approaches are used to handle these challenges such as incremental learning methods [34], which work on adapting and retuning the parameters of the general model based on the newly collected data. Another approach is the localized learning, which is based on developing a local model for each test point or subset of the test set [35]. In the present paper, the KNN-LS-SVM localized learning approach is used because of its simplicity and efficiency. Two techniques were used to test the localized models, the first based on LOSO testing approach, and the second approach was based on leave-one-out (LOO) testing approach.

3.3.1. Developing Personalized Models Using the Selected 12 Features and Different Class-Configurations Based on LOSO Testing Approach

As explained earlier, to develop a personalized classification model the new personal data were not considered in the training set to compare the performance with the global model. In other words, the new subject (the subject data that left out of the training set) is completely unknown to the model, which simulates the case when the model is dealing with an unknown test subject. The used localized learning approach of KNN-LS-SVM searches for the most similar (based on the similarity criterion, see (3)) training points to the new test point (from the new subject) in the input space by which a local model is developed to classify this test point. The resulted error performance (precision, sensitivity, F1-score, and accuracy) of the KNN-LS-SVM classifier based on LOSO testing approach and $K = 5$ is presented in Table 7.

**Table 7.** The error performance (precision, sensitivity, F1-score, and accuracy) of the localized model KNN-LS-SVM model for the three different 3-class configurations based on leave-one-subject-out (LOSO) testing approach.

| Configurations | Classes | Precision | Sensitivity | F1-Score | Accuracy |
|---|---|---|---|---|---|
| Conf. 1 | Class 1 | 0.47 | 0.36 | 0.41 | 0.83 |
| | Class 2 | 0.84 | 0.90 | 0.87 | |
| | Class 3 | 0.83 | 0.71 | 0.77 | |
| Conf. 2 | Class 1 | 0.84 | 0.95 | 0.89 | 0.81 |
| | Class 2 | 0.74 | 0.68 | 0.70 | |
| | Class 3 | 0.84 | 0.83 | 0.83 | |
| Conf. 3 | Class 1 | 0.87 | 0.94 | 0.90 | 0.85 |
| | Class 2 | 0.88 | 0.89 | 0.88 | |
| | Class 3 | 0.86 | 0.74 | 0.79 | |

3.3.2. Developing Personalized Models Using the Selected 12 Features and Different Class-Configurations Based on Leave-One-Out (LOO) Approach

In contrast with the first approach, for each subject one data-point is tested and the rest of the same subject data-pointdata-points are integrated with the training data. This approach mimics online personalized streaming modelling, since the new streaming personal data is considered in the training dataset and a dedicated classifier is developed online for each new test data-point. The obtained error performance of the KNN-LS-SVM classifier based on LOO testing approach and $K = 5$ is depicted in Table 8.

**Table 8.** The error performance (precision, sensitivity, F1-score, and accuracy) of the localized model KNN-LS-SVM model for the three different 3-class configurations based on leave-one-out (LOO) testing approach.

| Configurations | Classes | Precision | Sensitivity | F1-Score | Accuracy |
|---|---|---|---|---|---|
| Conf. 1 | Class 1 | 0.75 | 0.56 | 0.64 | 0.86 |
| | Class 2 | 0.87 | 0.93 * | 0.90 * | |
| | Class 3 | 0.86 | 0.78 | 0.82 | |
| Conf. 2 | Class 1 | 0.84 * | 0.95 * | 0.89 * | 0.79 |
| | Class 2 | 0.71 | 0.62 | 0.66 | |
| | Class 3 | 0.81 | 0.83 * | 0.82 | |
| Conf. 3 | Class 1 | 0.84 * | 0.91 | 0.87 | 0.87 * |
| | Class 2 | 0.89 * | 0.88 | 0.88 | |
| | Class 3 | 0.89 * | 0.80 | 0.84 * | |

* indicates the highest error performance value for each class in the different configurations.

For the proposed personalized models, the first approach of LOSO is mimicking the case that the model is applied to an unknown subject to predict individual's thermal sensation level based on the measured variables. The localized model is searching for the most similar (nearest) training points to each test point, of this subject, that to train the classification model for each test point. This approach could be useful in case of having a large amount of data with a diversity of subjects especially in the absence of streaming data from new subjects. The second approach of LOO mimics the case of having a prior knowledge about the test subject through personally labelled data. The localized model in this approach is also searching for the most similar training points, which may include this subject personal data. This approach can be efficient in the presence of streaming personal data that is labelled by the test subject.

*3.4. Streaming Algorithm Approach for Personalized Thermal Sensation Monitoring*

In this paper, we introduce the main framework of streaming algorithm for personalized classification model to predict individual's thermal sensation based on streaming data obtained from wearable sensors. The main framework of the proposed streaming algorithm approach is depicted in Figure 8.

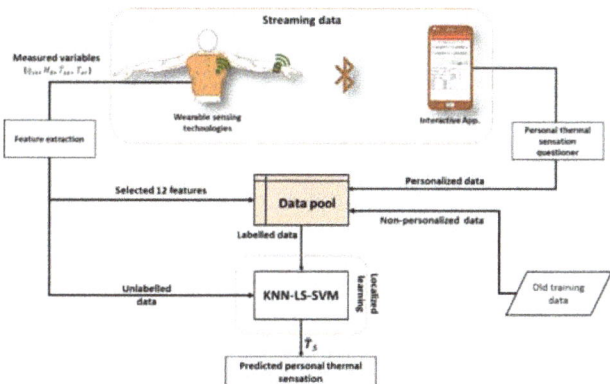

**Figure 8.** Schematic representation of the proposed streaming algorithm for online personalized thermal sensation monitoring.

The main components of the proposed algorithm (Figure 8) are explained in the following:

- *Streaming data*

The availability of the real-time sensors data, from the wearable technologies, has given the possibility of streaming data, which processed via the proposed online streaming algorithm to adapt and personalize the classifier model. The streaming data includes:

I. Wearable sensor data, which consists of the continuously measured variables, namely, individual's heart rate, skin heat flux, skin temperature, ambient temperature and aural temperature.
II. Data obtained from the interactive mobile App., which consists of personal data, namely, age and gender. Additionally, the individual's thermal sensation vote is to be obtained via mobile application-based questioner.

The workflow procedures of streaming data acquisition and labelling are depicted by the flowchart shown in Figure 9.

- *Feature extraction*

As shown earlier, the selected 12 features are extracted from the continuously measured variables, namely, $H_R$, $T_{er}$, $T_{sk}$, $\Delta \overline{T}$, $\overline{q}_{sk}$, the *rms* of ($H_r$, $T_c$, $T_{sk}$, $\dot{q}$), and $\frac{d\overline{q}_{sk}}{dt}$. Other personal futures, namely, age and gender are to be obtained via the interactive mobile App. from individual users.

- *Labelled data*

All training data must be labelled, either the old training data or the new personal data. Personal data is labelled manually via the questionnaire provided by the mobile App.

- *Unlabelled data*

Unlabelled data is the new data points to be labelled by the classifier, these unlabelled data points include the extracted features from the measured variables.

- *Localized Learning Algorithm*

The localized learning algorithm (i.e., KNN-LS-SVM) is the classifier that receives the unlabelled data points and train a dedicated model with the $K$ nearest training points in order to label the unlabelled ones. The output of this process is a predicted label of personal thermal sensation ($\hat{T}_S$).

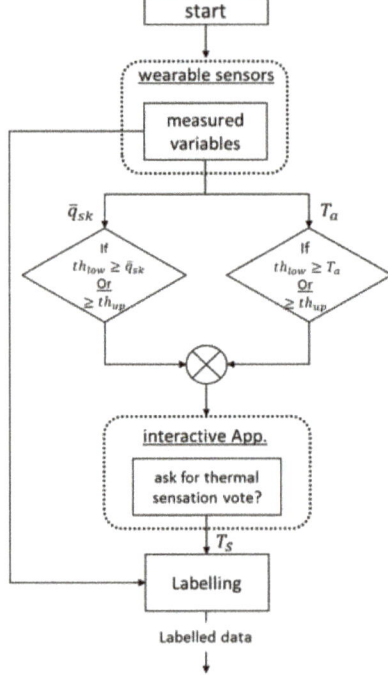

**Figure 9.** Flowchart represents the main workflow of the streaming data acquisition and labeling process.

## 4. Discussion

The main advantage of the proposed classification model in the present work, in comparison with other proposed models in recent studies (e.g., [17,22,25,28]), is its capability to handle the requirements for adaptive personalization and online streaming modelling. Moreover, the proposed model is reduced-dimension, with the minimum possible number of features, which makes it computationally suitable for smart wearable technologies.

The main results and findings of the present study is compared with recent studies that treat the prediction of the thermal sensation/comfort as a classification problem using machine-learning techniques.

In their study [27], Ghahramani et al. used HMM classification technique, in which three classes of thermal comfort, namely, comfortable, uncomfortably cool and uncomfortably warm are used. An important point to be considered in the work of Ghahramani et al. [27] is the class imbalance in their used experimental data between the positive class (comfortable), which represents 81% of the data and the negative class (uncomfortable), which represents only 19% of the data. Therefore, using the classification accuracy (reported 82.8 %) is considered misleading in this case. Hence, it is much more suitable in their case to compare the precision and sensitivity of this model and our general model (Model III Conf. 3). The reported results [27] of Ghahramani et al. showed a precision of 93.3% and sensitivity of 56.22% without clarifying the precision and sensitivity of the uncomfortable states of warm and cool. On the other hand, our results of (Model III Conf. 3), which is the closest to the compared approach, show a precision of 88% for all classes and sensitivity of 88%, 91%, and 78% for Class 1, Class 2, and Class 3, respectively. These results show more balance between precision and sensitivity for each class. Moreover, personalization and streaming algorithm compatibility is missing in their study.

Another relevant study [28], by Jiang et al., attempted to develop a personalized classification model, as for each subject, a classification model is trained with 50% of that subject data and tested with the rest. The reported result of this study [28] showed an average accuracy over all subjects of 89.82%. However, there is no clarification of the class distribution; hence, it is not clear whether the accuracy is efficient enough for evaluation. Moreover, it is not consistent to compare our final personalized model with that model as the latter is learned with seven classes; however, the former is learned with three classes.

In another comparable study [25] to our present work, Farhan et al., predicted individual thermal comfort using machine learning classifier. In their study Farhan et al., used publicly available dataset from which a balanced number of each class is chosen to train and test the classification model. Their developed classification model is trained with three classes that represent the three thermal comfort states of uncomfortably cool, neutral and uncomfortably warm divided based on predefined comfort thresholds. In contrast to our proposed classification model, the proposed classifiers in [25] do not consider model personalization or streaming online modelling. The best-obtained results amongst their developed models are of the SVM classifier as follows: precisions of (76.92, 62.8, and 94.2%) and sensitivities of (67.5, 89.8, and 75.7%) for classes −1, 0, and 1 respectively. On the other hand, our obtained results of (Model III conf. 3) are precisions of (88, 88, and 88%) and sensitivities of (88, 91, and 78%) of classes 1, 2, and 3 respectively. It is observed that the precisions of our developed classification model are more consistent for all classes, and the sensitivities are higher in total. Ultimately, their approach [25] does not consider personalizing the model or streaming online modelling.

In another recent study [17], a personal model is discussed; however, it is strictly applied to two subjects (male and female), unlike the case in the present study where we test the model on 25 test subjects.

After comparing our methodology and results with number of relevant and comparable studies, it is obvious that the presented study tackled number of classification and modeling challenges unlike many of the aforementioned relevant works. These challenges included the feature selection and dimension reduction, considering new streaming personal data into the training set with keeping the model complexity, rigidness against the problem of class imbalance, and ultimately personalizing the classification model using easily measured variable obtained from wearable sensors.

## 5. Conclusions

In this present paper, 25 participants are subjected to three different environmental temperatures, namely 5 °C (cold), 20 °C (moderate) and 37 °C (hot) at two different activity levels, namely, at low level (rest) and high level (cycling at 80 W power). Metabolic rate, heart rate, average skin temperature (from three different body locations), heat flux and aural temperature are measured continuously during the course of the experiments. The thermal sensation votes are collected from each test subject based on ASHRAE 7-points questioner. A general classification model based on LS-SVM technique is developed to predict the individual's thermal sensation. A localized learning algorithm based on KNN-LS-SVM approach is used to develop a personalized classification model to predict the individual's thermal sensation for 3-classes classification model. The developed classification model has the advantage of using a reduced-dimension input-space, which is suitable for wearable applications and online streaming algorithm. The developed personalized model showed an overall accuracy result of 86%. Additionally, we introduced the main framework of streaming algorithm based on the developed personalized classification model to predict individual's thermal sensation based on streaming data obtained from wearable sensors. In the present work, we believe that it is the first time to utilize the localized learning approach in the thermal state classification problem. One of the main advantages of the proposed approach, in this paper, that it is suitable for streaming algorithm and online modelling as the computational cost is not influenced by increasing the number of data-points. However, the newly obtained data-points is to be considered to develop the online model, which is the main advantage of the KNN-LSSVM. Furthermore, the localized learning approach enables personalization of the classification model by considering either the personally labelled data-points or the most similar data-points of other persons. On the other hand, number of limitations, concerning the developed model, should be acknowledged here. One important limitation to the developed classification model is regarding to the data size, as the number of data-points per person and in total are generally limited. Moreover, the 7-classes labeling is unbalanced, which made the class reduction is necessary to enhance the overall prediction performance during the course of this study. Otherwise, this study would be extended to be applied to a 7-classes classification problem. The data balance and data size can be enhanced by asking for more frequent votes during the experiment and considering more than three environment temperature levels. Finally, another limitation regards the proposed KNN-LSSVM modeling approach, in which an extra hyperparameter (i.e., $K$) is to be optimized, which adds an extra computational cost to the overall streaming algorithm.

**Author Contributions:** Conceptualisation, A.Y., J.-M.A. and A.Y.A.A.; methodology, A.Y., A.Y.A.A. and N.C.; software, A.Y. and A.Y.A.A.; validation, A.Y. and A.Y.A.A.; formal analysis, A.Y., N.C. and A.Y.A.A.; investigation, A.Y., N.C. and A.Y.A.A.; resources, J.-M.A.; data curation, A.Y., N.C. and A.Y.A.A.; writing—original draft preparation, A.Y., N.C. and A.Y.A.A.; writing—review and editing, A.Y., J.-M.A. and A.Y.A.A.; visualisation, A.Y. and A.Y.A.A.; supervision, J.-M.A. and A.Y.; project administration, J.-M.A.; funding acquisition, J.-M.A.

**Funding:** This research received no external funding.

**Acknowledgments:** The Author Ahmed Youssef Ali Amer is funded by a European Union Grant through the Interreg V-A Euregio Meuse-Rhine wearIT4health project.

**Conflicts of Interest:** The authors declare no conflict of interest.

### References

1. ASHRAE. *Thermal Environmental Conditions for Human Occupancy*; American Society of Heating, Refrigeration and Air Conditioning Engineers, Inc.: Atlanta, GA, USA, 2004.
2. ISO-10551. *Ergonomics of the Thermal Environmen—Assessment of the Influence of the Thermal Environment Using Subjective Judgement Scales*; ISO: Brussels, Belgium, 1995.
3. Fanger, P.O. *Thermal Comfort: Analysis and Applications In Environmental Engineering*, 1st ed.; Danish Technical Press: Lyngby, Denmark, 1970.
4. Koelblen, B.; Psikuta, A.; Bogdan, A.; Annaheim, S.; Rossi, R.M. Thermal sensation models: A systematic comparison. *Indoor Air* **2017**, *27*, 680–689. [CrossRef] [PubMed]
5. Enescu, D. Models and Indicators to Assess Thermal Sensation Under Steady-state and Transient Conditions. *Energies* **2019**, *12*, 841. [CrossRef]
6. Kenneth, K.C.; Parsons, C. *Human Thermal Environments: The Effects of Hot, Moderate and Cold Environments on Human Health, Comfort and Performance*, 3rd ed.; CRC Press: Boca Raton, FL, USA, 2014.
7. Nikolopoulou, M.; Steemers, K. Thermal comfort and psychological adaptation as a guide for designing urban spaces. *Energy Build.* **2003**, *35*, 95–101. [CrossRef]
8. Gagge, A.P.; Stolwijk, J.A.J.; Nishi, Y. An Effective Temperature Scale Based on a Simple Model of Human Physiological Regulatory Response. *ASHRAE Trans.* **1971**, *77*, 247–262.
9. Takada, S.; Matsumoto, S.; Matsushita, T. Prediction of whole-body thermal sensation in the non-steady state based on skin temperature. *Build. Environ.* **2013**, *68*, 123–133. [CrossRef]
10. Fiala, D. *Dynamic Simulation of Human Heat Transfer and Thermal Comfort*; De Montfort University: Leicester, UK, 1998.

11. Lomas, K.J.; Fiala, D.; Stohrer, M. First principles modeling of thermal sensation responses in steady-state and transient conditions. *ASHRAE Trans.* **2003**, *109*, 179–186.
12. Zhang, H. *Human Thermal Sensation and Comfort in Transient and Non-Uniform Thermal Environments*; University of California, Berkeley: Berkeley, CA, USA, 2003.
13. Guan, Y.; Hosni, M.H.; Jones, B.W.; Gielda, T.P. Investigation of Human Thermal Comfort Under Highly Transient Conditions for Automotive Applications-Part 2: Thermal Sensation Modeling. *ASHRAE Trans.* **2003**, *109*, 898–907.
14. Guan, Y.; Hosni, M.H.; Jones, B.W.; Gielda, T.P. Investigation of Human Thermal Comfort Under Highly Transient Conditions for Automotive Applications-Part 1: Experimental Design and Human Subject Testing Implementation. *ASHRAE Trans.* **2003**, *109*, 885–897.
15. Nilsson, H.O.; Holmer, I. Comfort climate evaluation with thermal manikin methods and computer simulation models. *Indoor Air* **2003**, *13*, 28–37. [CrossRef] [PubMed]
16. Kingma, B.R.M.; Schellen, L.; Frijns, A.J.H.; Lichtenbelt, W.D.V. Thermal sensation: A mathematical model based on neurophysiology. *Indoor Air* **2012**, *22*, 253–262. [CrossRef] [PubMed]
17. Lu, S.; Wang, W.; Wang, S.; Hameen, E.C. Thermal Comfort-Based Personalized Models with Non-Intrusive Sensing Technique in Office Buildings. *Appl. Sci.* **2019**, *9*, 1768. [CrossRef]
18. de Dear, R.; Brager, G.S. Developing an adaptive model of thermal comfort and preference. *ASHRAE Trans.* **1998**, *104*, 145–167.
19. Rijal, H.B.; Gumphreys, M.; Tuohy, P.; Nicol, F. Development of adaptive algorithms for the operation of windows, fans and doors to predict thermal comfort and energy use in Pakistani buildings. *ASHRAE Trans.* **2008**, *114*, 555–573.
20. Humphreys, M. Outdoor temperatures and comfort indoors. *Batim. Int. Build. Res. Pract.* **1978**, *6*, 92. [CrossRef]
21. Lee, S.; Bilionis, I.; Karava, P.; Tzempelikos, A. A Bayesian approach for probabilistic classification and inference of occupant thermal preferences in office buildings. *Build. Environ.* **2017**, *118*, 323–343. [CrossRef]
22. Ghahramani, A.; Castro, G.; Karvigh, S.A.; Becerik-Gerber, B. Towards unsupervised learning of thermal comfort using infrared thermography. *Appl. Energy* **2018**, *211*, 41–49. [CrossRef]
23. Kim, J.; Zhou, Y.; Schiavon, S.; Raftery, P.; Brager, G. Personal comfort models: Predicting individuals' thermal preference using occupant heating and cooling behavior and machine learning. *Build. Environ.* **2018**, *129*, 96–106. [CrossRef]
24. Chaudhuri, T.; Soh, Y.C.; Li, H.; Xie, L. Machine learning based prediction of thermal comfort in buildings of equatorial Singapore. In Proceedings of the 2017 IEEE International Conference on Smart Grid and Smart Cities (ICSGSC), Singapore, 23–26 July 2017; pp. 72–77.
25. Farhan, A.A.; Pattipati, K.; Wang, B.; Luh, P. Predicting individual thermal comfort using machine learning algorithms. In Proceedings of the 2015 IEEE International Conference on Automation Science and Engineering (CASE), Gothenburg, Sweden, 24–28 August 2015; pp. 708–713.
26. Dai, C.; Zhang, H.; Arens, E.; Lian, Z. Machine learning approaches to predict thermal demands using skin temperatures: Steady-state conditions. *Build. Environ.* **2017**, *114*, 1–10. [CrossRef]
27. Huang, C.C.; Yang, R.; Newman, M.W. The potential and challenges of inferring thermal comfort at home using commodity sensors. In Proceedings of the 2015 ACM International Joint Conference on Pervasive and Ubiquitous Computing, Osaka, Japan, 7–11 September 2015; pp. 1089–1100.
28. Jiang, L.; Yao, R. Modelling personal thermal sensations using C-Support Vector Classification (C-SVC) algorithm. *Build. Environ.* **2016**, *99*, 98–106. [CrossRef]
29. Hussain, S.; Kang, B.H.; Lee, S. A Wearable Device-Based Personalized Big Data Analysis Model. In *Lecture Notes in Computer Science*; Springer: Cham, Swizterland, 2014; Volume 8867, pp. 236–242.
30. Suykens, J.A.K.; van Gestel, T.; de Brabanter, J.; de Moor, B.; Vandewalle, J. *Least Squares Support Vector Machine*; World Scientific: Singapore, 2002.
31. Amer, A.Y.A. *Localized Least Squares Support Vector Machines with Application to Weather Forecasting*; KU Leuven: Leuven, Belgium, 2016.
32. Ashrae, *Ashrae Standard 55*; American Society of Heating, Refrigerating and Air-Conditioning Engineers Inc.: Atlanta, GA, USA, 2017.

33. Dewhirst, M.W.; Viglianti, B.L.; Lora-Michiels, M.; Hanson, M.; Hoopes, P.J. Basic principles of thermal dosimetry and thermal thresholds for tissue damage from hyperthermia. *Int. J. Hyperth* **2003**, *19*, 267–294. [CrossRef]
34. Losing, V.; Hammer, B.; Wersing, H. Incremental on-line learning: A review and comparison of state of the art algorithms. *Neurocomputing* **2018**, *275*, 1261–1274. [CrossRef]
35. Bottou, L.; Vepnik, V. Local learning algorithms. *Neural Comput.* **1992**, *4*, 888–900. [CrossRef]

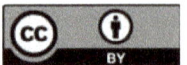

© 2019 by the authors. Licensee MDPI, Basel, Switzerland. This article is an open access article distributed under the terms and conditions of the Creative Commons Attribution (CC BY) license (http://creativecommons.org/licenses/by/4.0/).

Article

# Feature Extraction and Evaluation for Driver Drowsiness Detection Based on Thermoregulation

Jasper Gielen and Jean-Marie Aerts *

Department of Biosystems, Division Animal and Human Health Engineering, M3-BIORES: Measure, Model & Manage of Bioresponses Laboratory, KU Leuven, Kasteelpark Arenberg 30, 3001 Heverlee, Belgium
* Correspondence: jean-marie.aerts@kuleuven.be

Received: 19 July 2019; Accepted: 28 August 2019; Published: 30 August 2019

**Abstract:** Numerous reports state that drowsiness is one of the major factors affecting driving performance and resulting in traffic accidents. In the past, methods to detect driver drowsiness have been developed based on physiological, behavioral, and vehicular features. In this pilot study, we test the use of a new set of features for detecting driver drowsiness based on physiological changes related to thermoregulation. Nineteen participants successfully performed a driving simulation, while the temperature of the nose ($T_{nose}$) and wrist ($T_{wrist}$) as well as the heart rate (HR) were monitored. On average, an initial increase in temperature followed by a gradual decrease was observed in drivers who experienced drowsiness. For non-drowsy drivers, no such trends were observed. In addition, HR decreased on average in both groups, yet the decrease in the drowsy group was more distinct. Next, a classification based on each of these variables resulted in an accuracy of 68.4%, 88.9%, and 70.6% for $T_{nose}$, $T_{wrist}$, and HR, respectively. Combining the information of all variables resulted in an accuracy of 89.5%, meaning that ultimately the state of 17 out of 19 drivers was detected correctly. Hence, we conclude that the use of physiological features related to thermoregulation shows potential for future research in this field.

**Keywords:** driver drowsiness; thermoregulation; distal skin temperature; decision tree

## 1. Introduction

Driver drowsiness is one of the major factors causing traffic accidents. Dependent on the source, between 10%–20% of all accidents are claimed to be caused by driver drowsiness [1,2]. Besides, the majority of this kind of accidents occur during the night or right after noon [3]. This is not surprising since our physiological clock is programmed to facilitate sleep onset at these moments [4]. Furthermore, drowsiness and sleep are by definition very closely related. For instance, Johns defines drowsiness as "the intermediate state between wakefulness and being asleep" [5]. More so, experiencing drowsiness is used as a synonym for fighting against falling asleep.

In the literature, different methods for monitoring the driver's state have been presented and are based on features extracted from physiological, behavioral, or vehicular signals [6,7]. Physiological signals are measured directly or indirectly on the driver self. The relation between signals such as an electroencephalogram (EEG), electrocardiogram (ECG), electrooculogram (EoG), electromyogram (EMG), and sleep have been described in many studies [8]. Moreover, in polysomnography (PSG), these electrophysiological signals are interpreted according to the guidelines of the American Academy of Sleep Medicine (AASM) [9] for a gold standard reference measure of sleep and sleep quality [8]. Especially brain activity (EEG) shows the most distinct changes according to the state of the driver. Although, EEG technology has significantly evolved over the past years, setting up the devices still requires a lot of know-how and caution to obtain accurate measurements [10]. In addition, artifacts due to movement and other disturbing signals completely deteriorate the quality of the signal in less controlled setups. Alternatively, the driver's behavior is also monitored for drowsiness detection. Features such as eye closure, blinking frequency, yawning, and head-nodding can be extracted by applying camera vision and face recognition techniques (e.g., [11,12]). The advantage of using cameras is that the measurements are completely unobtrusive. When the camera is placed near the sun visor or the rear mirror, the driver's field of view is not obstructed at all. However, issues with lighting conditions have been associated with these techniques [7]. Thirdly, features extracted from the vehicle itself are also widely used to monitor driver drowsiness. The angle of the steering wheel, the pressure applied to the acceleration and brake pedal, distance to the vehicle in front and a lot of other vehicular features have been used in recent studies [13–15]. Currently, commercial applications built into cars, busses, and trucks are already available on the market. These so-called advanced driver assistance systems (ADAS) are designed to automate, adapt, and enhance vehicles for safer and better driving.

Along with these ADAS, there is an ongoing evolution towards autonomous driving. Apart from the technical aspects of self-driving vehicles, the component of human attention and control should not be neglected. For instance, commercial and transport airplanes fly autonomously for the majority of the time, yet the pilots still have to monitor the plane's status continuously and must be ready for intervention to assure a smooth and safe flight. Similarly, low levels of autonomous driving also requires an attentive driver [16]. Moreover, legal implications related to fully autonomous driving are expected to influence integration on the market more than the technical challenges [17].

In this paper, we focus on a new set of features to monitor driver drowsiness based on physiological changes related to thermoregulation. The functional link between temperature regulation and sleep onset has been studied for a long time. In regulating temperature, the body is typically considered in terms of a core and an outer shell [18]. The core body temperature ($T_C$) is maintained within a specific narrow range (around 37 °C), whereas the outer shell can vary over multiple degrees. To illustrate, in thermo-neutral conditions, distal skin temperature is reported to be 7–8 °C below the core [19]. However, at a room temperature of 35 °C, the hands and feet are only 3–4 °C cooler. Furthermore, it is a well-known phenomenon that $T_C$ varies periodically in a circadian way. Throughout the day, the temperature peaks in the evening around 21:00, followed by a gradual decrease overnight with a minimum around 05:00 [20]. To facilitate these temperature changes, heat production and dissipation are closely regulated. In thermo-neutral, sedentary conditions, this heat balance is mainly regulated by autonomous control of vasodilation and vasoconstriction of the arterioles in the skin. Accordingly, controlling blood flow to the skin is crucial for managing the human heat balance. Moreover, Rowel [21] states that skin blood flow takes up between 5% and 60% of our cardiac output depending on the environmental conditions. With respect to sleep and sleep onset, Gilbert et al. [19] presented the hypothesis that heat loss via the extremities is linked in feedback with activation of the sleep-promoting areas in the brain. More specifically, efferent warm sensitive neurons (WSN) in the preoptic anterior hypothalamus (PoAH) innervate and stimulate somnogenic brain structures, while other thermo-sensitive neurons innervating wake-promoting brain areas are inhibited. Quanten et al. [22] experimentally tested this hypothesis and showed that in conditions of unwanted sleepiness in active subjects there is a negative feedback connection between the distal-to-proximal temperature gradient and sleep onset.

In this work, we aim to investigate the use of features extracted from peripheral skin temperatures of the nose and wrist (heat dissipation) as well as the heart rate (heat production) to distinguish between subjects experiencing drowsiness while driving and subjects that remain alert.

## 2. Materials and Methods

### 2.1. Study Design and Participants

The data of 19 healthy subjects between 20 years old and 27 years old who volunteered to perform a driving test were used in this study. Each participant was asked to drive in a driving simulator while physiological variables related to thermoregulation were monitored. To simulate a monotonous driving experience, a PlayStation 3 and racing game (Gran Tourismo 5) were used together with a compatible steering wheel as well as acceleration and brake pedals (Logitech Driving Force EX). The race track named "Special Stage 7" was selected because it represents an empty highway at night. Additionally, a speed limit of 80 km/h was imposed. This setup was installed in a climate-controlled room of 2.3 by 3.6 m, where the temperature was held constant at 23 °C and the relative humidity kept at 50%. The constant thermal environment was deemed realistic since similar conditions have been reported in experimental measurements performed on the road [23].

Every participant arrived at the test facility at around 21:00. After an introduction to the setup and the purpose of this study, the volunteer was equipped with the different sensors (see Section 2.2. Data Collection). Subsequently, the driving simulation started between 21:30 and 22:15. The subjects performed the driving test in either one of the following conditions. In a first series of experiments, the lights inside the climate-controlled room were dimmed and there was no communication between the subject and the researcher present to follow up the measurements and the driver's state. The driving simulation was stopped after a maximum duration of 2.5 h or until the driver was too sleepy to continue driving in a normal way. In a second set of experiments, the lights inside the room were left on and communication between the researcher and the participant was allowed. It has been shown that exposure to light elicits acute physiological effects in humans such as an increase in alertness, suppression of melatonin, and an increase in $T_C$ [24]. In line with the hypothesis by Gilbert et al. [19], the thermoregulatory changes are thought to be related to the alerting effects instead of a direct relation between light exposure and thermoregulation. Evidently, the purpose of this second protocol was to increase the chances of staying alert during the simulation. However, the participants were not forced to stay alert. For these measurements, a maximum duration of 1.5 h was set in advance. The maximum duration was set to 1.5 h because this was the average in the first set of experiments. In other words, the first group of participants became-on average-too sleepy to drive after 1.5 h under the first conditions. Figure 1 visualizes the timing of the experiments and shows the driving simulator that was set up in the climate-controlled room.

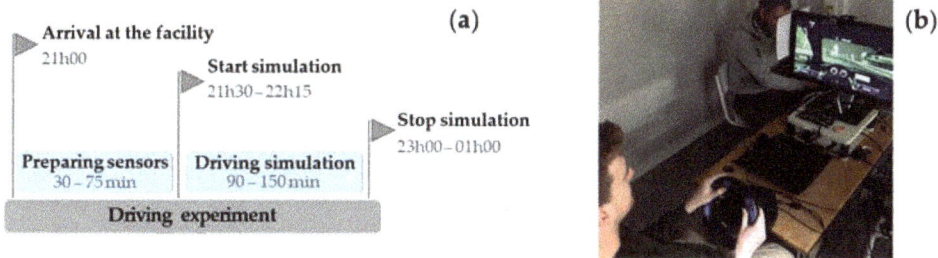

**Figure 1.** Timing of the driving experiment (**a**) and a photo of the driving simulator installed in the climate-controlled room (**b**).

In total, 26 people completed the driving simulation. However, the data of 7 participants were excluded due to missing sensor data (i.e., in 3 simulation data collection were not stored correctly) and/or limited duration of the driving simulation (i.e., 5 participants were falling asleep within 40 min to 60 min after the start). In case a participant became too drowsy to drive within 1 hour, it was assumed that the process of sleep onset started before entering the simulator. As a result, the analysis was applied to a dataset of 10 participants who performed the first protocol and 9 subjects who performed the second version. Afterwards, we checked whether this first group actually experienced drowsiness during the test and the second group did not (see Section 2.2. Data Collection).

The study was approved by the Social and Societal Ethics Committee (SMEC) of the KU Leuven (case number G-2019 04 1632) and all participants provided written informed consent before starting the driving test.

## 2.2. Data Collection

During the driving simulation, a number of different physiological variables were monitored. First, information about the state of the driver was obtained by means of a self-assessment of the mental state. The Stanford Sleepiness Scale (Stanford Sleepiness Scale: https://web.stanford.edu/~{}dement/sss.html) (SSS) was used for this purpose [25]. The SSS is a validated method for determining sleepiness and has been used in other studies on driver drowsiness [26,27]. The scale consists of 7 scores/levels to indicate the degree of sleepiness with '1' being the most alert and '7' being almost asleep. The driver was asked to score his/her mental state every 5 min based on this scale. The timing of these moments was indicated by the controlling researcher present in the room by a small hand gesture (i.e., slowly raising their right hand). This way, distraction from the driving task was minimal and the driver did not experience any abrupt changes in his/her mental state. When the highest score of 7 was given 2 times in a row, the experiment was terminated prematurely because we assumed the driver to be too drowsy to continue driving in a normal way. In the SSS, a score of 7 corresponds to the following state: "No longer fighting sleep, sleep onset soon; having dream-like thoughts". Secondly, the skin temperature of the tip of the nose ($T_{nose}$) was measured using a VarioCAM infrared thermal camera with a resolution of 640 by 480 pixels (InfraTec GmbH, Dresden, Germany). The camera pas pointed towards the face and from the thermal images, the position of the nose was manually determined. The frame rate of the camera was set to 1 frame per minute. Thirdly, the skin temperature at the wrist ($T_{wrist}$) was measured continuously with an Empatica E4 wristband at a sampling rate of 4 Hz (Empatica Inc., Cambridge, MA, USA). Fourth, the heart rate (HR) was monitored using a Zephyr HxM chest strap (MedTronic, Annapolis, MD, USA). The HR, expressed in beats per minute (bpm), was sampled every second with a smartphone and app for logging the data (Samsung Galaxy J1). In this research, we did not consider raw ECG measurements because it was decided beforehand that only the HR would be used in the analyses (see Section 2.4. Data Analysis). Lastly, the ratings of the SSS were used to check whether participants who performed the first protocol actually became drowsy during the driving test and the second group of subjects remained alert. This decision was based on the sleepiness scores. If a score of 5 was given at any point during the test, the participant was labeled as "drowsy". If this was not the case, the subject was labeled as "non-drowsy".

During one simulation, the data of $T_{wrist}$ were not stored correctly. Hence, only 18 measurements are available. In addition, the data of the heart rate were missing for 2 simulations.

## 2.3. Data Pre-Processing

Since there was a difference in the length of the driving simulations and sampling frequency of the different variables, the first step in pre-processing was resampling the data to a fixed number of observations for each participant. To do so, all measurements ($T_{nose}$, $T_{wrist}$, HR, and SSS) were subdivided in a fixed number of 9 windows. This specific number was chosen based on the average duration of the driving test (90 min) and the average number of SSS ratings (18 per simulation). Below, Figure 2 visualizes this first pre-processing step schematically.

Afterwards, the mean value for the data inside each window was calculated. Subsequently, the data for each person were scaled by subtracting the average temperature or heart rate. This step was performed to account for inter-individual variability in the baseline of the variables. For instance, the heart rate of one participant fluctuated around 50 bpm, whereas this was 70 bpm for someone else. Furthermore, the slope of the data inside each window was also determined by means of least squares linear regression. These slopes will be used as the main features to distinguish between drowsy and non-drowsy drivers. A positive value corresponds to an increase in the variable in a certain window. Conversely, a negative value indicates a decrease. All operations described above were executed using MATLAB® software (The Math works Inc., Natick, MA, USA).

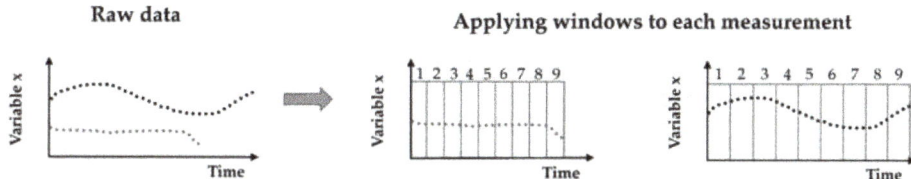

**Figure 2.** Visualization of pre-processing the data by subdividing each measurement into 9 windows. The black and grey dotted lines represent two fictional measurements for a certain variable x. Although the sampling frequency is the same for both measurements, the number of data points (i.e., length of the measurement) is not fixed. Accordingly, the number of data points inside the windows varies as well between the measurements.

### 2.4. Data Analysis and Classification

The first step in analyzing the data was looking for significant changes of $T_{nose}$, $T_{wrist}$, and HR for drowsy and non-drowsy subjects. The average trend over time was calculated for each variable as well as the distribution for each window. In addition, a Welch's ANOVA test was performed to check whether the data of the 9 windows were significantly different in their mean. The significance level ($\alpha$) was set to 5%, meaning that a p-value smaller than 0.05 indicated a significant difference. The Welch's test was chosen because it does not assume an equal variance in both distributions.

Secondly, in our attempt to distinguish between drowsy and non-drowsy subjects, we applied a decision tree approach based on changes in skin temperature and heart rate. This methodology aims to start from biological knowledge for building our classifier, which is in contrast to traditional data-based approaches. The latter type of methods focused mainly on accuracy or performance but did not lead to physiological insights per se. In essence, this approach was inspired by the methodology described in patent EP 2 842 490 B1 published in 2016 [28] as well as the observed trends in the data. More specifically for the skin temperatures, we expected an initial increase to facilitate heat loss for lowering the core body temperature ($T_C$). Afterwards, a gradual decrease in skin temperature was anticipated. On the other hand, a decrease in the heart rate was expected because energy and heat production in the body was supposed to go down. Based on this background, 3 univariate classifiers were built, which made their decisions based on the increases and decreases in the data. Hence, the classifications were performed based on $T_{nose}$, $T_{wrist}$, and HR. For the classification based on one of the temperature variables, a decision tree with 2 nodes was designed. The first nodes check whether an initial increase in the temperature occurred by evaluating the slope in the selected initial window (number 1, 2 or 3). Subsequently, the second node evaluated whether there was a decrease in temperature by looking at the slope in windows 4 to 9. Accordingly, the thresholds for both decision nodes were set to zero. Positive values for the slope corresponded to an increase in temperature and negative values to a decrease. On the other hand, for classification based on the heart rate, a decision tree with only one node assessed if HR was significantly decreasing over time. Figure 3 shows a schematic overview of both structures for the decision tree. For the decision tree based on the temperature variables, every combination of each 2 windows was tested. For the decision tree based on HR, all windows were tested separately. Information extracted from specific windows was used for classification to indicate the position of the most valuable information present in the data. The choice for a (combination of) window(s) was based on the performance of the corresponding decision tree. For this purpose, the sensitivity, specificity, and accuracy for each combination were determined. Here a "positive" test referred to a participant being labeled as "drowsy" by the classification algorithm. The windows that were used in the decision tree with the highest accuracy were selected in the end. The receiver operating characteristic (ROC) curves and corresponding area under the curve (AUC) values were calculated as well by changing the threshold from zero. The advantage of this method is that the results allow for a meaningful interpretation since the approach is based on physiological knowledge.

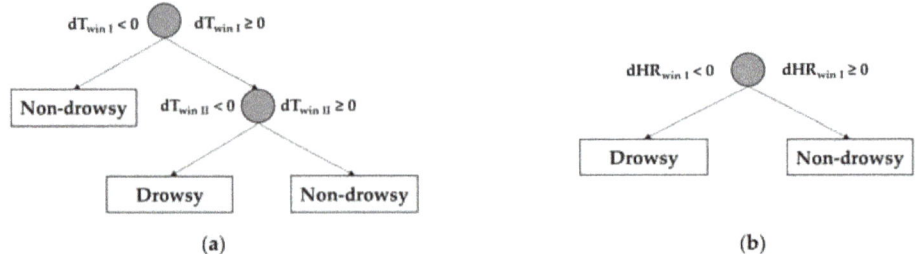

**Figure 3.** Schematic overview of the structure for the decision tree classification. (**a**) dT$_{win\ I}$ refers to the slope of the temperature in one of the initial windows of the measurement (number 1, 2, or 3). Accordingly, dT$_{win\ II}$ refers to the slope in either one of windows 4 to 9. As a result, the driver is labeled as "drowsy" when an increase in temperature is followed by a decrease. (**b**) dHR$_{win\ I}$ indicates the slope of the heart rate inside one of the nine windows.

In the final part of the analysis, classification was performed based on all 3 variables. For this, no predetermined structure was imposed. The only constraints were that the features (the sign of the slope inside a certain window) from the univariate classifications were used. Similarly, the sensitivity, specificity, and accuracy were used to evaluate the performance. However, it was not possible to determine ROC curves for this multivariate approach.

## 3. Results

### 3.1. Data Trends

As described above, the average trend in the distal skin temperatures, heart rate, and sleepiness score was calculated for both the group of drowsy and non-drowsy subjects. These trends and the corresponding 95% confidence interval are visualized in Figure 4. We note that on average T$_{nose}$ and T$_{wrist}$ increased over the first three windows (+0.55 and +0.91 °C, respectively), followed by a decrease (−1.05 °C and −2.01 °C, respectively) in the drowsy subjects. The skin temperatures of the non-drowsy subjects showed no such pattern. When looking at the heart rate, we observed that there was a decreasing trend for both the drowsy and the non-drowsy subjects, yet the trend appeared to be more distinct for drowsy drivers with an average decrease of 10 bpm compared to 3 bpm for the group of non-drowsy drivers. The sleepiness scores showed a linear increase from on average 2.5 to 6.7 and 2.3 to 3.1 for the drowsy and non-drowsy group, respectively. Furthermore, the results of the Welch's ANOVA are presented in Table 1. From these tests, we note that for drowsy subjects, the means of the windows differed significantly from each other in each of the four variables ($p$ <0.001). For the group of non-drowsy subjects, there was a significant difference in the mean of the heart rate between all nine windows, which indicated that the observed decreasing trend was significant ($p$ = 0.008). For the other three variables (T$_{nose}$, T$_{wrist}$, and SSS), the hypothesis that the means of all windows were equal was accepted.

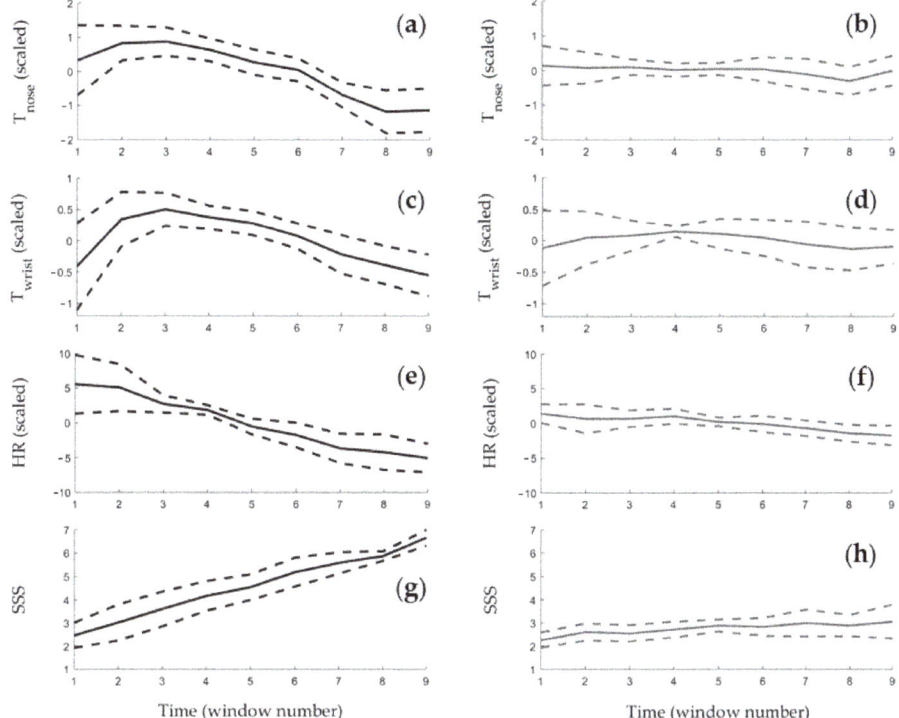

**Figure 4.** Average trend of $T_{nose}$, $T_{wrist}$, heart rate (HR), and Stanford sleepiness scale (SSS) in drowsy and non-drowsy subjects. (**a**) $T_{nose}$ in drowsy subjects, (**b**) $T_{nose}$ in non-drowsy subjects, (**c**) $T_{wrist}$ in drowsy subjects, (**d**) $T_{wrist}$ in non-drowsy subjects, (**e**) HR in drowsy subjects, (**f**) HR in non-drowsy subjects, (**g**) SSS in drowsy subjects, (**h**) SSS in non-drowsy subjects.

**Table 1.** Statistics of the Welch's ANOVA tests. The "degrees of freedom" for each test are indicated by dF. F indicates the corresponding F-statistic. "D" refers to the group of drowsy drivers and "ND" to the non-drowsy drivers.

| Welch's ANOVA | $T_{nose}$ | | $T_{wrist}$ | | HR | | SSS | |
|---|---|---|---|---|---|---|---|---|
| | D | ND | D | ND | D | ND | D | ND |
| dF | 9 | 8 | 8 | 8 | 8 | 7 | 9 | 8 |
| F | 11.8 | 0.5 | 7.9 | 0.9 | 15.7 | 3.5 | 54.2 | 1.9 |
| $p$-value | <0.001 | 0.820 | <0.001 | 0.493 | <0.001 | 0.008 | <0.001 | 0.097 |

### 3.2. Decision Tree Classification

Based on these observed trends, a decision tree classification was tested to distinguish between drowsy and non-drowsy participants. Afterwards, information about both the distal temperatures and the heart rate was used in a multivariate classifier.

3.2.1. Univariate Classification

The performance measures, as well as the selected window numbers for the three univariate decision trees, are presented in Table 2, and the corresponding ROC curves and AUC-values are shown in Figure 5. Firstly, a combination of the slope inside window 1 and 6 performs the best for the decision tree based on $T_{nose}$. In total, the condition of 13 out of 19 drivers was classified correctly.

Additionally, in case the classification was solely based on the information from window 6, this resulted in a sensitivity, specificity, and accuracy of 90.0%, 66.7%, and 79.0%, respectively. Secondly, when analyzing the temperature measured at the wrist, the combination of windows 2 and 4 came out on top. As mentioned, the data of 18 drivers were available. All participants that did not experience drowsiness were classified correctly, as well as 7 out of 9 "drowsy" drivers. For $T_{wrist}$ we did not observe an increase in the performance when the data of only one window were used. Third, the decision tree based on the information of the heart rate inside window 6 resulted in an overall accuracy of 70.6%. Here, these results are based on the data of 17 driving simulations.

**Table 2.** Performance of the different classifications based on information about $T_{nose}$, $T_{wrist}$, and HR. The "strict" multivariate classification refers to the fact that for all three variables, the imposed constraints must hold for a driver to be classified as drowsy. The "mild" classification represents the case when a driver is labeled as drowsy when only two out of three constraints are met. The sensitivity, specificity, and accuracy are expressed as a percentage. $N_{drowsy}$ and $N_{non-drowsy}$ indicate the number of samples used in each case.

| Classification | Windows | Sens. (%) | Spec. (%) | Acc. (%) | $N_{drowsy}$ | $N_{non-drowsy}$ |
|---|---|---|---|---|---|---|
| Univariate: $T_{nose}$ | 1 & 6 | 60.0 | 77.8 | 68.4 | 10 | 9 |
| Univariate: $T_{wrist}$ | 2 & 4 | 77.8 | 100.0 | 88.9 | 9 | 9 |
| Univariate: HR | 6 | 88.9 | 50.0 | 70.6 | 9 | 8 |
| Multivariate: "strict" | 6, 4 & 6 * | 50.0 | 100.0 | 75.0 | 8 | 8 |
| Multivariate: "mild" | 6, 4 & 6 * | 100.0 | 77.8 | 89.5 | 10 | 9 |

* Window number for $T_{nose}$, $T_{wrist}$, HR respectively.

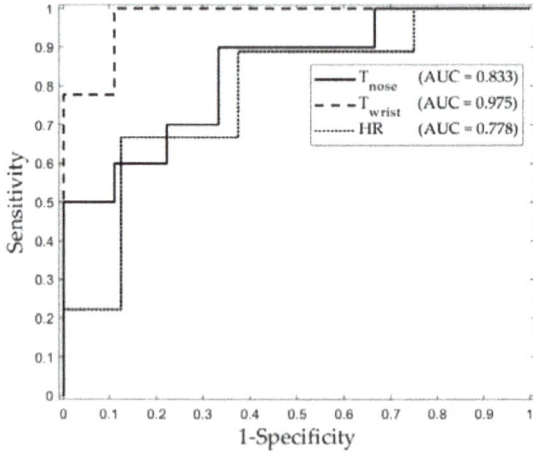

**Figure 5.** Receiver operating characteristic (ROC) curve and corresponding area under the curve (AUC) for the univariate classification based on $T_{nose}$, $T_{wrist}$, and HR.

3.2.2. Multivariate Classification

In the second classification approach, insights from the univariate classifications are combined to improve accuracy and robustness. Accordingly, the best performance was obtained by classifying the data based on the slope inside window 6 for $T_{nose}$, window 4 for $T_{wrist}$, and window 6 for HR. In a first, very strict classification approach, we imposed that for a certain simulation, the slope inside each of these windows had to be negative to classify the driver as drowsy. Accordingly, the order of the decisions was not of importance to this approach. In a second, milder classification approach, we assigned the label "drowsy" when at least two out of these three constraints were met. The performance of both classification types was also presented in Table 2 above. We note that the number of observations was not the same for both analyses. As mentioned in Section 2.2., the data of three simulations were missing information about $T_{wrist}$ or HR. Therefore, the first classification considered 16 out of 19 simulations. However, simulations with missing data can be considered in the second classification if the two available variables had the same sign of the slope inside the respective windows. Since this was the case for all three incomplete datasets, all 19 simulations were considered. Accordingly, we note that applying the strict constraints resulted in a specificity of 100.0% but also a relatively low sensitivity of 50.0%. Furthermore, an accuracy of 89.5% was observed under the mild constraints.

## 4. Discussion

### 4.1. Data Trends

From the first results presented in this study, it is clear that there are significant trends in the physiological variables of participants who became drowsy during the driving simulation. Moreover, these trends were not observed in participants that did not experience drowsiness. As expected, we observe an increase in both temperature variables in the first period of the driving simulation. This is in accordance with the fact that prior to sleep onset, the body dissipates heat via the extremities to lower the temperature of the core [29]. During this process, blood flow to the extremities is increased (vasodilation), which in turn increases the skin temperature. The result is an increased thermal gradient with the surrounding air to facilitate heat transfer to the environment. The subsequent decrease in skin temperature is also in line with the expectations. To avoid losing too much body heat, blood flow to the skin decreases again (vasoconstriction). Besides, the heart rate of drowsy drivers decreased on average more than that of non-drowsy drivers. We hypothesize that the decreasing trend rate can be interpreted as a secondary mechanism to control $T_C$, which is in accordance to the statements by Kräuchi and Wirz-Justice [20]. The human energy balance namely consists of energy producing and energy consuming (or reducing) components. Hence, the heart rate can be seen as a measure for providing energy to the body. Accordingly, lowering the heart rate means lowering the input to the energy balance. Nevertheless, we keep in mind that other physiological processes (e.g., stress) affect the heart rate and its dynamics as well. With respect to the SSS, we can infer that the test subjects evolved to a high sleepiness score in the first protocol, whereas this score did not increase significantly in the second protocol and fluctuated on average between two and three.

### 4.2. Decision Tree Classification

The first univariate classification based on information about the skin temperature of distal body parts (nose and wrist) shows promising results. The rather straightforward, predetermined structure of the decision trees, results in an accuracy between 68.4% and 88.9%. Moreover, AUC-values between 0.833 and 0.975 were observed. For both temperature variables, the specificity is higher than the sensitivity. This can be explained because two constraints have to be met for labeling the driver as "drowsy", whereas he/she can be labelled as "non-drowsy" after only one decision in the decision tree (see Figure 3). Moreover, we note that the performance for the classification based on $T_{wrist}$ are better than the performance of $T_{nose}$. When analyzing the raw data of both variables, we observed smaller changes in $T_{wrist}$ from sample to sample. Obviously, this was related to the much higher sampling frequency of $T_{wrist}$ (see Section 2.2. Data Collection). On the other hand, it has been shown that the temperature of the nose is also more variable. For example, it has been shown that the nose temperature changes periodically due to respiration [30]. Alternatively, an increased sensitivity and accuracy is observed when we only consider the information of window 6 for $T_{nose}$. From this, we conclude that the decrease in temperature is a more prominent feature for distinguishing between drowsy and non-drowsy drivers. Nevertheless, only considering this feature leads to more incorrect "drowsy" classifications, which is not surprising since the physiology behind temperature changes in relation to sleep onset suggests that both an increase and decrease occur. When considering the heart rate, a negative slope in window 6 is observed for 8 out 9 drivers who reached the SSS threshold and were labelled as "drowsy". In addition, such a decrease was also observed in half of the "non-drowsy" participants. Given the simplicity of the decision criterion, an overall accuracy of 70.6% stresses the significance of the decreasing trend in HR in our test population.

In the last section of the results, two classifications based on $T_{nose}$, $T_{wrist}$ and HR are presented. When the constraints for all three variables have to be met in order to label a driver as "drowsy", only four out of eight drivers who actually experienced drowsiness were labeled correctly. In contrast, no drivers were falsely labelled as being drowsy. Accordingly, the use of such stringent constraints can be applied to situations where false positive classifications are unacceptable. In other words, this methodology can be used when it is important to be certain that a driver labelled as drowsy, is actually drowsy. Nevertheless, a sensitivity of only 50.0% is not sufficient to distinguish between drowsy and non-drowsy drivers consistently. Evidently, using less stringent constraints results in a larger number of "drowsy" labels. Hence, all 10 drowsy drivers were labeled correctly. While the specificity is now decreased, we note that still 7 out of 9 non-drowsy drivers are correctly identified. This last classification resulted in an accuracy of 89.5%.

When comparing the different classification approaches, we note that the univariate classification for $T_{wrist}$ and the second multivariate classification resulted in similar accuracies (88.9% and 89.5%). Moreover, both results cannot be compared directly because the number of samples differs. The fact that a single temperature variable performs equally well as the multivariate classification indicates that including the heart rate for classifying the data does not add significant value to the current analysis.

*4.3. Comparison to State-of-the-Art Methods for Drowsiness Detection*

When comparing the performance of these classifications to related work on detecting driver drowsiness, we first note that, to our knowledge, no other studies make use of distal skin temperatures in their classification. Furthermore, only the patent by Berckmans et al. [28] presents a method based on similar signals, namely distal ear temperature and heart rate. Here, different conceptual approaches are described as well as the performance of one such method for a training and validation set; respective accuracies of 87.5% and 72.7% were obtained. On the other hand, multiple studies present methodologies to detect or monitor drowsiness based on information about the heart rate. More specifically, features related to heart rate variability (HRV) are most often used. For instance, Li and Chung [31] present a detection algorithm with an accuracy, sensitivity, and specificity of 95% each. In this study, two-minute-long drowsy and alert events were classified based on the ratio of low (0.04–0.15 Hz) to high frequency (0.15–0.40 Hz) variability in the heart rate obtained from photoplethysmography. In another study, ECG measurements were used to detect drowsiness based on HRV as well as respiratory frequency [32]. Here, a positive predictive value (PPV), sensitivity, and specificity of 96%, 59%, and 98%, respectively, was reported. In addition, an accuracy of around 78% corresponds to these results. In contrast to the two prior studies which used behavioral signs as a reference for the state of the driver, Fujiwara et al. validated their HRV-based drowsiness detection with EEG measurements [33]. Here, the algorithm was successful if drowsiness was indicated in a period of 15 min before sleep onset (NREM sleep stage 1). In 12 out of 13 subjects, sleep onset was detected in this timeframe. In comparison to these studies, our classification based on only the heart rate performs less well (an accuracy of 70.6%). However, HRV is interpreted as a measure for the dynamic control of the heart by different parts of the nervous system. In this study, the heart rate was interpreted as a part of the heat balance inside the human body. More specifically, HR represents the rate of aerobic heat production inside the body. Therefore, we also consider HR in combination with other components of the heat balance. Nonetheless, using ECG measurements in future research could make it possible to combine or compare these different approaches.

To put our own results further into perspective to the state-of-the-art, a couple of recent studies that used completely different variables and features are discussed hereafter. Firstly, Li et al. [34] present a smartwatch-based wearable EEG system for driver drowsiness detection. They designed a headband with three dry electrodes, instead of 21 electrodes used in the standard 10–20 system. In their analysis, they distinguished between "alert" and "drowsy" epochs that were labelled based on the percentage of eye closure (PERCLOS) and the number of adjustments on the steering wheel. The authors reported an average accuracy of 91.25% and 91.92% for detecting the alert and drowsy epochs, respectively. Secondly, Mandal et al. [12] developed a method to determine PERCLOS from images of a dome camera in a bus. Their results showed a matching rate between their method and a ground truth measure for PERCLOS of 85.02% and 95.18% for normal and fatigued drivers, respectively. Since their method was based on commercial technology that is already implemented in busses, monitoring bus drivers can be done unobtrusively. Thirdly, the work by Li et al. [13] presents yet a completely different approach. The fatigue level, scored by experts, was linked with data about the steering wheel angles (SWA) recorded under real driving conditions. The system was able to run on-line and performed with an accuracy of 78.01% in distinguishing drowsy from non-drowsy participants. In this research, we obtained accuracies between 70% and 90%, which is below the performances of the related state-of-the-art. Nevertheless, the results show potential for future research.

Lastly, it should be noted that each study applies different protocols and builds their classifier on different events or epochs. This makes it even more difficult to compare all results directly.

*4.4. Current Limitations and Future Perspectives*

Given the preliminary nature of this pilot study, several limitations and suggestions for future work are listed in this section. Firstly, more advanced methodologies and equipment will improve the quality of the obtained measurements. For instance, now a simple driving simulator is used as a basis for the experiments. Nowadays, there are simulators available with a driving experience very close to driving a real car. Nevertheless, when working with a simulator, lacking the danger of causing an accident is thought to affect the driver in his behavior [35]. On the other hand, purposely sending out drowsy drivers on the road would be unethical and illegal. Using wearable technology for ambulatory monitoring of the driver in real-life conditions might be a good alternative for this issue. Furthermore, applying a crossover study design in which each participant performs the driving test in drowsy and non-drowsy conditions would allow for a pairwise comparison of the individual direction and magnitude of the changes in thermoregulation. This is not possible with the current data since each driver only performed the test one time. Another way to improve the experimental work is by working with more advanced measures for determining the state of the driver. Now, each driver evaluates his/her state of alertness based on the SSS. Presumably, individual differences in the interpretation of each level of the SSS causes variability in the data. The use of EEG measurements (brain activity) could provide a solution to this issue. As mentioned, EEG is used as a gold standard in sleep research. Alternatively, scoring the driver's state based on an expert's opinion is also done in the literature. An expert can be trained in scoring the driver based on behavioral expressions. Although such a score is also the result of human interpretation, the variability due to a difference in the scorer is eliminated. A final remark on the applied methodology is the timing of the simulations. Currently, one fixed moment throughout the day is selected to perform the driving simulation. By executing the measurements at different moments, a generalization of the results is possible. For instance, Fujiwara et al. [33] used data collected at 11:00 and after lunch. However, we have to keep in mind that the theory behind this method is related to actual sleep onset and does not relate directly to short drops in attention throughout the day. Accordingly, future research on the proposed methodology will focus on this specific type of event. Related to the timing of these events, we expect that the observed physiological changes do not only occur at night. For instance, night shift workers have an altered sleep-wake cycle. In general, diurnal changes in body temperature and heart rate follow the daily activity-rest cycle [36].

Secondly, we discuss a number of limitations related to data analysis. At the moment, we applied a very straightforward method to determine significant differences in drowsy and non-drowsy drivers. Subdividing the measurements in a fixed amount of time windows was an inevitable part of the analysis. As mentioned, this is due to a difference in the length of the experiments. By applying the windows to the data and extracting the average value and the slope, a lot of detail, as well as information about the timing is lost. Nevertheless, this did not prevent us from identifying significant trends in the data and successfully distinguishing between drowsy and non-drowsy drivers. A follow-up study could either perform experiments of the same length or apply a time series approach to detect drowsiness over time and pinpoint key moments in the transition from an alert state to a drowsy one. Additionally, to allow for such a methodology to be applied in real-time and real-world situations, future research has to focus on using techniques such as recursive estimation and online time-series analysis to determine the increases and decreases in the variables in real-time. Overall, the current methodology for distinguishing between drowsy and non-drowsy drivers is elegant in its simplicity, allowing for a physiological interpretation of the results and indicates the potential of using thermoregulatory features for drowsiness detection. A final remark on the analysis is related to the lack of data for validation. Due to the limited number of measurements, no proper validation technique could be applied to the current dataset. Leave-one-out cross validation was briefly considered, however, this resulted in the same results for the training and test set. More specifically, only the selected window number could vary when using the decision tree classification. The selection for a (combination of) certain window(s), did not vary when only leaving out one observation at a time. Naturally, the lack of validation is identified as one of the most important limitations of the current communication.

## 5. Conclusions

In this work, the use of features extracted from distal skin temperatures and heart rate is tested for detecting drowsiness in driving simulations. In the first part of the analysis, we demonstrated that $T_{nose}$, $T_{wrist}$, and HR vary throughout the measurement in a specific pattern in participants who became drowsy. Initially, the temperature measured at the nose and the wrist increased to a maximal value. Subsequently, a gradual decrease in these temperature variables was observed. When studying the heart rate of the driver throughout each simulation, a significant decrease was observed in both drowsy and non-drowsy participants. However, the decreasing trend was more distinct in the group of drowsy drivers. Secondly, we showed that both populations of drivers (drowsy and non-drowsy) could be classified based on these observed trends in the data of $T_{nose}$, $T_{wrist}$, and HR. Despite the simplicity of these classifications, their performance indicates the potential for future research. The main advantage of the applied methodology is that it is based on knowledge about physiological processes related to sleep onset. Specifically, heat loss via the extremities and controlling of the heart rate regulates the decrease in core body temperature before and during sleep. A secondary classification approach was tested by using the information of all three different variables at the same time. From this analysis, we conclude that including the heart rate in our classification approach does not improve the performance significantly. Lastly, the current results were compared to the state-of-the-art in drowsiness monitoring and several limitations and suggestions for future research have been discussed.

**Author Contributions:** Conceptualization, J.G. and J.-M.A.; methodology, J.G.; formal analysis, J.G.; writing—original draft preparation, J.G. and J.-M.A.; writing—review and editing, J.G. and J.-M.A.; visualization, J.G.; supervision, J.-M.A.

**Funding:** This research received no external funding.

**Acknowledgments:** We would like to thank Steve De Raedt, Michiel De Vis, Arthur Devlieger, Robbert Jacobs, Jasmine Lalanto, Avitaj Mitra, Rahmath B. Paravakkal, Maarten Schoolmeesters, Laura Smets, Laura Verhelst, Wouter Verschueren, and Noor Vidts for their contribution to the experimental set-up and measurements, which was part of their students' project at the faculty of bio-science engineering at the KU Leuven.

**Conflicts of Interest:** The authors declare no conflict of interest.

## References

1. Tefft, B.C. *Prevalence of Motor Vehicle Crashes Involving Drowsy Drivers, United States, 2009–2013*; AAA Foundation for Traffic Safety: Washington, DC, USA, 2014.
2. Diependaele, K. *Sleepy at the Wheel. Analysis of the Extent and Characteristics of Sleepiness Among Belgian Car Drivers*; BRSI-KCRI: Brussels, Belgium, 2015.
3. Higgins, S.J.; Michael, J.; Austin, R.; Akerstedt, T.; Van Dongen, H.P.; Watson, N.; Czeisler, C.; Pack, A.I.; Rosekind, M.R. *Asleep at the Wheel: A National Compendium of Efforts to Eliminate Drowsy Driving*; NHTSA: Washington, DC, USA, 2017.
4. Waterhouse, J.; Fukuda, Y.; Morita, T. Daily rhythms of the sleep-wake cycle. *J. Physiol. Anthropol.* **2012**, *31*, 5. [CrossRef] [PubMed]
5. Johns, M.W. A sleep physiologist's view of the drowsy driver. *Transp. Res. Part F Traffic Psychol. Behav.* **2000**, *3*, 241–249. [CrossRef]
6. Sahayadhas, A.; Sundaraj, K.; Murugappan, M. Detecting driver drowsiness based on sensors: A review. *Sensors* **2012**, *12*, 16937–16953. [CrossRef] [PubMed]
7. Sikander, G.; Anwar, S. Driver Fatigue Detection Systems: A Review. *IEEE Trans. Intell. Transp. Syst.* **2018**, *20*, 2339–2352. [CrossRef]
8. Van De Water, A.T.M.; Holmes, A.; Hurley, D.A. Objective measurements of sleep for non-laboratory settings as alternatives to polysomnography—A systematic review. *J. Sleep Res.* **2011**, *20*, 183–200. [CrossRef] [PubMed]
9. Iber, C. *The AASM Manual for the Scoring of Sleep and Associated Events: Rules, Terminology and Technical Specifications*; American Academy of Sleep Medicine: Darien, IL, USA, 2007.
10. Grummett, T.S.; Leibbrandt, R.E.; Lewis, T.W.; DeLosAngeles, D.; Powers, D.M.W.; Willoughby, J.O.; Pope, K.J.; Fitzgibbon, S.P. Measurement of neural signals from inexpensive, wireless and dry EEG systems. *Physiol. Meas.* **2015**, *36*, 1469–1484. [CrossRef] [PubMed]
11. Choi, I.H.; Jeong, C.H.; Kim, Y.G. Tracking a driver's face against extreme head poses and inference of drowsiness using a hidden Markov model. *Appl. Sci.* **2016**, *6*, 137. [CrossRef]
12. Mandal, B.; Li, L.; Wang, G.S.; Lin, J. Towards Detection of Bus Driver Fatigue Based on Robust Visual Analysis of Eye State. *IEEE Trans. Intell. Transp. Syst.* **2017**, *18*, 545–557. [CrossRef]
13. Li, Z.; Li, S.E.; Li, R.; Cheng, B.; Shi, J. Online detection of driver fatigue using steering wheel angles for real driving conditions. *Sensors* **2017**, *17*, 495. [CrossRef] [PubMed]
14. Wakita, T.; Ozawa, K.; Miyajima, C.; Igarashi, K.; Itou, K.; Takeda, K.; Itakura, F. Driver identification using driving behavior signals. In Proceedings of the 8th International IEEE Conference on Intelligent Transportation Systems, Vienna, Austria, 13–16 September 2005.
15. Dehzangi, O.; Masilamani, S. Unobtrusive Driver Drowsiness Prediction Using Driving Behavior from Vehicular Sensors. In Proceedings of the 2018 24th International Conference on Pattern Recognition (ICPR), Beijing, China, 20–24 August 2018.
16. Taxonomy and Definitions for Terms Related to Driving Automation Systems for On-Road Motor Vehicles. Available online: https://www.sae.org/standards/content/j3016_201806/ (accessed on 15 July 2019).
17. Joan, C.; Shaun, K. Autonomous vehicles: No driver . . . no regulation? *Nature* **2018**, *361*, 2016–2018.
18. Aschoff, J.; Wever, R. Kern und Schale im Wärmehaushalt des Menschen. *Naturwissenschaften* **1958**, *45*, 477–485. [CrossRef]
19. Gilbert, S.S.; Van Den Heuvel, C.J.; Ferguson, S.A.; Dawson, D. Thermoregulation as a sleep signalling system. *Sleep Med. Rev.* **2004**, *8*, 81–93. [CrossRef]
20. Krauchi, K.; Wirz-Justice, A. Circadian rhythm of heat production, heart rate, and skin and core temperature under unmasking conditions in men. *Am. J. Physiol. Integr. Comp. Physiol.* **1994**, *38*, 819–829. [CrossRef] [PubMed]
21. Rowell, L.B. Human cardiovascular adjustments to exercise and thermal stress. *Physiol. Rev.* **1974**, *54*, 75–159. [CrossRef] [PubMed]
22. Quanten, S.; De Valck, E.; Cluydts, R.; Aerts, J.M.; Berckmans, D. Individualized and time-variant model for the functional link between thermoregulation and sleep onset. *J. Sleep Res.* **2006**, *15*, 183–198. [CrossRef] [PubMed]

23. Fiser, J.; Pokorny, J.; Podola, D.; Jıcha, M. Experimental Investigation of Car Cabin Environment During Real Traffic Conditions. *Eng. Mech.* **2013**, *20*, 229–236.
24. Cajochen, C.; Münch, M.; Kobialka, S.; Kräuchi, K.; Steiner, R.; Oelhafen, P.; Orgül, S.; Wirz-Justice, A. High sensitivity of human melatonin, alertness, thermoregulation, and heart rate to short wavelength light. *J. Clin. Endocrinol. Metab.* **2005**, *90*, 1311–1316. [CrossRef]
25. Hoddes, E.; Zarcone, V.; Smythe, H.; Phillips, R.; Dement, W.C. Quantification of Sleepiness: A New Approach. *Psychophysiology* **1973**, *10*, 431–436. [CrossRef]
26. Ting, P.H.; Hwang, J.R.; Doong, J.L.; Jeng, M.C. Driver fatigue and highway driving: A simulator study. *Physiol. Behav.* **2008**, *94*, 448–453. [CrossRef]
27. Brown, T.; Johnson, R.; Milavetz, G. Identifying Periods of Drowsy Driving Using EEG. *Ann. Adv. Automot. Med.* **2013**, *57*, 99–108.
28. Berckmans, D.; Aerts, J.-M.; Exadaktylos, V.; Taelman, J. Method and Device for Accurate Real-Time Detection of Drowsiness in Operators Using Physiological Responses. European Patent 2,842,490, 1 June 2016.
29. Krauchi, K.; Deboer, T. The interrelationship between sleep regulation and thermoregulation. *Front. Biosci.* **2010**, *15*, 604–625. [CrossRef]
30. Boccanfuso, L.; O'Kane, J.M. Remote measurement of breathing rate in real time using a high precision, single-point infrared temperature sensor. In Proceedings of the 2012 4th IEEE RAS & EMBS International Conference on Biomedical Robotics and Biomechatronics, Rome, Italy, 24–27 June 2012; pp. 1704–1709.
31. Li, G.; Chung, W.Y. Detection of driver drowsiness using wavelet analysis of heart rate variability and a support vector machine classifier. *Sensors* **2013**, *13*, 16494–16511. [CrossRef] [PubMed]
32. Vicente, J.; Laguna, P.; Bartra, A.; Bailón, R. Drowsiness detection using heart rate variability. *Med. Biol. Eng. Comput.* **2016**, *54*, 927–937. [CrossRef] [PubMed]
33. Fujiwara, K.; Abe, E.; Kamata, K.; Nakayama, C.; Suzuki, Y.; Yamakawa, T.; Hiraoka, T.; Kano, M.; Sumi, Y.; Masuda, F.; et al. Heart Rate Variability-Based Driver Drowsiness Detection and Its Validation With EEG. *IEEE Trans. Biomed. Eng.* **2019**, *66*, 1769–1778. [CrossRef] [PubMed]
34. Li, G.; Lee, B.L.; Chung, W.Y. Smartwatch-Based Wearable EEG System for Driver Drowsiness Detection. *IEEE Sens. J.* **2015**, *15*, 7169–7180. [CrossRef]
35. Hallvig, D.; Anund, A.; Fors, C.; Kecklund, G.; Karlsson, J.G.; Wahde, M.; Åkerstedt, T. Sleepy driving on the real road and in the simulator—A comparison. *Accid. Anal. Prev.* **2013**, *50*, 44–50. [CrossRef] [PubMed]
36. Zulley, J.; Wever, R.; Aschoff, J. The dependence of onset and duration of sleep on the circadian rhythm of rectal temperature. *Pflügers Arch. Eur. J. Physiol.* **1981**, *391*, 314–318. [CrossRef] [PubMed]

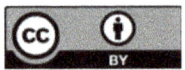

© 2019 by the authors. Licensee MDPI, Basel, Switzerland. This article is an open access article distributed under the terms and conditions of the Creative Commons Attribution (CC BY) license (http://creativecommons.org/licenses/by/4.0/).

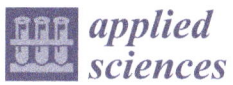 

*Article*

# Feature Engineering for ICU Mortality Prediction Based on Hourly to Bi-Hourly Measurements

**Ahmed Y. A. Amer** [1,2], **Julie Vranken** [3,4], **Femke Wouters** [3,4], **Dieter Mesotten** [3,4], **Pieter Vandervoort** [3,4], **Valerie Storms** [3,4], **Stijn Luca** [5], **Bart Vanrumste** [1] **and Jean-Marie Aerts** [2,*]

1. KU Leuven, E-MEDIA, Department of Electrical Engineering (ESAT) STADIUS, (ESAT) TC, Campus Group T, 3000 Leuven, Belgium
2. KU Leuven, Measure, Model & Manage Bioresponses (M3-BIORES), Department of Biosystems, 3000 Leuven, Belgium
3. Faculty of Medicine and Life Sciences, Hasselt University, 3500 Hasselt, Belgium
4. Ziekenhuis Oost-Limburg, Department of Anesthesiology, Department of Cardiology and Department Future Health, 3600 Genk, Belgium
5. Department of Data Analysis and Mathematical Modelling, Ghent University, 9000 Ghent, Belgium
* Correspondence: jean-marie.aerts@kuleuven.be

Received: 19 July 2019; Accepted: 24 August 2019; Published: 27 August 2019

**Abstract:** Mortality prediction for intensive care unit (ICU) patients is a challenging problem that requires extracting discriminative and informative features. This study presents a proof of concept for exploring features that can provide clinical insight. Through a feature engineering approach, it is attempted to improve ICU mortality prediction in field conditions with low frequently measured data (i.e., hourly to bi-hourly). Features are explored by investigating the vital signs measurements of ICU patients, labelled with mortality or survival at discharge. The vital signs of interest in this study are heart and respiration rate, oxygen saturation and blood pressure. The latter comprises systolic, diastolic and mean arterial pressure. In the feature exploration process, it is aimed to extract simple and interpretable features that can provide clinical insight. For this purpose, a classifier is required that maximises the margin between the two classes (i.e., survival and mortality) with minimum tolerance to misclassification errors. Moreover, it preferably has to provide a linear decision surface in the original feature space without mapping to an unlimited dimensionality feature space. Therefore, a linear hard margin support vector machine (SVM) classifier is suggested. The extracted features are grouped in three categories: statistical, dynamic and physiological. Each category plays an important role in enhancing classification error performance. After extracting several features within the three categories, a manual feature fine-tuning is applied to consider only the most efficient features. The final classification, considering mortality as the positive class, resulted in an accuracy of 91.56%, sensitivity of 90.59%, precision of 86.52% and $F_1$-score of 88.50%. The obtained results show that the proposed feature engineering approach and the extracted features are valid to be considered and further enhanced for the mortality prediction purpose. Moreover, the proposed feature engineering approach moved the modelling methodology from black-box modelling to grey-box modelling in combination with the powerful classifier of SVMs.

**Keywords:** feature engineering; intensive care unit; mortality prediction; hard-margin support vector machines

## 1. Introduction

Intensive care unit (ICU) patients are admitted because of an acute critical illness or because of the high need for intensive continuous monitoring. In addition, critical ICU patients are prone to rapid deterioration, resulting in a possibly fatal outcome when not monitored closely. Hence, the main challenge at the ICU is to reduce the morbidity of the admitted patients and prevent mortality which has a high likelihood due to severe illness [1]. Mortality prevention requires an intensive monitoring of vital signs, such as heart and respiration rate, oxygen saturation, non-invasive or arterial blood pressure, and so forth, that can capture clinical deterioration earlier and thus improve patient outcome. In the past, multiple scoring systems have been developed (e.g., Acute Physiology, Age, Chronic Health Evaluation II, Simplified Acute Physiology Score, Sequential Organ Failure Assessment) to provide insights and even predictions regarding ICU patient mortality [2]. However, these scoring systems are population-based and often use summarised nongranular data. This calls for the need for an in-depth investigation of vital signs and associated indicators preceding any deterioration using granular continuous data. This investigation can be handled by time-series analytics to understand the behaviour and interaction of different signals.

Most of the ICU mortality prediction studies focus on developing powerful mortality prediction models [3–16] in which the higher priority is to provide an accurate label or score about the admitted patients' status. One drawback of such an objective is paying less attention to features' simplicity and interpretability, which is the case with deep learning approaches [7–13]. The key approach in these studies is black-box modelling focusing mainly on predictive model error performance, regardless the interpretability of the features. Hence, the useful information that can be provided to the medical staff is strictly the prediction output. Moreover, a considerable number of relevant studies focus on investigating the continuously recorded vital signs of ICU patients in order to predict the mortality–risk of those patients [3–16]. A frequently used database in these studies is the medical information mart for intensive care (MIMIC) in its three releases (MIMIC, MIMIC II and III) with different versions [17,18]. These databases provide a diverse and very large population of ICU patients and contain high temporal resolution data including lab results, electronic documentation and bedside monitor trends and waveforms. In contrast, another approach that is used in investigating critically ill patients in the ICU is mechanistic modelling [19,20]. Mechanistic modelling is used to describe the system from mathematical and physical dynamics perspective. The main focus of mechanistic modelling is on the system dynamics, the interaction between the different variables and the way they interact from a system perspective taking into account biological and physiological laws [21]. A mechanistic modelling approach is used in investigating biological systems by developing mathematical models [22–24].

The main focus in this presented study is to engineer features that can provide clinical insight by which the medical staff is guided through the different parameters. However, prediction accuracy is used in this study to assess the relevancy of the extracted features to the mortality events. Moreover, the dataset in our study is a low frequently measured data (i.e., hourly to bi-hourly) as it is a daily-life dataset that is not generated for research purpose. Moreover, the set of variables, parameters and the investigated population here is limited compared to the ones provided by the MIMIC databases. In the light of the given approaches (Black-box predictive models and mechanistic models) and reviewed studies, our study stands between the two approaches (i.e., pure black-box modelling and mechanistic modelling), as the main focus of the study is to achieve an efficient and informative set of physiologically meaningful features (mechanistic aspect) by means of enhancing the predictive model error performance (black-box aspect) that could be representable for European ICU departments.

From an analytical perspective, the series of recordings for each vital sign is considered a time-series that is sampled by a specific sampling rate. During ICU monitoring, different vital signs are measured and recorded simultaneously, in which the simultaneity facilitates studying correlation, interaction and behaviour between and within the different vital signs. Moreover, the time-series of recorded vital signs enable extraction of different features (typically statistical and dynamic) within segmented time windows, showing the dynamic behaviour of the recorded sign.

Many features can be extracted within consecutive or overlapping time windows for different vital signs, either individually or in combination. This option provides a large number of dimensions that have to be evaluated and adjusted to inform the decision making of the algorithm, which requires an exhaustive investigation. However, such an investigation including a large number of numerical features is not an easy task for medical experts. Due to the high dimensionality issue, it is required to conduct such an investigation via a computational algorithm. In order to cope with these challenges, a simple and powerful classifier is used to explore the features. Ideally, this classifier should handle the problem of classification intuitively with the optimal margin hypothesis [25] which maximises the separability between the different classes. Moreover, the classifier should be capable of dealing with high dimensional data efficiently.

The proposed classifier for this purpose is the linear hard margin support vector machine (SVM) classifier which represents the simplest version of the powerful SVMs. The reason for using SVMs that it is relying on the maximum margin hypothesis. For linear hard margin SVM, it restrictively works efficiently once the input features provide linearly separable data points. With this property, it is feasible to extract features that may have a medical interpretation or physiological ground as the classifier would deal with the features as they are presented in the input space. In other words, it is required to have an acceptable performance only if the data points in the presented feature space are linearly separable with minimum misclassification error [25,26]. This error intolerance (or minimum tolerance) ensures that the introduced features provide a clear separation between the different classes (i.e., mortality and survival). Moreover, utilising such a linear classifier controls the dimensionality of the solution as it would only find a solution in the introduced dimensions. In other words, using a more sophisticated classifier (e.g., Radial Basis Function (RBF) SVM) would find a solution in an uncontrolled dimensionality, for instance, RBF SVM reaches infinite dimensionality due to the characteristics of the Gaussian kernel [26].

In this study, the problem is presented as integration between time-series prediction and classification. This integration is obtained by extracting features from the time-series and considering the dynamic behaviour of the time-series to construct the input space of the model. On the other hand, the output of the model is represented by the labels mortality/survival. The prediction is obtained by predicting the state (label) after the final record (last moment at ICU) on average 1.5 days ahead. The final record is the record preceding the patient's death (mortality label) or transfer to a lower care ward (survival label).

The objective of this study is to present a proof of concept for exploring features that can provide clinical insight through a feature engineering approach in order to improve the ICU mortality prediction in field conditions with low frequently measured data. The feature engineering approach is based on the hypothesis that utilising the linear hard margin SVM would provide a controllable and interpretable feature extraction approach.

This paper is arranged as follows: After the introduction, the second section of materials and methods comprises data description and an introduction to linear hard margin support vector machines. The third section includes the feature engineering process and results. The fourth section includes the discussion and the final section gives the conclusion.

## 2. Materials and Methods

### 2.1. Data

Data used for testing and evaluating the features were collected at the hospital Ziekenhuis Oost-Limburg (Genk, Belgium) during the period of 2015–2017. In detail, data were collected from patients hospitalised at the ICU and coronary care unit who were at these wards for at least ten days. Data consisted of vital parameters which were recorded continuously by Philips Intellivue monitors (Philips Electronics Nederland B.V., Amsterdam, The Netherlands), that recorded continuously and was annotated on average hourly to bi-hourly by the nursing staff. The recorded data was extracted from the electronic medical record for a total of 447 different patients, three of them readmitted to the unit again, hence, in total 450 recorded admissions annotated with either mortality or survival by discharge. The age of the patients was 65 ($\pm$16) years old, 305 of patients were males and 142 were females. The average duration of stay at the ICU is 20.96 days with a minimum of 10 days, maximum of 97 days, median of 30 days and IQR of 20–53 days of ICU stay. The vital parameter data consisted of the heart rate, the respiration rate, oxygen saturation, arterial blood pressure (ABP), non-invasive blood pressure (if ABP was not measured) and body temperature (not frequently). The patient population of the study has different reasons for ICU admission as shown in Figure 1. The local Ethical Committee was notified and approval was obtained (19/0023R).

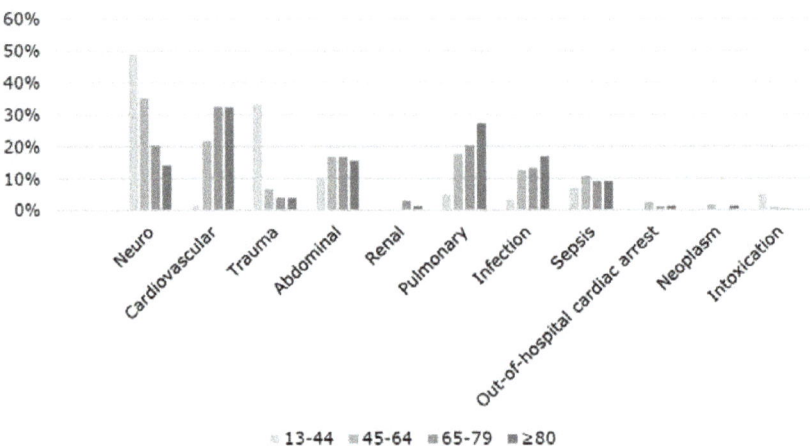

**Figure 1.** Distribution of the patient population and their reason for admission. The population was divided into age categories of 13–44, 45–64, 65–79 and >80 years of age.

*2.2. Hard-Margin SVM*

SVMs are originally presented as binary classifiers, that assign each data instance $\mathbf{x} \in \mathbb{R}^d$ to one of two classes described by a class label $y \in \{-1, 1\}$ based on the decision boundary that maximises the margin $2/||w||_2$ between the two classes as shown in Figure 2. The margin is determined by the distance between the decision boundary and the closest data point from each class [25–28].

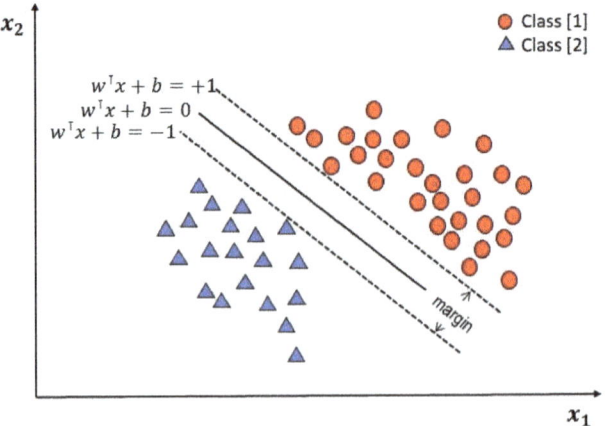

**Figure 2.** Schematic representation of a two-dimensional dataset consisting of two linearly separable classes. The dotted lines indicate the boundaries where the margin is maximised without tolerating any misclassifications (adapted from Reference [28]).

Generally, a feature map $\boldsymbol{\phi}: \mathbb{R}^d \mapsto \mathbb{R}^p$, where $d$ is the number of input space dimensions and $p$ is the number of feature space dimensions, is used to transform the geometric boundary between the two classes to a linear boundary $L: \mathbf{w}^\top \boldsymbol{\phi}(\mathbf{x}) + b = 0$ in feature space, for some weight vector $\mathbf{w} \in \mathbb{R}^{p \times 1}$ and $b \in \mathbb{R}$. The class of each instance can then be found by $y = \text{sgn}\,(w^\top \phi(x) + b)$, where sgn refers to the sign function.

The estimation of the boundary $L$ is performed based on a set of training examples $\mathbf{x}_i$ ($1 \leq i \leq N$) with corresponding class labels $y_i \in \{-1, 1\}$, where $N$ is the number of data points. An optimal boundary is found by maximising the margin that is defined as the smallest distances between $L$ and any of the training instances. In particular, one is interested in constants $\mathbf{w}$ and $b$ that minimise a loss-function [28]:

$$\min_{\mathbf{w}, b} \frac{1}{2} \mathbf{w}^\top \mathbf{w},$$

and are subject to:

$$y_i(\mathbf{w}^\top \boldsymbol{\phi}(x_i) + b) \geq 1, \qquad i = 1, 2, ..., N.$$

By applying the lagrangian to the problem we get

$$\mathcal{L}(\mathbf{w}, b; \alpha) = \frac{1}{2}\|\mathbf{w}\|_2^2 - (\sum_{i=1}^{N} \alpha_i (y_i [\mathbf{w}^\top \boldsymbol{\phi}(x_i) + b] - 1),$$

where $\alpha_i \geq 0$ are the Lagrangian multipliers for $i^{th}$ data point. By solving the optimisation problem

$$\max_{\alpha} \min_{\mathbf{w}, b} \mathcal{L}(\mathbf{w}, b; \alpha),$$

the following optimisation conditions are obtained:

$$\frac{\partial \mathcal{L}}{\partial \mathbf{w}} = 0 \longrightarrow \mathbf{w} = \sum_{i=1}^{N} \alpha_i y_i \phi(x_i),$$

$$\frac{\partial \mathcal{L}}{\partial b} = 0 \longrightarrow \sum_{i=1}^{N} \alpha_i y_i = 0,$$

$$\frac{\partial \mathcal{L}}{\partial \alpha} = 0 \longrightarrow y_i(\mathbf{w}^\top \boldsymbol{\phi}(x_i) - b) = 1,$$

The resulting classifier in both primal space and dual space are

$$f(\mathbf{x}) = \text{sgn}\,(\mathbf{w}^\top \boldsymbol{\phi}(x) + b),$$

$$f(\mathbf{x}) = \text{sgn}(\sum_{i=1}^{N} \alpha_i y_i \phi(x_i)^\top \boldsymbol{\phi}(\mathbf{x}) + b).$$

The dot product $\phi(x_i)^\top \boldsymbol{\phi}(\mathbf{x})$ is computationally expensive, hence, it is replaced with the *kernel* function $k(x_i, \mathbf{x})$, this replacement is known as the *kernel* trick. With the *kernel* trick, there is no need to execute the step of feature map as it is implicitly done by the *kernel* function. Hence, the dual space classifier with the *kernel* trick is

$$f(\mathbf{x}) = \text{sgn}(\sum_{i=1}^{N} \alpha_i y_i k(x_i, \mathbf{x}) + b).$$

For practical reasons, we suggest to obtain the linear hard margin SVM from the standard SVM formula that tolerate misclassifcation errors [29]

$$\min_{\mathbf{w},b;\xi} \frac{1}{2}\mathbf{w}^\top\mathbf{w} + C\sum_{i=1}^{N}\xi_i,$$

subject to:

$$y_i(\mathbf{w}^\top\boldsymbol{\phi}(\mathbf{x}_i) + b) \geq 1 - \xi_i \quad \text{and} \quad \xi_i \geq 0, \quad i = 1, 2, ..., N.$$

where the constant C denotes the *penalty term* that is used to penalise misclassification through the slack variables $\xi_i$ in the optimisation process. The linear hard margin SVM can be obtained via penalising the error extremely by giving C a very high value (e.g., $10^{10}$). With this trick, we can get a solution with misclassified instances to be investigated through the feature engineering phase.

## 3. Feature-Engineering

The process of feature engineering is implemented in an interactive way between extracting new features and the classifier error performance as shown in Figure 3. This process is executed in three phases: feature-extraction, evaluation and feature fine-tuning. This process has a closed-loop nature as shown in Figure 3, since the three phases influence each other. The proposed three categories of features are statistical features, dynamic features, physiological features. The following sections describe the different feature engineering phases and the extracted features per category.

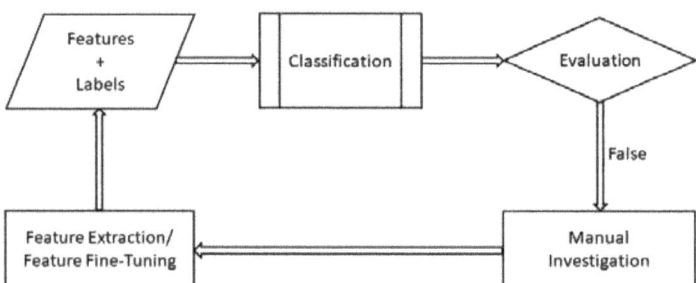

**Figure 3.** A flow chart illustrating the feature engineering methodology.

### 3.1. Evaluation

The engineered features are evaluated by feeding them into a linear hard-margin SVM classifier to predict mortality or survival of a subject. For this purpose, a leave-one-out procedure is used to produce a confusion matrix showing the true positives (TP), the true negatives (TN), the false positives (FP) and the false negatives (FN). The positive class is the mortality state and the negative class is the survival one. Using these numbers, different error performance metrics are calculated (i.e., sensitivity, precision, accuracy and $F_1$-score). Furthermore, we evaluate the features by looking at the effect on the number of true positives and true negatives when they are added to the model.

### 3.2. Feature Extraction

Firstly, all features are extracted within the last 84 observations which represent on average five days before the patient's discharge. The first 60 observations (3.5 days on average) out of 84 are considered for feature extraction to predict mortality/survival 24 observations ahead (1.5 days on average) at discharge (i.e., after observation 84). This period is determined after different test trials with different periods and is found to be the most efficient and informative period based on the classification performance. Moreover, this average period of 3.5 days agrees with the experience of clinical experts in the field. This agreement is based on the fact that there is no standard at the moment that refers to a minimum or maximum of observations to use, in order to provide the best of the care. As it is a human/medical judgement which made based on a combination of patient-specific prognosis and trends, clinical expertise and experience and often corresponds to 3–4 days. The scheme of the feature extraction process is shown in Figure 4. Three categories of features are extracted, as described below.

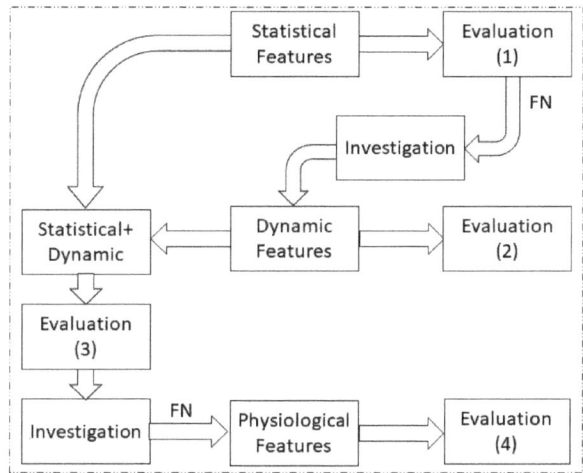

**Figure 4.** A flow chart illustrating the feature extraction process including the three feature categories (i.e., statistical, dynamic and physiological) and the sequence of the process marked by the evaluation steps. Also, in the process, the investigation is applied to the false negative patients only.

3.2.1. Statistical Features

The first category of features to be extracted is the set of statistical features which represent the basic characteristics of each time-series within segmented, non-overlapping time windows: *minimum, maximum, mean, median, standard deviation, variance,* and *energy*.

Statistical features are extracted within windows whose sizes are defined by the number of observations and not by a specific time period due to the nonuniform sampling rate (hourly to bi-hourly) as mentioned before. Extraction is based on the raw measurements of the vital signs and their first derivatives as well as the calculated standard early warning scores (EWS) of these measurements based on ZOL hospital standards. A weak point about statistical features is the static nature of these features as they do not reveal the dynamic behaviour of the time-series. Therefore, another category of features is required to be explored, namely dynamic features.

3.2.2. Dynamic Features

The extracted dynamic features are *Pearson correlation coefficients, crossing-the-mean count, outlier-occurrence count,* and *outlier indicator*. *Correlation coefficient* is computed between each pair of vital signs within each window. For this feature, it is necessary to be applied to the *z-score* of the vital signs. *Crossing-the-mean count* of a vital sign is determined by counting the number of times that the recorded vital sign crosses its mean value within each window. This feature indicates the abrupt changes in the vital sign from one observation to another. *Outlier-occurrence count* is computed by counting the number of outliers detected within each window. An outlier is detected by the statistical definition: any point outside the range $\mu \pm 3\sigma$ for a normally distributed variable is an outlier. For this feature, it is not expected to work with the vital sign of oxygen saturation ($SpO_2$) as it is negatively skewed, however, it will be tested as a feature to prove the concept. Finally, the *outlier indicator* is determined by the difference between the mean and the median of the records within each window.

### 3.2.3. Physiological Features

In order to enhance the classification performance, a manual investigation of the misclassified instances (based on the statistical and dynamic features) is required. The investigation is focusing on the false negative patients (i.e., deceased patients classified as survived) as the main objective is relevant to a reliable mortality prediction which is inversely proportional to the false negative count. This manual investigation is based on the measured physiological vital signs and uses physiological process knowledge resulting in physiological features. The different physiological features are described hereafter. By investigating the time-series of false negative patients, a consistent behaviour is noticed within the period of interest, in which the systolic blood pressure (SBP) approaches the diastolic blood pressure (DBP) as shown in Figure 5a.

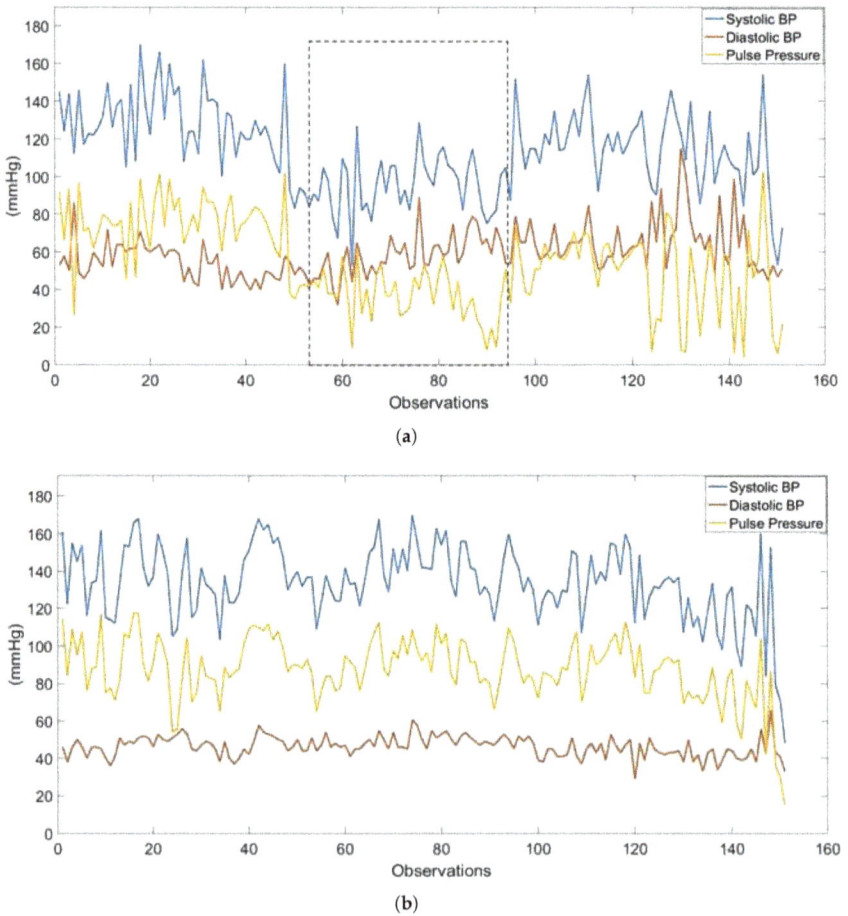

**Figure 5.** (a) Systolic blood pressure (BP), diastolic BP and pulse pressure (PP) of the last 150 observations (approximately the last nine days) of one false negative patient. The dashed window refers to the region where the systolic BP and diastolic BP measurements approach closely. (b) Systolic BP, diastolic BP and PP of the last 150 observations of another false negative patient. The mean value of the pulse pressure is 87.4 mmHg and median 88 mmHg.

It is found that the difference (SBP-DBP) within certain measurement periods is smaller than 20 mmHg. A relevant observation that is noticed with other false negative patients is that this difference is relatively high (i.e., greater than 60 mmHg) during certain measurement periods as shown in Figure 5b. This difference between SBP and DBP is also known as the pulse pressure ($PP$) and varies normally in a range between 40–60 mmHg [30,31]. As the $PP$ is a linear combination between two vital signs, it can be considered as a new variable from which both statistical and dynamic features can be extracted. By reviewing medical literature focusing on $PP$ and its effect on the mortality prediction (e.g., References [32,33]), our finding is partially consistent with their conclusion.

By further investigating the data, another behaviour is noticed with false negative patients, namely a frequent drop in respiration rate ($RR$) as shown in Figure 6a. Due to this behaviour, a new feature is proposed to represent this drop and the count of its occurrence. This feature is defined as the number of times the RR drops below a specific threshold within each window and is further referred as *low-RR count*. For this feature, two parameters are selected: the threshold and the window size. Both of them are searched exhaustively by maximising the classification performance by considering the new feature. The best-found combination is a threshold of 5 bpm and a window size of 60 observations.

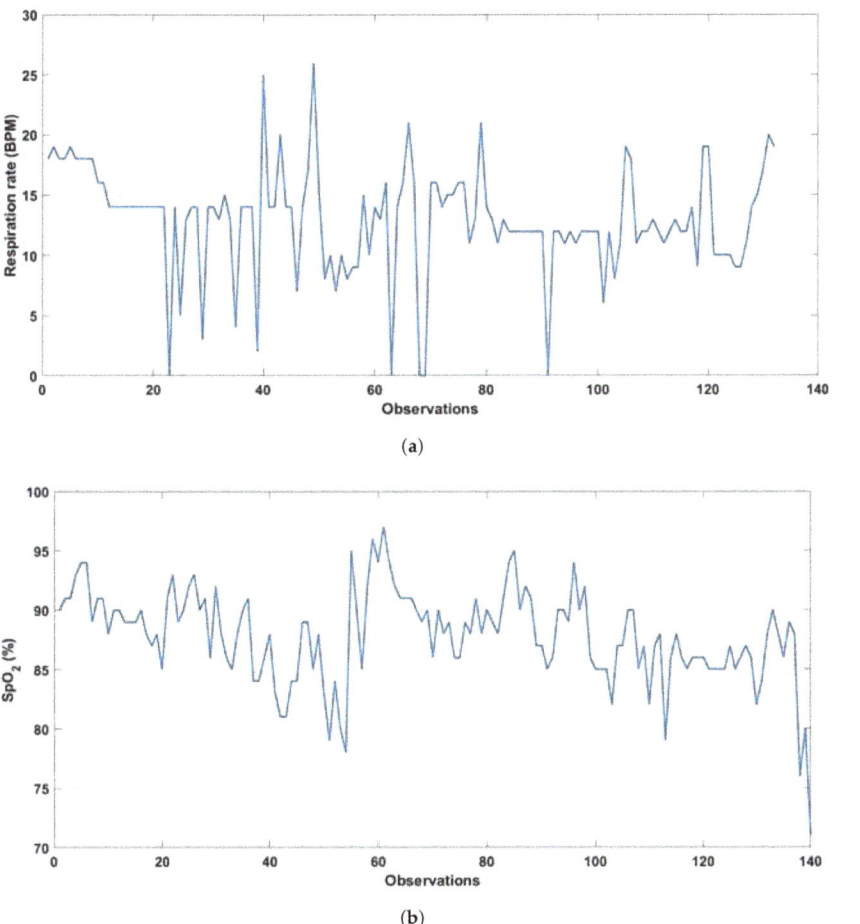

**Figure 6.** (**a**) Respiration rate of a deceased patient with an obvious drop at specific observations below the normal range (12–20 BPM) (**b**) Oxygen saturation ($SpO_2$) of another deceased patient that drops frequently (minimum 78% during the stay).

Another observation in some false negative patients' vital signs is a physiological feature related to a frequent drop of oxygen saturation $SpO_2$ as shown in Figure 6b. Similar to *low-RR count*, this feature is defined as the number of times the $SpO_2$ drops below a specific threshold within each window. Moreover, the threshold and window size combination affects the influence of the feature on the performance. The best-found combination is a threshold of 77% and a window size of 60. This feature is further referred to *low-$SpO_2$ count*.

Both, *low-$SpO_2$ count* and *low-RR count* created only an added value to the classification performance after the fine-tuning step.

Finally, a physiological feature that is imported directly from the patients' medical record is their positive and negative diagnosis with cardiovascular diseases ($CVD$). By considering this feature exclusively in the input space, no single positive class is recognised. However, by adding this feature to the optimal combination of features, a remarkable enhancement is achieved as will be discussed later.

### 3.3. Feature Fine-Tuning

After defining three different categories of features, it is necessary to fine-tune the proposed features in order to obtain the most efficient combination and representation of them. As will be shown in Section 4, the error performance can drop after combining features from different categories. One interpretation of this drop is that some features are strictly efficient for a group of patients and confusing for the rest. In order to limit this effect a fine-tuning step is performed.

The feature fine-tuning phase is based on the selection of vital signs instead of the selection of dimensions which is in contrast with existing automatic and conventional feature-selection techniques. Indeed, the rows of the input matrix of our data correspond with the different subjects in the study and contain the different features calculated on multiple windows (e.g., the statistical feature of mean is extracted from $m$ vital signs within $n$ time-windows resulting in $mn$ columns for each subject). Conventional feature-selection techniques select the columns of the matrix that are most representative for the study. However, in this way feature values within a specific time-window can be excluded leading to features that are hard to interpret. For this reason, we propose a backward selection approach where a feature (corresponding to multiple columns in the input matrix) can be excluded from the set of features. Moreover, prior knowledge is used in order to reduce the randomness in the selection process of the features. For instance, we will exclude the statistical and dynamic features of the $HR$ guided by the prior knowledge that the heart is a main actuator in the control system of a human body that responds to different excitations (e.g., medication), not only critical events [34]. The effect on the performance score of this selection will be discussed in Section 4.

The procedure of feature fine-tuning that we propose in this work starts with exploring whether statistical and dynamic features are providing high performance when extracted from all vital signs or strictly from a subset of these vital signs. Moreover, we assess the effect on the classification performance of using aggregate features which are calculated on a group of vital signs together rather than on individual vital signs. Furthermore, feature values can be presented as either real or absolute. This procedure is applied exhaustively to the statistical and dynamic features and is assessed by the error performance. The resulting fine-tuning (FT) steps are as follows:

1. FT1: For $HR$ extracted features, it is found that excluding both statistical and dynamic features enhances the error performance.
2. FT2: The *correlation coefficients* feature is found more efficient when presented in both real and absolute values.
3. FT3:*Outlier-occurrence count*, is found most efficient when applied to $SBP$, $MAP$, $RR$ and $PP$ excluding $DBP$ and $SpO_2$. Moreover, the *outlier-occurrence count* is found more efficient when presented in an aggregate form instead of individually except for the vital sign $SBP$.

4. FT4: The *correlation coefficients* feature is providing the best performance when computed only between $HR$ and $SBP$. Together with considering the features *low-$SpO_2$ count* and *low-RR count* the classification performance is improved.
5. FT5: *crossing-the-mean count* is found more efficient when applied only to $SBP$ and $RR$ and represented in the aggregate form.
6. FT6: The dynamic feature of *outlier indicator* is more efficient when applied only to $SBP$ and $DBP$.
7. FT7: Ultimately, considering the physiological feature of $CVD$ enhanced the performance.

## 4. Results

The obtained results based on the previously mentioned evaluation metrics for each category and for each fine-tuning step are explained below.

Starting with the statistical features, the resulting classification output is 83 TP's, 148 TN's, 87 FN's and 132 FP's. This result is fixed over the different test trials score-wise and patient-wise. In other words, the correctly classified patients are fixed over the different test trials because of using the linear hard margin SVM.

For dynamic features, the resulting classification output considering only the dynamic features is 32 TP's, 247 TN's, 138 FN and 33 FP's. Despite the remarkable reduction in the number of TP's, 18 new TP's are recognised by the dynamic features that are not recognised by the statistical features, in addition to 116 new TN's. This result is again fixed over the different test trials score-wise and patient-wise. With both statistical and dynamic features, the classifier performance is improved slightly compared to only statistical features with 2.8% increment in the accuracy. As the resulting classification output after combining both categories is 85 TP's, 159 TN's, 85 FN and 121 FP's. Despite the weak performance at this stage, the correctly classified instances are fixed with each test trial. This means that extracted features at this level are able to discriminate clearly between the correctly classified patients.

For physiological features, namely the $PP$, the resulting classification output with exclusively the extracted statistical and dynamic features of $PP$ is 45 TP's, 222 TN's, 125 FN's and 58 FP's. It is important to note that the investigated FN's at the earlier stage are correctly classified by the $PP$ extracted features. However, adding the $PP$ extracted features to both statistical and dynamic features provided the following results: 83 TP's, 118 TN's, 87 FN's and 162 FP's. The classification output of the different feature-categories combinations are shown in Figure 7a. Moreover, feature extraction results are combined and depicted in Table 1.

Table 1. Feature Extraction results.

| Feature Combination | TP | TN | FN | FP | Sensitivity (%) | Precision (%) | F1-Score | Accuracy (%) |
|---|---|---|---|---|---|---|---|---|
| Statistical (Stat) | 83 | 148 | 87 | 132 | 48.88 | 38.60 | 43.14 | 51.33 |
| Dynamic (Dyn) | 32 | 247 | 138 | 33 | 18.82 | 49.23 | 27.23 | 62.00 |
| Stat+Dyn | 85 | 159 | 85 | 121 | 50.00 | 41.26 | 45.21 | 54.22 |
| Physiological (Phy) | 45 | 222 | 125 | 58 | 26.47 | 43.69 | 32.97 | 59.33 |
| Phy+Stat+Dyn | 83 | 118 | 87 | 162 | 48.88 | 33.88 | 40.02 | 44.67 |

Before showing the results of the fine-tuning phase, we present the results of using the feature selection and ranking technique of automatic relevance determination (ARD) [28] based on backward selection method. The classification output of the ARD selected dimensions is 92 TP's, 218 TN's, 78 FN's and 62 FP's.

For the fine-tuning phase, the results are depicted in Table 2 and Figure 7b in a cumulative way.

Table 2. Feature Fine-tuning results.

| Cumulative Fine-Tuning Steps | Results | | | | | | | |
|---|---|---|---|---|---|---|---|---|
| | TP | TN | FN | FP | Sensitivity (%) | Precision (%) | F1-Score | Accuracy (%) |
| ARD | 92 | 218 | 78 | 62 | 54.12 | 59.74 | 56.80 | 68.89 |
| FT1 | 99 | 164 | 71 | 116 | 58.23 | 46.04 | 51.42 | 58.44 |
| +FT2 | 101 | 179 | 69 | 101 | 59.41 | 50.00 | 54.30 | 59.41 |
| +FT3 | 106 | 185 | 64 | 95 | 62.35 | 52.74 | 57.14 | 64.67 |
| +FT4 | 129 | 219 | 41 | 61 | 75.88 | 67.89 | 71.66 | 82.67 |
| +FT5 | 143 | 243 | 27 | 37 | 84.11 | 79.44 | 81.70 | 85.78 |
| +FT6 | 147 | 251 | 23 | 29 | 86.47 | 83.52 | 84.97 | 88.44 |
| +FT7 | 154 | 256 | 16 | 24 | 90.59 | 86.52 | 88.50 | 91.56 |

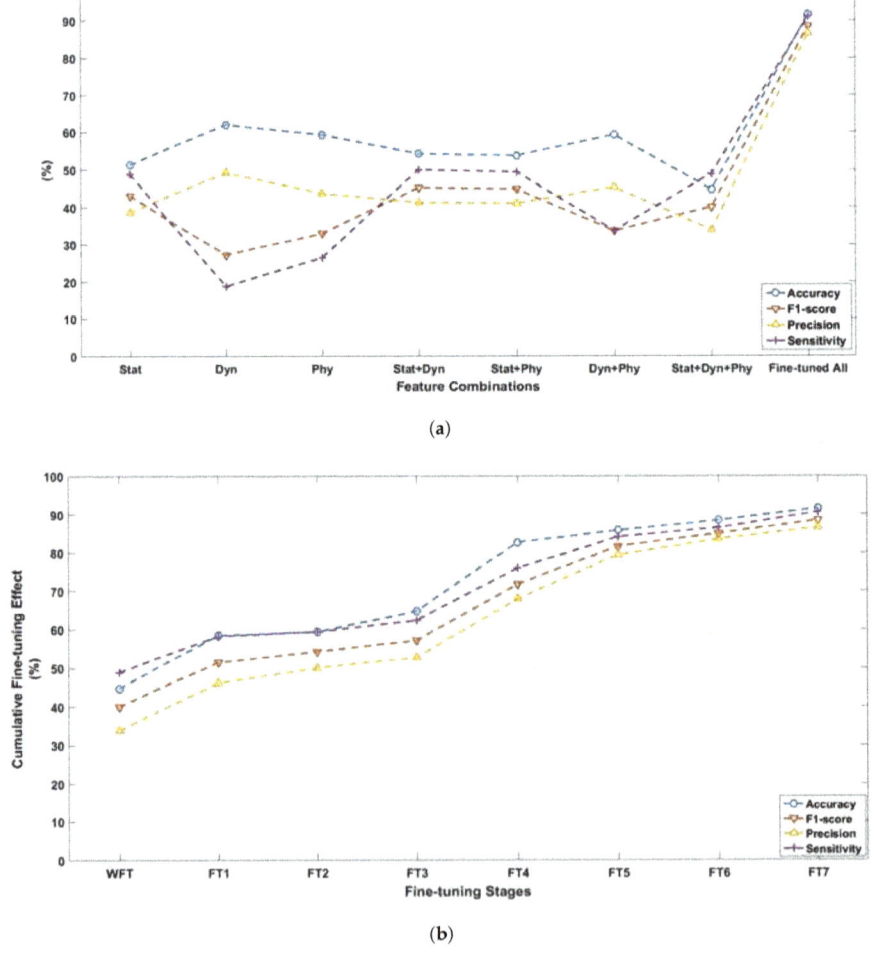

(a)

(b)

**Figure 7.** (a) $F_1$-score, accuracy, sensitivity and precision of the classifier with all possible combinations of the three feature categories in addition to the fine-tuned combination. (b) The cumulative effect of the different fine-tuning stages on the classification accuracy, $F_1$-score, precision, and sensitivity. WFT refers to 'without fine-tuning', FTx refers to the xth stage of fine-tuning as illustrated in the text.

## 5. Discussion

Many studies are using the area under receiver operating characteristics curve (AUC) as an evaluation metric. In this study, we prefer to use the confusion matrix for evaluation and direct quantification of error metrics of concern (e.g., sensitivity, precision). However, the calculated AUC for our optimised classifier is 0.91 for comparison purposes. This result, when compared to several recent studies is satisfactory. For instance, a recent study focusing on a special profile of ICU patients reported an AUC of 0.70 using a developed novel mortality prediction SOFA-RV [35]. Another study [12] that evaluates the Super ICU Learner Algorithm (SICULA) and its predictive power applied to MIMIC II database reported an AUC of 0.88 on average under specific conditions and 0.94 on average when applied to an external validation set with calibration. The study of Luo Y. et al. [11] reported an AUC of 0.848. Luo Y. et al. proposed an unsupervised feature learning algorithm that extracts features automatically from the clinical multivariate time-series. Luo Y. et al. applied their algorithm to the MIMIC-II [17] dataset with a prediction horizon extending to 30 days. The study in Reference [8] that developed a convolutional neural network (CNN) as a deep learning approach to predict mortality risk at ICU reported, as the highest performance, an AUC of 0.87, a precision of 0.7443 and a recall of 0.8188. The developed model used the variables of heart and respiration rate, systolic and diastolic blood pressure obtained from the MIMIC-III dataset [18]. Landon et al. [8] referred to the difficulties and limitations of using electronic medical report (EMR) data, similar to our dataset, for the purpose of mortality prediction at ICU. Nemati et al. in their study [36] of sepsis early prediction, which is a lead cause of morbidity and mortality of ICU patients, developed a machine learning model that reported an AUC of 0.83–0.85 for a prediction horizon of 12 down to 4 h prior to clinical recognition. Nemati et al. used an EMR data with high-resolution vital signs time-series obtained from the MIMIC-III dataset [18]. Two medical studies [32,33] reported an observed relevance between the low pulse pressure and mortality risk. Which is consistent with our finding of considering the pulse pressure as an independent variable from which both statistical and dynamic features can be extracted to inform mortality prediction. Moreover, the medical study in Reference [37] concludes the relevance between the widened (high) pulse pressure and the mortality risk for a special profile of critically ill patients. This conclusion as well is consistent with our finding, as we referred to the statistical and dynamic features of the pulse pressure which will indicate either abnormally high or low levels of pulse pressure. It is important to note that each study has different conditions, different objectives, different datasets, parameters and variables and predictive models.

At the feature extraction phase, the variation of results with different categories shows that a set of features can be efficient with a group of patients (i.e., correctly classified) but the same set of features can be inefficient or confusing to another group of patients (i.e., misclassified). For instance, statistical features classified correctly 83 TP's and 148 TN's, on the other hand, dynamic features classified correctly 32 TP's and 247 TN's. Considering the patient identity, it is found that dynamic features correctly classified 18 TP's and 116 TN's that the statistical features misclassified. The same observation is noticed with *PP* extracted features (45 TP's and 222 TN's) and those features extracted from both *SBP* and *DBP* together (72 TP's and 199 TN's). The difference in this situation is that *PP* is a result of a linear combination between *SBP* and *DBP*, however, *PP* extracted features correctly classified 14 TP's and 58 TN's that are misclassified by *SBP*/*DBP* extracted features. Hence, the influence of features should be evaluated on a subject-basis in addition to error metrics. Another observation is that the physiological features of *low-RR* and *low-SPO2 count* do not correctly classify any true positive patient despite their physiological basis when presented as the only input features. However, their contribution is significant when combined with the consistent set of features as shown at the feature fine-tuning phase. Therefore, excluding a feature has to be done after that it has been tested in combination with different groups of features especially if the extracted feature has a physiological basis.

At the fine-tuning phase, we have to note that this process is based on feature-vector-level not dimension-level as a single extracted feature may include multiple dimensions (e.g., the mean within each window for a specific vital sign). Which is in contrast with conventional feature selection techniques that rely on selecting the most relevant dimensions regardless of the interpretation of the selected dimensions. The initial modification is excluding both statistical and dynamic features extracted from $HR$ in order to enhance the performance. This modification is required as many of the cardiovascular patients in this study have common cardiac diseased behaviour, which confuses the classifier. Moreover, the heart acts as one of the main actuators in the human control system responding to different types of excitations. Hence, $HR$ disturbances might not be sufficient to predict mortality, leading to a high false alarm rate. Ultimately, considering the cardiovascular patients specifically, HR statistical characteristics, as well as their HR dynamic features are both technically confusing to mortality prediction. Moreover, the enhancement of detecting more TP's by presenting some dynamic features in an aggregate form can be interpreted by the fact that the concurrence of vital signs deterioration is partially a sufficient mortality indicator but not a necessary one. In other words, total deterioration implies mortality but not vice versa. Introducing the *correlation coefficients* feature with absolute values in addition to real values provides an improvement. Both absolute and real values help the linear classifier to distinguish between the instances based on the correlation strength and correlation sign respectively. Restricting the *crossing-the-mean count* to $SBP$ and $RR$ caused an improvement. Thus, observation-to-observation variability of both vital signs even for a relatively low sampling rate (i.e., 0.5–1 sample/hour) is more informative than the other vital signs for resting patients such as ICU patients.

As the main objective of this study is to engineer feature that can provide clinical insight about mortality prediction, it is important to refer to the decision tree classifiers. As one of the decision trees advantages is model interpretability in terms of the input attributes. However, some shortages are present in decision trees in contrast with SVM's that supported the choice of the latter. These shortages are mainly the greedy nature of the algorithm, local optimisation, prone to overfitting and expensive computational cost compared to linear hard margin SVM in which there are no hyperparameters to optimise. Moreover, we based our study on the optimal margin hypothesis which is not provided by decision trees in contrast with SVM's. For comparison reasons, a decision tree analysis is applied to the final set of features. A CART algorithm decision tree (MATLAB 2017) is used with the following settings: the splitting criterion of *gdi*, minimum parent size of 368, minimum leaf size of 184, maximum splits of 450 and pruning based on classification error criterion. The classification output of the optimised decision tree is as follows: sensitivity of 41.2% precision of 42.42%, F1-score 41.80% and accuracy of 52.22%. It is obvious that the results are poor compared to the results of linear hard margin SVM. The poor performance is quite expected because of the conceptual differences between the two classification techniques (i.e., Decision trees and SVMs). It is possible that if the whole feature engineering process is designed based on the decision tree classifier properties, the results can be better.

Model development, feature extraction and fine-tuning are implemented on observation-basis instead of time-basis (hourly/daily). We hypothesise that observation-basis are more realistic as the events (observations) within a specific time period are more informative than time period regardless of the number of observations. Ideally, the number of observations is fixed along a specific period for all patients and uniformly distributed as well which is not the case with our dataset. However, for a proof of concept, we evaluate the classification performance based on extracting the same features on time-basis. Time-basis is implemented by considering the last 7 days before discharge, considering the first 5 days for feature extraction to predict mortality 2 days ahead. These periods are defined based on the observation-basis analysis. By extracting statistical, dynamic and physiological features without fine-tuning, the output classification performance is 88 TP's, 163 TN's, 82 FN's and 117 FP's. In comparison with the classification performance on observation-basis (83 TP's, 118 TN's, 87 FN's and 162 FP's) the error performance is higher.However, by following the same feature fine-tuning steps the final classification output (82 TP's, 160 TN's, 88 FN's and 120 FP's) is dropped compared to that obtained by an observation-based approach (154 TP's, 256 TN's, 16 FN's and 24 FP's). This drop can be interpreted by the fact that the fine-tuning phase is a manual crafting of the feature combination which is sensitive to the features setup (i.e., observation-basis or time-basis).

## 6. Conclusions

In this study, we proposed a proof of concept for a feature engineering approach to explore features that can provide clinical insight in order to enhance the mortality prediction of ICU patients using the machine learning algorithm of linear hard margin SVM. The optimal combination of features that provided the best classification performance comprises the following features:

1. Statistical features of the raw physiological variables, their first derivative of $SBP$, $DBP$, $MAP$, $RR$, $SpO_2$ and $PP$. Moreover, the statistical features extracted from the EWS of $SBP$, $RR$ and $SpO_2$. A window size of 15 observations.
2. Real and absolute values of *correlation coefficients* between $HR$ and $SBP$ in a window size of 30 observations.
3. *Outlier-occurrence count* of $SBP$, $MAP$, $RR$ and $PP$. represented in an aggregate form except for the $SBP$ represented individually as well. A window size of 60 observations.
4. *crossing-the-mean count* of $SBP$ and $RR$, it is presented in the aggregate form. A window size of 60 observations.
5. *Outlier indicator* of $SBP$ and $DBP$. A window size of 60 observations.
6. *Low-$SpO_2$ count* less than 77% and *low-RR count* less than 5 $BPM$. A window size of 60 observations.

The proposed approach allows moving from black-box to grey-box modelling, starting from a powerful black-box technique such as SVMs. Moreover, in this case study, low frequently measured vital signs (hourly to bi-hourly) enabled us to extract efficient features for the purpose of relatively long term analysis.

From a feature engineering perspective, some features or variables are individually unable to distinguish between the two classes (i.e., mortality and survival). However, by combining such features in suitable feature combinations, their use becomes beneficial. Furthermore, combining different efficient features might cause a drop in performance. Therefore, a feature fine-tuning phase is essential in order to synthesise efficient feature-combination.

From the medical perspective, we can conclude that the heart rate as an individual variable can be confusing to predict the mortality. This conclusion is supported by improving the error performance by excluding the heart rate features. Moreover, we can recommend paying more attention to the pulse pressure explicitly, either high or low level, since both levels are found associated with the mortality of a group of patients. Watching the pulse pressure requires implicitly to consider the diastolic blood pressure which is excluded from the EWS standards. Finally, we conclude that different profiles of patients require a different set of features to handle the mortality prediction efficiently.

For future work, we propose to test the developed model with the extracted features along the stay of the ICU patients. In other words, we can scan the complete period of stay with the moving window of 60 observations for feature extraction to predict the mortality-risk 24 observations ahead. Despite the fact that along the stay the patients will be labelled as survival, the medical doctors may label any upcoming events with possible mortality-risk.

**Author Contributions:** Conceptualization, A.Y.A.A., P.V., S.L., B.V. and J.-M.A.; Data curation, J.V., F.W. and V.S.; Formal analysis, A.Y.A.A.; Investigation, A.Y.A.A.; Methodology, A.Y.A.A.; Resources, D.M. and P.V.; Software, A.Y.A.A.; Supervision, S.L., B.V. and J.-M.A.; Validation, A.Y.A.A.; Visualization, A.Y.A.A., J.V.; Writing—original draft, A.Y.A.A.; Writing—review and editing, A.Y.A.A., J.V., S.L., B.V. and J.-M.A.

**Funding:** This research is funded by a European Union Grant through wearIT4health project. The wearIT4health project is being carried out within the context of the Interreg V-A Euregio Meuse-Rhine programme, with EUR 2,3 million coming from the European Regional Development Fund (ERDF). With the investment of EU funds in Interreg projects, the European Union directly invests in economic development, innovation, territorial development, social inclusion and education in the Euregio Meuse-Rhine.

**Conflicts of Interest:** The authors declare no conflict of interest. The funders had no role in the design of the study; in the collection, analyses, or interpretation of data; in the writing of the manuscript, or in the decision to publish the results.

## References

1. Braber, A.; van Zanten, A.R. Unravelling post-ICU mortality: Predictors and causes of death. *Eur. J. Anaesthesiol.* **2010**, *27*, 486–490. [CrossRef] [PubMed]
2. Goldhill, D.R.; McNarry, A.F.; Mandersloot, G.; McGinley, A. A physiologically-based early warning score for ward patients: The association between score and outcome. *Anaesthesia* **2005**, *60*, 547–553. [CrossRef] [PubMed]
3. Lokhandwala, S.; McCague, N.; Chahin, A.; Escobar, B.; Feng, M.; Ghassemi, M.M.; Stone, D.J.; Celi, L.A. One-year mortality after recovery from critical illness: A retrospective cohort study. *PLoS ONE* **2018**, *13*, e0197226. [CrossRef] [PubMed]
4. Celi, L.A.; Galvin, S.; Davidzon, G.; Lee, J.; Scott, D.; Mark, R. A database-driven decision support system: Customized mortality prediction. *J. Pers. Med.* **2012**, *2*, 138–148. [CrossRef] [PubMed]
5. Celi, L.A.; Tang, R.J.; Villaroel, M.; Davidzon, G.A.; Lester, W.T.; Chueh, H.C. A clinical database-driven approach to decision support: Predicting mortality among patients with acute kidney injury. *J. Healthc. Eng.* **2011**, *2*, 97–110. [CrossRef] [PubMed]
6. Johnson, A.E.W.; Mark, R.G. Real-time mortality prediction in the Intensive Care Unit. *AMIA Ann. Symp. Proc.* **2017**, *2017*, 994–1003.
7. Alves, T.; Laender, A.; Veloso, A.; Ziviani, N. Dynamic Prediction of ICU Mortality Risk Using Domain Adaptation. *IEEE Int. Conf. Big Data* **2018**, 1328–1336. [CrossRef]
8. Landon, B.; Aditya, P.; Izzatbir, S.; Clayton, B. Real Time Mortality Risk Prediction: A Convolutional Neural Network Approach. *Int. Conf. Health Inf.* **2018**, 463–470. [CrossRef]
9. Zhu, Y.; Fan, X.; Wu, J.; Liu, X.; Shi, J.; Wang, C. Predicting ICU Mortality by Supervised Bidirectional LSTM Networks. In Proceedings of the IJCAI 2018 Joint Workshop on Artificial Intelligence in Health (AIH 2018), Stockholm, Sweden, 13–19 July 2018; pp. 49–60.
10. Johnson, A.E.; Pollard, T.J.; Mark, R.G. Reproducibility in critical care: A mortality prediction case study. *Mach. Learn. Healthc. Conf.* **2017**, *2017*, 361–376.
11. Luo, Y.; Xin, Y.; Joshi, R.; Celi, L.; Szolovits, P. Predicting ICU Mortality Risk by Grouping Temporal Trends from a Multivariate Panel of Physiologic Measurements. In Proceedings of the AAAI Conference on Artificial Intelligence, Phoenix, AZ, USA, 12–17 February 2016.
12. Pirracchio, R.; Petersen, M.L.; Carone, M.; Rigon, M.R.; Chevret, S.; van der Laan, M.J. Mortality prediction in intensive care units with the Super ICU Learner Algorithm (SICULA): A population-based study. *Lancet Respir. Med.* **2015** *3*, 42–52. [CrossRef]
13. Mayaud, L.; Lai, P.S.; Clifford, G.D.; Tarassenko, L.; Celi, L.A.; Annane, D. Dynamic data during hypotensive episode improves mortality predictions among patients with sepsis and hypotension. *Crit. Care Med.* **2013**, *4*, 954–962. [CrossRef]
14. Verplancke, T.; Van Looy, S.; Benoit, D.; Vansteelandt, S.; Depuydt, P.; De Turck, F.; Decruyenaere, J. Support vector machine versus logistic regression modeling for prediction of hospital mortality in critically ill patients with haematological malignancies. *BMC Med. Inform. Dec. Mak.* **2008**, *8*, 56–63. [CrossRef]
15. Kim, S.; Kim, W.; Park, R.W. A Comparison of Intensive Care Unit Mortality Prediction Models through the Use of Data Mining Techniques. *Healthc. Inform. Res.* **2011** *17*, 232–243. [CrossRef]
16. Vieira, S.M.; Mendonça, L.F.; Farinha, G.J.; Sousa, J.M. Modified binary PSO for feature selection using SVM applied to mortality prediction of septic patients. *Appl. Soft Comput.* **2013**, *13*, 3494–3504. [CrossRef]
17. Saeed, M.; Villarroel, M.; Reisner, A.T.; Clifford, G.; Lehman, L.W.; Moody, G.; Heldt, T.; Kyaw, T.H.; Moody, B.; Mark, R.G. Multiparameter Intelligent Monitoring in Intensive Care II (MIMIC-II): A public-access intensive care unit database. *Crit. Care Med.* **2011**, *39*, 952–960. [CrossRef] [PubMed]
18. Johnson, A.E.W.; Pollard, T.J.; Shen, L.; Li-Wei, H.L.; Feng, M.; Ghassemi, M.; Moody, B.; Szolovits, P.; Celi, L.A.; Mark, R.G. MIMIC-III, a freely accessible critical care database. *Sci. Data* **2016**, *3*, 160035. [CrossRef] [PubMed]
19. Aerts, J.M.; Haddad, W.M.; An, G.; Vodovotz, Y. From data patterns to mechanistic models in acute critical illness. *J. Crit. Care* **2014**, *29*, 604–610. [CrossRef]
20. Young, P.C. *Recursive Estimation and Time-Series Analysis: An Introduction*; Springer Science and Business Media: Berlin, Germany, 2012.

21. Vodovotz, Y.; Csete, M.; Bartels, J.; Chang, S.; An, G. Translational systems biology of inflammation. *PLoS Comput. Biol.* **2008**, *4*, e1000014. [CrossRef]
22. Kumar, R.; Clermont, G.; Vodovotz, Y.; Chow, C.C. The dynamics of acute inflammation. *J. Theor. Biol.* **2004**, *230*, 145–155. [CrossRef]
23. Reynolds, A.; Rubin, J.; Clermont, G.; Day, J.; Vodovotz, Y.; Ermentrout, G.B. A reduced mathematical model of the acute inflammatory response: I. Derivation of model and analysis of anti-inflammation. *J. Theor. Biol.* **2006**, *242*, 220–236. [CrossRef]
24. Day, J.; Rubin, J.; Vodovotz, Y.; Chow, C.C.; Reynolds, A.; Clermont, G. A reduced mathematical model of the acute inflammatory response II. Capturing scenarios of repeated endotoxin administration. *J. Theor. Biol.* **2006**, *242*, 237–256. [CrossRef]
25. Boser, B.E.; Guyon, I.M.; Vapnik, V.N. A training algorithm for optimal margin classifiers. In Proceedings of the Fifth Annual Workshop on Computational Learning Theory, Pittsburgh, PA, USA, 27–29 July 1992; pp. 144–152.
26. Cortes, C.; Vapnik, V. Support-vector networks. *Mach. Learn.* **1995**, *20*, 273–297. [CrossRef]
27. Suykens, J.A.K.; Vandewalle, J. Least Squares Support Vector Machine Classifiers. *Neural Process. Lett.* **1999**, *9*, 293–300. [CrossRef]
28. Suykens, J.A.K.; Van Gestel, T.; De Brabanter, J.; De Moor, B.; Vandewalle J. *Least Squares Support Vector Machines*; World Scientific Publishing Co.: Singapore, 2002.
29. Abu-Mostafa, Y.S.; Malik, M.-I.; Hsuan-Tien, L. *Learning from Data*; AMLBook: New York, NY, USA, 2012.
30. Homan, T.D.; Cichowski, E. *Physiology, Pulse Pressure*; StatPearls [Internet]; StatPearls Publishing: Treasure Island, FL, USA, 2018.
31. Stergiopulos, N.; Segers, P.; Westerhof, N. Use of pulse pressure method for estimating total arterial compliance in vivo. *Am. J. Physiol.-Heart Circ. Physiol.* **1999**, *276*, H424–H428. [CrossRef]
32. Yildiran, T.; Koc, M.; Bozkurt, A.; Sahin, D.Y.; Unal, I.; Acarturk, E. Low pulse pressure as a predictor of death in patients with mild to advanced heart failure. *Texas Heart Inst. J.* **2010**, *37*, 284–290.
33. Voors, A.A.; Petrie, C.J.; Petrie, M.C.; Charlesworth, A.; Hillege, H.L.; Zijlstra, F.; McMurray, J.J.; van Veldhuisen, D.J. Low pulse pressure is independently related to elevated natriuretic peptides and increased mortality in advanced chronic heart failure. *Eur. Heart J.* **2005**, *26*, 1759–1764. [CrossRef]
34. Grodins Fred, S. *Control Theory and Biological Systems*; Columbia University Press: New York, NY, USA, 1963.
35. Akin, S.; Caliskan, K.; Soliman, O.I.; Muslem, R.; Guven, G.; Van Thiel, R.J.; Struijs, A.; Gommers, D.; Zijlstra, F.; Bakker, J.; et al. A novel mortality risk score predicting intensive care mortality in cardiogenic shock patients treated with veno-arterial extracorporeal membrane oxygenation. *Eur. Heart J.* **2018**, *39*, 5690. [CrossRef]
36. Nemati, S.; Holder, A.; Razmi, F.; Stanley, M.D.; Clifford, G.D.; Buchman, T.G. An Interpretable Machine Learning Model for Accurate Prediction of Sepsis in the ICU. *Crit. Care Med.* **2018**, *46*, 547–553. [CrossRef]
37. Al-Khalisy, H.; Nikiforov, I.; Jhajj, M.; Kodali, N.; Cheriyath, P. A widened pulse pressure: A potential valuable prognostic indicator of mortality in patients with sepsis. *J. Community Hosp. Intern. Med. Perspect.* **2015**, *5*, 29426. [CrossRef]

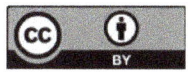

© 2019 by the authors. Licensee MDPI, Basel, Switzerland. This article is an open access article distributed under the terms and conditions of the Creative Commons Attribution (CC BY) license (http://creativecommons.org/licenses/by/4.0/).

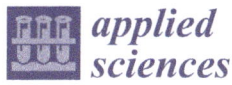 

*Article*

# Real-Time Model Predictive Control of Human Bodyweight Based on Energy Intake

Alberto Peña Fernández [1], Ali Youssef [1], Charlotte Heeren [1], Christophe Matthys [2,3] 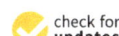 and Jean-Marie Aerts [1,*]

[1] Department of Biosystems, Division Animal and Human Health Engineering, M3-BIORES: Measure, Model & Manage of Bioresponses Laboratory, KU Leuven, Kasteelpark Arenberg 30, 3001 Heverlee, Belgium
[2] Nutrition & Obesity, Clinical and Experimental Endocrinology, Department of Chronic Diseases, Metabolism and Aging, KU Leuven, UZ Herestraat 49, 3000 Leuven, Belgium
[3] Clinical Nutrition Unit, Department of Endocrinology, University Hospitals Leuven, 3000 Leuven, Belgium
* Correspondence: jean-marie.aerts@kuleuven.be

Received: 3 June 2019; Accepted: 25 June 2019; Published: 27 June 2019

**Featured Application:** *This work sets the basis for developing a control system that allows managing, in an automated and individualized manner, human bodyweight in terms of energy intake, by taking advantage of the real-time monitoring capabilities of the ever-growing wearable technology sector.*

**Abstract:** The number of overweight people reached 1.9 billion in 2016. Lifespan decrease and many diseases have been linked to obesity. Efficient ways to monitor and control body weight are needed. The objective of this work is to explore the use of a model predictive control approach to manage bodyweight in response to energy intake. The analysis is performed based on data obtained during the Minnesota starvation experiment, with weekly measurements on body weight and energy intake for 32 male participants over the course of 27 weeks. A first order dynamic auto-regression with exogenous variables model exhibits the best prediction, with an average mean relative prediction error value of 1.01 ± 0.02% for 1 week-ahead predictions. Then, the performance of a model predictive control algorithm, following a predefined bodyweight trajectory, is tested. Root mean square errors of 0.30 ± 0.06 kg and 9 ± 3 kcal day$^{-1}$ are found between the desired target and simulated bodyweights, and between the measured energy intake and advised by the controller energy intake, respectively. The model predictive control approach for bodyweight allows calculating the needed energy intake in order to follow a predefined target bodyweight reference trajectory. This study shows a first possible step towards real-time active control of human bodyweight.

**Keywords:** weight loss; mHealth; dynamic model; adaptive control

---

## 1. Introduction

Managing one's own weight can be a difficult task to perform [1]. In order to assist people in managing their weight, it is important to know the required calorie intake. An imbalance in energy intake versus energy expenditure over a longer period can lead to severe changes in body weight [2]. A positive energy balance, meaning that the energy intake is higher than the energy expenditure, results in an increase in body fat [3]. A long-term positive energy balance can lead to overweight (body mass index (BMI) = 25–29.9 kg·m$^{-2}$) or even obesity (BMI ≥ 30 kg·m$^{-2}$), a syndrome that negatively affects the cardiovascular system [4]. Obesity is associated with different clinical manifestations such as diastolic dysfunction [5], cancers [6], atrial fibrillation due to pericardial fat [7], hypertension and coronary heart diseases [4]. In 2010, obesity caused more than 3 million deaths worldwide [8]. In 1975, the total number of obese men and women amounted up to 34 million and 71 million, respectively. These numbers rose up to 266 million men and 375 million women in 2014 [4], reaching more than 1.9 billion overweight people in 2016 [9]. Furthermore, the most worrisome trend is the rising rates of obesity in children and adolescents, the prevalence of which tripled between 1971 and 2002 [10]. By contrast, a negative energy balance leads to being underweight. Its prevalence in developed nations is increasing due to voluntary and involuntary caloric restriction [3]. Therefore, a prolonged imbalance in energy intake is a risk factor for several diseases (e.g., diabetes, anorexia of ageing) and affects a large number of people. Thus, it is important to find new and more efficient ways to monitor and control body weight [11].

Health professionals (e.g., dietitians, physical trainers) are qualified to assist individuals in their quest to obtain an optimized energy balance. Based on our own research, we have proven that digital applications (e.g., use of smartphone, wearables . . . ) can assist in optimizing the energy balance and the health professionals are considered as buddies [12]. Nowadays, smartphones and wearables are suitable tools to collect and process information. The built-in digital cameras, sensors, storage capabilities and wireless connectivity of smartphones can be beneficial for automatic dietary monitoring [13,14]. In addition, smartphone applications are able to give direct feedback and are already used as tools to monitor physical health [15]. Currently, there are numerous smartphone applications available to track in an individualized and objective manner weight, physical activity and dietary energy intake [16,17]. However, studies show that the engagement of individuals with these apps decreases after some time, even when personalized suggestions are provided [15,18,19]. One of the contributing aspects to this may rely on the fact that nowadays, empirical equations describing the nutrition process are used to predict weight loss and/or to advise dietary energy intake levels. Although these equations are extremely relevant to gather knowledge about the nutrition process, their parameters are estimated at a population-based level. Therefore, inaccurate predictions or suggestions are obtained when applied to data from a single individual. This can diminish the trust in the smartphone app, leading to a loss of engagement and adherence to the suggestions, finally quitting its use [18–20].

Past and current theoretical models describing the nutrition process are based on the first thermodynamics law on energy conservation [2,21]. Based on some of the earliest models proposed, still nowadays, many health institutions recommend reducing daily calorie intake with 2 MJ to lose 0.5 kg in 1 week, known as the 3500 kcal rule [21]. However, comparisons between weight loss predicted by the 3500 kcal rule and dynamic models are performed, confirming the invalidity of this rule [22,23]. The human body has its own feedback system to regulate body mass, meaning that an increase or decrease of energy intake does not directly relate to a change in body mass [24,25]. Decades ago, multiple dynamic models describing changes in bodyweight based on changes in energy expenditure and energy intake were already proposed to account for this [24–28]. Even models applied during starvation were proposed with the aim of characterizing how the body stores and metabolizes energy in the absence of food [29,30]. Besides, more complex models attempting to refine the description of the adaptation process of the human body during weight loss, as perturbations to the macronutrients metabolization and energy flux balances, have been proposed [2,31–33]. The main drawbacks of these models are their high complexity and the fact that they rely on several a priori assumptions and parameter estimates based on population-based averages. These drawbacks are highlighted in [11,34] and reduced models are proposed, although the parameter estimates still rely on population-averaged values. It is also proposed that previous models addressed the body adaptation process as an open-loop systems instead as a closed-loop one [11].

Therefore, although theoretical models provide a good insight in weight control process, there are other external and internal factors, which affect macronutrient metabolization and energy flux balances and that should be considered. For instance, new insights from the domain of chrono-nutrition indicate that, the rate of energy absorption varies in time [35,36]. These recent insights determine the best time to consume meals and the suitable meal proportions and its impact on bodyweight status [37,38]. Therefore, the main limitation of the current models is that the algorithms are developed at population-based level and cannot account for the individual time-variant characteristics of each individual person. Biological systems, such as the human body, should be considered as complex, individual, time-varying and dynamic (CITD) systems [39]. Data-based mechanistic (DBM) models can be suitable for modelling such systems. While DBM models are based on a simple model structure, they allow coping with non-linear characteristics of the process by estimating the model parameters in real-time, which are only accepted if they can be interpreted in meaningful physical/physiological terms [40]. Even though real-time monitoring of weight is still at its early stages in humans, other sectors such as the farming industry already use real-time monitoring of weight to optimize feeding and breeding activities. Data-based modelling has already proven useful in the emerging precision feeding control in livestock [41,42]. In [41], an algorithm to control the growth trajectory of broiler chickens based on an adaptive dynamic process model is developed. In [43], this model predictive growth control is tested in a real broiler farm. In farm conditions, the mean relative error (MRE) between actual and target weight trajectories was 7.3%. Besides, the model proved to be beneficial in broiler farms, suggesting the possibility of using the model predictive control for other purposes such as for weight control in human beings [41].

Therefore, the aim of this work is to test the capabilities of DBM models to develop a model predictive control (MPC) system, which allows estimating individualized dietary energy intake needed to achieve a desired change in bodyweight. Such a system could be implemented easily in current smartphone applications for tracking weight, energy intake and physical activity in real time. Automatic, individualized and accurate dietary energy intake suggestions are expected to increase the engagement to the application and the adherence to the suggestions of the users, as well to assist dietitians in the individualized treatment of patients.

## 2. Materials and Methods

### 2.1. Data Collection

The dataset used in this work is retrieved from an on-line accessible experimental dataset from the Minnesota starvation experiment, described by [30]. In this study, the energy intake of 32 male participants (age between 20 and 33 years old) is reduced to resemble the weight loss in undernourished prisoners of war. Prior to the 24 weeks of energy restriction (S1–S24), a 12-week control phase (C1–C12) is used to bring all participants as close to the group norm as possible. Information on daily energy intake for each participant during the control phase is available for only the last three weeks (C10–C12). For each participant, an average of daily energy intake for each week of the starvation period is specified. The starvation phase is followed with a recovery phase of 20 weeks (R1–R20). However, no information on daily energy intake is obtained during this last phase of the Minnesota starvation experiment. Physical activity is mandatory during both, control and starvation phases, and includes at least 35 km of walking per week. Total energy expenditure (TEE) is not directly measured but estimated based on resting energy expenditure (REE) and energy expended during physical activity (EEPA). REE is calculated the week prior to the starvation phase and at the end of the starvation phase. Therefore, no weekly estimation on TEE is provided. During the entire study, each participant is weighed once every week. Therefore, the dataset is comprised by the averages of body weight and daily energy intake from the last 3 weeks of the control phase and the entire starvation phase for the 32 test participants. The average height of the participants present in the dataset is $H = (1.79 \pm 0.06)$ m. The average initial and final bodyweights are $BW_i = (69.50 \pm 0.10)$ kg and $BW_f = (53 \pm 4)$ kg. Finally, the average energy intake during the last three weeks of the control phase is $EI_c = (3.5 \pm 0.3) \cdot 10^3$ kcal day$^{-1}$, and the average energy intake during the starvation experiment is $EI_s = (1.6 \pm 0.2) \cdot 10^3$ kcal day$^{-1}$.

## 2.2. Modelling

A description of the basis for the data-based mechanistic framework tested is given in [40]. In essence, the data-based mechanistic approach firstly infers the deterministic model structure inductively from the data. Afterwards, this model structure, and associated parameters, are only accepted if they can be interpreted in physically meaningful terms according to the process under study [40]. Thus, in this study, firstly a time-invariant parameters single-input, single-output (SISO) transfer function (TF) modelling approach is used to identify the transfer function model structure, which allows characterizing the relation between the energy intake and bodyweight for each individual subject. Afterwards, in line with the aim of this study, the forecasting properties of time-variant parameters models, dynamic linear regression (DLR) and dynamic auto-regression with exogenous variables (DARX) models are studied in order to evaluate their potential to monitor in real-time and forecast the time-varying bodyweight development of the participants. Finally, the model selected as best, according to its performance in terms of the minimal mean relative prediction error (MRPE), is used to develop a model predictive controller and to simulate the energy intake advice by it. MATLAB® (MATLAB 2015b, The Mathworks, Inc.) Software and the CAPTAIN Toolbox is used to perform the data-based mechanistic approach [44,45].

### 2.2.1. Time-Invariant Single-Input, Single-Output (SISO) Transfer Function (TF) Model

For the system identification process, a SISO TF model with time-invariant parameters is tested. The model has the following general structure [46],

$$y(k) = \frac{B(z^{-1})}{A(z^{-1})} u(k-\delta) + \xi(k) \qquad (1)$$

where $y(k)$ and $u(k)$ are the output (bodyweight [kg]), and the input (energy intake [kcal day$^{-1}$]) of the model, respectively; $\xi(k)$ is additive noise assumed to be zero mean, serially uncorrelated sequence of random variables with variance $\sigma^2$, accounting for measurement noise, modelling errors and effects of unmeasured inputs to the process; $k$ is the sample of the measurement; $\delta$ is the time delay of the input, expressed in number of time intervals; $A(z^{-1})$ and $B(z^{-1})$ are two series given by:

$$A(z^{-1}) = 1 + a_1 z^{-1} + a_2 z^{-2} + \ldots + a_{n_a} z^{-n_a} \qquad (2)$$

$$B(z^{-1}) = b_0 + b_1 z^{-1} + b_2 z^{-2} + \ldots + b_{n_b} z^{-n_b} \qquad (3)$$

where $a_j$ and $b_j$ are the model parameters to be estimated; $z^{-1}$ is the backward shift operator, i.e., $z^{-1} y(k) = y(k-1)$, with $y$ and $k$ defined as in Equation (1); $n_a$ and $n_b$ are the orders of the respective $A$ and $B$ polynomials. The model parameters are estimated using a refined instrumental variable (RIV) approach [46]. Normally, the model is referred to as the triad [$n_a$ $n_b$ $\delta$].

In order to test the fitting accuracy of the different models estimated, the goodness of fit is quantified using the coefficient of determination, $R_T^2$. Its general expression is given by [46],

$$R_T^2 = 1 - \frac{\sigma_e^2}{\sigma_y^2} \qquad (4)$$

where $\sigma_e^2$ is the variance of the residuals, when comparing the model estimations with the output measured values, and $\sigma_y^2$ is the variance in the output. In addition, the Young information criterion (YIC) is estimated. It is given by the following expression [46],

$$YIC = \log_e\left(\frac{\sigma_e^2}{\sigma_y^2}\right) + \log_e\left(\frac{1}{h} \sum_{i=1}^{h} \frac{\sigma_e^2 \cdot \hat{p}_{ii}}{\hat{a}_i^2}\right) \qquad (5)$$

where $\sigma_e^2$ is the variance of the residuals, $\sigma_y^2$ is the variance of the output, $h$ is the number of estimated parameters, $\hat{p}_{ii}$ are the diagonal elements of the covariance matrix from the parameters estimations and $\hat{a}_i^2$ is the square value of the $i$-th parameter. The first term of YIC is simply a relative measure of how well the model explains the data. The smaller the model residuals the more negative the term becomes. The second term provides a measure of the conditioning of the instrumental variable cross product matrix. If the model is over-parameterized, then it can be shown that this matrix will tend to singularity and, because of its ill conditioning, the elements of its inverse will increase in value, often by several orders of magnitude. Then, the second term in YIC tends to dominate the criterion function, indicating over-parameterization [46].

2.2.2. Time-Variant Parameters Models

As it is expected that the relationship between energy intake and bodyweight varies throughout the monitored period (i.e., behaves in a time-varying way), a dynamic auto-regression with exogenous variables (DARX) modelling approach is tested further. The model structure is similar to that described in Equation (1) but allowing the model parameters in the $A$ and $B$ series to vary over time [46]. The DARX expression is given by,

$$y_t = \frac{B(z^{-1}, t)}{A(z^{-1}, t)} u_{t-\delta} + \frac{1}{A(z^{-1}, t)} e_t \qquad (6)$$

in which the previous $A$ and $B$ series described by Equations (2) and (3) are now expressed as,

$$A(z^{-1}, t) = 1 + a_{1,t} z^{-1} + a_{2,t} z^{-2} + \ldots + a_{n_a,t} z^{-n_a} \qquad (7)$$

$$B(z^{-1}, t) = b_{0,t} + b_{1,t} z^{-1} + b_{2,t} z^{-2} + \ldots + b_{n_b,t} z^{-n_b} \qquad (8)$$

In order to estimate the time-variable model parameters, $a_{i,t}$ and $b_{i,t}$, it is necessary to make some assumptions about the nature of their temporal variability. In this approach, it is assumed that they show a stochastic evolution described by a general random walk process [46] and they are estimated using a sliding window approach, similarly to the work of [47]. By this sliding window approach, the effect of obsolete data is minimized. In terms of the biological process, this time variation of the parameters allows the modelling approach accounting for external influences to the process, such as environmental or health aspects, which are not explicitly taken into account in the model [47].

Following a similar procedure, a dynamic linear regression modelling approach is also tested. The DLR is the simplest state space model using time-variant parameters. Its general expression is given by:

$$y_t = T_t + \sum_{i=1}^{m} b_{i,t} u_{i,t} \qquad (9)$$

where $y_t$ is the output or dependent variable (bodyweight); $T_t$ is a trend or low frequency component; $b_{i,t}$ are time-varying parameters over the observational interval which reflect possible changes in the regression relationship; and $u_{i,t}$ are the inputs of the model (energy intake), which are assumed to affect the dependent variable $y_t$ [46]. In this study, on each discrete time instant $t$, for feed amount or composition the linear relation can be written as:

$$BW_t = c_{1,t} + c_{2,t} EI_t \qquad (10)$$

with BW the measured bodyweight (kg) and EI the energy intake (kcal day$^{-1}$) at time $t$. $c_{1,t}$ (kg) and $c_{2,t}$ (kg·kg$^{-1}$) are the time-variant model parameters estimated at time $t$. More specifically, the parameter $c_{1,t}$ is expected to resemble the general bodyweight trend exhibited by each individual. Also, the parameter $c_{2,t}$, is expected to resemble the energy efficiency at time $t$ (defined as change of bodyweight per change of energy intake). The fitting agreement is tested using the normalized root mean square error (NRMSE) given by,

$$NRMSE = 1 - \frac{\|BW_{ref} - BW_{fit}\|}{\|BW_{ref} - avg(BW_{ref})\|} \quad (11)$$

where $BW_{ref}$ is the weight curve used as reference, $BW_{fit}$ is the weight curve obtain by the model and $avg(BW_{ref})$ is the average value of the bodyweight reference curve. The NRMSE provides a value in the range $(-\infty, 1]$, being 1 a perfect fitting agreement.

Besides, the prediction accuracy of the DARX and DLR models is also tested. The accuracy of the model predictions is investigated by applying the recursive estimation algorithm combining different window sizes $S$ and prediction horizons $F$ to each dataset. In this work, window sizes ranging from 3 to 15 weeks and a prediction horizons ranging from 1 to 7 weeks have been tested. As a result, for each dataset, 91 (13 × 7) combinations of window size and prediction horizon are evaluated. Then, the goodness of the predictions is quantified by means of the mean relative prediction error (MRPE), which is given by,

$$MRPE = \frac{1}{N} \sum_{t=1}^{N} \sqrt{\left(\frac{W_t - \widehat{W_t}}{W_t}\right)^2} \cdot 100 \quad (12)$$

where MRPE is expressed as a percentage; $N$ is the number of samples; $W_t$ (kg) is the bodyweight measured at time $t$ and $\widehat{W_t}$ (kg) is the predicted weight at time $t$ [47].

### 2.3. Model Predictive Control (MPC)

After selecting in the previous steps the best time-invariant parameters and time-variant parameters models, a model predictive control (MPC) system is developed. An MPC solves an optimization problem to advise the dependent variable or input needed to the system in order to achieve an output or independent variable, according to the model included in the controller, the closest to the desired or reference output. The standard cost function is generally described as function of four terms, each one focusing on a particular aspect of the controller performance [48],

$$J(z_k) = J_y(z_k) + J_u(z_k) + J_{\Delta u}(z_k) + J_\epsilon(z_k) \quad (13)$$

where $J_y(z_k)$ is related to the output reference tracking performance,

$$J_y(z_k) = \sum_{j=1}^{n_y} \sum_{i=1}^{p} \left\{ \frac{w_{i,j}^y}{s_j^u} [r_j(k+i|k) - y_j(k+i|k)] \right\}^2 \quad (14)$$

where $k$ is the current control interval, $p$ the prediction horizon, $n_y$ the number of outputs, $z_k$ is the suggested input, given by $z_k^T = [u(k|k)^T \ u(k+1|k)^T \ \cdots \ u(k+p-1|k)^T \ \epsilon_k]$; $y_j(k+i|k)$ and $r_j(k+i|k)$ is the predicted $j$-th output value and the reference value, respectively, at the $i$-th prediction horizon step. Finally, $w_{i,j}^y$ and $s_j^y$ are the tuning weight and scale factor, respectively, for the predicted $j$-th output at the $i$-th prediction horizon step.

Also, $J_u(z_k)$ is related to the dependent variable tracking performance and is given by,

$$J_u(z_k) = \sum_{j=1}^{n_u} \sum_{i=0}^{p-1} \left\{ \frac{w_{i,j}^{\Delta u}}{s_j^u} [u_j(k+i|k) - u_j(k+i-1|k)] \right\}^2 \quad (15)$$

where $k$, $p$, and $z_k$ are defined as before. $n_u$ the number of inputs, $u_j(k+i|k)$ and $u_{j,target}(k+i|k)$ is the predicted $j$-th input and target input, respectively, at the $i$-th prediction horizon step. Finally, $w_{i,j}^u$ and $s_j^u$ are the tuning weight and scale factor, respectively, for the predicted $j$-th input at the $i$-th prediction horizon step.

Besides, $J_{\Delta u}(z_k)$ accounts for the changes in the dependent variable in consecutive realisations, given by,

$$J_{\Delta u}(z_k) = \sum_{j=1}^{n_u} \sum_{i=0}^{p-1} \left\{ \frac{w_{i,j}^u}{s_j^u} \left[ u_j(k+i|k) - u_{j,target}(k+i|k) \right] \right\}^2 \quad (16)$$

where $k$, $p$, $n_u$, and $z_k$ are defined as before. $u_j(k+i|k)$ and $u_{j,target}(k+i|k)$ is the predicted $j$-th input and target input, respectively, at the $i$-th prediction horizon step. Finally, $w_{i,j}^{\Delta u}$ is the tuning weight for the predicted $j$-th input movement at the $i$-th prediction horizon step and $s_j^u$ the scale factor for the $j$-th input.

Finally, $J_y(z_k)$ addresses the violation of constraints when these are included in the controller,

$$J_\epsilon(z_k) = \rho_\epsilon \epsilon_k^2 \quad (17)$$

where $z_k$ is defined as before. $\rho_\epsilon$ is the constraint violation penalty weight and $\epsilon_k^2$ the slack variable at control interval $k$.

In this work, the input variable is the energy intake and the output the bodyweight. This MPC approach is tested when using time-invariant parameters and time-variants parameters models using constrains and without them. The constraints simply account for the minimum and maximum values allowed for bodyweight and energy intake. The minimum and maximum bodyweight are, $BW_{min}$ = 52.2 kg and $BW_{max}$ = 69.8 kg, respectively. In addition, the minimum and maximum energy intake are, $EI_{min}$ = 1223 kcal day$^{-1}$ and $EI_{max}$ = 3556 kcal day$^{-1}$, respectively.

The controller's performance and robustness are tested. Firstly, the bodyweight measured curve from each test participant in the Minnesota starvation experiment is used as reference curve and the energy intake suggested by the MPC is compared with the energy intake actually measured to evaluate the performance. Afterwards, the robustness is tested by performing 100 Monte Carlo simulations. In each simulation, the average values of the $a$- and $b$-parameters are disturbed with random noise and the impact on the performance is evaluated. Finally, the MPC is applied using theoretical curves as bodyweight reference curves. Since no ideal target trajectory is suggested in literature, three different target body weight trajectories are proposed. In [49], it is recommended to decrease bodyweight by 5–10% within 6 months. The study, performed on obese women, concludes that a weight loss of 5–10% of the total body weight results in improvements in blood glucose levels and hypertension [49]. The initial and final body weight for the three targeted body weight trajectories are set to the same values. The initial body weight is defined as the average maximum body weight over all participants prior to the start of the starvation phase, which is 69.36 kg. The final body weight is set to 59.36 kg and has to be reached after one year or 52 weeks. This means that the initial body weight is decreased with 14.4%. The first and second trajectories gradually decrease the body weight in even steps, holding these steps constant for 3 or 8 weeks, respectively. The third body weight trajectory follows an exponential trend with equation $BW_t = BW_0 \cdot 0.95^t$ ($t$ = 1,..., 52 weeks) where the desired bodyweight at the start of the simulation is reduced more rapidly than near the end of the simulation. The MPC algorithm used to test the three trajectories has different constraints. The maximum value of the output is defined as the average maximum body weight over all participants prior to the start of the starvation phase, which is 69.36 kg. The minimum output value is the target body weight at the end of the trajectory of 59.36 kg. The maximum input or energy intake is the average maximum energy intake of 3538.72 kcal day$^{-1}$ prior to the starvation phase. The minimum energy intake is calculated using the Henry equations based on the average height, age, target bodyweight and gender [50]. These equations estimate the basal metabolic rate (BMR) and defines the minimum energy intake to account for daily energy expenditure in rest. As the age of the male participants from the Minnesota starvation experiment varies between 20 and 33 years, the following equation is used for the estimation of the minimum energy:

$$BMR \text{ (kcal day}^{-1}) = 14.4 \cdot BW(kg) + 313 \cdot H(m) + 113 \quad (18)$$

where $BW$ is the target body weight of 59.36 kg and $H$ is the average height of 1.79 m of all participants. This equation results in a minimum energy intake of 1672.05 kcal day$^{-1}$.

Both, the $NMRSE$, given by Equation (11), and the root mean square error ($RMSE$) are used to quantify the deviation between the desire targeted (reference) and simulated, using the MPC, energy intake or bodyweight curves. The $RMSE$ is given by the expression:

$$RMSE = \sqrt{\frac{\|y_{ref} - y_{sim}\|^2}{N_s}} \qquad (19)$$

where $N_s$ is the number of samples, $y_{ref}$ is the reference energy (or bodyweight) curve and $y_{sim}$ is the simulated energy intake (or bodyweight) curve by the MPC.

## 3. Results and Discussion

### 3.1. Time-Invariant SISO TF Models

In Figure 1, the gathered energy intake and bodyweight curves from the 32 participants are displayed.

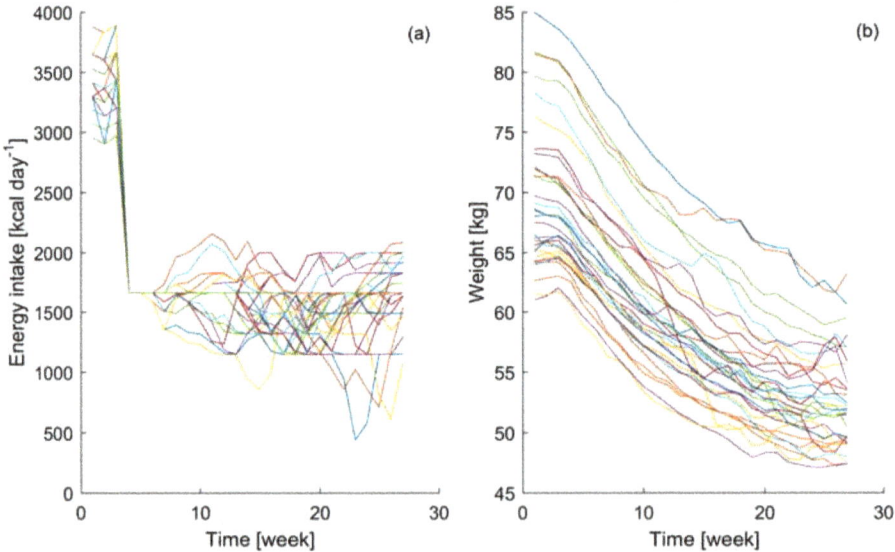

**Figure 1.** Energy intake in kcal day$^{-1}$ (**a**) and bodyweight in kg (**b**) curves collected for each one of the 32 participants in the Minnesota starvation.

The obtained data have shown clear interpersonal differences between participants in their energy intake and bodyweight curves during the course of the experiment. Even though during the control phase it is attempted to reduce the variability in the bodyweight among the participants, it can be seen that the individual variability in energy intake during the starvation stage of the experiment induced different responses in the bodyweight time course. Similar energy intake patterns lead to different bodyweight time courses, which highlights the individual characteristics of the biological process, emphasizing the importance of the aim of this study.

Therefore, using the Minnesota starvation experiment dataset, 32 sub-datasets are created using the bodyweight and energy intake from each individual participant. Using each sub-dataset, a system identification procedure is performed to define the best time-invariant parameters model structure needed to relate energy intake and bodyweight. In Table 1, a summary is shown of the first and second order model performances in terms of $YIC$ and the goodness of fit, $R_T^2$. Table 2 shows the Pearson correlation coefficients ($r$), to assess the similarity between the model outputs and the weight curves from the participants. A representative example of the agreement between the measured and estimated bodyweight curves for one individual test participant (participant 8) in the Minnesota starvation experiment is displayed in Figure 2.

**Table 1.** Average Young information criterion ($YIC$) and coefficient of determination, $R_T^2$, together with their standard deviation, obtained during the system identification process for each of the 32 sub-datasets created from the Minnesota starvation excel spreadsheet used in the work of [31]. [$n_a$ $n_b$ $\delta$] indicates the different combinations (24 in total) of time –invariant first and second order models: number of $a$-parameters ($n_a$) ranging from 1 to 2 (Equation (2)), number of $b$-parameters ($n_b$) ranging from 1 to 2 (Equation (3)) and delays ($\delta$) ranging from 0 to 5 samples.

|  | [1 1 0] | [1 2 0] | [2 1 0] | [2 2 0] |
|---|---|---|---|---|
| $YIC$ | −12 ± 2 | −5 ± 3 | −6 ± 4 | −1 ± 5 |
| $R_T^2$ | 0.99 ± 0.01 | 0.99 ± 0.01 | 0.93 ± 0.24 | 0.83 ± 0.34 |
|  | [1 1 1] | [1 2 1] | [2 1 1] | [2 2 1] |
| $YIC$ | −11 ± 2 | −6 ± 2 | −1 ± 6 | 2 ± 6 |
| $R_T^2$ | 0.99 ± 0.01 | 0.99 ± 0.01 | 0.60 ± 0.47 | 0.53 ± 0.49 |
|  | [1 1 2] | [1 2 2] | [2 1 2] | [2 2 2] |
| $YIC$ | −9 ± 1 | −6 ± 2 | 5 ± 3 | 7 ± 6 |
| $R_T^2$ | 0.97 ± 0.01 | 0.98 ± 0.01 | 0.09 ± 0.28 | 0.21 ± 0.39 |
|  | [1 1 3] | [1 2 3] | [2 1 3] | [2 2 3] |
| $YIC$ | −8 ± 1 | −4 ± 2 | 5 ± 2 | 5 ± 4 |
| $R_T^2$ | 0.96 ± 0.02 | 0.96 ± 0.02 | 0.03 ± 0.17 | 0.24 ± 0.36 |
|  | [1 1 4] | [1 2 4] | [2 1 4] | [2 2 4] |
| $YIC$ | −6 ± 2 | 1 ± 4 | 6 ± 2 | 6 ± 4 |
| $R_T^2$ | 0.90 ± 0.16 | 0.84 ± 0.27 | 0.03 ± 0.14 | 0.18 ± 0.30 |
|  | [1 1 5] | [1 2 5] | [2 1 5] | [2 2 5] |
| $YIC$ | −2 ± 4 | 1 ± 3 | 4 ± 3 | 7 ± 5 |
| $R_T^2$ | 0.75 ± 0.34 | 0.72 ± 0.37 | 0.15 ± 0.31 | 0.19 ± 0.35 |

**Table 2.** Mean and standard deviation of the Pearson correlation coefficient obtained when comparing the first and second orders time-invariant models with no delay ([$n_a$ $n_b$ 0]) output and each one of the weight curves collected for the 32 participants in the experiment.

| [1 1 0] | [1 2 0] | [2 1 0] | [2 2 0] |
|---|---|---|---|
| 0.999 ± 0.001 | 0.999 ± 0.001 | 0.999 ± 0.001 | 0.999 ± 0.001 |

The results have shown that a first order model is sufficient to characterize the impact of energy intake in bodyweight, as reflected by the superior $YIC$, $R_T^2$, and a high Pearson correlation coefficient results (see Tables 1 and 2). During the system identification process, the presence of delay was allowed, but the best results were always obtained when no delay (i.e., $\delta$ = 0) was present in the models. From a biological viewpoint this make sense, as metabolizing the ingested energy takes about 12 h, while the used time interval is one week (i.e., 168 h). Thus, the time delay between energy intake and bodyweight change reduces to nearly zero in terms of the used measurement interval of one week.

In addition, the $YIC$ value also indicates that the parameters estimation when using a first order model is reliable. Ideally, it would be possible to define a first order model, using the average values of the different estimations of $a$- and $b$-parameters obtained for each subject, which would allow estimating the impact of bodyweight of a given energy intake. When the $a$- and $b$-parameters from the individual estimations are averaged together, the following model is obtained,

$$BW_t = a_1 \cdot BW_{t-1} + b_0 \cdot EI_t = (0.92 \pm 0.03) \cdot BW_{t-1} + (9 \pm 3) \cdot 10^{-4} \cdot EI_t \qquad (20)$$

where $BW$ is bodyweight in kg, $EI$ is the energy intake in kcal day$^{-1}$ and $t$ is the time sample in weeks. It can be seen that the $b$-parameter exhibits more variability than the $a$-parameter. This is expected, taking into account the biological process under study. Translating the model to the biological process, it states that the bodyweight at time $t$ is the bodyweight of the time sample before plus a contribution of a certain percentage of the energy intake at time sample $t$. Therefore, on one hand it is expected that the $a$-parameter should be close to one and should not show too much variability between participants. On the other hand, the $b$-parameter should resemble energy efficiency and thus it is expected to vary between the different individuals. From Equation (20), it can be the seen that the results matched perfectly this hypothesis. Running this average model in all datasets results in an average coefficient of determination of $R_T^2 = 0.3 \pm 0.2$. Therefore, by defining an average model in which an average $b$-parameter value is set, the performance of the model drops drastically. In several previous studies [24–28,31–33], models were developed to estimate bodyweight changes in response to changes in the energy balance, taking into account energy intake and physical activity. These models are mechanistic models, using population-based average estimations of parameters to describe the energy balance equations. This explains the high standard deviation exhibited in the results of these models. The same is observed in this work, when an average time-invariant parameters model is developed. This clearly indicates the need for accurately estimating the proper $b$-parameter value for each individual.

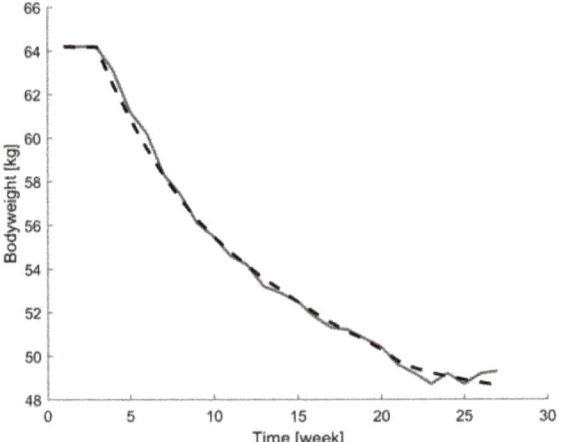

**Figure 2.** Comparison between the bodyweight curved collected for test participant 8 in the Minnesota starvation experiment (solid line) and the bodyweight curve simulated by a first order time-invariant parameters transfer function model (dashed line).

Therefore, from the system identification step it can be concluded that a first order transfer function model is sufficient to characterize the impact of energy intake on the bodyweight time course. However, it is necessary to use $b$-parameters that resemble the energy efficiency of the individual, and thus developing an average model is not a suitable approach. Moreover, it is expected that this energy efficiency would not only be individually different, but also change throughout the experimental period. Internal and external factors are expected to affect how a person translates the energy intake into a bodyweight change throughout the weight intervention process. Therefore, by including time-variant parameters in the model, it is expected to cope with these dynamic characteristic of the process. Thus, in the next section the results of the time-variant parameters modelling approach are described.

*3.2. Time-Variant Parameters Models*

By allowing the parameters to vary in time, it is expected to capture the changes induced in the energy efficiency by factors not taken explicitly into account in the model and, hence, obtain a more accurate estimation of bodyweight.

Firstly, the modelling accuracy is evaluated when modelling the complete experiment. In the previous section, it was shown that a first order transfer function model is sufficient to describe the relation between the energy intake and the bodyweight. Thus, a first order DARX model and a DLR model are tested. In Table 3, the results from the modelling performance for the complete experiment, in terms of the *NRMSE* and *r*, are shown for both time-varying modelling approaches.

**Table 3.** Normalized root mean square error (*NRMSE*) and Pearson correlation coefficient (*r*) evaluating the fitting agreement between the experimental data and the model output of the dynamic linear regression (DLR) model and a first order dynamic auto-regression with exogenous variables (DARX).

|   | DLR | DARX |
|---|---|---|
| *NRMSE* | 0.997 ± 0.003 | 0.941 ± 0.031 |
| *r* | 0.999 ± 0.001 | 0.997 ± 0.003 |

These results indicate that the DLR model provides a better and more consistent fitting agreement than the DARX model. Thus, from these results it seems that the DLR model outperforms the DARX approach. One of the reasons, which can explain this finding, could be the higher stochasticity behavior in the DLR model. Stochastic models can account for the variability among individuals in populations. Thus, a combination of deterministic and stochastic parts in the model allows quantifying both, the trend and the variability present in the process [51]. Besides, in the work of [2], weight loss is modelled by energy deficit, using energy flux balances. They found that when a stochastic component is added to the model the results improved. This is in line with the results obtained in this analysis. Allowing the time –variant model parameters to have a stochastic behavior, in order to characterize their time-evolution, improves the modelling performance. However, this analysis just confirms that a first order model with time-variant parameters allows characterizing the relation between energy intake and bodyweight time-course more accurately than using time-invariant parameters models, as expected. In order to develop a control system in the next phase, the model should not only describe the process accurately but also should exhibit suitable forecasting properties. Therefore, the forecasting capabilities of both time-variant parameters models are tested. In Tables 4 and 5, the forecasting performance for the DLR and DARX models is displayed in terms of *MRPE*.

**Table 4.** Mean relative prediction error (*MRPE*), in percentage, for different combinations of time window (*TW*) and prediction horizon (*PH*) sizes, measured in weeks, when applying the dynamic linear regression (DLR) model.

|   |   | TW [Week] | | | | | | | | | | | | |
|---|---|---|---|---|---|---|---|---|---|---|---|---|---|---|
|   |   | 3 | 4 | 5 | 6 | 7 | 8 | 9 | 10 | 11 | 12 | 13 | 14 | 15 |
| PH [week] | 1 | 2.82 | 1.96 | 1.81 | 1.75 | 1.66 | 1.66 | 1.57 | 1.51 | 1.39 | 1.36 | 1.31 | 1.33 | 1.24 |
|  | 2 | 4.54 | 3.57 | 3.37 | 3.20 | 3.09 | 3.00 | 2.87 | 2.70 | 2.50 | 2.41 | 2.35 | 2.28 | 2.13 |
|  | 3 | 5.86 | 5.09 | 4.73 | 4.54 | 4.29 | 4.15 | 3.99 | 3.75 | 3.43 | 3.34 | 3.21 | 3.09 | 2.98 |
|  | 4 | 7.22 | 6.44 | 5.98 | 5.65 | 5.37 | 5.21 | 4.99 | 4.65 | 4.39 | 4.23 | 4.01 | 3.91 | 3.77 |
|  | 5 | 8.30 | 7.66 | 7.10 | 6.73 | 6.50 | 6.31 | 5.99 | 5.71 | 5.32 | 5.06 | 4.81 | 4.67 | 4.39 |
|  | 6 | 9.31 | 8.73 | 8.22 | 7.89 | 7.65 | 7.35 | 7.06 | 6.68 | 6.17 | 5.99 | 5.71 | 5.44 | 5.15 |
|  | 7 | 10.24 | 9.92 | 9.43 | 9.08 | 8.67 | 8.44 | 8.05 | 7.53 | 7.26 | 7.02 | 6.59 | 6.34 | 6.03 |

**Table 5.** Mean relative prediction error (*MRPE*), in percentage, for different combinations of time window (*TW*) and prediction horizon (*PH*) sizes, measured in weeks, when applying the dynamic auto-regression with exogenous variables (DARX) model. The values >100 indicate an extremely low forecasting performance of the model.

| | | TW [week] | | | | | | | | | | | | |
|---|---|---|---|---|---|---|---|---|---|---|---|---|---|---|
| | | 3 | 4 | 5 | 6 | 7 | 8 | 9 | 10 | 11 | 12 | 13 | 14 | 15 |
| PH [week] | 1 | 2.05 | 1.23 | 1.15 | 1.11 | 1.04 | 1.04 | 1.00 | 0.97 | 1.01 | 0.98 | 0.99 | 1.02 | 1.05 |
| | 2 | 6.02 | 2.13 | 1.83 | 1.70 | 1.56 | 1.51 | 1.46 | 1.45 | 1.48 | 1.45 | 1.46 | 1.53 | 1.52 |
| | 3 | 24.64 | 3.45 | 2.69 | 2.35 | 2.06 | 1.95 | 1.91 | 1.86 | 1.90 | 1.85 | 1.91 | 1.91 | 1.90 |
| | 4 | >100 | 4.94 | 3.50 | 2.92 | 2.53 | 2.38 | 2.30 | 2.31 | 2.33 | 2.27 | 2.27 | 2.25 | 2.28 |
| | 5 | >100 | 6.35 | 4.22 | 3.44 | 3.07 | 2.84 | 2.79 | 2.77 | 2.79 | 2.70 | 2.67 | 2.67 | 2.74 |
| | 6 | >100 | 8.36 | 5.02 | 4.05 | 3.55 | 3.30 | 3.21 | 3.15 | 3.19 | 3.07 | 3.06 | 3.12 | 3.18 |
| | 7 | >100 | 11.21 | 5.85 | 4.66 | 4.08 | 3.74 | 3.64 | 3.57 | 3.59 | 3.50 | 3.53 | 3.54 | 3.53 |

Besides, in Figure 3, the results obtained for the different combinations of time window and prediction horizon sizes tested for both time-variant parameters models are displayed, together with a representative example for the one-week ahead prediction horizon forecasting results.

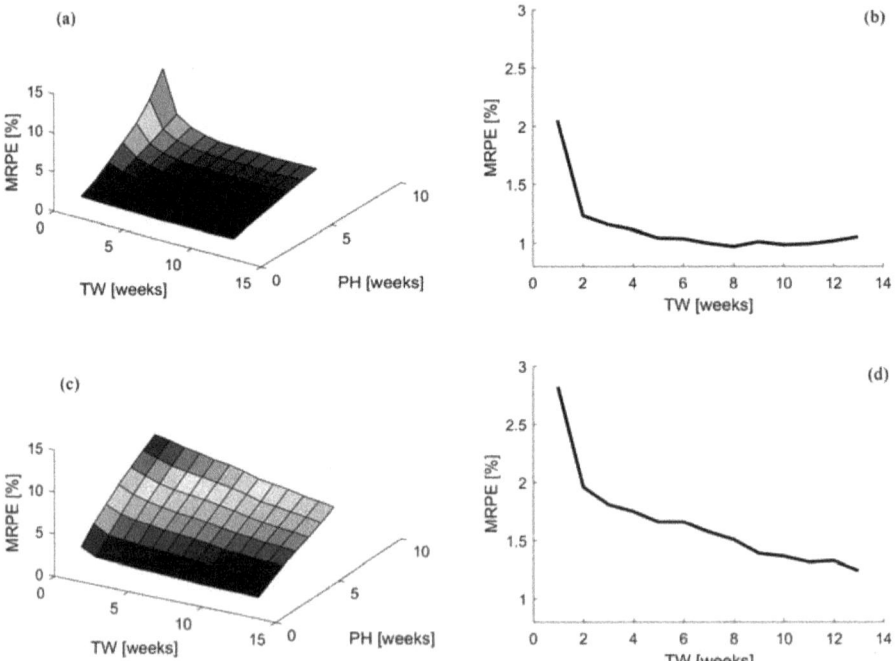

**Figure 3.** Average mean relative prediction error (*MRPE*) from the 32 test participants in the Minnesota starvation experiment for different combinations of time window (*TW*) and prediction horizon (*PH*) sizes for the DARX (**a**) and DLR (**c**) models. Besides, the *MRPE* for one-week ahead prediction according to different time window sizes is shown for the DARX (**b**) and DLR (**d**) models.

It is clear from the aforementioned results that the DARX model is able to achieve the best forecasting performance. Time window sizes ranging between 7 and 12 weeks lead to a *MRPE* of 1.01 ± 0.02%, on average, when using the DARX model. In the same range, the average *MRPE* for the DLR model is 1.53 ± 0.12%. Thus, there is a difference of 0.52% in favor of the DARX model prediction capabilities. Besides, the evolution of the *MRPE* among the different time window and prediction horizon sizes in the DLR model improves, as more data is included in the time window. Biologically, it is expected that the energy efficiency will vary with time and the current efficiency should be more relevant than the efficiency in past instances. Thus, it seems that the DLR model is not capturing fully the expected biological behavior of the process.

In contrast, the DARX model shows that increasing the window size improves the forecasting performance, but only until a certain range. Once this range is exceeded, the forecasting properties worsen again. This is expected, as the sliding time window with a fixed size should help in removing the impact of obsolete data in the model [47]. Thus, this is more in line with what it is expected in terms of the biological process under study. Furthermore, it can be seen that the optimal time window size changes according to the prediction horizon size. For instance, if the prediction horizon is raised to 4–5 weeks, thus over a month time, the MRPE error ranges between 2.5–3% and the optimal time window size range increases to 10–14 weeks.

The prediction of bodyweight using a recursive linear regression approach based on time-variant parameters has been already tested on broiler chickens [47]. In that study, the lowest *MRPE* reaches a value of 1.4% for a prediction horizon of 1 day and the highest *MRPE* is 4.1% for a prediction horizon of 7 days, when broiler chickens are fed ad libitum [47]. These results illustrate that using time-variant parameters models to predict human bodyweight is highly accurate, improving the previous results.

Lastly, it is important to mention that because little information on energy expenditure is known, the bodyweight predictions are based solely on energy intake. The data from the Minnesota starvation experiment include merely estimations of the resting energy expenditure on the week prior to the starvation phase and at the end of the starvation phase. Thus, calculating the weekly energy balance is not possible. There are several models in literature that attempt to address this characteristic during a weight program intervention by using complex mechanistic models based on systems of one dimensional differential equations [28,29,31,32]. Although these theoretical models resemble accurately the dynamic process of bodyweight change, the large amount of model parameters are estimated based on averages from population studies [32] and do not take into account the changes in the values of the model parameters throughout the experimental period [11]. In the modelling framework proposed in this study, not only the dynamic evolution through time, but also the dynamics induced by the impact of internal and external factors in the model parameters are taken into account implicitly by the model. This allows designing more compact models, reducing greatly their complexity while capturing the most relevant dynamics of the process. In future, if both energy intake and expenditure would be available, a time-variant model in which both are used as inputs could be developed. Moreover, gathering regular information about the time course of fat body mass and lean body mass would allow developing a time-variant model, whose model parameters could be related to existing mechanistic equations describing bodyweight component changes in response to changes in energy intake and energy expenditure. On one hand, this would help dietitians to develop further the current mechanistic expressions to describe more accurately the bodyweight change process. On the other hand, it would enable them to evaluate and adapt in real-time the impact of the suggested dietary energy intake to achieve a desire bodyweight change at individualized patient level.

In summary, these results show that a time-variant parameters model allows characterizing accurately the dynamics of a body weight change induced by a change in dietary energy intake. Using a window size of seven weeks of dietary energy intake allows forecasting bodyweight one-week ahead with a MRPE of 1.04% and four-weeks ahead with a MRPE of 2.53%. Therefore, from this analysis with time-variant models, it seems that a first order DARX model is the best model choice when balancing fitting agreement and forecasting performance. Besides, it seems to describe more accurately the biological process under study. Therefore, this model is considered the best option to develop a model-predictive control to estimate the energy intake needed to achieve a desired bodyweight change. In the next section, the model predictive controller is developed and tested. When using the time-variant parameters model in the controller, the time window size of seven weeks is selected. It should be noted that even though in this study the time window size is fixed, it would be possible to perform a similar analysis as the one described in this section to estimate in real-time which would be the optimal time window size to be used in the controller's model for each individual.

### 3.3. Simulation Model Predictive Control

Several MPC systems are developed using both the time-invariant and time-variant parameters transfer function models tested in the previous sub-sections. In order to test the capabilities of the controller for each individual participant, the bodyweight collected during the experiment is used as reference bodyweight curve and then the energy intake advised by the controller is compared with the measured energy intake. First, simulations are performed without any constraint to the system. Next, simulations with constraints are performed as well. In Figure 4, a comparison between the energy intake suggested by the different controllers and the energy intake collected during the experiments is displayed.

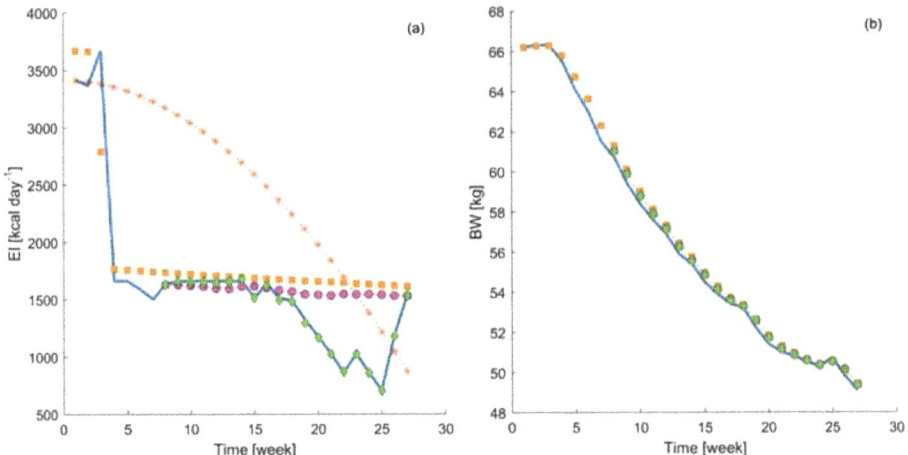

**Figure 4.** In (**a**), the energy intake curves suggested by the model predictive control (MPC) (dashed colored lines) compared with the energy intake measured (solid blue line) during the Minnesota starvation experiment are shown for participant 15. In (**b**), the bodyweight time course obtained following the MPC suggestions (dash colored lines) compared with the bodyweight measured (solid blue line) during the Minnesota starvation experiment is shown for participant 15. The different MPCs tested are the MPC using a time-invariant parameters transfer function model, without (red *) and with constraints (yellow square), and the MPC using the time-variant parameters DARX model, without (purple circle) and with constraints (green diamond).

The results have shown that the developed MPC, using the time-variant parameters DARX model, suggested an energy intake which is closest (see Table 6) to the actual energy intake collected during the experiment in comparison to that suggested by the MPC developed using time-invariant models. The MPC developed using the time-invariant model with constraints and the one using the DARX model without constraints perform similarly. Finally, the MPC developed using the time-invariant model and without constraints suggests an energy intake, which follows completely different dynamics. In addition, all MPC systems tested generate similar bodyweight curves, which follow closely the reference bodyweight curve. In order to quantify this visual inspection, Table 6 shows a summary of the *NRMSE*, *RMSE* and *r* values when comparing the measured energy intake and bodyweight curves with those estimated from the different controller simulations. Besides, the *RMSE* between the final weight achieved by the participant and the final weight obtained in the different controller simulations is summarized in Table 7.

**Table 6.** Normalized root mean square error (*NRMSE*), root mean square error (*RMSE*) and Pearson correlation coefficient (*r*) when comparing the MPC suggestions for energy intake and bodyweight outcome, with the energy intake and body weight from the Minnesota starvation experiment. The MPC systems tested are the one using the time-invariant parameters model without constraints (TI), the same one but with constraints (TIC), the MPC system using the time-variant parameter DARX model without constraints (TV) and this one with constraints (TVC). The RMSE for bodyweight has kg as units and the RMSE for energy intake has kcal day$^{-1}$ units. The NRMSE value is set to 0 when the energy intake suggested by the MPC and the measured energy intake curves follow diverging dynamics.

|  | Bodyweight [kg] | | | | Energy Intake [kcal day$^{-1}$] | | | |
| --- | --- | --- | --- | --- | --- | --- | --- | --- |
|  | TI | TIC | TV | TVC | TI | TIC | TV | TVC |
| NRMSE | 0.92 ± 0.01 | 0.92 ± 0.01 | 0.90 ± 0.03 | 0.91 ± 0.02 | 0 | 0 | 0 | 0.92 ± 0.04 |
| RMSE | 0.46 ± 0.19 | 0.46 ± 0.19 | 0.33 ± 0.08 | 0.32 ± 0.08 | 1278 ± 875 | 726 ± 324 | 232 ± 121 | 13 ± 10 |
| r | 0.99 ± 0.01 | 0.99 ± 0.01 | 0.99 ± 0.01 | 0.99 ± 0.01 | 0.43 ± 0.12 | 0.95 ± 0.03 | 0.41 ± 0.27 | 0.99 ± 0.01 |

**Table 7.** Root mean square error (*RMSE*) when comparing the MPC end value of bodyweight outcome for all MPCs tested and final energy intake suggestion for the MPC using the time-variant parameter DARX model with constraints (TVC) with the final bodyweight and energy intake values from the Minnesota starvation experiment. The MPC systems tested are the one using the time-invariant parameters model (TI), the same one but adding constraints (TIC), and the MPC system using the time-variant parameter DARX model (TV) and this one with constraints (TVC). The *RMSE* for bodyweight has kg as units and the *RMSE* for energy intake has kcal day$^{-1}$ units.

|  | Bodyweight [kg] | | | | Energy Intake [kcal day$^{-1}$] |
| --- | --- | --- | --- | --- | --- |
|  | TI | TIC | TV | TVC | TVC |
| RMSE | 0.38 ± 0.06 | 0.38 ± 0.06 | 0.26 ± 0.06 | 0.26 ± 0.03 | 9 ± 3 |

It can be seen that the best performance is obtained when using the DARX model in the controller with constraints in the simulation. The *RMSE* for bodyweight and energy intake is only 260 g and 9 kcal day$^{-1}$, respectively. Moreover, the difference between the final bodyweight and energy intake values from all MPC's and the measured ones during the experiment are, on average, lower than 440 g and 12 kcal day$^{-1}$, respectively.

These results highlight again the need to use individualized time-variant parameters models to develop a MPC capable to manage automatically the individualized advice of energy intake to achieve a desire bodyweight change. However, this does not necessarily mean that the other MPCs are suggesting completely wrong energy intake levels. As it can be seen in Figure 4, all outcome bodyweight curves from the MPCs follows closely the reference one. Thus, these suggested energy intake curves should be understood as alternative possibilities that, in principle, would have taken the participant to similar end bodyweight without lowering suddenly the energy intake, but by lowering the energy intake following another pattern. When starting to lower the energy intake following one of these alternative curves, it would be still needed to develop a time-variant model to monitor the performance of the test subject in real-time and adapt the suggested curves to the new conditions. In this regard, these capabilities can be exploited by dietitians to determine which is the healthier alternative for an individual patient to achieve the desire bodyweight change according to its response to the initial treatment through time.

Thus, in order to test the MPC system capabilities to follow theoretical reference curves, three different theoretical bodyweight curves are defined according to the procedure described in Section 2.3 of the Material and Methods section. In Figure 5, the different energy intake curves suggested by the controller are displayed. In addition, the resulting estimated weight curves obtained when following these suggestions, compared with the defined theoretical ones, are displayed as well. In order to perform these simulations, the average time-invariant model obtained in Section 3.1 of this section is used as model for the controller. This approach cannot be tested with the time-variant parameters DARX models, as there is no actual data collection from the participants following these theoretical curves.

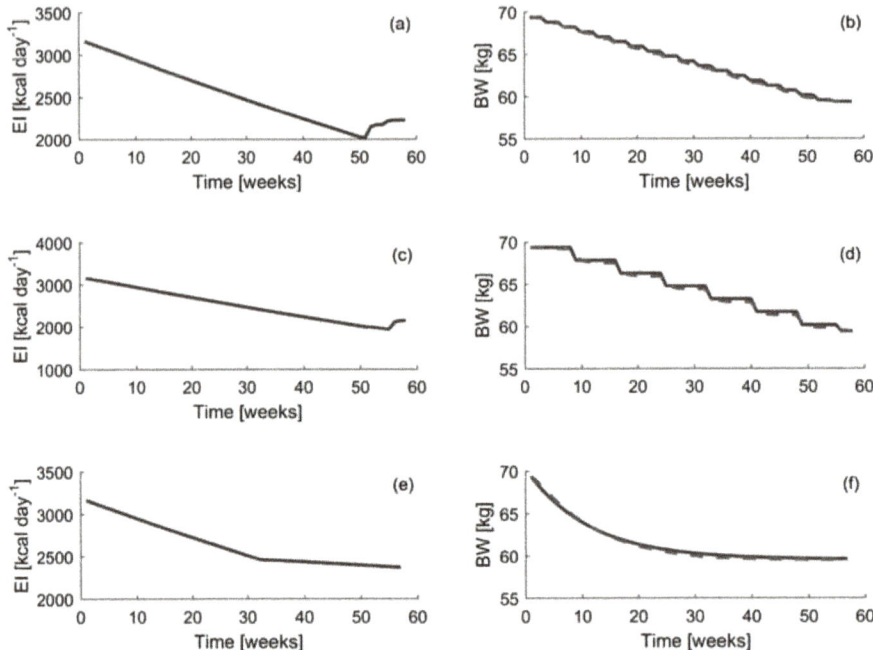

**Figure 5.** Energy intake curves suggested by the MPC controller using the time-invariant averaged TF model in order to follow the theoretical bodyweight curves 1, 2 and 3, (**a**), (**c**) and (**e**), respectively. The reference bodyweight curves 1, 2 and 3 (solid lines) and bodyweight curves obtained with the MPC simulation (dashed lines) are display in (**b**), (**d**) and (**f**), respectively.

It can be seen that the energy intake curves suggested by the controller are similar. The main difference is the energy intake change rate over consecutive weeks. Depending on the theoretical bodyweight curve used as reference, the energy intake suggested for an average individual decreases faster or slower in consecutive weeks. The $NRMSE$, $RMSE$ and $r$ describing the differences between the reference bodyweight curve and the bodyweight curves achieved with the control simulation are summarized in Table 8. Table 9 shows the $RMSE$ between the final bodyweight value from the controllers and the one from the theoretical reference curve.

**Table 8.** Normalized root mean square error ($NRMSE$), root mean square error ($RMSE$), in kg, and Pearson correlation coefficient ($r$) for the comparison between the bodyweight curve obtain following the suggestions from the MPC systems using the time-invariant parameters transfer function model, without (TI) and with constraints (TIC) and the three theoretical bodyweight reference curves generated.

|   | Reference Curve 1 | | Reference Curve 2 | | Reference Curve 3 | |
|---|---|---|---|---|---|---|
|   | TI | TIC | TI | TIC | TI | TIC |
| NRMSE | 0.968 ± 0.004 | 0.969 ± 0.003 | 0.941 ± 0.002 | 0.941 ± 0.003 | 0.943 ± 0.002 | 0.951 ± 0.010 |
| RMSE | 0.10 ± 0.05 | 0.10 ± 0.04 | 0.19 ± 0.05 | 0.19 ± 0.05 | 0.15 ± 0.04 | 0.13 ± 0.08 |
| r | 0.999 ± 0.001 | 0.998 ± 0.002 | 0.999 ± 0.001 | 0.999 ± 0.001 | 0.998 ± 0.002 | 0.999 ± 0.001 |

**Table 9.** Root mean square error (*RMSE*), in kg, for the comparison between the end bodyweight from the curves obtain following the suggestions from the MPC systems using the time-invariant parameters transfer function model, without (TI) and with constraints (TIC) and the three theoretical bodyweight reference curves generated.

|  | Reference Curve 1 | | Reference Curve 2 | | Reference Curve 3 | |
| --- | --- | --- | --- | --- | --- | --- |
|  | TI | TIC | TI | TIC | TI | TIC |
| *RMSE* | 0.010 ± 0.003 | 0.010 ± 0.003 | 0.034 ± 0.012 | 0.006 ± 0.003 | 0.065 ± 0.38 | 0.065 ± 0.036 |

It can be seen that the *RMSE* errors, when comparing the complete curves or just the final values, are small, less than 200 g on average, in all cases. Thus, the MPC controller is able to follow closely a predefined theoretical bodyweight curve. Therefore, the MPC developed in this study may be used to set a theoretical bodyweight reference curve and evaluate the energy intake curve suggested to follow the given bodyweight curve in order to achieve the desired final weight.

Finally, as the last part of the analysis, the robustness of the controller is tested. A random contribution, at the level of the standard error in the parameters estimations (10%), is added as uncertainty to the *a*- and *b*-parameters of the time-invariant model. Using Monte Carlo simulations, the robustness of the model is tested, generating 100 realizations varying *a*- or *b*-parameter estimations. In Figure 6, examples of the suggested energy intake and bodyweight curves obtained from these 100 Monte Carlo simulations, adding uncertainty in the *a*- and *b*-parameters, respectively, are shown.

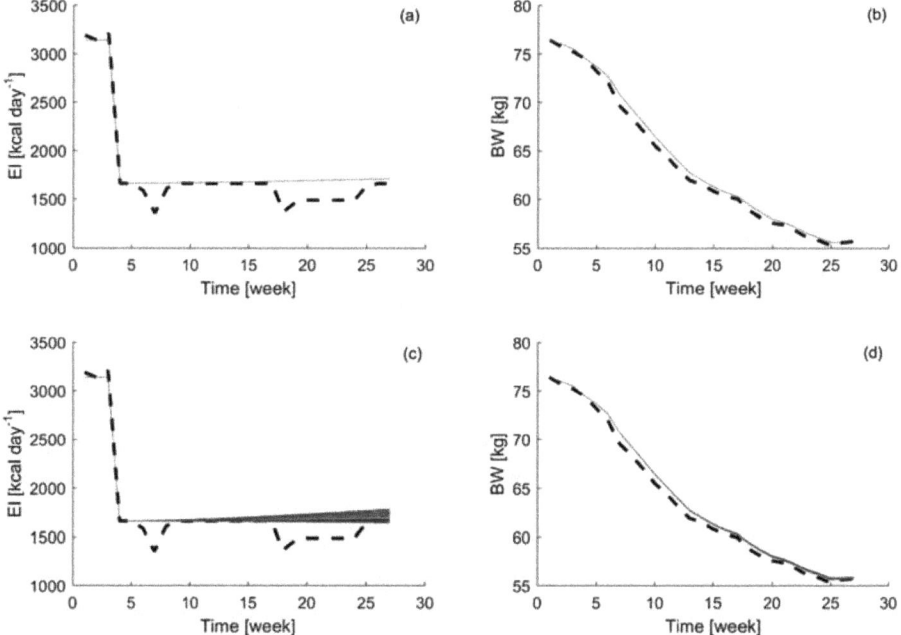

**Figure 6.** Energy intake curves suggested by the MPC system based on the time-invariant parameters TF model when uncertainty is added to the a-parameter estimation (**a**) or in b-parameter estimation (**c**) and the obtained bodyweight curves when following these respective energy curves (**b**) and (**d**), after 100 Monte Carlo simulations are performed.

The results have shown how the controller's suggestions for energy intake are much less sensitive to the uncertainty in the *a*-parameter than in the *b*-parameter. This is expected as the *b*-parameter represents the energy intake efficiency; thus, slight changes in this parameter induce changes in the energy required to achieve a target bodyweight. However, uncertainty in the $a$-parameter should be limited as well, because an increase in uncertainty may lead to an unstable model. Therefore, these results point out again towards the need to use time-variant parameters models, such the DARX model tested in this study, to obtain accurate estimations of the model parameters and their time evolution for individual participants. Accounting in the model parameters for this variability improves considerably the capabilities of the MPC to suggest energy intake levels which take the individuals variability into account, enabling it to get the closest possible to the targeted bodyweight.

In [41], the growth trajectory of broiler chickens is controlled based on an adaptive dynamic model. Here, the performance of the MPC algorithm is quantified by calculating the mean relative error (MRE) between the actual and target weight trajectory of the broiler chickens. The MRE values ranged between 3.7% and 7.0%. For broiler chickens, it is important that the actual growth trajectory resembles the target trajectory, in order to suppress negative effects associated with fast growing broiler chickens. Examples of negative effects include decreased reproduction capacity of the breeder stock, increased body fat deposition and metabolic diseases, such as sudden death syndrome [41]. In [43], the MPC developed in [41] was tested in commercial broiler settings. In this case, the MRE ranged between 6% and 11% under these conditions. Translating the NRMSE and RMSE results from this work to MRE values, obtains, on average, a MRE of 0.65 ± 0.07% and 0.34 ± 0.06% when comparing the experimental measured bodyweight curve for each participant and the bodyweight curve obtained following the suggestions from the MPC using time-invariant parameters and time-variant parameters models, respectively. Moreover, MRE of 0.12 ± 0.01%, 0.18 ± 0.02% and 0.15 ± 0.03% are obtained when comparing the theoretical bodyweight reference trajectory curves and those obtained when following the MPC suggestions for the theoretical reference trajectories 1, 2 and 3, respectively. Therefore, the MPC's developed in this work show that they are capable of following different bodyweight reference trajectories accurately. Similarly as in the case of the time-variant parameters models, the MPC's developed in this work exhibit a high accuracy when compared with the ones developed for livestock applications. Thus, this enables dietitians to develop a theoretical bodyweight curve and test the energy intake suggested to fulfill this goal in an individualized manner for their patients. Besides, taking advantage of the adaptive capabilities of the MPC, it is possible to modify in real-time this bodyweight reference trajectory according to the performance of the patient and health considerations.

In [11,34], dynamic models are developed to control bodyweight dynamics. These models are dynamic in the sense of accounting for the time evolution of the bodyweight and energy processes. However, these models do not account for the time evolution of the model parameters or the individualized estimation of those parameters working in real-time. These dynamic models still rely on average mechanistic descriptions of the bodyweight and energy flux dynamics. Thus, these approaches lack the adaptability characteristics of the MPC developed in this work. However, a MPC as developed in this work has still some drawbacks to be taken into account in the future. No information on the ratio of carbohydrates, lipids and proteins with respect to the total energy intake is provided. In addition to the total energy intake, further optimization of the MPC algorithm can include suggestions on the ratio of carbohydrates, lipids and proteins based on the recommended dietary allowances. An important factor influencing the dietary behavior is the degree of saturation. Food with a high energy density usually ensures a low degree of satiety. Therefore, food with a low energy density is usually recommended, as it provides a longer period of satiety [52]. In [12], it is shown that combining current methods to deal with bodyweight changes with mHealth applications may enhance the performance of the first ones. Therefore, on the one hand, the current applications may benefit from including such a MPC as developed in this work. By providing more individual accurate estimations of energy intake and bodyweight change levels, it is expected to enhance the engagement to the mHealth technology and the adhesion to its suggestions, improving weight management [33]. On the other hand, if further development of apps and wearables enhance the characterization of the energy intake, physical activity and other related physiological variables, the MPC developed in this work can be extended to manage more accurately the metabolization and energy flux balances processes. In such a situation, a comparison with the existing mechanistic models would allow extracting more biological and physical information while keeping the real-time and automatic properties of the controller.

To sum up, it can be seen that such a MPC system may help people to manage and control their bodyweight in real time. Taking advantage of the new possibilities offered by wearables and smartphones, an individual can gather real-time information about their energy intake, bodyweight and activity. Then, mHealth applications may exploit such compact and accurate MPC algorithms to manage body weight change taking advantage of the data gathered. This enables a target bodyweight or bodyweight reference curve to be defined and suggestions for the energy intake needed to achieve this goal to be made. Besides, the MPC system may be a useful tool for dietitians as well. They can develop theoretical bodyweight curves for losing weight using biological and medical information and simulate the energy intake suggested to follow this curve at individual patient level as close as possible. Moreover, at certain points in the treatment, this theoretical curve can be adapted according to the performance of the patient and medical considerations. Thus, the MPC system can be used not only to simulate an energy intake pattern according to a predefined bodyweight curve, but also to monitor the impact of the strategy in individual patients and adapt the strategy accordingly throughout the bodyweight change process.

*3.4. Current Limitations and Future Perspectives*

The Minnesota starvation experiment was performed in 1944 to investigate the psychological and physiological effects of severe dietary restriction [53]. The experiment was designed to mimic the dietary conditions of prisoners during World War II. Therefore, due to both the period in which the experiment was performed and the focus, only male participants were selected. This restriction in energy intake is not a recommended method to lose weight, as the energy intake is lower than the minimum requirements. However, this abrupt change in energy intake presents the perfect conditions to perform an analysis of the system's dynamics and the modelling of body weight in response to energy intake. Unfortunately, the experiment has some limitations with respect to age, gender, size of the study population, and BMI category. The population of the Minnesota starvation experiment counted 32 male participants. The size of the population was small and the population did not represent differences in gender, BMI category and age. A study, performed on male and female mice, showed that the metabolic processes during bodyweight dynamics are gender-dependent [54]. Therefore, it is necessary to verify and model the body weight dynamics of both males and females. The age of the participants varied between a limited range of 20 and 33 years. Metabolic processes are not only dependent on the gender but also on the age. To estimate the basal metabolic rate (BMR), the equations in [49] are often used and are different depending on gender and age. Calculation of BMR is based on height and weight. In the Minnesota starvation experiment, the average body weight and BMI of the participants prior to the starvation phase were 69.36 kg and 21.7, respectively. All participants apart from one had a BMI in the normal category. Only one subject was slightly overweight with a BMI of 25.4. The aim of this study is to make a first step towards designing a controller to help overweight or obese people lose body weight. However, the constructed controller is based on data of 32 male participants within the normal BMI category. Regardless of the limited subject variation, the controller should eventually depend on time-variant parameters opposed to time-invariant parameters. The benefit of using time-variant parameters is that if the underlying metabolic processes are changed due to unknown factors, the parameters are updated in order to predict future body weight more accurately.

The modelling framework also has certain limitations. It is known that the weight loss intervention strategies will be affected by external factors [55], such as psychological [56–59], occupational [60–63], and metabolic factors [64,65], besides their combined effects [66,67]. These external factors will affect the weight loss intervention, as well as its maintenance in the long term [68,69]. Besides, there is a high degree of heterogeneity in the impact of these factors both, during and after a weight intervention [70]. In principle, the modelling framework developed in this study cannot provide directly any information about this matter during its application throughout the weight intervention. However, there is an aspect in the proposed modelling approach, which can actually allow getting some insight in this regard. One of the reasons for allowing the parameters to vary with time is to capture the contribution of external factors, which impact the process under study but which are not taken explicitly into account in the model. Therefore, the time evolution of the model parameters can be understood as a summary of the contribution of each individual external factor, besides the inherent time evolution related to the process input (energy intake in this study). This is the reason why, although we use a simple compact model based solely on energy intake and bodyweight, this allows describing accurately the weight loss intervention.

This, at first sight, model limitation actually provides one of the most interesting aspects for future improvement and development of the modelling approach. More specifically, it opens the possibility to use the time evolution of the model parameters as data-based reference to describe the impact of these external factors. If experiments, in which in a controlled manner a weight intervention is taking place and only one or a limited number of its external factors are allowed to vary, then the output from the current mechanistic expression can be tested against the time-variant model parameters. This would allow not only quantifying the impact of one or several of these external factors, but also gaining insight in how to refine the proposed mechanistic relations assumed for them. Yet, the validity of the proposed model could be validated too. Finally, the development of novel features in smartphone and wearable technologies continues growing exponentially. Therefore, it is expected that soon it will become possible to have available real-time measurements of more variables playing a role in the weight intervention. Thus, the model and controller proposed in this study could be expanded and refined in order to describe more accurately and gain more insight in the weight intervention.

## 4. Conclusions

In this work, a data-based mechanistic (DBM) model is tested to describe the individual dynamic responses of bodyweight to changes in the energy intake. During the course of this study, time-invariant and time-variant parameters models are tested. A DARX time-variant parameters model exhibits on average a *NRMSE* of 0.94 ± 0.03. Furthermore, this model allows forecasting bodyweight one week ahead with a *MRPE* of 1.01 ± 0.02%, on average. Moreover, a model predictive controller is developed using this DARX model. This allows suggesting dietary energy intake needed to follow a predefined bodyweight reference trajectory. Targeting experimentally measured bodyweight trajectories, the controller managed to calculate the needed energy intake accurately (*RMSE* = 9 ± 3 kcal day$^{-1}$ between the actual energy intake and the suggested energy intake by the controller). Additionally, it was able to accurately follow the bodyweight reference trajectory (*RMSE* = 0.30 ± 0.06 kg between the actual reference bodyweight and the bodyweight following energy intake suggestions from the controller). Therefore, it can be concluded that in the light of the aforementioned results and findings the developed modeling and MPC algorithms suggested by this paper form a potential solution for real-time bodyweight monitoring and management.

**Author Contributions:** Conceptualization, A.P.F., A.Y., C.M. and J.-M.A.; methodology, A.P.F., A.Y. and J.-M.A.; formal analysis, A.P.F., A.Y. and C.H.; writing—original draft preparation, A.P.F. and A.Y.; writing—review and editing, A.P.F., A.Y., C.M. and J.-M.A.; visualization, A.P.F. and A.Y.; supervision, C.M. and J.-M.A.

**Funding:** This research received no external funding.

**Conflicts of Interest:** The authors declare no conflict of interest.

## References

1. Higginson, A.D.; McNamara, J.M. An adaptive response to uncertainty can lead to weight gain during dieting attempts. *Evol. Med. Public Heal.* **2016**, *2016*, 369–380. [CrossRef] [PubMed]
2. Chow, C.C.; Hall, K.D. The dynamics of human body weight change. *PLoS Comput. Biol.* **2008**, *4*, 1–11. [CrossRef] [PubMed]

3. Mantzoros, C.S. *Nutrition and Metabolism*; 2009 ed.; Humana press, Springer Science & Business Media: New York, NY, USA, 2009.
4. Di Cesare, M.; Bentham, J.; Stevens, G.A.; Zhou, B.; Danaei, G.; Lu, Y.; Bixby, H.; Cowan, M.J.; Riley, L.M.; Hajifathalian, K.; et al. Trends in adult body-mass index in 200 countries from 1975 to 2014: A pooled analysis of 1698 population-based measurement studies with 19.2 million participants. *Lancet* **2016**, *387*, 1377–1396.
5. Russo, C.; Jin, Z.; Ph, D.; Homma, S.; Rundek, T.; Elkind, M.S.V.; Sacco, R.L.; Di Tullio, M.R. Effect of obesity and overweighton left ventricular diastolic function: A community-based study in an elderly cohort. *J. Am. Coll. Cardiol.* **2011**, *57*, 1368–1374. [CrossRef] [PubMed]
6. Taubes, G. Unraveling the obesity-cancer connection. *Science* **2004**, *335*, 28–32. [CrossRef] [PubMed]
7. Wong, C.X.; Abed, H.S.; Molaee, P.; Nelson, A.J.; Brooks, A.G.; Sharma, G.; Leong, D.P.; Lau, D.H.; Middeldorp, M.E.; Roberts-Thomson, K.C.; et al. Pericardial fat is associated with atrial fibrillation severity and ablation outcome. *J. Am. Coll. Cardiol.* **2011**, *57*, 1745–1751. [CrossRef] [PubMed]
8. Ng, M.; Fleming, T.; Robinson, M.; Thomson, B.; Graetz, N.; Margono, C.; Mullany, E.C.; Biryukov, S.; Abbafati, C.; Abera, S.F.; et al. Global, regional and national prevalence of overweight and obesity in children and adults during 1980–2013: A systematic analysis. *Lancet* **2014**, *384*, 766–781. [CrossRef]
9. Skolnik, R. *Noncommunicable Diseases Country Profiles 2018*; World Health Organization: Geneva, Switzerland, 2018; ISBN 9789241514620.
10. Altman, M.; Wilfley, D.E. Evidence Update on the Treatment of Overweight and Obesity in Children and Adolescents. *J. Clin. Child Adolesc. Psychol.* **2015**, *44*, 521–537. [CrossRef]
11. Laila, D.S. A note on human body weight dynamics and control based on the macronutrient and energy flux balance. In Proceedings of the 2010 American Control Conference, Baltimore, MD, USA, 30 June–2 July 2010; pp. 3580–3585.
12. Hurkmans, E.; Matthys, C.; Bogaerts, A.; Scheys, L.; Devloo, K.; Seghers, J. Face-To-face versus mobile versus blended weight loss program: Randomized clinical trial. *JMIR mHealth uHealth*. **2018**, *6*, e14. [CrossRef]
13. Zhu, F.; Bosch, M.; Woo, I.; Kim, S.; Boushey, C.J.; Ebert, D.S.; Delp, E.J. The use of mobile devices in aiding dietary assessment and evaluation. *IEEE J. Sel. Top. Signal Process.* **2010**, *4*, 756–766. [PubMed]
14. Amft, O.; Tröster, G. Recognition of dietary activity events using on-body sensors. *Artif. Intell. Med.* **2008**, *42*, 121–136. [CrossRef] [PubMed]
15. Pellegrini, C.A.; Duncan, J.M.; Moller, A.C.; Buscemi, J.; Sularz, A.; Demott, A.; Pictor, A.; Pagoto, S.; Siddique, J.; Spring, B. A smartphone-supported weight loss program: Design of the ENGAGED randomized controlled trial. *BMC Public Health* **2012**, *12*, 1041. [CrossRef] [PubMed]
16. Steele, R. An Overview of the State of the Art of Automated Capture of Dietary Intake Information. *Crit. Rev. Food Sci. Nutr.* **2015**, *55*, 1929–1938. [CrossRef] [PubMed]
17. Zaidan, S.; Roehrer, E. Popular Mobile Phone Apps for Diet and Weight Loss: A Content Analysis. *JMIR mHealth uHealth* **2016**, *4*, e80. [CrossRef] [PubMed]
18. Gilmore, L.A.; Duhé, A.F.; Frost, E.A.; Redman, L.M. The technology boom: A new era in obesity management. *J. Diabetes Sci. Technol.* **2014**, *8*, 596–608. [CrossRef] [PubMed]
19. Patel, M.L.; Hopkins, C.M.; Brooks, T.L.; Bennett, G.G. Comparing Self-Monitoring Strategies for Weight Loss in a Smartphone App: Randomized Controlled Trial. *JMIR mHealth uHealth* **2019**, *7*, e12209. [CrossRef] [PubMed]
20. Pellegrini, C.A.; Pfammatter, A.F.; Conroy, D.E.; Spring, B. Smartphone application to support weight loss: Current perspectives. *Adv Health Care Technol.* **2015**, *1*, 13–22. [CrossRef] [PubMed]
21. Wishnofsky, M. Caloric equivalents of gained or lost weight. *Am. J. Clin. Nutr.* **1958**, *6*, 542–546. [CrossRef]
22. Hall, K.D.; Sacks, G.; Chandramohan, D.; Chow, C.C.; Wang, Y.C.; Gortmaker, S.L.; Swinburn, B.A. Quantification of the effect of energy imbalance on bodyweight. *Lancet* **2011**, *378*, 826–837. [CrossRef]
23. Thomas, D.M.; Martin, C.K.; Lettieri, S.; Bredlau, C.; Kaiser, K.; Church, T.; Bouchard, C.; Heymsfield, S.B. Can a weight loss of one pound a week be achieved with a 3500-kcal deficit? Commentary on a commonly accepted rule. *Int. J. Obes.* **2013**, *37*, 1611–1613. [CrossRef]
24. Antonetti, V.W. The equations governing weight change in human beings. *Am. J. Clin. Nutr.* **1973**, *26*, 64–71. [CrossRef] [PubMed]
25. Westerterp, K.R.; Donkers, J.H.; Fredrix, E.W.; Boekhoudt, P. Energy intake, physical activity and body weight: A simulation model. *Br. J. Nutr.* **1995**, *73*, 337–347. [CrossRef] [PubMed]

26. Leibel, R.L.; Rosenbaum, M.; Hirsch, J. Changes in energy expenditure resulting from altered body weight. *J. Occup. Environ. Med.* **1995**, *38*, 621–628.
27. Hall, K.D. What is the required energy deficit per unit weight loss? *Int. J. Obes. (Lond.)* **2008**, *32*, 573–576. [CrossRef] [PubMed]
28. Christiansen, E.; Garby, L. Prediction of body weight changes caused by changes in energy balance. *Eur. J. Clin. Investig.* **2002**, *32*, 826–830. [CrossRef] [PubMed]
29. Song, B.; Thomas, D.M. Dynamics of starvation in humans. *J. Math. Biol.* **2007**, *54*, 27–43. [CrossRef]
30. Hargrove, J.L.; Heinz, G.; Heinz, O. Modeling transitions in body composition: The approach to steady state for anthropometric measures and physiological functions in the Minnesota human starvation study. *Dyn. Med.* **2008**, *7*, 1–11. [CrossRef]
31. Hall, K.D. Body fat and fat-free mass inter-relationships: Forbes's theory revisited. *Br. J. Nutr.* **2007**, *97*, 1059–1063. [CrossRef]
32. Hall, K.D. Predicting metabolic adaptation, body weight change, and energy intake in humans. *Am. J. Physiol. Metab.* **2009**, *298*, E449–E466. [CrossRef]
33. Thomas, D.M.; Schoeller, D.A.; Redman, L.A.; Martin, C.K.; Levine, J.A.; Heymsfield, S.B. A computational model to determine energy intake during weight loss. *Am. J. Clin. Nutr.* **2010**, *92*, 1326–1331. [CrossRef] [PubMed]
34. Thomas, D.M. A simple model predicting individual weight change in humans. *J. Biol. Dyn.* **2011**, *5*, 579–599. [CrossRef] [PubMed]
35. Oike, H.; Oishi, K.; Kobori, M. Nutrients, Clock Genes, and Chrononutrition. *Curr. Nutr. Rep.* **2014**, *3*, 204–212. [CrossRef] [PubMed]
36. Tahara, Y.; Shibata, S. Chrono-biology, Chrono-pharmacology, and Chrono-nutrition. *J. Pharmacol. Sci.* **2014**, *124*, 320–335. [CrossRef] [PubMed]
37. Almoosawi, S.; Vingeliene, S.; Karagounis, L.G.; Pot, G.K. Chrono-nutrition: A review of current evidence from observational studies on global trends in time-of-day of energy intake and its association with obesity. *Proc. Nutr. Soc.* **2016**, *75*, 487–500. [CrossRef]
38. Vilela, S.; Oliveira, A.; Severo, M.; Lopes, C. Chrono-Nutrition: The Relationship between Time-of-Day Energy and Macronutrient Intake and Children's Body Weight Status. *J. Biol. Rhythms* **2019**, *34*, 1–11. [CrossRef] [PubMed]
39. Berckmans, D. Automatic on-line monitoring of animals by precision livestock farming. In Proceedings of the 2004 ISAH Conference, Saint-Malo, France, 6–10 September 2004; pp. 27–30.
40. Young, P.C. The data-based mechanistic approach to the modelling, forecasting and control of environmental systems. *Annu. Rev. Control* **2006**, *30*, 169–182. [CrossRef]
41. Aerts, J.M.; Van Buggenhout, S.; Vranken, E.; Lippens, M.; Buyse, J.; Decuypere, E.; Berckmans, D. Active control of the growth trajectory of broiler chickens based on online animal responses. *Poult. Sci.* **2003**, *82*, 1853–1862. [CrossRef]
42. Hauschild, L.; Lovatto, P.A.; Pomar, J.; Pomar, C. Development of sustainable precision farming systems for swine: Estimating real- time individual amino acid requirements in growing- fi nishing pigs. *J. Anim. Sci.* **2012**, *90*, 2255–2263. [CrossRef]
43. Cangar, O.; Aerts, J.M.; Vranken, E.; Berckmans, D. Effects of different target trajectories on the broiler performance in growth control. *Poult. Sci.* **2008**, *87*, 2196–2207.
44. Taylor, C.J.; Pedregal, D.J.; Young, P.C.; Tych, W. Environmental time series analysis and forecasting with the Captain toolbox. *Environ. Model. Softw.* **2007**, *22*, 797–814. [CrossRef]
45. Young, P.C.; Taylor, C.J.; Tych, W.; Pedregal, D.J. *The CAPTAIN Toolbox*; Centre for Research on Environmental Systems and Statistics, Lancaster University: Lancashire, UK, 2007. Available online: http://captaintoolbox.co.uk/Captain_Toolbox.html/Captain_Toolbox.html (accessed on 10 May 2019).
46. Young, P. *Recursive Estimation and Time-Series Analysis*, 2nd ed.; Spring: Berlin/Heidelberg, Germany, 1984; ISBN 9783642219801.
47. Aerts, J.M.; Lippens, M.; De Groote, G.; Buyse, J.; Decuypere, E.; Vranken, E.; Berckmans, D. Recursive prediction of broiler growth response to feed intake by using a time-variant parameter estimation method. *Poult. Sci.* **2003**, *82*, 40–49. [CrossRef] [PubMed]
48. Bemporad, A.; Morari, M.; Ricker, N.L. *MathWorks Model Predictive Control Toolbox$^{TM}$ User's Guide*; Mathworks: Natick, MA, USA, 2015.

49. LeCheminant, J.D.; Jacobsen, D.J.; Bailey, B.W.; Kirk, E.P.; Donelly, J.E. Is greater than 10 percent weight loss associated with further risk reduction in obese women? *Med. Sci. Sports Exerc.* **2004**, *36*, S82.
50. Henry, C.J.K. Basal metabolic rate studies in humans: Measurement and development of new equations. *Public Health Nutr.* **2005**, *8*, 1133–1152. [CrossRef] [PubMed]
51. Strathe, A.B.; Sørensen, H.; Danfær, A. A new mathematical model for combining growth and energy intake in animals: The case of the growing pig. *J. Theor. Biol.* **2009**, *261*, 165–175. [CrossRef] [PubMed]
52. Duncan, K.H.; Bacon, J.A.; Weisner, R.L. The effects of high and low energy density diets on satiety, energy intake and eating time on obese and nonobese subjects. *Am. J. Clin. Nutr.* **1983**, *37*, 763–767. [CrossRef]
53. Keys, A.; Brozek, J.; Henschel, A.; Mickelsen, O.; Taylor, H.L. *The Biology of Human Starvation*; University of Minnesota Press: Minneapolis, MN, USA, 1950.
54. Benz, V.; Bloch, M.; Wardat, S.; Böhm, C.; Maurer, L.; Mahmoodzadeh, S.; Wiedmer, P.; Spranger, J.; Foryst-Ludwig, A.; Kintscher, U. Sexual dimorphic regulation of body weight dynamics and adipose tissue lipolysis. *PLoS ONE* **2012**, *7*. [CrossRef]
55. Blüher, M. Obesity: Global epidemiology and pathogenesis. *Nat. Rev. Endocrinol.* **2019**, *15*, 288–298. [CrossRef]
56. Teixeira, P.J.; Carraça, E.V.; Marques, M.M.; Rutter, H.; Oppert, J.M.; De Bourdeaudhuij, I.; Lakerveld, J.; Brug, J. Successful behavior change in obesity interventions in adults: A systematic review of self-regulation mediators. *BMC Med.* **2015**, *13*, 1–16. [CrossRef]
57. Brockmeyer, T.; Simon, J.J.; Becker, A.; Friederich, H.C. Reward-related decision making and long-term weight loss maintenance. *Physiol. Behav.* **2017**, *181*, 69–74. [CrossRef]
58. Teixeira, P.J.; Marques, M.M. Health Behavior Change for Obesity Management. *Obes. Facts* **2018**, *10*, 666–673. [CrossRef] [PubMed]
59. Harcourt, B.E.; Pons, A.; Kao, K.T.; Twindyakirana, C.; Alexander, E.; Haberle, S.; McCallum, Z.; Sabin, M.A. Psychosocial measures and weight change in a clinical paediatric population with obesity. *Qual. Life Res.* **2019**, *28*, 1555–1564. [CrossRef] [PubMed]
60. Østbye, T.; Stroo, M.; Brouwer, R.J.N.; Peterson, B.L.; Eisenstein, E.L.; Fuemmeler, B.F.; Joyner, J.; Gulley, L.; Dement, J.M. The steps to health employee weight management randomized control trial: Rationale, design and baseline characteristics. *Contemp. Clin. Trials* **2013**, *35*, 68–76. [CrossRef] [PubMed]
61. Ott, U.; Stanford, J.B.; Greenwood, J.L.J.; Murtaugh, M.A.; Gren, L.H.; Thiese, M.S.; Hegmann, K.T. Stages of weight change among an occupational cohort. *J. Occup. Environ. Med.* **2015**, *57*, 270–276. [CrossRef] [PubMed]
62. Haynes, P.L.; Silva, G.E.; Howe, G.W.; Thomson, C.A.; Butler, E.A.; Quan, S.F.; Sherrill, D.; Scanlon, M.; Rojo-Wissar, D.M.; Gengler, D.N.; et al. Longitudinal assessment of daily activity patterns on weight change after involuntary job loss: The ADAPT study protocol. *BMC Public Health* **2017**, *17*, 1–11. [CrossRef]
63. Gudzune, K.A.; Alexander, E.; Tseng, E.; Durkin, N.; Jerome, G.J.; Dalcin, A.; Appel, L.J.; Clark, J.M. Influence of subsidies and promotional strategies on outcomes in a beneficiary-based commercial weight-loss programme. *Clin. Obes.* **2019**, *9*, e12307. [CrossRef] [PubMed]
64. Horton, E.S. Metabolic aspects of exercise and weight reduction. *Med. Sci. Sports Exerc.* **1986**, *18*, 10–18. [CrossRef]
65. Anton, S.D.; Moehl, K.; Donahoo, W.T.; Marosi, K.; Lee, S.A.; Mainous, A.G.; Leeuwenburgh, C.; Mattson, M.P. Flipping the Metabolic Switch: Understanding and Applying the Health Benefits of Fasting. *Obesity* **2018**, *26*, 254–268. [CrossRef]
66. Gram Quist, H.; Christensen, U.; Christensen, K.B.; Aust, B.; Borg, V.; Bjorner, J.B. Psychosocial work environment factors and weight change: A prospective study among Danish health care workers. *BMC Public Health* **2013**, *13*, 21–23. [CrossRef]
67. Guerrero-Vargas, N.N.; Espitia-Bautista, E.; Buijs, R.M.; Escobar, C. Shift-work: Is time of eating determining metabolic health? Evidence from animal models. *Proc. Nutr. Soc.* **2018**, *77*, 199–215. [CrossRef]
68. Montesi, L.; El Ghoch, M.; Brodosi, L.; Calugi, S.; Marchesini, G.; Grave, R.D. Long-term weight loss maintenance for obesity: A multidisciplinary approach. *Diabetes, Metab. Syndr. Obes. Targets Ther.* **2016**, *9*, 37–46.

69. Pedersen, S.; Sniehotta, F.F.; Sainsbury, K.; Evans, E.H.; Marques, M.M.; Stubbs, R.J.; Heitmann, B.L.; Lähteenmäki, L. The complexity of self-regulating food intake in weight loss maintenance. A qualitative study among short- and long-term weight loss maintainers. *Soc. Sci. Med.* **2018**, *208*, 18–24. [CrossRef] [PubMed]
70. Ryder, J.R.; Kaizer, A.M.; Jenkins, T.M.; Kelly, A.S.; Inge, T.H.; Shaibi, G.Q. Heterogeneity in Response to treatment of adolescents with severe obesity: The need for precision obesity medicine. *Obesity* **2019**, *27*, 288–294. [CrossRef] [PubMed]

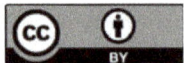

© 2019 by the authors. Licensee MDPI, Basel, Switzerland. This article is an open access article distributed under the terms and conditions of the Creative Commons Attribution (CC BY) license (http://creativecommons.org/licenses/by/4.0/).

*Article*

# Novel Design and Lateral Stability Tracking Control of a Four-Wheeled Rollator

Xin Zhang [1], Jiehao Li [2], Zhenhuan Hu [1], Wen Qi [3], Longbin Zhang [4], Yingbai Hu [5], Hang Su [1,3,*], Giancarlo Ferrigno [3] and Elena De Momi [3]

1. College of Art and Design, Guangdong University of Technology, Guangzhou 510000, China; zx474099@gmail.com (X.Z.); hu18813291455@gmail.com (Z.H.)
2. Key Laboratory of Intelligent Control and Decision of Complex Systems, Beijing Institute of Technology, Beijing 100081, China; 3120185447@bit.edu.cn
3. Dipartimento di Elettronica, Informazione e Bioingegneria, Politecnico di Milano, 20133 Milano, Italy; wen.qi@polimi.it (W.Q.); giancarlo.ferrigno@polimi.it (G.F.); elena.demomi@polimi.it (E.D.M.)
4. BioMEx Center & KTH Mechanics, KTH Royal Institute of Technology, SE-100 44 Stockholm, Sweden; longbin@kth.se
5. Department of Informatics, Technical University of Munich, 85748 Munich, Germany; yingbai.hu@tum.de
* Correspondence: hang.su@polimi.it; Tel.: +39-338-750-6165

Received: 25 April 2019; Accepted: 4 June 2019; Published: 6 June 2019

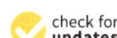

**Featured Application:** A rollator is an integrated functional application used clinically to empower and assist natural human mobility for the elderly or disabled users. In this paper, an integrated system of four-wheeled rollator is designed by introducing a novel mechanical design theory and a lateral stability tracking control is performed to validate the control feasibility of the four-wheeled rollator, providing an optimized procedure for further development of rollators.

**Abstract:** Design and control of smart rollators have attracted increasing research interests in the past decades. To meet the requirements of the elderly or disabled users, this paper proposes a novel design and tracking control scheme for empowering and assisting natural human mobility with a four-wheeled rollator. Firstly, by integrating the advantages of Kano Model Analysis and the Theory of Inventive Problem Solving (TRIZ), we introduce a novel Kano-TRIZ industrial design method to design and optimize its mechanical structure. The demand and quality characteristics of the clinical rollator are analyzed according to the Kano model. The Quality Function Deployment (QFD) and TRIZ are adopted to integrate industrial product innovations and optimize the function configuration. Furthermore, a lateral stability controller based on Model Predictive Control (MPC) scheme is introduced to achieve good tracking control performance with the lateral deviation and the heading angle deviation. Finally, the feasibility of the design and control method is verified with a simulation study. The simulation results indicate that the proposed algorithm keeps the lateral position error in a reasonable range. In the co-simulation of ADAMS-MATLAB, the trajectory of the rollator is smooth with constrained position error within 0.1 m, the turning angle and speed can achieve stable tracking control within 5 s and the heading angle is accurate and the speed is stable. A compared experiment with MPC and SMC show that MPC controller has faster response, higher tracking accuracy and smoother trajectory on the novel designed rollator. With the increasing demand for rollators in the global market, the methodology proposed in this paper will attract more research and industry interests.

**Keywords:** Kano-TRIZ design theory; quality function deployment; four-wheeled rollator; model predictive control

## 1. Introduction

With the aging population, the physiological changes of organs and its consequent loss of function lead to the increased physical disability, which limits human mobility of the elderly. This has been one of the main reasons for the loneliness, and it affects the mental health of the elderly [1–3]. A four-wheeled rollator is a tool that assists human with motor dysfunction to walk. As a life partner for the elderly, the four-wheeled rollator creates a relative old-age lifestyle by empowering and assisting natural human mobility [4] and improves the quality of life in later life, allowing older people with motion system limitation to go out with the assistance from the four-wheeled rollator, which is beneficial to the physical and mental health of users.

In recent years, the research in the design and control of smart rollators has attracted many interests [5–8]. However, most of the research in the literature adopt questionnaires, interviews, observations and other methods to obtain user needs [9], without analyzing the type and importance of the requirements. They directly designed the mechanical structure according to the original demand. Functions of the design and the requirement that needs to be solved are still not satisfied. The solving the problem invention theory (TRIZ) [10–12] has been successfully applied in several domains such as aeronautics, car industry, and electronics, etc. It is known as using the TRIZ problem model to describe the design problem and then using TRIZ tool to solve the described problem. TRIZ is capable of modeling and converting the simulation solution into the practical solution of the industry domain. Kano model is a non-linear relationship between customer satisfaction and product objective quality. By integrating the advantages of Kano Model Analysis and TRIZ, the Kano-TRIZ design theory [13,14] presents an effective methodology to study and to provide design principles of the four-wheeled rollator, which take account of the physical and mental characteristics of the elderly. Quality Function Deployment (QFD) is a user-driven quality function configuration method. However, in the research of rollator design [15–19], the popularity of TRIZ to solve the problems of four-wheeled rollator design is still relatively limited, basically in the germination stage.

Except for the mechanical design of the four-wheeled rollator, its mobility is also of vital of importance for its market feasibility. The lateral motion stability control of four-wheeled rollator is the main challenge in terms of safety, especially for the elderly lacking motion ability. Hence it is necessary to develop a stable controller to validate the feasibility of motion control of the rollator. Since the longitudinal movement of the four-wheeled rollator can be controlled by handbrake and human traction, this paper focuses on its lateral motion stability. The purpose of the lateral stability control of the four-wheel rollator is to design an advanced controller to achieve the smooth trajectory tracking control of the rollator. According to the literature, the lateral control approaches of the rollators mainly include proportional-integral-derivative (PID) control, fuzzy adaptive control, sliding mode variable structure control, neural network control, etc. Wu et al. [20] proposed a parameter self-tuning fuzzy PID control method to effectively reduce the yaw rate and slip rate. Based on the rollator model and steering system model, Han et al. [21] designed a neural network PID controller with good real-time and robustness. In order to overcome the problems of nonlinearity, parameter uncertainty, and time-varying external disturbance, ref. [22] proposed an adaptive fuzzy sliding mode control strategy to achieve adaptive control. The performance in terms of smooth is considered in [23], a fuzzy control algorithm based on iterative genetic algorithm is proposed. Ref. [24] proposed a trajectory optimization algorithm to formulate the lateral vehicle guidance task along a reference trajectory, which is with optimized efficiency. Ref. [25] proposed a two-layer model predictive control controller to optimize the required longitudinal force and yaw moment adjustments and to achieve the minimized error of the steady state tracking objective. A combined control algorithm was designed in [26] by taking the yaw rate and the centroid slip angle error as input variables and using the braking torque as the steering angle of the control objectives. In [27], a novel fusion feed-forward neural network controller for task decomposition was proposed to realize the lateral control of autonomous vehicles. In [28], a robust output feedback vehicle lateral motion control strategy considering network-induced delay and tire force saturation was proposed to overcome the uncertainty of tire turning stiffness and external disturbance.

In this paper, we introduce a QFD model and Kano-TRIZ industrial design method to design a novel four-wheeled rollator and adopt a model predictive control algorithm to achieve the lateral trajectory tracking control of the rollator. A simulation was conducted to validate its feasibility in terms of the trajectory tracking error of the proposed design and control methodology.

The remainder of this paper is structured as follows: Section 2 describes the novel rollator design with Kano-Triz theory; Section 3 discusses the kinematic and dynamic model of the designed rollator and introduces lateral stability tracking control for its controller development; simulation and validation is performed and the corresponding results and discussions are drawn in Section 4. The conclusion and future work are presented in Section 5.

## 2. Novel Rollator Mechanical Design with Kano-TRIZ

This chapter focuses on the development of a four-wheeled elderly rollator application based on the new Kano-TRIZ industrial design approach. The main idea is to analyze the characteristics of the target users and the problems of using rollators for elderly people in daily life. The Kano model is applied to construct the demand function. Further, the QFD method is used to optimize the technical features, and the TRIZ industrial design method is utilized to design the function of a rollator to meet the characteristics of the elderly user. By taking account of the motion system, material weight, human weight and ground counterforce, the optimized functional diagram design of the four-wheeled rollator is shown in Figure 1.

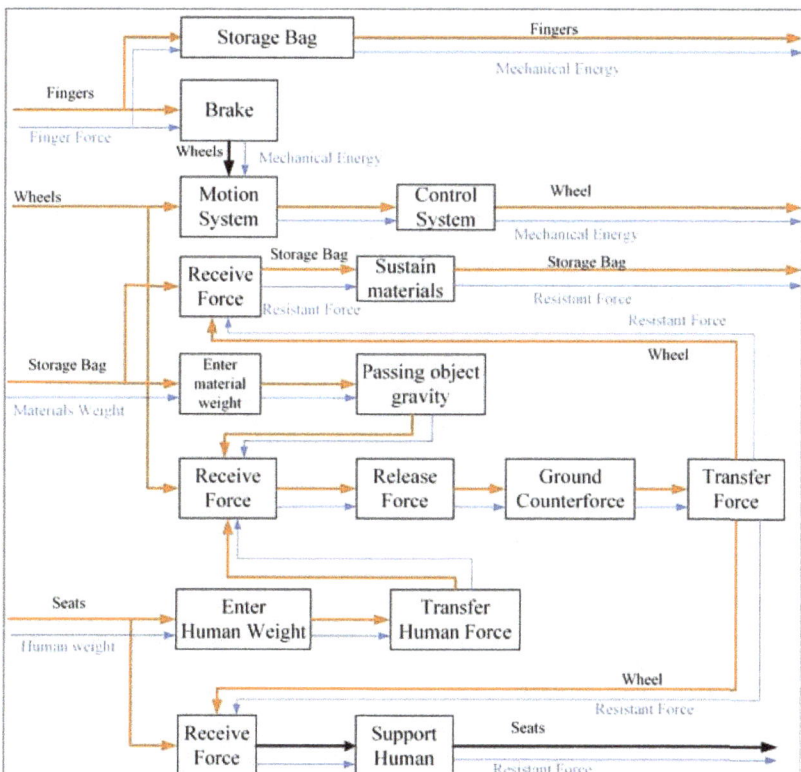

**Figure 1.** A functional diagram for rollator design.

## 2.1. Functional Mechanical Design

The main functions of the four-wheeled elderly rollator are assisted walking, rest, storage and safety control. Similar to the functions of bicycle operation, this rollator is divided into three sub-functions: adjusting the height, moving forward and stopping the movement. The function diagram for the rollator mechanical design shown in Figure 1.

## 2.2. Kano Model Analysis

Firstly, the questionnaires of the demand for the products to analyze the needs of the target users is conducted after product analysis. A sorting rule of the questionnaires is chosen as:

The average composite score of the sorting questions is automatically calculated according to the ranking of all the candidates' options. It reflects the comprehensive ranking of the options. The higher the score is, the higher the overall ranking will be. The calculation method is to calculate the option average comprehensive score and its weight is determined by where the options are arranged. For example, if there are 3 candidates to participate in sorting, the rank has a weight of 3 in the first position, the second position has a weight of 2, and the third position has a weight of 1. If a topic is filled in 12 times, option A is selected and ranked in the first position 2 times, while the second position is 4 times and the third position is 6 times. The average comprehensive score of option $A = (2 \times 3 + 4 \times 2 + 6 \times 1)/12 = 1.67$ points.

It is should be noticed that the score here is related to the number of options. For example, there are 3 options for sorting and the first score is 3 points. If there are 30 options, the first score is 30 points, and this score won't be affected. If the sorting option is a multiple-choice question that refers to the previous question, the first score in that row is the number of options for the multiple-choice question.

The survey method is adopted and a conclusion of the questionnaires is made and shown in Figure 2. Then we compared all the collected Kano attribute questionnaires with the Kano model analysis table, and obtain the Kano category membership of demand indicators in questionnaires filled out by each user. The corresponding analysis principle diagram of TRIZ solving problem is shown in Figure 3. TRIZ tools for electronic data processing allow building a specific idea and database. A criterion proposed in the literature is adapted to allow automatic update of the Knowledge Base [29,30].

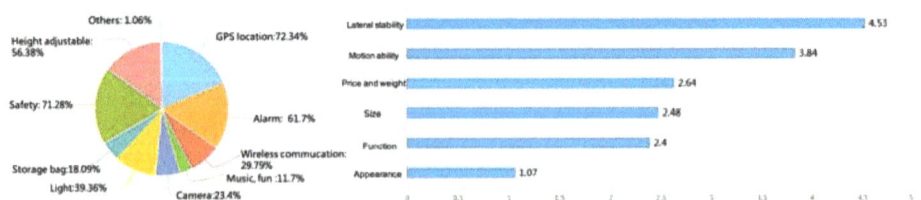

**Figure 2.** Demand analysis of Kano attribute questionnaires.

TRIZ theory is a creative method to solve the inherent contradictions of products, which can produce breakthrough innovations and fundamentally eliminate the problems of navigation design for elderly rollators. The designer ignores the type and importance of the demand and directly designs the product according to the original requirements, which leads to some of the functions are not what the user is currently demanding. The Kano model can be used to classify users' needs and determine the relative importance. The QFD evaluation is used to convert customer requirements into effective product demand after the Kano analysis. Therefore, the process of using TRIZ-KANO-DQF industrial design new method is shown in Figure 3:

1. TRIZ translates specific product technical features into technical features that engineering designers can understand;

2. The Kano model is used to analyze the function demand after the survey of user requirements;
3. The QFD evaluation method with the design of the quality house (HOQ) is carried out to transform the user's requirements to product demand.

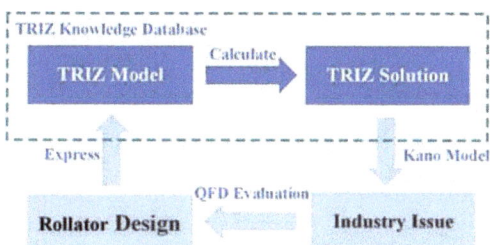

**Figure 3.** Principle diagram of TRIZ solving problem.

Figure 4 exhibits the specific process of the four-wheeled rollator. In the original manuscript, the roundness combined with the block shape makes the user feel more energetic, but it lacks diplomatic feeling. Then an improved manuscript that combining the lines and block shape is designed. This manuscript gives a steady feeling but it makes the user feel heavy with fatigue. We finally decided to combine the line style, and strengthen the structural performance of the bottom, making users feel that the product is stable and reliable.

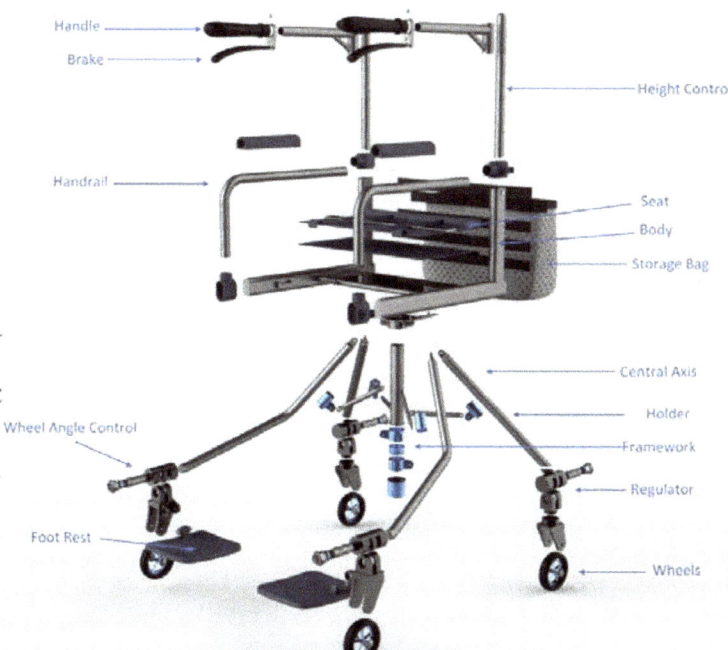

**Figure 4.** Novel design of four-wheeled rollator.

### 2.3. Structural Details of Modeling, Structure and Materials

With the increase of age, the physical function of the elderly continues to deteriorate, resulting in a weakened memory and cognitive disability. From the Kano questionnaires, the product with simple and intuitive feelings is more suitable for elderly users. Therefore, the simple geometric shape is used as the modeling foundation, and the common object design form in daily life is applied, which can meet the needs of safety and reliability. The seat adjuster is designed to meet the needs of different users while planning a simple replacement structure for the tire. The frame is mainly made of aluminum alloy. The handle is in direct contact with the user for a long time, which requires the soft material and air permeability, so we select the permeability rubber. The seat and storage bag materials are made of nylon fabric, for weight, durable and easy to install.

## 3. Lateral Stability Tracking Control of Designed Rollator

Because of the high safety requirement of rollator for the elderly, it is necessary to design the lateral motion control of the auxiliary driving system [31]. In this chapter, a tracking controller of the four-wheel rollator is carried out by the model prediction algorithm in term of the trajectory error.

### 3.1. Rollator Kinematic Model

Figure 5 exhibits the kinematic model of the rollator. $(X_r, Y_r)$ and $(X_f, Y_f)$ are the center coordinates of the rear axis and the front axis, respectively. $\varphi$ is the yaw angle, $\delta_f$ the steering angle of front wheels, $v_r$ the velocity of the rear axle center, $v_f$ the velocity of front axle center, L is the wheel track, R is the radius, P is the center of rotation, M is the center of the rear axis, and N is the center of the front axis.

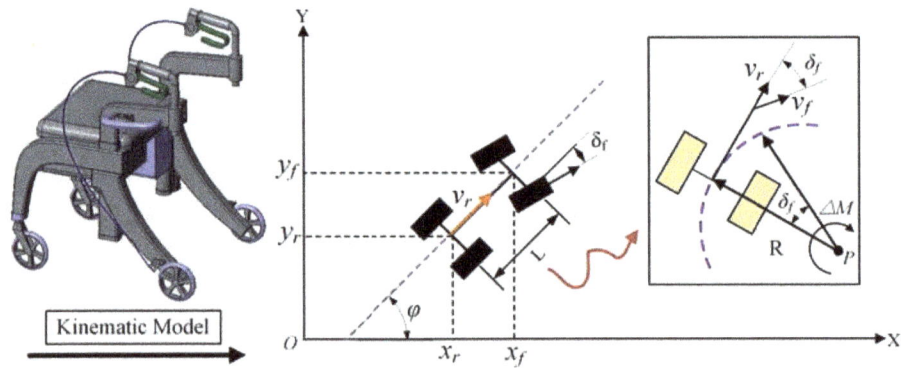

**Figure 5.** Kinematic model of four-wheeled rollator.

Assuming that the steering radius and the radius of road curvature are the same in the steering process, the velocity of the rear axis $v_r$ can be described as:

$$v_r = \dot{X}_r \cos \varphi + \dot{Y}_r \sin \varphi \qquad (1)$$

The kinematic model of the rollator is presented as:

$$\begin{array}{l} \dot{X}_f \sin\left(\varphi + \delta_f\right) - \dot{Y}_f \cos\left(\varphi + \delta_f\right) = 0 \\ \dot{X}_r \cos \varphi - \dot{Y}_r \sin \varphi = 0 \end{array} \qquad (2)$$

According to Equation (2), we can define:

$$\begin{array}{l} \dot{X}_r = v_r \cos \varphi \\ \dot{Y}_r = v_r \sin \varphi \end{array} \qquad (3)$$

where $v_r$ is the robot speed, $(X_r, Y_r)$ and $(X_r, Y_r)$ are the coordinate of rear-wheel and front-wheel, respectively, and $\varphi$ and $\delta_f$ are the course angle and turning angle of front-wheel, respectively. From the mathematical relationship between the front and rear wheels, the following can be obtained as:

$$X_f = X_r + L \cos \varphi$$
$$Y_f = Y_r + L \sin \varphi \tag{4}$$

Furthermore, the angle rate $\omega$ is obtained as:

$$\omega = \frac{v_r \tan \delta_f}{L} \tag{5}$$

where $L$ is the wheel base of front and rear wheels.

Therefore, the kinematic model of rollator could be written as:

$$\begin{bmatrix} \dot{X}_r \\ \dot{Y}_r \\ \dot{\varphi} \end{bmatrix} = \begin{bmatrix} \cos \varphi \\ \sin \varphi \\ 0 \end{bmatrix} v_r + \begin{bmatrix} 0 \\ 0 \\ 1 \end{bmatrix} \omega \tag{6}$$

where $\zeta_s = [X_r, Y_r, \varphi]^T$ is the system state and $u_S = [v_r, \omega]^T$ is the control value.

### 3.2. Rollator Dynamic Model and Tire Model

Figure 6 demonstrates the dynamic model and tire model of the rollator.

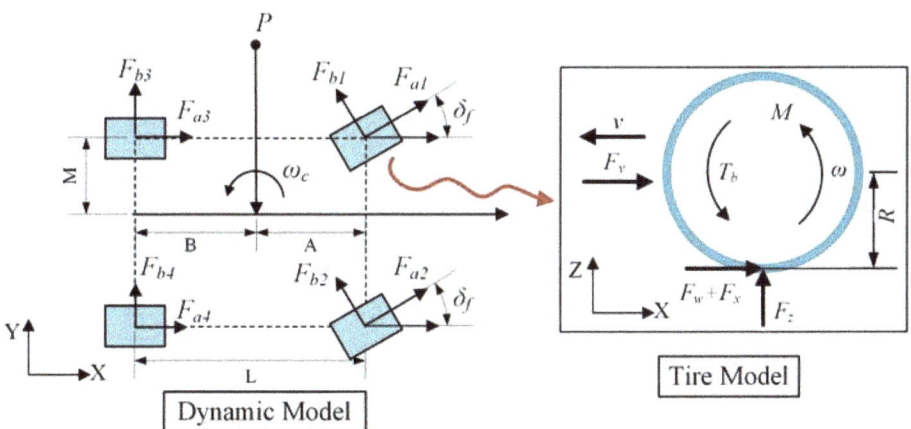

**Figure 6.** Dynamic model and tire model.

In order to insure the high safety requirement of the elderly rollator, we design longitudinal motion, lateral motion and transverse motion, separately [32–34]. According to the Newton's laws, the dynamic model can be described as:

$$\begin{aligned} m\ddot{x} &= m\dot{y}\omega_c + F_{a1} \cos \delta_f + F_{a2} \cos \delta_f + F_{a3} + F_{a4} \\ m\ddot{y} &= -m\dot{x}\omega_c + F_{b1} \cos \delta_f + F_{b2} \cos \delta_f + F_{b3} + F_{b4} \\ I_z \ddot{\varphi} &= A \left( F_{b1} \cos \delta_f + F_{b2} \cos \delta_f \right) - B \left( F_{b3} + F_{b4} \right) + M \left( -F_{a1} \cos \delta_f + F_{a2} \cos \delta_f - F_{a3} + F_{a4} \right) \end{aligned} \tag{7}$$

where $F_{a1}$, $F_{a2}$, $F_{a3}$ and $F_{a4}$ are the wheel force of left front, right front, left rear and right front respectively in X-axis. $F_{b1}$, $F_{b2}$, $F_{b3}$ and $F_{b4}$ are the wheel force of left front, right front, left rear and right front respectively in Y-axis. $I_Z$ is the rotational inertia and $\omega_c$ the center yaw velocity.

Assuming that the lateral force of the tire during the regular tire movement is proportional, there are:

$$\begin{aligned} F_{b1} &= \psi_{\delta F} \Gamma_{\delta F} \\ F_{b2} &= \psi_{\delta R} \Gamma_{\delta R} \\ \psi_{\delta F} &= \beta + \frac{M\omega_r}{v_x} - \delta_f \\ \psi_{\delta R} &= \beta + \frac{M\omega_r}{v_x} \end{aligned} \tag{8}$$

where $\psi_{\delta F}$ and $\psi_{\delta R}$ are tire cornering angle of front-wheel and rear-wheel, respectively. $\Gamma_{\delta F}$ and $\Gamma_{\delta B}$ of front-wheel and rear-wheel, respectively. $\beta$ is the slip angle.

Slip ratio is the key issue of the tire in maintaining stable motion. In Figure 6, the tire model can be presented as:

$$\begin{aligned} J\dot{\omega} &= RF_x - RF_\omega - T_b \\ M\dot{v} &= -F_x - \mu F_v \end{aligned} \tag{9}$$

where $R$ is the rolling radius, $v$ is rollator speed, $T_b$ is the braking torque, $F_x$ is the friction, $F_v$ is the air resistance, $F_\omega$ is the rolling resistance, $F_z$ is the ground reaction force, $M$ is the rollator quality and $J$ is the rotational inertia At the same time, the slip rate $S$ and the friction $F_x$ can be defined as:

$$\begin{aligned} S &= \frac{v - \omega R}{v} \\ F_x &= \mu F_z \end{aligned} \tag{10}$$

where $\mu$ is the adhesion coefficient.

We assume that the system state is $x_1 = \frac{v}{R}$, $x_2 = \omega$ and $x_3 = S$, then the tire function can be transformed as:

$$\begin{aligned} \dot{x}_1 &= -\frac{F_v + F_Z \mu}{MR} \\ \dot{x}_2 &= \frac{F_z R \mu - F_w R - T_b}{J} \\ \dot{x}_3 &= \frac{1}{v} \left[ \frac{(S-1)(F_v + F_z + \mu F_z)}{M} + \frac{F_z R^2 (T_b - \mu)}{J} \right] \end{aligned} \tag{11}$$

### 3.3. Lateral Controller Development

Figure 7 exhibits the MPC controller structure for lateral trajectory tracking. MPC scheme is mainly composed of a trajectory error function, system constraint and optimization objective function [35]. The error equation is the mathematical description of the tracking control system and the basis of the control algorithm. System constraints include rollator actuator constraints, control smooth constraints and stability constraints. The design of the objective function is based on the stability and rapidity of trajectory tracking.

#### 3.3.1. Trajectory Error Function

According to the kinematic model in Equation (6) and tracking error model in Figure 8, we can obtain the relationship as:

$$\begin{bmatrix} \dot{X}_r \\ \dot{Y}_r \\ \dot{\varphi} \end{bmatrix} = \begin{bmatrix} \cos \varphi \\ \sin \varphi \\ \tan \delta / L \end{bmatrix} v_r \tag{12}$$

where $(x, y)$ is the center coordinate, $\varphi$ is yaw angle, and $v$ is the velocity. Then the rollator control system can be seen as input variable $u(v, \delta)$ and state variable $\chi(x, y, \varphi)$:

$$\dot{\mathcal{X}} = \mathcal{W}(\mathcal{X}, u) \tag{13}$$

To facilitate the MPC controller [36], we define the expected equation of motion trajectory as:

$$\dot{X}_d = \mathcal{W}(X_d, u_d) \tag{14}$$

where expected state variable is $X_d = [x_d, y_d, \varphi_d]^T$ and the expected input variable is $u_d = [v_d, \delta_d]$. We transform the Equation (13) according to the Taylor formulation and ignore the high-order term, then:

$$\dot{x} = w(x_d, u_d) + \left.\frac{\partial \mathcal{W}(x,u)}{\partial x}\right|_{\substack{x=x_d \\ u=u_d}} (x - x_d) + \left.\frac{\partial w(x,u)}{\partial u}\right|_{\substack{x=x_d \\ u=u_d}} (u - u_d) \tag{15}$$

Therefore, we can get the lateral error function according to Equations (14) and (15).

$$\begin{aligned}
\dot{x}_e &= (\dot{x} - \dot{x}_d) = -v_d \sin\varphi_d (x - x_d) + \cos\varphi_d (v - v_d) \\
\dot{y}_e &= (\dot{y} - \dot{y}_d) = v_d \cos\varphi_d (y - y_d) + \sin\varphi_d (v - v_d) \\
\dot{\varphi}_e &= (\dot{\varphi} - \dot{\varphi}_d) = \frac{\tan\delta_d}{L}(v - v_d) + \frac{v_d}{L\cos^2\delta_d}(\delta - \delta_d)
\end{aligned} \tag{16}$$

Furthermore, to discretize the error function, we can obtain the model as follow

$$\tilde{X}(k+1) = \mathcal{H}_{k,t}\tilde{X}(k) + \mathcal{K}_{k,t}\tilde{u}(k) \tag{17}$$

Among them, $\mathcal{H}_{k,t} = \begin{bmatrix} 1 & 0 & -v_d T \sin\varphi_d \\ 0 & 1 & v_d T \cos\varphi_d \\ 0 & 0 & 1 \end{bmatrix}$, $\mathcal{K}_{k,t} = \begin{bmatrix} T\cos\varphi_d & 0 \\ T\sin\varphi_d & 0 \\ \frac{\tan\delta_d}{L}T & \frac{v_d}{L\cos^2\delta_d}T \end{bmatrix}$ and $T$ is the sampling time.

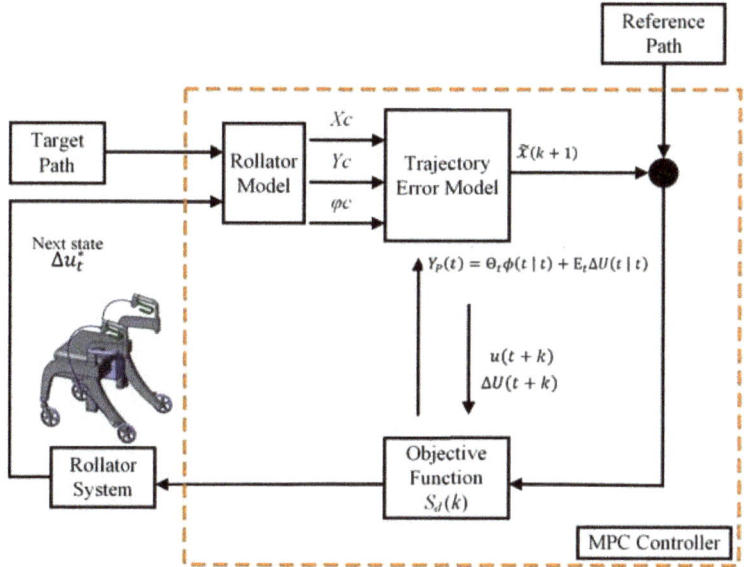

**Figure 7.** MPC controller structure.

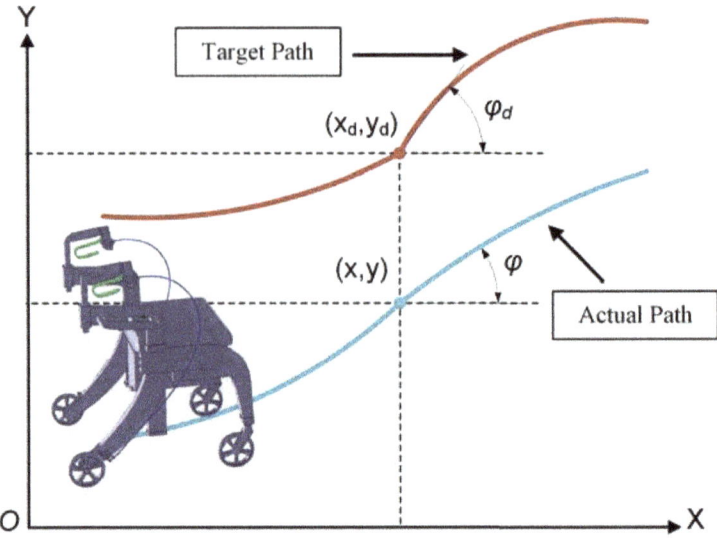

**Figure 8.** Tracking error model.

3.3.2. Objective Function Design

The objective function requires that elderly rollator can track the desired trajectory safely and quickly, so it is necessary to optimize the state error and control variable. We set the objective function as follows:

$$S(k) = \sum_{j=1}^{N} \tilde{X}^T(k+j|k)\mathcal{L}(k+j) + \tilde{u}^T(k+j-1)\mathcal{M}\tilde{u}(k+j-1) \quad (18)$$

where $\mathcal{L}$ and $\mathcal{M}$ are weighting factors.

As can be seen form the objective function, $\sum_{j=1}^{N} \tilde{X}^T(k+j|k)\mathcal{L}\tilde{X}(k+j)$ reflects the ability of the control system to follow the desired trajectory, and $\tilde{u}^T(k+j-1)\mathcal{M}\tilde{u}(k+j-1)$ represents the constraints of control variables. The objective function can be transformed into the standard quadratic form, but the control increment cannot be controlled. Therefore, we design an improved objective function using relaxation factors as follows:

$$S_d(k) = \sum_{i=1}^{N_p} \|Y(k+i|t) - Y_{\text{ref}}(k+i|t)\|_{\mathcal{L}}^2 + \sum_{i=1}^{N_e-1} \|\Delta U(k+i|t)\|_{\mathcal{L}}^2 + \sigma\psi^2 \quad (19)$$

Among them, $N_p$ is the prediction horizon, $N_e$ is the control horizon, $\sigma$ is the weight coefficient, and $\psi$ is the weighting factor. Then, we can transform the trajectory error model as:

$$\phi(k|t) = [\tilde{X}(k|t), \tilde{u}(k-1|t)]^T \quad (20)$$

The state function can be described as:

$$\phi(k+1|t) = \tilde{\mathcal{H}}_{k,t}(k|t) + \tilde{\mathcal{F}}_{k,t}\Delta U(k|t) \\ Y(k|t) = \tilde{z}_{k,t}\phi(k|t) \quad (21)$$

where $\tilde{\mathcal{H}}_{k,t} = \begin{bmatrix} \mathcal{H}_{k,t} & \mathcal{K}_{k,t} \\ 0_{m \times n} & I_m \end{bmatrix}$, $\tilde{\mathcal{K}}_{k,t} = [\mathcal{X}_{k,t}, I_m]^T$, $n$ is the state degree and $m$ is the control variable degree. To simplify the calculation, we assume

$$\begin{aligned} \mathcal{H}_{k,t} &= \mathcal{H}_{l,t} \\ \mathcal{X}_{k,t} &= \mathcal{X}_{t,t} \end{aligned} \qquad (22)$$

where $k = 1, 2, \cdots, t + N - 1$. Based on the above analysis, the model prediction output can be obtained as follows:

$$Y_P(t) = \Theta_t \phi(t|t) + E_t \Delta U(t|t) \qquad (23)$$

which subjects to $Y_P(t) = \begin{bmatrix} Y(t+1|t) \\ Y(t+2|t) \\ \cdots \\ \gamma(t+N_c|t) \\ \cdots \\ \gamma(t+N_P|t) \end{bmatrix}, \Theta_t = \begin{bmatrix} \tilde{Z}_{t,t} \tilde{\mathcal{H}}_{t,t} \\ \tilde{Z}_{t,t} \tilde{\mathcal{F}}_{t,t}^2 \\ \cdots \\ \tilde{Z}_{t,t} \tilde{\mathcal{F}}_{t,t}^{N_c} \\ \cdots \\ \tilde{Z}_{t,t} \tilde{\mathcal{F}}_{t,t}^{N_P} \end{bmatrix}, \Delta U = \begin{bmatrix} \Delta u(t|t) \\ \Delta u(t+1|t) \\ \cdots \\ \Delta u(t+N_c|t) \end{bmatrix}$, and $E_t =$

$$\begin{bmatrix} \tilde{Z}_{t,t} \tilde{\mathcal{H}}_{t,t} & 0 & 0 & 0 \\ \tilde{Z}_{t,t} \tilde{\mathcal{F}}_{t,t} \tilde{\mathcal{K}}_{t,t} & \tilde{Z}_{t,t} \tilde{\mathcal{K}}_{t,t} & 0 & 0 \\ \cdots & \cdots & \ddots & \cdots \\ \tilde{Z}_{t,t} \tilde{\mathcal{H}}_{t,t}^{N_c-1} \tilde{\mathcal{K}}_{t,t} & \tilde{Z}_{t,t} \tilde{\mathcal{H}}_{t,t}^{N_c-2} \tilde{\mathcal{K}}_{t,t} & \cdots & \tilde{Z}_{t,t} \tilde{\mathcal{K}}_{t,t} \\ \vdots & \vdots & \ddots & \vdots \\ \tilde{Z}_{t,t} \tilde{\mathcal{H}}_{t,t}^{N_P-1} \tilde{\mathcal{K}}_{t,t} & \tilde{Z}_{t,t} \tilde{\mathcal{H}}_{t,t}^{N_P-2} \tilde{\mathcal{K}}_{t,t} & \cdots & \tilde{Z}_{t,t} \tilde{\mathcal{H}}_{t,t}^{N_P-N_c-1} \tilde{\mathcal{K}}_{t,t} \end{bmatrix}.$$

### 3.3.3. Control Constraint Design

In the previous section, an improved optimization function is designed for the trajectory tracking error model. Considering the safety and stability of the rollator, it is necessary to restrict the control limit and control increment, as following:

$$\begin{aligned} u_{\min}(t+k) &\le u(t+k) \le u_{\max}(t+k) \\ \Delta U_{\min}(t+k) &\le \Delta U(t+k) \le \Delta U_{\max}(t+k) \end{aligned} \qquad (24)$$

where $k = 1, 2, \cdots, t + N_c - 1$. To transform the Equation (24), we can get

$$u(t+k) = u(t+k-1) + \Delta U(t+k) \qquad (25)$$

Define the following vectors: $U_\lambda = 1_{N_c} \otimes u(k-1)$ and $H = I_m \otimes \begin{bmatrix} 1 & 0 & \cdots & \cdots & 0 \\ 1 & 1 & 0 & \cdots & 0 \\ 1 & 1 & 1 & \ddots & 0 \\ \vdots & \vdots & \ddots & \ddots & 0 \\ 1 & 1 & \cdots & 1 & 1 \end{bmatrix}$.

The optimization objective function can be represented as

$$\delta[\phi(t), u(t), \Delta U(t)] = \mathcal{F}_t \begin{bmatrix} \Delta U(t)^T, \psi \end{bmatrix}^T + \begin{bmatrix} \Delta U(t)^T, \psi \end{bmatrix}^T \mathcal{D}_t \begin{bmatrix} \Delta U(t)^T, \psi \end{bmatrix}^T \qquad (26)$$

where $|\mathcal{F}_t = [2e_t^T \mathcal{L} E_t, 0]$ and $\mathcal{D}_t = \begin{bmatrix} E_t^T \mathcal{L} E_t + \mathcal{M} & 0 \\ 0 & \sigma \end{bmatrix}$. Therefore, the prediction horizon error can be obtained:

$$\begin{aligned} e_t &= \Theta_t \phi(t|t) - Y_{\text{ref}}(t) \\ Y_{\text{ref}}(t) &= [Y_{\text{ref}}(t+1|t), \cdots, Y_{\text{ref}}(t+N_P|t)]^T \end{aligned} \qquad (27)$$

When the model predictive control completes the optimization objective function each time, the control input increment of the system in the control horizon is:

$$\Delta U_t^* = \left[\Delta u_t^*, \Delta u_{t+1}^*, \cdots, \Delta u_{t+N_c-1}^*\right]^T \qquad (28)$$

Finally, the first element of the control increment (Equation (28)) is applied to the control system as the actual control input increment

$$u(t) = u(t-1) + \Delta u_t^* \qquad (29)$$

In order to achieve the ability of stability and smoothness for tracking performance, we define the constraint condition of control variable as

$$\begin{bmatrix} -0.3 \\ -25 \end{bmatrix} \leq u \leq \begin{bmatrix} 0.3 \\ 25 \end{bmatrix}$$
$$\begin{bmatrix} -0.02 \\ -0.04 \end{bmatrix} \leq \Delta U \leq \begin{bmatrix} 0.02 \\ 0.04 \end{bmatrix} \qquad (30)$$

## 4. Results and Discussion

In order to verify the lateral stability control of the MPC algorithm proposed in the previous chapter, simulation experiments are performed using ADAMS-MATLAB.

We set up two different experiments, including tracking a desired line with MPC algorithm and following a sinusoid with MPC and SMC.

The initial condition of the simulation is set as follows: the rollator starts from the coordinate origin and tracks the expected curve $y = 2$ with the desired longitudinal velocity $v = 1$ m/s. The sampling time is 50 ms and the simulation time is 20 s. The simulation process includes areference trajectory generation, variable initialization, system matrix definition and controller design. The simulation results are shown in Figures 9–12.

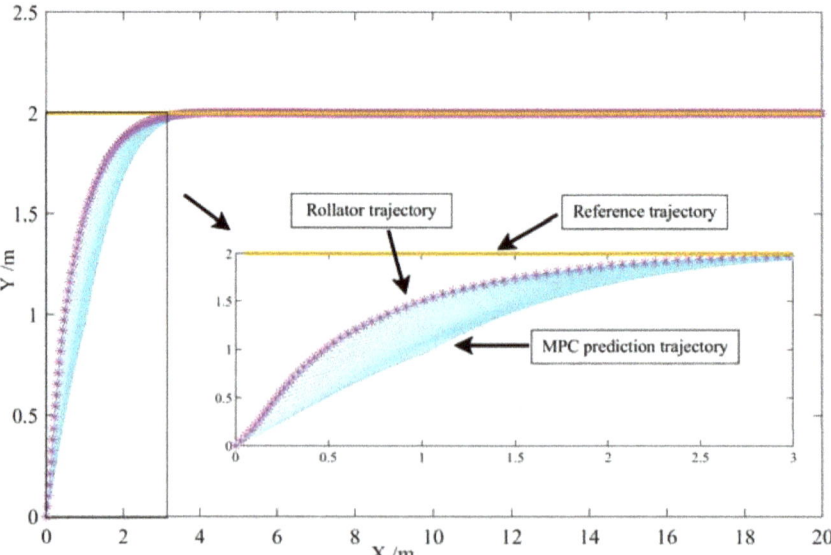

**Figure 9.** Results of MPC-based Predicted Trajectory.

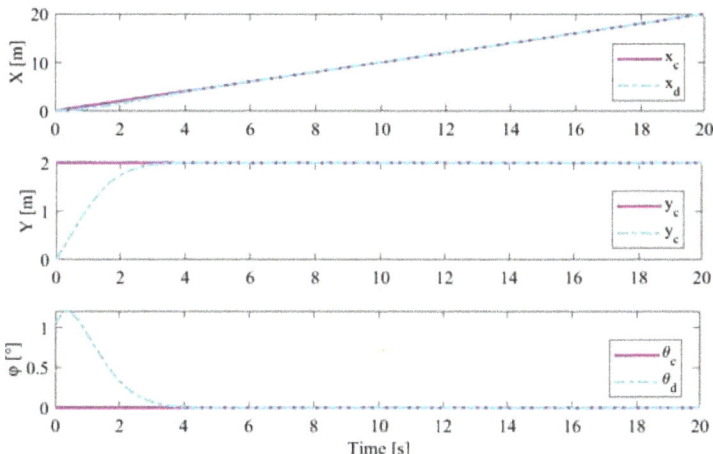

**Figure 10.** Longitudinal position, lateral position and yaw angle.

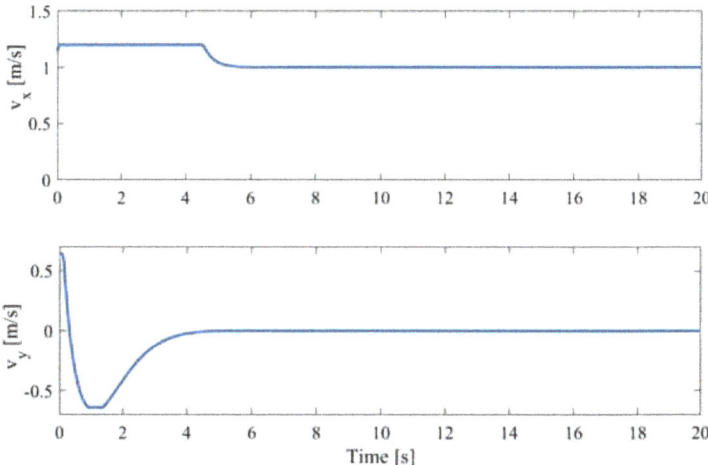

**Figure 11.** Longitudinal velocity and lateral velocity.

Figures 9–12 present the trajectory control performance of the elderly rollator based on the model prediction controller. The reference trajectory is a straight line as shown in Figure 9. The four-wheeled rollator is moved at a uniform speed of 1 m/s. The tracking performance of longitudinal position, lateral position and yaw angle to follow the desired trajectories are shown in Figure 10 based on the MPC control method. Figure 11 shows the longitudinal speed and lateral speed. Figure 12 demonstrates the longitudinal error, lateral error and leading angle error. It can be seen from Figures 9–12 that the rollator can quickly track the reference trajectory at 0–4 s as well as at 4–20 s. The curve is smooth and the fluctuation is small. The position control is within the constraint range, and the yaw angle is within the constraint range in particular. Therefore, the MPC algorithm proposed in this rollator system can be used to improve the stability of elderly rollator.

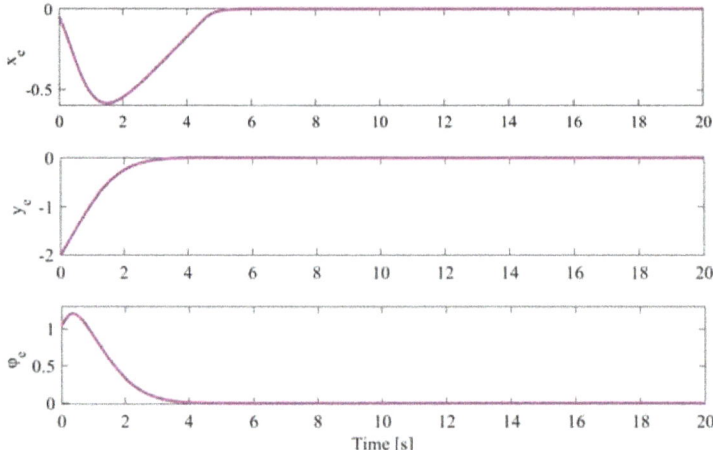

**Figure 12.** Longitudinal error, lateral error and yaw angle error.

In order to demonstrate how the controller response and the accuracy of thealgorithm, the co-simulation of rollator for ADAMS-MATLAB are carried out. The reference path is a circle shape with a radius of 25 m, and Figures 13 and 14 show the control effect of the rollator based on the MPC algorithm to track the circular trajectory. Figure 13 shows the tracking performance, and Figure 14 exhibits the longitudinal position, lateral position, angle relationship, speed change and heading angle of the rollator. It can be seen from the co-simulation results that the proposed MPC strategy can track the reference path well, and the rollator responds smoothly with position error within 0.1 m. The turning angle and speed can achieve stable tracking control within 5 s. There are no fluctuations in lateral position and longitudinal position. In addition, the heading angle is accurate and the speed is stable. Thus, the MPC algorithm can be used to improve the efficiency of the rollator system.

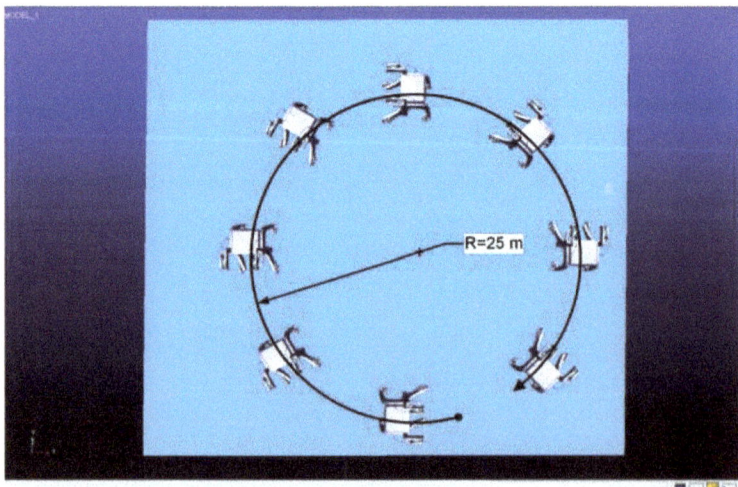

**Figure 13.** The tracking results of circle path.

To further illustrate the effectiveness of the proposed algorithm, a contrastive experiment of trajectory tracking is designed. The reference trajectory is set to a 5 m straight line and then a sinusoidal curve. The model predictive control algorithm and the sliding mode control algorithm are used for simulation respectively. The comparison results are shown in Figure 15. It can be concluded that both MPC and SMC can track the reference path well in a straight direction, but the MPC algorithm has a better effect in tracking the reference curve than SMC control in sinusoidal curve section. The deviation error of MPC control is almost zero, while the SMC is 0.3 m. Obviously, the MPC controller has faster response, higher tracking accuracy and smoother trajectory, meeting the travel requirements of the elderly rollator.

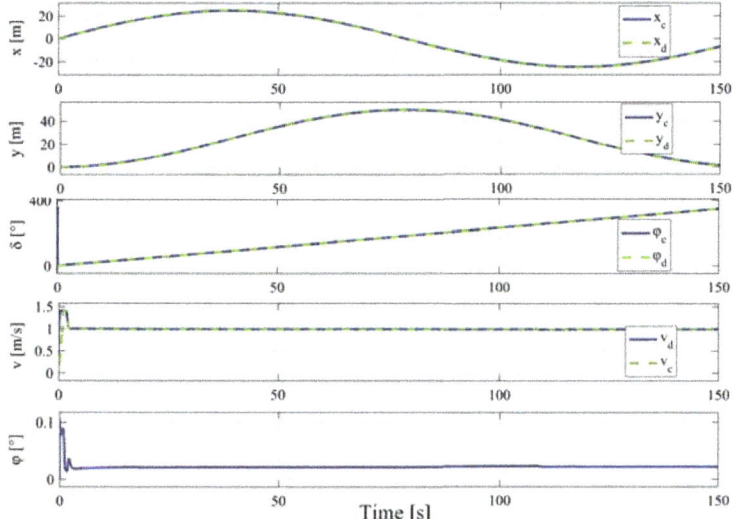

**Figure 14.** Longitudinal position, lateral position and heading angle, slip angle, yaw rate and heading angle.

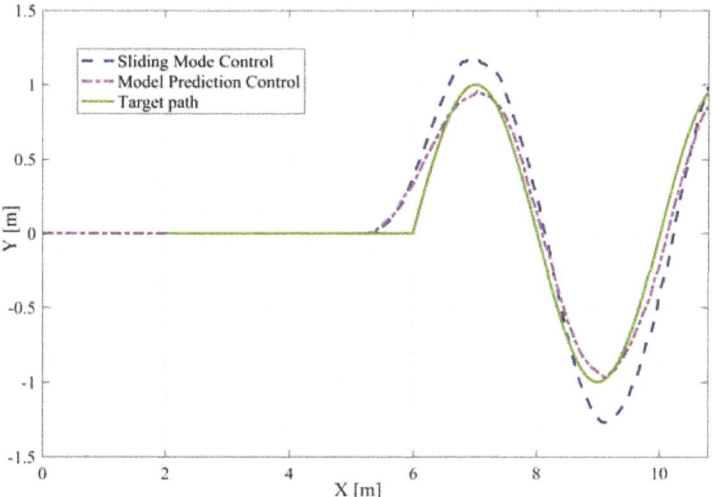

**Figure 15.** Tracking performance of MPC and SMC.

Since the four-wheeled rollator is an integrated functional application for empowering and assisting human mobility for the elderly or disabled users. The design must consider the practical demand of the elderly or disabled users. As the conclusion of the questionnaires, functions of the rollator, such as height adjustable, safety, GPS location, and wireless communication, etc., has been reorganized. A Kano model analysis is conducted and the TRIZ theory is utilized to redesign a novel rollator for meeting the requirements of the elderly. Compared to the designed rollator in the state of art [3,37–39], the novel rollator is more suitable for elderly users, featured with a simple geometric shape, the adjustable seat, and suitable materials, etc.

Furthermore, safety [40,41] and reliability are also important factors for the rollator. Uncertain human-robot interactions [42–45] cannot be avoided during the usage of the rollator. However, there are few studies achieving lateral stability control of the systems of the rollator using MPC. Hence, we validate the novel designed rollator with the lateral stability tracking control, which is a main challenge of the commercial rollator. Hence, we try to design the lateral stability of an active control system for the elderly walker. In this paper, we have presented an MPC based path-tracking controller to improve the safety of elderly rollator. The simulation results indicate that the proposed algorithm keeps the lateral position error in a reasonable range. In the co-simulation of ADAMS-MATLAB, the trajectory of the rollator is smooth with constrained position error within 0.1 m, the turning angle and speed can achieve stable tracking control within 5 s and the heading angle is accurate and the speed is stable. In addition, a compared experiment with MPC and SMC show that MPC controller has faster response, higher tracking accuracy and smoother trajectory on the novel designed rollator. Thus, the novel designed rollator can be available in practical life. The research on the rollator focuses on the novel design and balance control of the novel rollator, while the main issue in this paper is to design the stability system of the novel designed elderly rollator for practical engineering.

The characteristics of the novel rollator are with high security, low-speed stability and reliability. Adopting the MPC algorithm in the actual engineering application of rollator system is to meets the requirements of the low-speed stability of the elderly rollator. At the same time, MPC has the advantages of higher tracking accuracy, lower position error, and robustness, which meet the requirements of high security.

## 5. Conclusions and Future Work

To facilitate the development of the elderly or disabled users, this paper presents a novel design and tracking control scheme for empowering and assisting natural human mobility with a four-wheeled rollator. The main contributions of this paper are listed as follows:

1. An integrated system of four-wheeled rollator is designed to meet the requirements of the elderly by introducing a novel mechanical design theory that integrates the advantages of Kano Model Analysis with the Theory of Inventive Problem Solving (TRIZ).
2. A lateral stability tracking control approach based on an MPC scheme is performed to validate the control feasibility of the novel designed four-wheeled rollator, which is introduced to achieve the high safety requirements of the elderly walker.

The contributions of this paper mentioned above provides an optimized procedure for further development of rollators. At present, the rollator designed for the elderly is being industrialized in China and European, providing convenience for the users to travel safely. For future works, extensive experiments will be performed to verify the effectiveness of the proposed MPC approach on the actual rollator system. We will consider more challenging problems (e.g., dead-zone and time-delay) [46–49] in our proposed control framework. The system stability and tracking accuracy might not be guaranteed under these situations. It will mainly focus on the improvement of the intelligent level of the rollator for walking aids.

**Author Contributions:** Conceptualization, X.Z. and H.S.; methodology, X.Z. and J.L.; software, J.L. and Z.H.; validation, L.Z. and Y.H.; formal analysis, J.L.; investigation, W.Q.; data curation, Y.H. and W.Q.; writing—original draft preparation, X.Z.; writing—review and editing, L.Z., J.L. and W.Q.; supervision, X.Z., G.F. and E.D.M.; project administration, X.Z., H.S., G.F. and E.D.M.

**Funding:** This study was supported in part by Nation Social Science Foundation of China under Grant15BG88, in part by Nation Natural Science Foundation of China under Grant 61773060, in part by the Chinese Scholarship Council Grant.

**Conflicts of Interest:** The authors declare no conflict of interest. The funders had no role in the design of the study; in the collection, analyses, or interpretation of data; in the writing of the manuscript, or in the decision to publish the results.

## Abbreviations

The following abbreviations are used in this manuscript:

QFD  Quality Function Deployment
MPC  Model Predictive Control
TRIZ  Theory of Inventive Problem Solving
PID  Proportional-Integral-Derivative

## References

1. Probst, V.S.; Troosters, T.; Coosemans, I.; Spruit, M.A.; de Oliveira Pitta, F.; Decramer, M.; Gosselink, R. Mechanisms of improvement in exercise capacity using a rollator in patients with COPD. *Chest* **2004**, *126*, 1102–1107. [CrossRef] [PubMed]
2. VanWye, W.R.; Hoover, D.L. Management of a patient's gait abnormality using smartphone technology in-clinic for improved qualitative analysis: A case report. *Physiother. Theory Pract.* **2018**, *34*, 403–410. [CrossRef] [PubMed]
3. Kulyukin, V.; Kutiyanawala, A.; LoPresti, E.; Matthews, J.; Simpson, R. iWalker: Toward a rollator-mounted wayfinding system for the elderly. In Proceedings of the 2008 IEEE International Conference on RFID, Las Vegas, NV, USA, 16–17 April 2008; pp. 303–311.
4. Su, H.; Li, Z.; Li, G.; Yang, C. EMG-Based neural network control of an upper-limb power-assist exoskeleton robot. In Proceedings of the 10th International Symposium on Neural Networks, Dalian, China, 4–6 July 2013; pp. 204–211.
5. Zhang, H.; Ye, C. RGB-D camera based walking pattern recognition by support vector machines for a smart rollator. *Int. J. Intell. Robot. Appl.* **2017**, *1*, 32–42. [CrossRef] [PubMed]
6. Lee, A.L.; Beauchamp, M.K.; Goldstein, R.S.; Brooks, D. Clinical and Physiological Effects of Rollators in Individuals with Chronic Obstructive Pulmonary Disease: A Systematic Review. *J. Cardiopulm. Rehabil. Prev.* **2018**, *38*, 366–373. [CrossRef] [PubMed]
7. Modise, T.D.; Steyn, N.; Hamam, Y. Human feet tracking in arranging the navigation of a robotic rollator. In Proceedings of the 2017 IEEE AFRICON, Cape Town, South Africa, 18–20 September 2017; pp. 88–93.
8. Ballesteros, J.; Urdiales, C.; Martinez, A.B.; Tirado, M. Automatic assessment of a rollator-user's condition during rehabilitation using the i-Walker platform. *IEEE Trans. Neural Syst. Rehabil. Eng.* **2017**, *25*, 2009–2017. [CrossRef] [PubMed]
9. Su, H.; Enayati, N.; Vantadori, L.; Spinoglio, A.; Ferrigno, G.; De Momi, E. Online human-like redundancy optimization for tele-operated anthropomorphic manipulators. *Int. J. Adv. Robot. Syst.* **2018**, *15*. [CrossRef]
10. Hu, M.; Yang, K.; Taguchi, S. Enhancing robust design with the aid of TRIZ and axiomatic design (Part I). *TRIZ J.* **2000**. [CrossRef]
11. Borgianni, Y.; Matt, D.T. Axiomatic design and TRIZ: Deficiencies of their integrated use and future opportunities. *Procedia CIRP* **2015**, *34*, 1–6. [CrossRef]
12. Lee, C.H.; Wang, Y.H.; Trappey, A.J. Service design for intelligent parking based on theory of inventive problem solving and service blueprint. *Adv. Eng. Inform.* **2015**, *29*, 295–306. [CrossRef]
13. Altshuller, G. *The Innovation Algorithm: TRIZ, Systematic Innovation and Technical Creativity*; Technical Innovation Center, Inc.: Worcester, MA, USA, 1999.
14. Zouaoua, D.; Crubleau, P.; Choulier, D.; Richir, S. Application of evolution laws. *Procedia Eng.* **2015**, *131*, 922–932. [CrossRef]
15. Vinodh, S.; Kamala, V.; Jayakrishna, K. Integration of ECQFD, TRIZ, and AHP for innovative and sustainable product development. *Appl. Math. Model.* **2014**, *38*, 2758–2770. [CrossRef]
16. Filippi, S.; Barattin, D. Exploiting TRIZ tools in interaction design. *Procedia Eng.* **2015**, *131*, 71–85. [CrossRef]

17. Pokhrel, C.; Cruz, C.; Ramirez, Y.; Kraslawski, A. Adaptation of TRIZ contradiction matrix for solving problems in process engineering. *Chem. Eng. Res. Des.* **2015**, *103*, 3–10. [CrossRef]
18. Brad, S.; Brad, E. Enhancing SWOT analysis with TRIZ-based tools to integrate systematic innovation in early task design. *Procedia Eng.* **2015**, *131*, 616–625. [CrossRef]
19. Van Pelt, A.; Hey, J. Using TRIZ and human-centered design for consumer product development. *Procedia Eng.* **2011**, *9*, 688–693. [CrossRef]
20. Wu, Y.; Wang, C.; Zhou, L.; Ou, L. A simulation of vehicle lateral stability based on fuzzy PID control. In Proceedings of the 2009 International Conference on Measuring Technology and Mechatronics Automation, Zhangjiajie, China, 11–12 April 2009; pp. 194–199.
21. Han, G.; Fu, W.; Wang, W.; Wu, Z. The lateral tracking control for the intelligent vehicle based on adaptive PID neural network. *Sensors* **2017**, *17*, 1244. [CrossRef] [PubMed]
22. Guo, J.; Li, L.; Li, K.; Wang, R. An adaptive fuzzy-sliding lateral control strategy of automated vehicles based on vision navigation. *Veh. Syst. Dyn.* **2013**, *51*, 1502–1517. [CrossRef]
23. Onieva, E.; Naranjo, J.E.; Milanés, V.; Alonso, J.; García, R.; Pérez, J. Automatic lateral control for unmanned vehicles via genetic algorithms. *Appl. Soft Comput.* **2011**, *11*, 1303–1309. [CrossRef]
24. Gutjahr, B.; Gröll, L.; Werling, M. Lateral vehicle trajectory optimization using constrained linear time-varying MPC. *IEEE Trans. Intell. Transp. Syst.* **2017**, *18*, 1586–1595. [CrossRef]
25. Nahidi, A.; Kasaiezadeh, A.; Khosravani, S.; Khajepour, A.; Chen, S.K.; Litkouhi, B. Modular integrated longitudinal and lateral vehicle stability control for electric vehicles. *Mechatronics* **2017**, *44*, 60–70. [CrossRef]
26. Zhao, S.; Li, Y.; Zheng, L.; Lu, S. Vehicle lateral stability control based on sliding mode control. In Proceedings of the 2007 IEEE International Conference on Automation and Logistics, Jinan, China, 18–21 August 2007; pp. 638–642.
27. Ho, M.; Chan, P.; Rad, A.B.; Shirazi, M.; Cina, M. A novel fused neural network controller for lateral control of autonomous vehicles. *Appl. Soft Comput.* **2012**, *12*, 3514–3525. [CrossRef]
28. Wang, R.; Jing, H.; Wang, J.; Chadli, M.; Chen, N. Robust output-feedback based vehicle lateral motion control considering network-induced delay and tire force saturation. *Neurocomputing* **2016**, *214*, 409–419. [CrossRef]
29. Vezzetti, E.; Moos, S.; Kretli, S. A product lifecycle management methodology for supporting knowledge reuse in the consumer packaged goods domain. *Comput. Aided Des.* **2011**, *43*, 1902–1911. [CrossRef]
30. Cascini, G.; Rissone, P. Plastics design: Integrating TRIZ creativity and semantic knowledge portals. *J. Eng. Des.* **2004**, *15*, 405–424. [CrossRef]
31. Yi, K.; Liang, X.; He, Y.; Yang, L.; Han, J. Active-Model-Based Control for the Quadrotor Carrying a Changed Slung Load. *Electronics* **2019**, *8*, 461. [CrossRef]
32. Gong, J.; Jiang, Y.; Xu, W. *Model Predictive Control for Self-Driving Vehicles*; Beijing Institute of Technology Press: Beijing, China, 2014.
33. Jiang, L. Path tracking of automatic parking system based on sliding mode control. *Trans. Chin. Soc. Agric. Mach.* **2019**, *50*, 356–364.
34. Shen, W.; Pan, Z.; Li, M.; Peng, H. A Lateral Control Method for Wheel-Footed Robot Based on Sliding Mode Control and Steering Prediction. *IEEE Access* **2018**, *6*, 58086–58095. [CrossRef]
35. Li, Z.; Yang, C.; Su, C.; Deng, J.; Zhang, W. Vision-Based Model Predictive Control for Steering of a Nonholonomic Mobile Robot. *IEEE Trans. Control Syst. Technol.* **2016**, *24*, 553–564. [CrossRef]
36. Ke, F.; Li, Z.; Yang, C. Robust Tube-Based Predictive Control for Visual Servoing of Constrained Differential-Drive Mobile Robots. *IEEE Trans. Ind. Electron.* **2018**, *65*, 3437–3446. [CrossRef]
37. Luo, J.; Liu, C.; Yang, C. Estimation of EMG-Based Force Using a Neural-Network-Based Approach. *IEEE Access* **2019**, *126*, 64856–64865. [CrossRef]
38. Alkjær, T.; Larsen, P.K.; Pedersen, G.; Nielsen, L.H.; Simonsen, E.B. Biomechanical analysis of rollator walking. *Biomed. Eng. Online* **2006**, *5*, 2. [CrossRef] [PubMed]
39. Su, H.; Li, S.; Manivannan, J.; Bascetta, L.; Ferrigno, G.; De Momi, E. Manipulability Optimization Control of a Serial Redundant Robot for Robot-assisted Minimally Invasive Surgery. In Proceedings of the 2019 IEEE International Conference on Robotics and Automation, Montreal, QC, Canada, 20–24 May 2008; pp. 303–310.

40. Su, H.; Sandoval, J.; Makhdoomi, M.; Ferrigno, G.; De Momi, E. Safety-enhanced human-robot interaction control of redundant robot for teleoperated minimally invasive surgery. In Proceedings of the 2018 IEEE International Conference on Robotics and Automation (ICRA), Brisbane, Australia, 21–25 May 2018; pp. 6611–6616.
41. Su, H.; Sandoval, J.; Vieyres, P.; Poisson, G.; Ferrigno, G.; De Momi, E. Safety-enhanced collaborative framework for tele-operated minimally invasive surgery using a 7-DoF torque-controlled robot. *Int. J. Control Autom. Syst.* **2018**, *16*, 2915–2923. [CrossRef]
42. Su, H.; Yang, C.; Ferrigno, G.; De Momi, E. Improved Human—Robot Collaborative Control of Redundant Robot for Teleoperated Minimally Invasive Surgery. *IEEE Robot. Autom. Lett.* **2019**, *4*, 1447–1453. [CrossRef]
43. Yang, C.; Luo, J.; Pan, Y.; Liu, Z.; Su, C.Y. Personalized variable gain control with tremor attenuation for robot teleoperation. *IEEE Trans. Syst. Man Cybern. Syst.* **2017**, *48*, 1759–1770. [CrossRef]
44. Li, Z.; Su, C.Y.; Li, G.; Su, H. Fuzzy approximation-based adaptive backstepping control of an exoskeleton for human upper limbs. *IEEE Trans. Fuzzy Syst.* **2014**, *23*, 555–566. [CrossRef]
45. Li, Z.; Xiao, S.; Ge, S.S.; Su, H. Constrained multilegged robot system modeling and fuzzy control with uncertain kinematics and dynamics incorporating foot force optimization. *IEEE Trans. Syst. Man Cybern. Syst.* **2015**, *46*, 1–15. [CrossRef]
46. Luo, J.; Yang, C.; Wang, N.; Wang, M. Enhanced teleoperation performance using hybrid control and virtual fixture. *Int. J. Syst. Sci.* **2019**, *50*, 451–462. [CrossRef]
47. Luo, J.; Yang, C.; Su, H.; Liu, C. A Robot Learning Method with Physiological Interface for Teleoperation Systems. *Appl. Sci.* **2019**, *9*, 2099. [CrossRef]
48. Zhang, L.; Li, Z.; Yang, C. Adaptive neural network based variable stiffness control of uncertain robotic systems using disturbance observer. *IEEE Trans. Ind. Electron.* **2016**, *64*, 2236–2245. [CrossRef]
49. Yang, J.; Su, H.; Li, Z.; Ao, D.; Song, R. Adaptive control with a fuzzy tuner for cable-based rehabilitation robot. *Int. J. Control Autom. Syst.* **2016**, *14*, 865–875. [CrossRef]

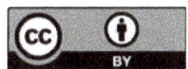

© 2019 by the authors. Licensee MDPI, Basel, Switzerland. This article is an open access article distributed under the terms and conditions of the Creative Commons Attribution (CC BY) license (http://creativecommons.org/licenses/by/4.0/).

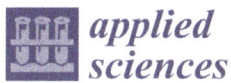 

*Article*

# Long-Term Effects of a Soft Robotic Suit on Gait Characteristics in Healthy Elderly Persons

Shanhai Jin [1], Xiaogang Xiong [2,*], Dejin Zhao [1], Changfu Jin [1] and Motoji Yamamoto [3,*]

1. School of Engineering, Yanbian University, Yanji 133002, China; jinshanhai@ybu.edu.cn (S.J.); djzhao@ybu.edu.cn (D.Z.); jincf9@163.com (C.J.)
2. School of Mechanical Engineering and Automation, Harbin Institute of Technology (Shenzhen), Shenzhen 518055, China
3. Faculty of Engineering, Kyushu University, Fukuoka 8190395, Japan
* Correspondence: xiongxg@hit.edu.cn (X.X.); yama@mech.kyushu-u.ac.jp (M.Y.)

Received: 10 March 2019; Accepted: 8 May 2019; Published: 13 May 2019

**Abstract:** As a walking assistive device for elderly persons, one of the major aims should be to improve and rehabilitate gait characteristics after long-term repeated use of the device. However, most of the existing research on walking assistive devices only emphasize their immediate effects, and there is limited research indicating the long-term effects. To address this gap, this paper experimentally validates the effects of our soft wearable robotic suit on gait characteristics of elderly persons after repeated use of the device for six weeks. Experimental results on four elderly subjects (age = $74.8 \pm 5.0$ year) show that, after six weeks of gait rehabilitation training by the robotic suit, the gait characteristics of the subjects were improved, leading to an increased walk ratio with an average of 9.8% compared with the initial state. The results of this research will benefit the potential use of the robotic suit in gait training and rehabilitation for elderly persons and also will be useful to the establishment of practical guidelines that maximize the training and rehabilitation effectiveness of the robotic suit.

**Keywords:** rehabilitation robotics; soft walking assistive robot; long-term effect; gait characteristics; elderly person

## 1. Introduction

The worldwide elderly population has increased to 12.3%, and the number will increase dramatically to an estimated 22% by the year 2050 [1,2]. One of the major age-related changes is the decline of walking performance that is featured by slow walking speed, rapid cadence, reduced step length, and decreased joint range of motion, as a consequence of lower limb skeletal muscle degradation [3–7]. Such declining walking performance may result in reduced daily physical activities, which in turn probably cause further muscle degeneration of the lower limbs. Finally, elderly persons may fall into a vicious cycle of skeletal muscle decline and daily physical activity reduction. Thus, for elderly persons, rehabilitating or at least maintaining walking performance is appealing.

In order to prevent this kind of vicious cycle, researchers have developed lower limb exoskeletons. For example, Cyberdyne Inc. [8] researched a walking-function-regaining exoskeleton. Honda Motor Co., Ltd. [9] studied a walking assistive device for improving walking ability in daily activities, and IHMC [10] presented a robotic orthosis for hip and knee assistance, as other examples. Besides these, many similar exoskeletons have also been reported in the literature [11–16]. One of the major advantages of these devices is that they are capable of generating large enough forces for assisting the human joints. Besides that, the full or a greater portion of the body weight of wearers can be shared by their rigid frames. Even so, before their practical applications, some critical issues regarding their design and implementation should be solved. 1. Joint misalignment between exoskeleton and wearer may result in resistive force [17] and, consequently, may result in increase of energy expenditure. 2. Rigid frames may constrain the motion range of the lower limb of the wearer [18], while conducting daily physical activities requires a sufficient motion range. 3. A massive power supply system is required for generating a large assistive force. This places additional payload on the wearer and also may lead to increased energy expenditure. 4. The procedures of mounting and removing an exoskeleton are complicated, even impossible in some cases without the help of a fully-trained assistant. Such issues perhaps are problematic when using exoskeletons in daily physical activities.

To avoid the limitations of exoskeletons, soft robotic devices have been researched for lower limb assistance, among which typical ones include Park et al.'s soft orthosis for ankle assistance [19,20], Asbeck et al.'s soft exosuit for ankle assistance [21], Ding et al.'s multi-joint soft exosuit for gait assistance [22,23], and our soft wearable robotic suit for hip assistance [24,25]. In such devices, exact joint alignment between wearer and device is not necessary. Additionally, because of the adoption of soft materials, wearers can walk with almost no kinematic constraints, and they can conduct interactions with devices in a biomechanically-compatible and safe way [26]. Moreover, a smaller and lighter power supply system can be applied because they usually provide relatively less assistive power compared with exoskeletons.

Specifically, in previous works [24,25], the author and his colleagues have presented a soft robotic suit, as shown in Figure 1, for walking assistance for elderly persons in daily physical activities. The device provides a small, yet effective assistive force for hip flexion. In addition, its weight is light, and it provides an almost full lower limb motion range for wearers. It has been reported [24] that, as an immediate effect on nine $74.2 \pm 3.7$ year-old elderly persons, the device significantly reduced energy expenditure in level walking with an average of 5.9% and significantly increased the walk ratio, which is a normalized measure of step length (i.e., stride length divided by cadence) [27], with an average of 8.9% in the condition of the device worn and powered on (PON) compared with the condition of worn, but powered off (POFF). It has also been reported [25] that energy expenditure was significantly reduced by 6.5% for inclined walking in the PON condition compared with the POFF condition.

One of the major aims of walking assistive devices should be to provide gait training and rehabilitation for elderly persons by repeated use of the device. However, most of the existing research only focuses on immediate effects of the devices, e.g., the differences between the POFF condition and the PON condition. There is limited research indicating the long-term effects, e.g., the differences of the POFF condition between the initial state and the state of after long-term repeated use, and only a few reports are available in the literature [28]. To address this gap, this paper experimentally validates the effects of our robotic suit on gait characteristics after six weeks' repeated use of the device for demonstrating its potential use in gait training and rehabilitation for elderly persons. It is hoped that the results of this research will be useful to the establishment of practical guidelines that maximize the training and rehabilitation effectiveness of the device.

The rest of the paper is provided as follows. An overview of the author and his colleagues' soft robotic suit is given in Section 2. The six weeks' effects of the device on gait characteristics are experimentally validated in Section 3. Section 5 discusses the experimental results, and Section 6 concludes the paper and suggests future work.

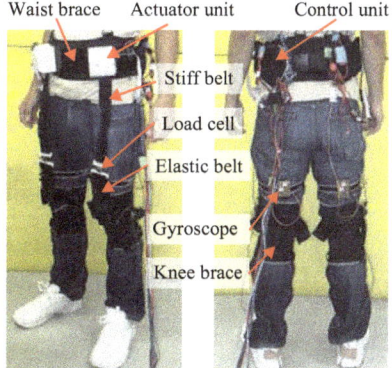

**Figure 1.** Entire design of a soft wearable robotic suit for hip flexion.

## 2. Overview of a Soft Wearable Robotic Suit

We have presented a soft wearable robotic suit for energy-efficient walking for elderly persons in daily physical activities. Figure 1 illustrates the entire design of the device, which consists of a waist support brace, knee braces, actuators, controllers, stiff and elastic belts, load cells, and gyroscopes. For each leg, one actuator and one controller were affixed to the front and the back sides of the waist support brace, respectively. The upper end of the stiff belt was pinned to the actuator, and the bottom two ends of the inverted Y-shaped elastic belt were attached to the lateral two sides of the knee brace, respectively. In addition, the bottom end of the stiff belt and the upper end of the elastic belt were connected through the load cell. Moreover, the gyroscope was attached to the thigh. The total mass of the device was 2.7 kg, excluding the power supply system (the power of the device was supplied by an external power supply by a power cable.).

The robotic suit assists hip flexion through a small, yet effective tension force, as shown in Figure 2. Specifically, a tension force is generated on the stiff and elastic belts by the winding up of the belts during the swing phase, and it is transmitted to the wearer's hip joint. In the case of stand phase, the device provides a small enough tension force that permits "creeping" of the belts along the thigh without influencing the hip extension.

Figure 3 shows the control architecture. The hip angle was calculated through the numerical integration of the hip angular velocity, which was obtained by the gyroscope. Estimations of average gait cycle and three events of heel contact, minimum hip angle, and maximum hip angle were conducted. Then, these estimated values were applied for the desired assistive force generation. In order to track the desired force smoothly and safely, a proxy-based sliding mode controller [29] was conducted with a control cycle of $T = 0.001$ s. Figure 4 illustrates the typical data of hip angle and assistive force.

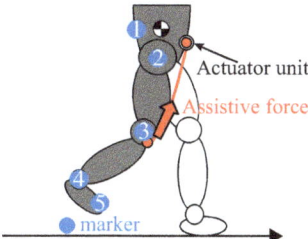

**Figure 2.** Assistance strategy for hip flexion. Blue-filled circles express reflective markers attached to the subjects in the experiment of Section 3 (1. approximation of the center of mass, 2. hip, 3. knee, 4. ankle, and 5. toe).

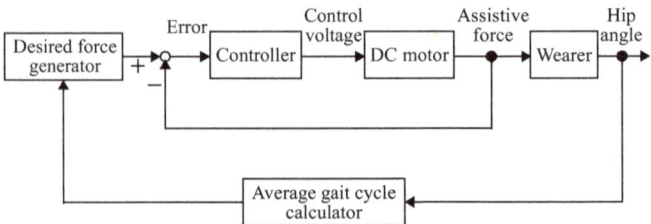

**Figure 3.** Control architecture of the robotic suit.

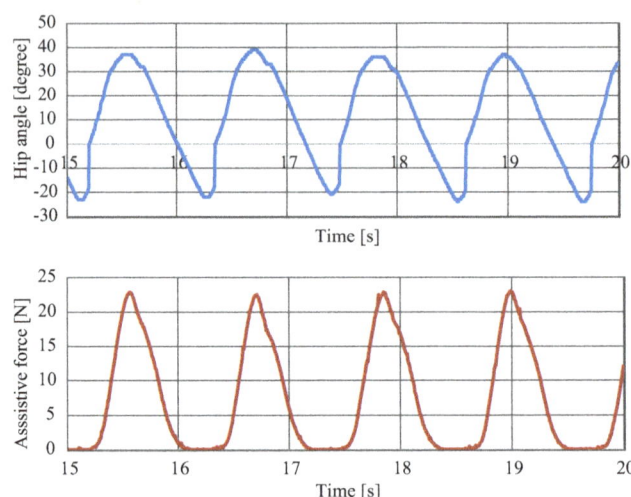

**Figure 4.** Measured hip angle and generated assistive force.

## 3. Experiment

A 6-week experiment was conducted for validating the long-term effects of the robotic suit on the gait characteristics of elderly persons. Here, it should be mentioned that the term "long-term effects" is a relative term. Specifically, it refers to the differences of the POFF condition between the initial state and the state of after 6 weeks' repeated use of the robotic suit and is used to distinguish it from "immediate effects", which refers to the comparison between the POFF condition and the PON condition. The Experiment Ethics Committee of the Faculty of Engineering of Kyushu University approved the experiment.

### 3.1. Subjects

Four healthy elderly subjects (two males, two females, age = 74.8 ± 5.0 years, weight = 60.0 ± 9.2 kg, height = 160.5 ± 7.5 cm) participated in the experiment.

### 3.2. Protocol

Each subject performed a preliminary exercise before conducting the main experiment. First, subjects were allowed to walk on a treadmill (SportsArt, FM-TR22F) for familiarizing with treadmill walking. Then, the procedure reported in [30] was applied for determining the preferred walking speed of each subject (3.8 ± 0.5 km/h). After that, at the preferred walking speed, each subject was instructed to walk in the PON condition with the maximum assistive force 23.3 ± 4.9 N for getting use to the device. Here, for each subject, the maximum assistive force was set as the value that the subject felt most comfortable with in the PON condition by considering individual differences [31]. Moreover, for all subjects, the assistance started at the event of minimum hip angle, reached its maximum value at the event of maximum hip angle, and ended at the event of heel contact.

The evaluation was conducted continuously over a period of 6 weeks. Each subject participated in the experiment at the same time (e.g., 9:00) on the same day (e.g., Monday) of each week. On each experimental day, each subject performed 4 trials of 6-min treadmill walking at the preferred walking speed, as shown in Figure 5. Among them, two trials were in the POFF condition, and the other two were in the PON condition. A 10-min rest was conducted after Trials 1 and 3, and a 20-min rest was provided after Trial 2. For excluding the influences of measurement errors and biomechanical variations, the order of the experimental conditions was reversed on each week. Specifically, for each subject, the trial order was randomly determined for Week 1 (i.e., either Trial Order A or Trial Order B, as depicted in Figure 5). Then, for the remaining 5 weeks, the reverse order of each previous week was applied.

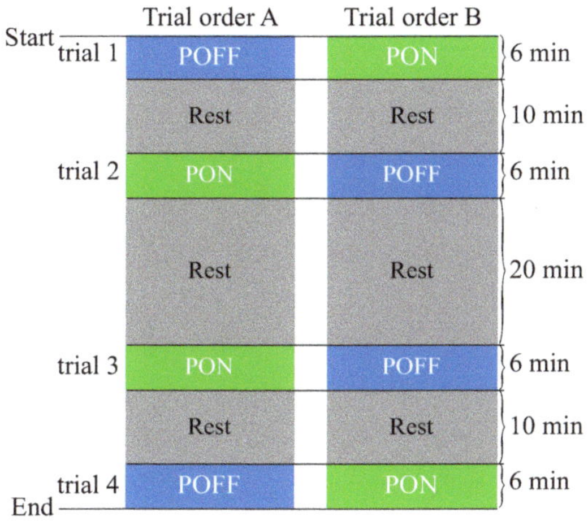

**Figure 5.** Protocol of each experimental day. PON, powered on; POFF, powered off.

For each trial, as illustrated in Figure 2, reflective markers were affixed to an approximation of the center of mass (COM), hip, knee, ankle, and toe. A 6-camera motion capture system (S250e, NaturalPoint, Inc., Oregon, USA) was used for tracking the reflective markers during the last 1-min period of walking with a frequency of 75 Hz.

*3.3. Data Analysis*

Missing marker frames (maximum 10 frames) of the measured data were filled by applying a third-degree polynomial interpolation provided by the Motive software (NaturalPoint, Inc.). Horizontal position data of the markers were measured in absolute coordinates, and then, they were converted to the relative coordinate data by setting the horizontal position of COM in the absolute coordinate as the horizontal origin of the relative coordinate system.

For all trials, joint angles were calculated by using the kinematic data. In addition, stride duration was obtained by detecting the period between two successive maximum horizontal positions of the toe. Then, cadence was computed by using the stride duration, and step length was calculated from cadence and walking speed. After that, the walk ratio was obtained by dividing the step length by cadence. The averages of all trials of each subject in each condition of each day were used for the analysis.

Paired *t*-tests were conducted for identifying the significant changes of maximum hip angles (flexion and extension), maximum knee angles (flexion and extension), maximum ankle angles (dorsiflexion and plantar flexion), and the walk ratio (i.e., stride length divided by cadence) in the POFF condition between Week 1 and Week 6. In addition, a paired *t*-test was also performed to determine the significant difference in the walk ratio between the POFF condition and the PON condition by using the average value of four subjects in each condition of each week. Standard deviations were calculated for all measures.

## 4. Results

Figure 6 compares average maximum hip, knee, and ankle angles of each week between the POFF condition and the PON condition. It is shown that the effects of assistance were mainly detected in hip flexion, knee flexion, and ankle dorsiflexion, with average increases of 10.5%, 1.9%, and 33.7%, respectively. In addition, the tendency of the values increased as the week progressed.

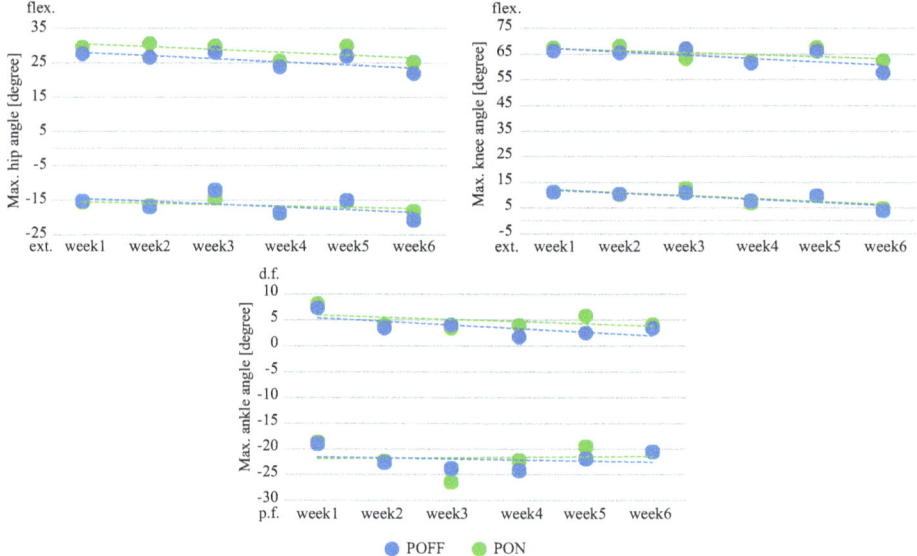

**Figure 6.** Comparison of average maximum joint angles of each week between the POFF condition and the PON condition. Here, flex.: flexion, ext.:extension, d.f.: dorsiflexion, and p.f.: plantar flexion.

Figures 7 and 8 compare the joint angles of hip, knee, and ankle achieved in the POFF condition between Week 1 and Week 6. It was observed that, after six weeks' use of the robotic suit, the gait characteristics were changed. Specifically, maximum hip flexion angle was reduced from 27.6 ± 3.1 degrees to 22.5 ± 3.2 degrees, while maximum hip extension angle was increased from 15.4 ± 9.1 degrees to 20.8 ± 5.2 degrees. For the knee joint, maximum extension angle reached 3.6 ± 3.9 degrees from 10.1 ± 9.0 degrees, while maximum flexion angle reduced to 58.3 ± 6.2 degrees from 66.5 ± 5.0 degrees. Besides that, in the case of ankle joint, the maximum dorsiflexion angle was reduced to 3.4 ± 5.8 degrees from 7.4 ± 5.0 degrees, while maximum plantar flexion angle was increased to 21.4 ± 5.6 degrees from 19.4 ± 6.1 degrees. Statistically-significant differences were found in maximum hip flexion, maximum knee flexion, and maximum ankle dorsiflexion, with an average reduction of 20.7%, 12.5%, and 54.3%, respectively, in Week 6.

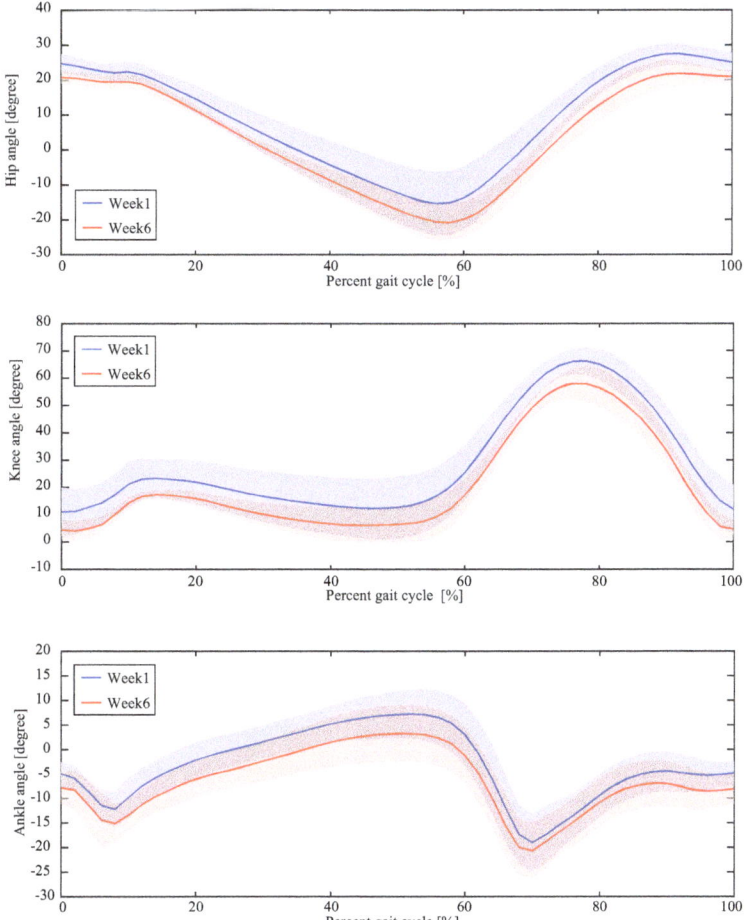

**Figure 7.** Comparison of joint angles achieved in the POFF condition between Week 1 and Week 6. On each graph, the solid curve represents the average value, and the shadowed region denotes one standard deviation.

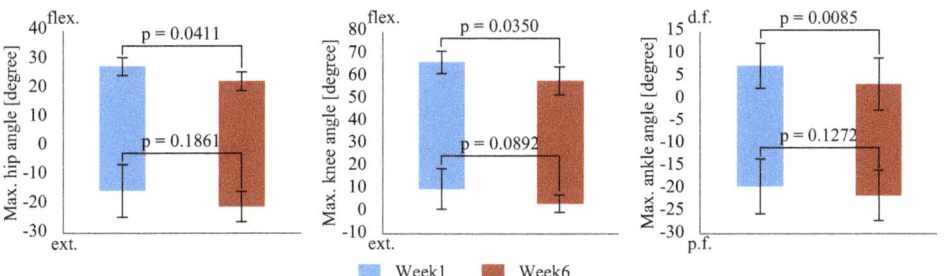

**Figure 8.** Comparison of maximum joint angles achieved in the POFF condition between Week 1 and Week 6. Here, flex.: flexion, ext.:extension, d.f.: dorsiflexion, and p.f.: plantar flexion. On each bar chart, the error bar denotes one standard deviation.

As a result of the above-mentioned changes, the walk ratio varied concurrently, as illustrated in Figure 9. It is shown that, for each week, the walk ratio of the PON condition was higher than that of the POFF condition. In addition, the tendencies of both conditions increased as the week progressed (POFF: $y = 0.00009148x + 0.00503251$, $R^2 = 0.623$; PON: $y = 0.00004885x + 0.00555119$, $R^2 = 0.397$), but the difference between the two conditions decreased.

Figure 10 shows statistical comparisons of the six weeks' average walk ratio between the POFF condition and the PON condition. It is shown that walk ratio of the PON condition was 0.0057 m/steps/min, while that of the POFF condition was 0.0054 m/steps/min. A statistically-significant difference was detected.

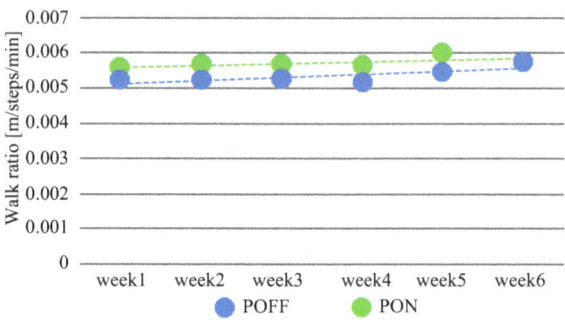

**Figure 9.** Comparison of the average walk ratio of each week between the POFF condition and the PON condition.

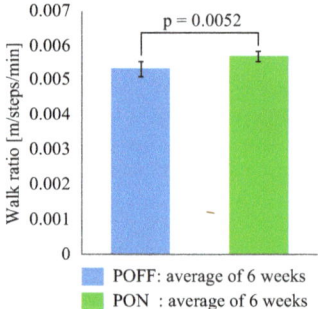

**Figure 10.** Comparison of the average walk ratio between the POFF condition and the PON condition. On each bar chart, the error bar denotes one standard deviation.

Figure 11 compares the individual walk ratio of the POFF condition between Week 1 and Week 6. It is shown that, compared with initial state, the walk ratio of three subjects increased 6.8%, 22.2%, and 13.7%, respectively, after six weeks' use of the robotic suit, while that of one subject slightly decreased 2.9%. Figure 12 shows statistical comparisons of the walk ratio achieved in the POFF condition between Week 1 and Week 6. It is shown that, although no significant difference was detected, after six weeks, the walk ratio increased from $0.0052 \pm 0.0013$ m/steps/min to $0.0057 \pm 0.0009$ m/steps/min in the POFF condition, with an average increase of 9.8%.

Figure 13 demonstrates typical motions around the timings of the toe off and the heel contact. One can observe that, compared with Week 1, the lower limb of Week 6 acted more like an inverted pendulum motion.

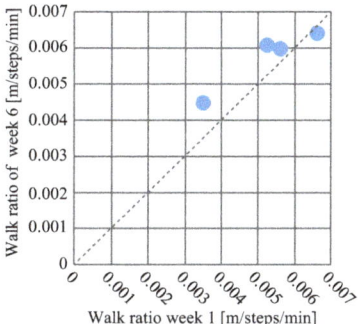

**Figure 11.** Comparison of the walk ratio of each subject achieved in the POFF condition between Week 1 and Week 6.

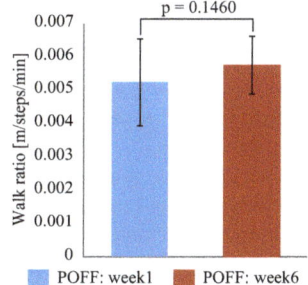

**Figure 12.** Comparison of the walk ratio achieved in the POFF condition between Week 1 and Week 6. On each bar chart, the error bar denotes one standard deviation.

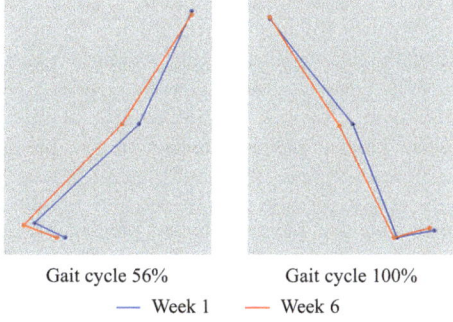

**Figure 13.** Comparison of the typical motions of the POFF condition around the timings of the toe off and the heel contact between Week 1 and Week 6.

## 5. Discussion

Motion ranges of hip, knee, and ankle joints increased in the PON condition compared with those in the POFF condition. Correspondingly, the walk ratio of the PON condition increased to 0.0057 m/steps/min from 0.0054 m/steps/min of the POFF condition, with an average increase of 6.9%. Toward this, we considered that the provided hip flexion assistance contributed to the hip flexion and consequently brought the swing leg to be positioned further forward compared with the case of the POFF condition. This result is consistent with our previous results [24] showing that the walk ratio in the PON condition was significantly increased to 0.0057 m/steps/min with an average increase of 8.9% compared with that in the POFF condition. It is recognized that healthy young persons walk at a walk ratio of approximately 0.0065 m/steps/min [32]. Thus, it can be confirmed that, as immediate effects (i.e., comparison between the POFF condition and the PON condition), the robotic suit improved gait characteristics of the elderly persons to a level closer to a healthy gait pattern.

On the other hand, after six weeks' use of the robotic suit, the walk ratio in the POFF condition reached $0.0057 \pm 0.0013$ m/steps/min from its initial state $0.0052 \pm 0.0009$ m/steps/min, with an average increase of 9.8%. Moreover, it was interestingly observed that elderly persons with a lower walk ratio may improve more by repeated use of the robotic suit. A similar study has also been conducted by Shimada et al. [28] to evaluate the long-term effects of a hip assistive device for three months. However, they reported that there was no increase of the walk ratio after three months' walking training with their device, while they found a significant increase of the walk ratio in an experiment for validating the immediate effects [33]. Thus, it can be argued that, as long-term effects (i.e., comparison in the POFF condition between Week 1 and Week 6), our device had the potential to make a contribution to gait rehabilitation of elderly persons.

However, it is also found that, different from the immediate effect of the improved walk ratio by mainly increasing hip flexion, knee flexion, and ankle dorsiflexion, the walk ratio increased with reduced hip flexion, knee flexion, and ankle dorsiflexion, but increased hip extension, knee extension, and ankle plantar flexion in the case of long-term effects. Toward such a difference, we considered that the provided hip flexion assistance may indirectly influence the dynamics of the lower limbs. The most potential contributor could be the improved pelvic rotation. It is known [34,35] that the pelvic rotation plays an important role in determining step length or, equivalently, the walk ratio. That is, the greater pelvic rotation allowed for a larger step length. It was also reported [36–38] that elderly persons walk in degraded pelvic rotation and hip extension, resulting in a declined walk ratio and walking speed. By considering these, in the case of using the device, we assumed that hip flexion assistance promoted the forward pelvis rotation of the elderly subjects. In turn, this promotion concurrently enhanced the standing leg muscles that were used for stabilizing the oppositely-rotating trunk, as pointed out in [39]. In such a way, after six weeks' repeated use of the device, it seems that muscles used for hip extension were reactivated and then softened, consequently leading to improved maximum hip extension. On the other hand, this improvement contributed to the improved gait characteristics with the increased walk ratio.

In addition, it was studied that energy expenditure of elderly persons during walking is higher than that of young persons [40]. Several researches have suggested that the possible reasons for such increase are decreased motion range of lower limb joints and shortened step length (i.e., walk ratio) [41–44]. It is also known [43] that a full knee extension (i.e., maximum knee extension angle with zero degrees) allows the lower limbs to behave like an inverted pendulum motion, with which a healthy person at preferred speed (i.e., the walk ratio was approximately 0.0065 m/steps/min) optimizes the potential energy and the kinetic energy exchange of COM, consequently leading to minimized energy expenditure. In our previous study [24], it has been observed that energy expenditure was significantly reduced 5.9% in the PON condition with a significant 8.9% increase of walk ratio. Thus, it can be inferred that, as immediate effects, the elderly subjects participating in this study probably walked more easily and comfortably with less energy in the PON condition owing to the improved gait characteristics, although the energy expenditure was not directly measured here. Similarly, as long-term effects, increased knee extension and increased walk ratio achieved after six weeks' repeated use of the device also probably improved energy efficiency of walking for the elderly subjects in the POFF condition.

As a whole, it can be concluded that the robotic suit is effective not only at improving gait characteristics as immediate effects, but also potentially useful for rehabilitating gait characteristics as long-term effects.

## 6. Conclusions and Future Work

This paper has experimentally validated the long-term effects of a soft robotic suit for walking assistance for elderly persons in daily activities. Experimental results illustrated that, after six weeks' use of the device, the gait characteristics of the subjects were improved to a level closer to a healthy gait pattern in the POFF condition, leading to an increased walk ratio with an average increase of 9.8% compared with the initial state. As was discussed, the promoted forward pelvis rotation and the correspondingly improved extensions of hip and knee joints were probably the major contributors for the rehabilitated gait characteristics. Such long-term effects of our robotic suit support its potential use in gait training and rehabilitation for elderly persons.

It also should be mentioned here that, although average improvements were found in some gait parameters, e.g., walk ratio, no significant differences were detected in these parameters probably due to the limit of the sample size of subjects and day-to-day variations.

As future research, the performance evaluation of the robotic suit for a longer period, e.g., a period longer than six months, is desirable for further supporting the effectiveness of the device in the long term. Future research also should include the development of effective training guidelines for maximizing rehabilitation effectiveness and the design of an adaptive control scheme for different walking patterns with the aim of achieving maximized effectiveness.

**Author Contributions:** Data curation, C.J.; Funding acquisition, S.J., X.X. and M.Y.; Project administration, M.Y.; Validation, D.Z.; Writing-original draft, S.J.; Writing-review and editing, X.X.

**Funding:** This research was funded by the Research Foundation of Jilin Province Development and Reform Commission (Grant No. 2019C048-2), the Shenzhen Peacock Technical Innovation Funding (Grant No. KQJSCX20170726103546683), the Science & Technology Development Foundation of Jilin Province (Grant No. 20180520019JH), the Science & Technology Research Foundation of the Education Department of Jilin Province (Grant No. JJKH20180883KJ), and the Grant-in-Aid for the Adaptable & Seamless Technology Transfer program through Target-driven R&D of the Japan Science and Technology Agency (Grant No. AS2415010K).

**Conflicts of Interest:** The authors declare no conflict of interest.

## References

1. United Nations Population Fund. Aging. 2015. Available online: Http://www.unfpa.org/ageing (accessed on 13 May 2019).
2. Herrmann, M.; Guzman, J.M.; Juran, S.; Schensul, D. Population Dynamics in the Least Developed Countries: Challenges and Opportunities for Development and Poverty Reduction. 2011. Available online: http://www.unfpa.org/publications/population-dynamics-ldcs (accessed on 13 May 2019).
3. Prince, F.; Corriveau, H.; Hebert, R.; Winter, D. Gait in the elderly. *Gait Posture* **1997**, *5*, 128–135. [CrossRef]
4. DeVita, P.; Hortobagyi, T. Age causes a redistribution of joint torques and powers during gait. *J. Appl. Physiol.* **2000**, *88*, 1804–1811. [CrossRef] [PubMed]
5. Watelain, E.; Barbier, F.; Allard, P.; Thevenon, A.; Angue, J. Gait pattern classification of healthy elderly men based on biomechanical data. *Arch. Phys. Med. Rehabil.* **2000**, *81*, 579–586. [CrossRef]
6. Menz, H.; Lord, S.; Fitzpatrick, C. Age-related differences in walking stability. *Age Ageing* **2003**, *32*, 137–142. [CrossRef] [PubMed]
7. Kirkwood, R.; Moreira, B.; Vallone, M.; Mingoti, S.; Dias, R.; Sampaio, R. Step length appears to be a strong discriminant gait parameter for elderly females highly concerned about falls: A cross-sectional observational study. *Physiotherapy* **2011**, *97*, 126–131. [CrossRef] [PubMed]
8. Yasuhara, K.; Shimada, K.; Koyama, T.; Ido, T.; Kikuchi, K.; Endo, Y. Walking assist device with stride management assist. *Honda R&D Techn. Rev.* **2009**, *21*, 54–62.
9. Kawamoto, H.; Hayashi, T.; Sakurai, T.; Eguchi, K.; Sankai, Y. Development of single leg version of HAL for hemiplegia. In Proceedings of the 31st Annual International Conference of the IEEE Engineering in Medicine and Biology Society, Minneapolis, MI, USA, 2–6 September 2009; pp. 5038–5043.
10. Raj, A.K.; Neuhaus, P.D.; Moucheboeuf, A.M.; Noorden, J.H.; Lecoutre, D.V. Mina: A sensorimotor robotic orthosis for mobility assistance. *J. Robot.* **2011**, *2011*, 284352. [CrossRef]

11. Yeh, T.; Wu, M.; Lu, T.; Wu, F.; Huang, C. Control of McKibben pneumatic muscles for a power-assist, lower-limb orthosis. *Mechatronics* **2010**, *20*, 686–697. [CrossRef]
12. Ikehara, T.; Tanaka, E.; Nagamura, K.; Tamiya, T.; Ushida, T.; Hashimoto, K.; Kojima, S.; Ikejo, K.; Yuge, L. Development of closed-fitting-type walking assistance device for legs with self-contained control system. *J. Robot. Mech.* **2010**, *22*, 380–390. [CrossRef]
13. Wu, Q.; Wang, X.; Du, F.; Zhang, X. Design and control of a powered hip exoskeleton for walking assistance. *Int. J. Adv. Robot. Syst.* **2015**, *12*, 18. [CrossRef]
14. Kong, K.; Jeon, D. Design and control of an exoskeleton for the elderly and patients. *IEEE/ASME Trans. Mech.* **2006**, *11*, 428–432. [CrossRef]
15. Hyon, S.; Morimoto, J.; Matsubara, T.; Noda, T.; Kawato, M. XoR: Hybrid drive exoskeleton robot that can balance. In Proceedings of the 2011 IEEE/RSJ International Conference on Intelligent Robots and Systems, San Francisco, CA, USA, 25–30 September 2011; pp. 3975–3981.
16. Nakamura, T.; Saito, K.; Wang, Z.; Kosuge, K. Realizing model-based wearable antigravity muscles support with dynamics terms. In Proceedings of the 2005 IEEE/RSJ International Conference on Intelligent Robots and Systems, Edmonton, AB, Canada, 2–6 August 2005; pp. 2694–2699.
17. Schiele, A. Ergonomics of exoskeletons: Subjective performance metrics. In Proceedings of the 2009 IEEE/RSJ International Conference on Intelligent Robots and Systems, St. Louis, MO, USA, 11–15 October 2009; pp. 480–485.
18. Cenciarini, M.; Dollar, A.M. Biomechanical considerations in the design of lower limb exoskeletons. In Proceedings of the 2011 IEEE International Conference on Rehabilitation Robotics, Zurich, Switzerland, 29 June–1 July 2011; pp. 1–6.
19. Park, Y.; Chen, B.; Young, D.; Stirling, L.; Wood, R.J.; Goldfield, E.; Nagpal, R. Bio-inspired active soft orthotic device for ankle foot pathologies. In Proceedings of the 2011 IEEE/RSJ International Conference on Intelligent Robots and Systems, San Francisco, CA, USA, 25–30 September 2011; pp. 4488–4495.
20. Park, Y.; Hen, B.C.; Perez-Arancibia, N.O.; Young, D.; Stirling, L.; Wood, R.J.; Goldfield, E.C.; Nagpal, R. Design and control of a bio-inspired soft wearable robotic device for ankle -foot rehabilitation. *Bioinspir. Biomim.* **2014**, *9*, 016007. [CrossRef] [PubMed]
21. Asbeck, A.T.; Rossi, S.M.M.D.; Holt, K.G.; Walsh, C.J. A biologically inspired soft exosuit for walking assistance. *Int. J. Robot. Res.* **2015**, *34*, 744–762. [CrossRef]
22. Asbeck, A.T.; Schmidt, K.; Galiana, I.; Wagner, D.; Walsh, C.J. Multi-joint soft exosuit for gait assistance. In Proceedings of the 2015 IEEE International Conference on Robotics and Automation, Seattle, WA, USA, 26–30 May 2015; pp. 6197–6204.
23. Ding, Y.; Galiana, I.; Asbeck, A.T.; Rossi, S.M.M.D.; Bae, J.; Santos, T.R.T.; Araujo, V.L.; Lee, S.; Holt, K.G.; Walsh, C. Biomechanical and Physiological Evaluation of Multi-joint Assistance with Soft Exosuits. *IEEE Trans. Neural Syst. Rehabil. Eng.* **2017**, *25*, 119–130. [CrossRef] [PubMed]
24. Jin, S.; Iwamoto, N.; Hashimoto, K.; Yamamoto, M. Experimental Evaluation of Energy Efficiency for a Soft Wearable Robotic Suit. *IEEE Trans. Neural Syst. Rehabil. Eng.* **2017**, *25*, 1192–1201. [CrossRef] [PubMed]
25. Jin, S.; Guo, S.; Hashimoto, K.; Xiong, X.; Yamamoto, M. Influence of a soft robotic suit on metabolic cost in long-distance level and inclined walking. *Appl. Bionics Biomech.* **2018**, *2018*, 9573951. [CrossRef]
26. Majidi, C. Soft robotics: A perspective current trends and prospects for the future. *Soft Robot.* **2014**, *1*, 5–11. [CrossRef]
27. Sekiya, N.; Nagasaki, H. Reproducibility of the walking patterns of normal young adults: Test-retest reliability of the walk ratio(step-length:step-rate). *Gait Posture* **1998**, *7*, 225–227. [CrossRef]
28. Shimada, H.; Hirata, T.; Kimura, Y.; Naka, T.; Kikuchi, K.; Oda, K.; Ishii, K.; Ishiwata, K.; Suzuki, T. Effects of a robotic walking exercise on walking performance in community-dwelling elderly adults. *Geriatr. Gerontol. Int.* **2009**, *9*, 372–381. [CrossRef]
29. Kikuuwe, R.; Yasukouchi, S.; Fujimoto, H.; Yamamoto, M. Proxy-based sliding mode control: A safer extension of PID position control. *IEEE Trans. Robot.* **2010**, *26*, 670–683. [CrossRef]
30. Holt, K.G.; Hamill, J.; Anders, R.O. Predicting the minimal energy costs of human walking. *Med. Sci. Sport. Exerc.* **1991**, *23*, 491–498. [CrossRef]

31. Jin, S.; Guo, S.; Hashimoto, K.; Yamamoto, M. Influence of maximum assistive force of a soft wearable robotic suit on metabolic cost reduction. In Proceedings of the 8th IEEE International Conference on Cybernetics and Intelligent Systems and the 8th IEEE International Conference on Robotics, Automation and Mechatronics, Ningbo, China, 19–21 November 2017; pp. 146–150.
32. Rota, V.; Perucca, L.; Simone, A.; Tesio, L. Walk ratio (step length/cadence) as a summary index of neuromotor control of gait: Application to multiple sclerosis. *Int. J. Rehabil. Res.* **2011**, *34*, 265–269. [CrossRef] [PubMed]
33. Shimada, H.; Suzuki, T.; Kimura, Y.; Hirata, T.; Sugiura, M.; Endo, Y.; Yasuhara, K.; Shimada, K.; Kikuchi, K.; Oda, K.; et al. Effects of an automated stride assistance system on walking parameters and muscular glucose metabolism in elderly adults. *Br. J. Sport. Med.* **2011**, *42*, 922–929. [CrossRef]
34. Kerrigan, D.; Lee, L.; Collins, J. Reduced hip extension during walking: Healthy elderly and fallers versus young adults. *Arch. Phys. Med. Rehabil.* **2001**, *82*, 26–30. [CrossRef] [PubMed]
35. Cristopoliski, F.; Barela, J.; Leite, N.; Fowler, N.; Rodacki, A. Stretching exercise program improves gait in the elderly. *Gerontology* **2009**, *55*, 614–620. [CrossRef]
36. Kerrigan, D.; Xenopoulos-Oddsson, A.; Sullivan, M.; Lelas, J.; Riley, P. Effect of a hip flexor-stretching program on gait in the elderly. *Arch. Phys. Med. Rehabil.* **2003**, *84*, 1–6. [CrossRef]
37. Watt, J.; Jackson, K.; Franz, J.; Dicharry, J.; Evans, J.; Kerrigan, D. Effect of a supervised hip flexor stretching program on gait in frail elderly patients. *PM&R* **2011**, *3*, 330–335.
38. Aboutorabi, A.; Arazpour, M.; Bahramizadeh, M.; Hutchins, S.; Fadayevatan, R. The effect of aging on gait parameters in able-bodied older subjects: A literature review. *Aging Clin. Exp. Res.* **2016**, *28*, 393–405. [CrossRef]
39. Kisner, C.; Colby, L. *Therapeutic Exercise: Foundations and Techniques*, 6th ed.; F. A Davis Company: Philadelphia, PA, USA, 2012.
40. Wert, D.; Brach, J.; Perera, S.; VanSwearingen, J. Gait biomechanics, spatial and temporal characteristics, and the energy cost of walking in older adults with impaired mobility. *Phys. Ther.* **2000**, *90*, 977–985. [CrossRef]
41. Waters, R.; Barnes, G.; Husserl, T.; Silver, L.; Liss, R. Comparable energy expenditure after arthrodesis of the hip and ankle. *J. Bone Jt. Surg. Am. Vol.* **1988**, *70*, 1032–1037. [CrossRef]
42. Donelan, J.; Kram, R. Mechanical and metabolic determinants of the preferred step width in human walking. *Proc. R. Soc. Lond. Ser. B Biol. Sci.* **2001**, *268*, 1985–1992. [CrossRef] [PubMed]
43. Gordon, K.E.; Ferris, D.P.; Kuo, A.D. Metabolic and mechanical energy costs of reducing vertical Center of Mass Movement During Gait. *Arch. Phys. Med. Rehabil.* **2009**, *90*, 136–144. [CrossRef] [PubMed]
44. Ellis, R.; Howard, K.; Kram, R. The metabolic and mechanical costs of step time asymmetry in walking. *Proc. R. Soc. B Biol. Sci.* **2013**, *280*, 1–7. [CrossRef] [PubMed]

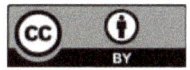

© 2019 by the authors. Licensee MDPI, Basel, Switzerland. This article is an open access article distributed under the terms and conditions of the Creative Commons Attribution (CC BY) license (http://creativecommons.org/licenses/by/4.0/).

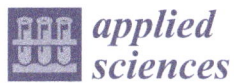 

*Article*

# Control Reference Parameter for Stance Assistance Using a Passive Controlled Ankle Foot Orthosis—A Preliminary Study

Dimas Adiputra [1,2,*,†], Mohd Azizi Abdul Rahman [1,*,†], Ubaidillah [3,4,*,†], Saiful Amri Mazlan [1], Nurhazimah Nazmi [1], Muhammad Kashfi Shabdin [1], Jun Kobayashi [5] and Mohd Hatta Mohammed Ariff [1]

1 Advanced Vehicle System Research Group, Universiti Teknologi Malaysia, 54100 Kuala Lumpur, Malaysia; amri.kl@utm.my (S.A.M.); nurhazimah2@live.utm.my (N.N.); dekashaf@gmail.com (M.K.S.); mohdhatta.kl@utm.my (M.H.M.A.)
2 Department of Electrical Engineering, Institut Teknologi Telkom Surabaya, 60234 Surabaya, Indonesia
3 Department of Mechanical Engineering, Universitas Sebelas Maret, 57126 Surakarta, Indonesia
4 National Center for Sustainable Transportation Technology, 40132 Bandung, Indonesia
5 Faculty of Computer Science and Systems Engineering, Kyushu Institute of Technology, 804-8550 Kitakyushu, Japan; jkoba@ces.kyutech.ac.jp
* Correspondence: adimas@ittelkom-sby.ac.id (D.A.); azizi.kl@utm.my (M.A.A.R.); ubaidillah_ft@staff.uns.ac.id (U.)
† These authors contributed equally to this work.

Received: 18 September 2019; Accepted: 6 October 2019; Published: 18 October 2019

**Featured Application:** The control reference parameter suggested in this study is implemented in a Passive-Controlled Ankle Foot Orthosis (PICAFO) equipped with magnetorheological (MR) brake on its ankle joint. Previously, the PICAFO has been shown to successfully deal with foot drop by locking the foot ankle position during the swing phase. By adding functions such as stance assistance, the user can get more benefits when using the PICAFO.

**Abstract:** This paper aims to present a preliminary study of control reference parameters for stance assistance among different subjects and walking speeds using a passive-controlled ankle foot orthosis. Four young male able-bodied subjects with varying body mass indexes (23.842 ± 4.827) walked in three walking speeds of 1, 3, and 5 km/h. Two control references, average ankle torque (aMa), and ankle angular velocity (aω), which can be implemented using a magnetorheological brake, were measured. Regression analysis was conducted to identify suitable control references in the three different phases of the stance. The results showed that aω has greater correlation (p) with body mass index and walking speed compared to aMa in the whole stance phase (p1(aω) = 0.666 > p1(aMa) = 0.560, p2(aω) = 0.837 > p2(aMa) = 0.277, and p3(aω) = 0.839 > p3(aMa) = 0.369). The estimation standard error (Se) of the aMa was found to be generally higher than of aω (Se1(aMa) = 2.251 > Se1(aω) = 0.786, Se2(aMa) = 1.236 > Se2(aω) = 0.231, Se3(aMa) = 0.696 < Se3(aω) = 0.755). Future studies should perform aω estimation based on body mass index and walking speed, as suggested by the higher correlation and lower standard error as compared to aMa. The number of subjects and walking speed scenarios should also be increased to reduce the standard error of control reference parameters estimation.

**Keywords:** control parameter reference; stance assistance; magnetorheological brake; body mass index; walking speed; ankle torque; ankle angular velocity

## 1. Introduction

Walking gait assistance is essential, especially for people with abnormal gaits such as a weak ankle, spasticity, or foot drop [1]. These symptoms are common in post-stroke patients doing rehabilitation. In such cases, therapists and ancillary devices such as Ankle Foot Orthosis (AFO) may be used in gait assistance [2]. The AFO is an L-shape brace that covers the lower limb from the foot to the calf [3]. Figure 1 illustrates the gait assistance for foot drop patient using AFO. The reduction of dorsiflexion (e.g., blue circle) resulted in unwanted plantarflexion, which may lead to abnormal gait [4] toe-drags when walking [5]. The patient should avoid toe-dragging, as this disturbs walking stability and increases the probability of a fall [6]. Here, the stiffness of the AFO joint restricts the unwanted plantarflexion, which then prevents the foot drop symptom occurrence, thus increasing walking stability. Because of this function, the post-stroke patients with foot drop symptom are usually suggested to use AFO to address their gait abnormalities in rehabilitation [7].

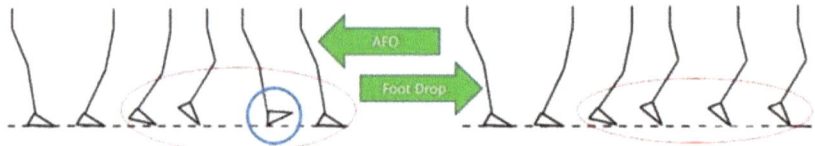

**Figure 1.** Illustration of foot drop treatment using Ankle Foot Orthosis (AFO).

The level of AFO restriction or AFO joint stiffness should be adjusted accordingly to achieve the maximum benefits [8]. For instance, sufficient work replacement by actuator will reduce muscle activity [9,10]. Different types of joints, such as rigid joint, flexible joint, and articulated joint, have different joint stiffnesses [11]. Rigid AFO has the highest possible joint stiffness, as the joint is fix and cannot rotate all. This AFO type is not suitable for treatment as it decreases the forward propulsion of the user by limiting the range of motion (ROM) [7,12]. A flexible AFO made from materials such as polypropylene [13] and carbon fiber [14] allows more ROM than a rigid AFO. However, the problem of a lack of forwarding propulsion remains [15]. Lastly, the articulated AFO allows maximum ROM as compared with the other two. It has electronic actuators (passive or active) and gait controller to control not only the joint stiffness but also ankle joint movement [11]. Therefore, an articulated AFO offers greater flexibility compared to rigid and flexible AFOs, and is capable of normal walking replication for intensive training purposes [16].

The previous study has developed a passive-controlled AFO (i.e., PICAFO in short). PICAFO is equipped with magnetorheological (MR) brake as a passive actuator for controlling the ankle joint stiffness using an electromyography (EMG) based Fuzzy Logic Controller (FLC) [17–19]. Surface electromyography or sEMG was used to classify the gait phases into two phases with a uniform threshold rather than a single threshold [20,21]. The two phases namely, Phase I runs from foot flat (FF) to heel off (HO), continuing to toe-off (TO), while phase II runs from TO to initial contact (IC) to FF. As shown in Figure 2, FLC also used additional information from ankle positions for controlling the MR brake stiffness. The result was that the controller could generate different joint stiffness in distinct gait phases [17], such as low and medium stiffness during the stance phase and high stiffness during the swing phase. The PICAFO successfully demonstrated foot drop prevention due to the high stiffness during the swing phase [18].

Despite that, the exact amount of joint stiffness, which was the control reference parameter, was pre-determined to be similar, even though different subjects and walking styles may require different joint stiffnesses during the stance and swing. Locking the ankle position during the swing phase could be done very straightforwardly by applying high stiffness, regardless of the subject and walking style [6]. However, the stiffness level during the stance phase, which prevents over dorsiflexion, was necessary to be adjusted accordingly [9]. Too much stiffness will distract the movement like rigid and flexible AFO did, but insufficient stiffness will result in insignificant gait assistance [8]. Several research questions were highlighted as follows:

(1) What is the suitable control reference parameter for stance assistance using PICAFO? Controlling the walking gait at the stance phase is not limited to the joint stiffness only. Other mechanical properties that can serve as the control reference parameter is also presented, such as motion parameter and assistive torque [11]. These mechanical properties are possible to be controlled using active actuators such as tracking and generation of the ankle motion path using electric motors [22–25], and assistive torque generation using pneumatics muscle [26–28] for balancing the body [29]. However, in this study, PICAFO was equipped only with MR brake as the actuator, which is not suitable for implementation of sophisticated control reference such as motion path. On the other hand, additional actuators are not a wise choice due to consideration of complex structure and overall weight of the PICAFO [30]. Because of that, mechanical properties such as ankle torque and ankle angular velocity were chosen to be investigated in this study since these can be controlled using an MR brake [31].

(2) What critical parameter is suitable for estimation of the control reference parameter? Estimating the desired control reference requires information such as ground terrains, walking styles, user's anthropometrics, and other factors. In the previous study on AFO with MR brake, the control reference estimation which associated with the walking style such as the walking speed has been reported [32,33]. However, without investigation on the effect of the user's anthropometric such as body mass index (BMI) to the control reference. BMI is commonly used to describe human identity [34]. Thus, an additional critical parameter such as the BMI is expected to increase the control reference estimation accuracy.

To sum up, this preliminary study investigates the control reference parameters for stance assistance using PICAFO. The chosen control reference parameters were ankle torque and ankle angular velocity. On the other hand, the chosen critical parameters were walking speed and BMI. Section 2 further discussed the research materials and methods. Meanwhile, Sections 3 and 4 discussed the research findings and analysis, respectively.

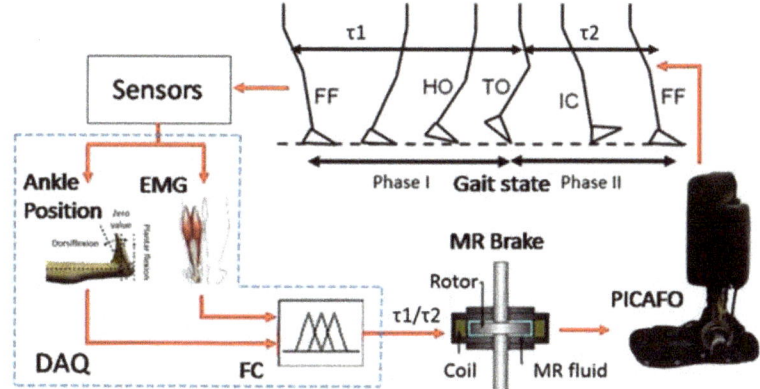

**Figure 2.** Passive-controlled AFO (PICAFO) system with fix ankle joint stiffness reference in distinct gait phases.

## 2. Materials and Methods

A walking experiment was conducted to answer the research questions. An advanced vehicle research group experiment was conducted in a rehabilitation engineering facility under Malaysia-Japan International Institute of Technology, Universiti Teknologi Malaysia, Kuala Lumpur, Malaysia.

Meanwhile, orthopedic doctors' committee, Institutional Review Board of Education Hospital of Universitas Sebelas Maret, Indonesia declared that the walking experiment in this study is safe for work involving human subjects (approval letter: No. 893/UN27.49/TU/2018). Young male subjects who could walk normally and had never suffered from any spasticity or foot symptoms in their life participated in a walking experiment. The subjects gave their written consent before experimenting. This section presents further details on the data collection, data processing, and data analysis for the walking experiment.

## 2.1. Data Collection

Four young male able-bodied subjects with body mass indexes (BMI) of 18.026, 23.072, 24.509, and 29.761, respectively, participated in the walking experiment. The setup was as shown in Figure 3. Subjects who could walk normally were selected for the experiment and each had never suffered from any spasticity and foot symptoms. Table 1 shows the details of the subjects anthropometric. The experiment was done by having the subjects walked on a treadmill using the PICAFO as a test measurement device, as shown in Figure 4. There were three sensors on the test device, namely a force sensor, rotary encoder, and accelerometer. Data from the sensors were sent to a personal computer through the USB-6211 data acquisition for data logging. Note that there was no applied controller for the PICAFO stiffness; thus, it had zero stiffness for the whole data collection. For each subject, there were three sessions of walking. The treadmill applied different walking speed, for instance, speeds (Sp) of 1 km/h, 3 km/h, 5 km/h represent slow, medium, and fast walking velocity, respectively. In each session, data of 20 steps of walking were collected and repeated two times. Therefore, there were a total of 480 walking steps observations for analysis.

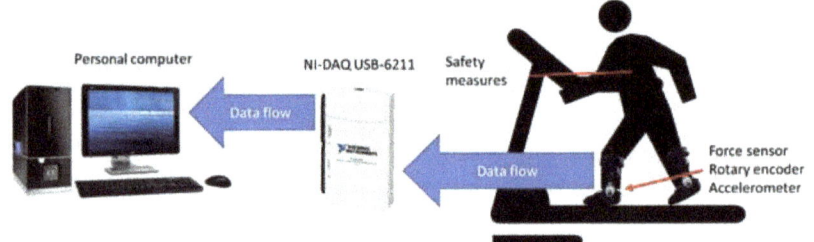

**Figure 3.** Experimental setup.

**Table 1.** Subject's anthropometric.

| Anthropometric Parameters | Subject, Sb | | | | Mean | Standard Deviation |
|---|---|---|---|---|---|---|
| | 1 | 2 | 3 | 4 | | |
| Body mass (kg) | 45 | 61.3 | 70 | 97.5 | 68.45 | 21.964 |
| Height (m) | 1.58 | 1.63 | 1.69 | 1.81 | 1.678 | 9.912 |
| BMI | 18.026 | 23.072 | 24.509 | 29.761 | 23.842 | 4.827 |
| Gender | Male | Male | Male | Male | - | - |
| Age (year) | 29 | 25 | 25 | 29 | 27 | 2.310 |
| Foot mass (kg) | 2.353 | 2.589 | 2.715 | 3.114 | 2.693 | 0.276 |
| Foot length (m) | 0.135 | 0.14 | 0.15 | 0.17 | 0.1488 | 0.0134 |

As illustrated in Figure 4, the sensor placement and walking steps data collected from the sensors are the followings:

1. Rotary encoder typed B1-106

Data collected: ankle position ($\theta$), ankle angular velocity ($\omega$), ankle angular acceleration ($\alpha$).

Sensor placement: at the ankle joint right after the MR brake in the same axis. The standing position is the neutral position, dorsiflexion is a positive direction, and plantarflexion is a negative direction [17].

2. 3-axis accelerometer ADXL-335

Data collected: linear ankle acceleration (a).

Sensor placement: near the ankle joint with x-axis on the horizontal sagittal plane and y-axis on the vertical sagittal plane.

3. Force sensor FLX-A201

Data collected: ground reaction force on the heel ($F_{heel}$) and toe ($F_{toe}$).

Sensor placement: inside the PICAFO insole with fix position such as 9 cm of toe distance and 6 cm of heel distance from the ankle joint axis in the sagittal plane.

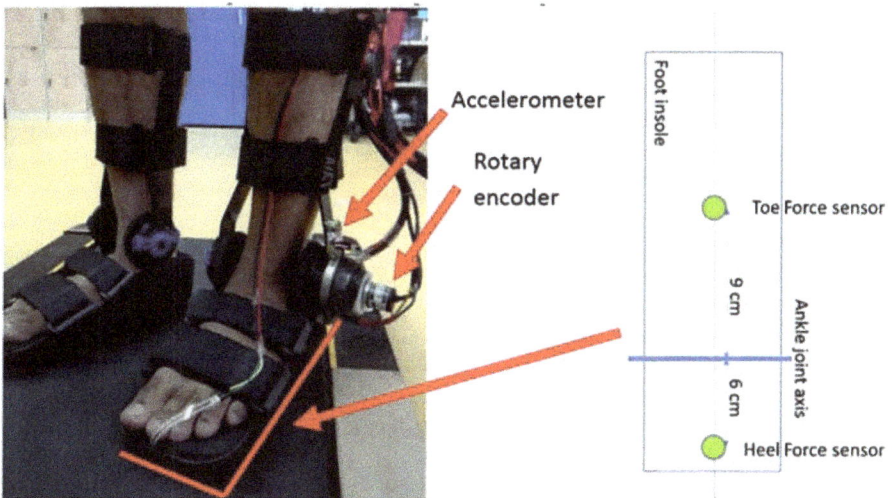

**Figure 4.** The PICAFO as testing device and sensors placement.

This research focused on the investigation of the ankle angular velocity and ankle torque. The ankle angular velocity could be measured directly from the rotary encoder. However, the ankle torque could not be measured directly. Therefore, the estimation of the ankle torque was conducted by using foot dynamic equations [35]. Free body diagram of a foot during walking is shown in Figure 5. Equations (1) and (2) described the net force equation on x-axis and y-axis. Equation (3) describes the net torque around the foot center of mass (CoM), in which Fa is the ankle force; Ma is the ankle torque; Ftoe is the GRF on toe; Fheel is the GRF on heel; m is the foot mass; I is the foot inertia around the center of gyration (CoG); R is the distance of the working force to the CoM, g is the gravity constant; a is a linear acceleration of the ankle; and α is the angular acceleration of the ankle. The up, right, and counterclockwise (dorsiflexion) vectors are denoted with a positive (+ve) sign. Additionally, down, left, and clockwise (plantarflexion) vectors are denoted with a negative (−ve) sign.

$$F_{ax} + F_{toex} + F_{heelx} = ma_x \tag{1}$$

$$F_{ay} + F_{toey} + F_{heely} - mg = ma_y \tag{2}$$

$$M_a - F_a R_a + F_{toe} R_{toe} - F_{heel} R_{heel} = I\alpha \tag{3}$$

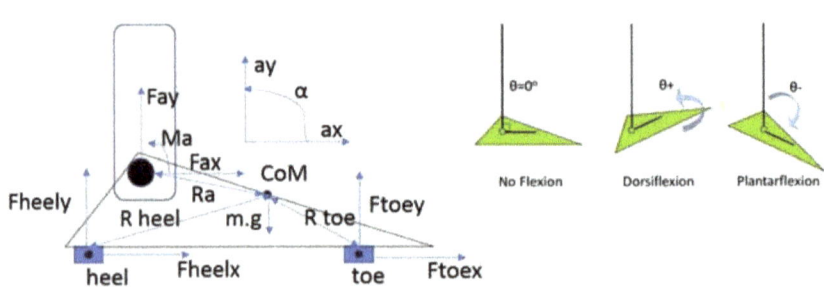

**Figure 5.** The foot dynamics.

Static and constant variables such as foot mass and foot length of the subject were measured before conducting the data collection. The foot mass was the total of the actual foot mass (1.45% of the body's mass) and the PICAFO's mass (1.7 kg) [35]. For example, subject 1 has a mass of 61.3 kg. Thus the foot mass for the dynamic calculation is (61.3 Kg × 1.45%) + 1.7 Kg = 2.589 Kg. Foot mass and foot length were further used to determine the foot inertia (I), CoM, foot CoG, $R_a$, $R_{toe}$, and $R_{heel}$, as shown in Table 2. After all the necessary parameters were determined, the estimation of the ankle force could be done by solving Equations (1) and (2). Finally, the ankle force was included in Equation (3) for estimating the ankle torque $M_a$.

**Table 2.** The subject's derived anthropometric.

| Anthropometric Parameters | Subject, Sb | | | | Mean | Standard Deviation |
|---|---|---|---|---|---|---|
| | 1 | 2 | 3 | 4 | | |
| I (kgm² × 10⁻²) | 0.967 | 1.144 | 1.378 | 2.030 | 1.380 | 0.403 |
| CoG (m) | 0.064 | 0.067 | 0.071 | 0.081 | 0.071 | 0.006 |
| CoM, $R_a$ (m) | 0.068 | 0.070 | 0.075 | 0.085 | 0.074 | 0.067 |
| $R_{toe}$ (m) | 0.028 | 0.018 | 0.015 | 0.015 | 0.019 | 0.005 |
| $R_{heel}$ (m) | 0.122 | 0.132 | 0.135 | 0.135 | 0.131 | 0.005 |

*2.2. Data Processing*

In this research, the region of interest for investigating the control reference parameter was the stance phase only. In preventing foot drop, the PICAFO can generate a maximum stiffness to lock the foot position regardless of the subject's anthropometric and walking style. Therefore, this study did not consider the swing phase for the investigation. Because of that, the collected data, such as the ankle torque and ankle angular velocity, were classified into three different phases of stance only such as IC to FF (1), FF to HO (2), and HO to TO (3). IC is when the foot contacts the ground on the heel first after the swing, while FF is when both toe and heel touch the ground while the body propelled forward. HO, as the name suggests, is when the heel is lifted, pushing the ground. TO starts when the foot begins to swing after being pushed off the ground. Measured data were divided into several phases to obtain the data average. The difference between the ankle position and the time-lapse defined the average ankle angular velocity (aω). On the other hand, the mean of all the data point presented in that phase defined the average ankle torque (a$M_a$). For illustration, see Figure 6.

*2.3. Data Analysis*

The goal of this preliminary research was to identify suitable control reference parameters (aω or a$M_a$) for estimation based on BMI and walking speed (WS) in three different phases of stance. Regression analysis such as multiple R, R-squared, adjusted R-squared, the standard of error, and t-test for critical parameter coefficients were the tools. The regression error was assumed to be independent one to another with constant variance; thus, it has a normal distribution. Therefore, the regression response (control reference) and the slope parameter (critical parameter coefficient) were also normally distributed. Table 3 presents the scenario for data analysis. The value of R explains the correlation between the critical parameter and control reference. A value for R near to one indicates better correlation. The standard error explains the relationship nature of the critical parameter and control reference. The less standard error means a better relationship. As for the t-test, it was conducted to see the probability of the critical parameter coefficient being zero (P-value > 0.05). Zero coefficient means that the critical parameter is insignificant for the control reference estimation.

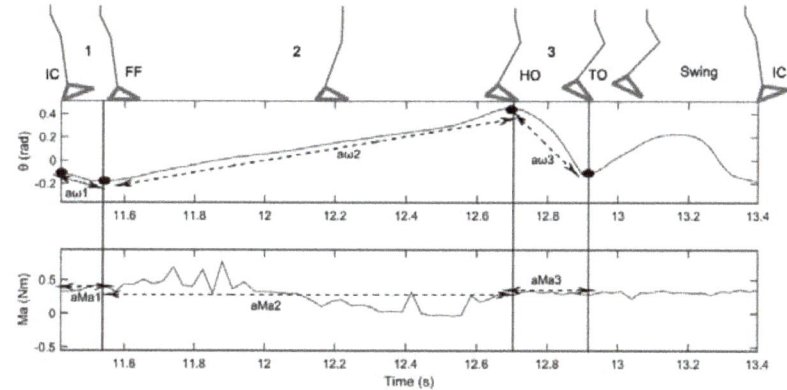

**Figure 6.** Average ankle torque and angular velocity in different stance phase (1, 2, 3).

Table 3. Data analysis scenario.

| Case | Stance Phase | Critical Parameter | | Control Reference | |
|---|---|---|---|---|---|
| | | BMI | WS | a$\omega$ | aM$_a$ |
| 1 | IC to FF | | √ | √ | |
| 2 | | | √ | | √ |
| 3 | | √ | | √ | |
| 4 | | √ | | | √ |
| 5 | | √ | √ | √ | |
| 6 | | √ | √ | | √ |
| 7 | FF to HO | | √ | √ | |
| 8 | | | √ | | √ |
| 9 | | √ | | √ | |
| 10 | | √ | | | √ |
| 11 | | √ | √ | √ | |
| 12 | | √ | √ | | √ |
| 13 | HO to TO | | √ | √ | |
| 14 | | | √ | | √ |
| 15 | | √ | | √ | |
| 16 | | √ | | | √ |
| 17 | | √ | √ | √ | |
| 18 | | √ | √ | | √ |

## 3. Result

This section describes the results of the data analysis. Figures 7–9 show the linear regression of control reference parameter a$\omega$ and aM$_a$ during IC to FF, FF to HO, and HO to TO respectively. The estimation of the actual value (blue dot) was conducted based on walking speed (grey dash line) only; BMI (yellow dash line) only; and a combination of both (orange dotted line). The left graph shows the actual and estimated values from the walking speed point of view, while the right graph shows the actual and estimation value from the BMI point of view. Table 4 presents the regression statistic result. Lastly, Table 5 presents the estimation value and *t*-test results of the critical parameter coefficient for multiple regression of control reference parameter a$\omega$ and aM$_a$.

The correlation of the control reference parameter with walking speed shows an inverse relationship. If aω has a positive correlation, then aM$_a$ has a negative correlation (Figure 8) and vice versa (Figures 7 and 9). Meanwhile, from a BMI point of view, a similar correlation behavior is also observed, however with a less steep gradient. The analysis considered only the absolute correlation value. Table 4 presents the correlation analysis results in terms of multiple R (p), and R-squared (p$^2$). The results show that the combination of walking speed and BMI to the control reference parameter has the highest correlation score compare to when they are just a stand-alone critical parameter in all stance phases. This result is also consistent for both the control reference parameter aω and aM$_a$. However, the highest correlation score belonged to aω instead of aM$_a$ (p1(aω) = 0.666 > p1(aM$_a$) = 0.560, p2(aω) = 0.837 > p2(aM$_a$) = 0.277, and p3(aω) = 0.839 > p3(aM$_a$) = 0.369).

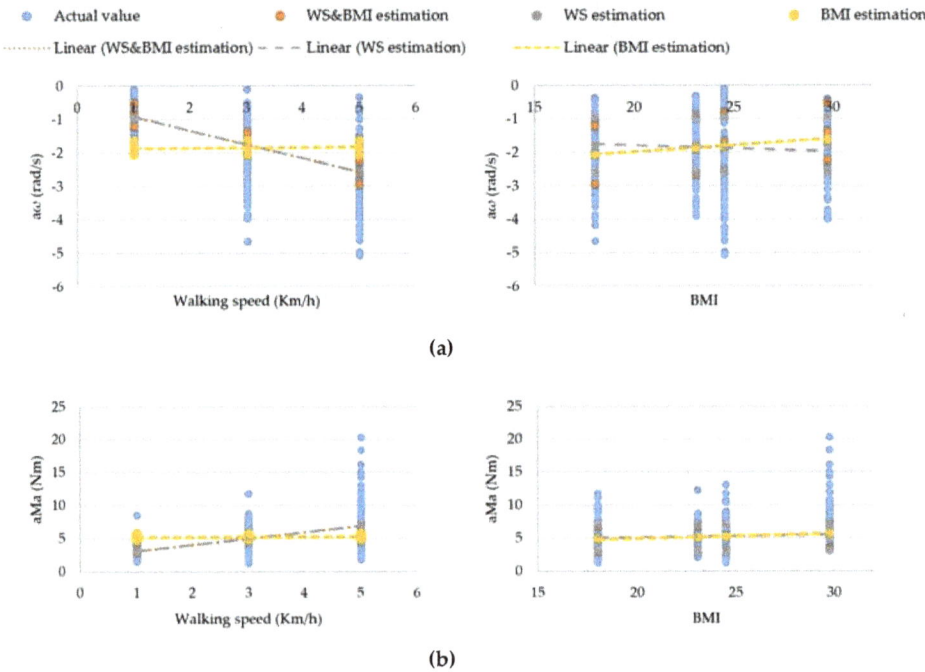

**Figure 7.** The regression of (**a**) average ankle velocity (aω) and (**b**) average ankle torque (aM$_a$) with different critical parameter during IC to FF phase.

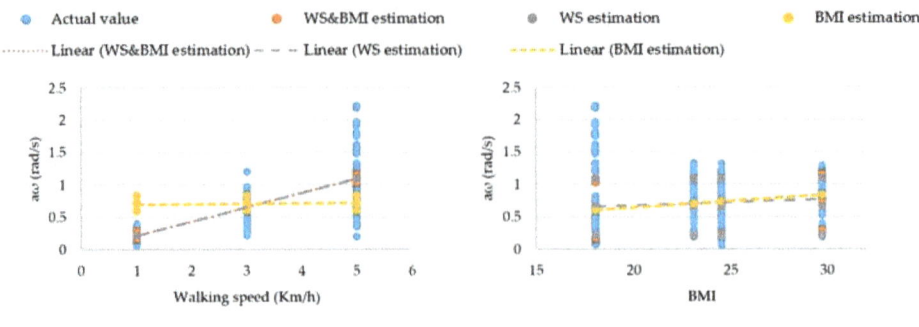

**Figure 8.** *Cont.*

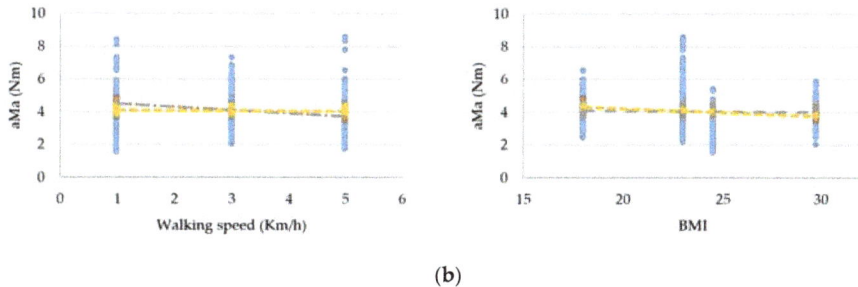

(b)

**Figure 8.** The regression of (**a**) average ankle velocity (aω) and (**b**) average ankle torque (aM_a) with different critical parameter during FF to HO phase.

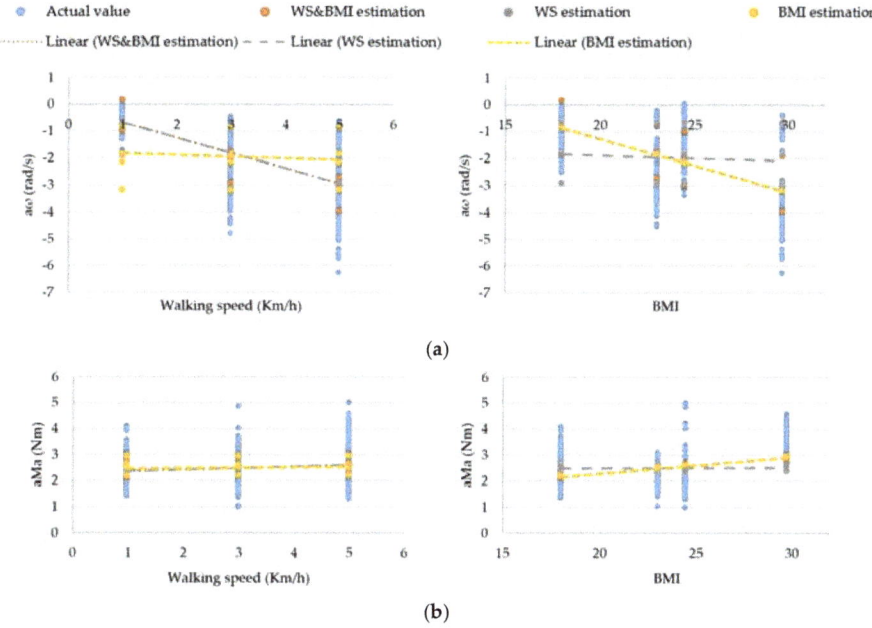

(b)

**Figure 9.** The regression of (**a**) average ankle velocity (aω) and (**b**) average ankle torque (aM_a) with different critical parameter during HO to TO phase.

Table 4. Regression statistic result.

| Phase | Regression Statistics | aω | | | aM_a | | |
|---|---|---|---|---|---|---|---|
| | | WS | BMI | WS & BMI | WS | BMI | WS & BMI |
| IC to FF | Multiple R (p1) | 0.625 | 0.159 | 0.666 | 0.558 | 0.117 | 0.560 |
| | R Square (p1²) | 0.391 | 0.025 | 0.444 | 0.311 | 0.014 | 0.314 |
| | Standard Error (Se1) | 0.822 | 1.040 | 0.786 | 2.253 | 2.695 | 2.251 |
| FF to HO | Multiple R (p2) | 0.830 | 0.199 | 0.837 | 0.246 | 0.154 | 0.277 |
| | R Square (p2²) | 0.689 | 0.039 | 0.700 | 0.060 | 0.024 | 0.077 |
| | Standard Error (Se2) | 0.235 | 0.413 | 0.231 | 1.245 | 1.270 | 1.236 |
| HO to TO | Multiple R (p3) | 0.645 | 0.607 | 0.839 | 0.130 | 0.357 | 0.369 |
| | R Square (p3²) | 0.416 | 0.368 | 0.705 | 0.017 | 0.128 | 0.136 |
| | Standard Error (Se3) | 1.060 | 1.103 | 0.755 | 0.742 | 0.699 | 0.696 |
| | Observations | 480 | 480 | 480 | 480 | 480 | 480 |

The standard error (Se) results in Table 4 show that in general, the estimation of $aM_a$ has higher Se compare to estimation of $a\omega$ (Se1($aM_a$) = 2.251 > Se1($a\omega$) = 0.786, Se2($aM_a$) = 1.236 > Se2($a\omega$) = 0.231, Se3($aM_a$) = 0.696 < Se3($a\omega$) = 0.755). BMI based estimation resulted in the highest estimated Se for each $a\omega$ and $aM_a$. On the other hand, the estimation based on walking speed only shows a smaller standard error, but the error reduced more when the two critical parameters were combined. For instance, during HO to TO, the standard error of $a\omega$ was 1.060 based on WS only, 1.103 based on BMI only, and 0.755 based on the combination of both. For illustrations of the reduced standard error, see Figures 7–9. The estimations based on both walking speed and BMI show wider coverage in hitting the actual value compare to estimation based on walking speed or BMI only.

The results of critical parameter coefficient estimation show that the WS coefficient consistently has the opposite sign between $a\omega$ and $aM_a$ estimation for the whole stance phase, similar to the correlation analysis result. BMI coefficient results also show agreement with the correlation analysis result. The $t$-test results reveal that all coefficients for $a\omega$ estimation were significantly not possible to be zero ($P$-value < 0.05). However, some coefficient for $aM_a$ estimation was insignificantly not possible to be zero. For instance, BMI coefficient has a confidence interval of −0.002 to 0.009 during IC to FF ($P$-value = 0.201), and WS coefficient has a confidence interval of 0.000 to 0.009 during HO to TO ($P$-value = 0.061).

**Table 5.** Critical parameter coefficient for multi regression of $a\omega$ and $aM_a$: estimation value and $t$-test result.

| | | | | | | |
|---|---|---|---|---|---|---|
| | | | $a\omega$ | | | |
| IC to FF | Coefficients | Standard Error | Lower 95% | Upper 95% | t Stat | P-value |
| Intercept | −1.807 | 0.234 | −2.266 | −1.347 | −7.735 | <0.05 |
| WS | −0.431 | 0.025 | −0.481 | −0.380 | −16.898 | <0.05 |
| BMI | 0.058 | 0.010 | 0.039 | 0.077 | 6.035 | <0.05 |
| FF to HO | Coefficients | Standard Error | Lower 95% | Upper 95% | t Stat | P-value |
| Intercept | −0.238 | 0.069 | −0.372 | −0.103 | −3.461 | <0.05 |
| WS | 0.216 | 0.007 | 0.202 | 0.231 | 28.889 | <0.05 |
| BMI | 0.011 | 0.003 | 0.005 | 0.016 | 3.740 | <0.05 |
| HO to TO | Coefficients | Standard Error | Lower 95% | Upper 95% | t Stat | P-value |
| Intercept | 3.841 | 0.224 | 3.400 | 4.282 | 17.126 | <0.05 |
| WS | −0.508 | 0.024 | −0.557 | −0.460 | −20.783 | <0.05 |
| BMI | −0.177 | 0.009 | −0.195 | −0.159 | −19.244 | <0.05 |
| | | | $aM_a$ | | | |
| IC to FF | Coefficients | Standard Error | Lower 95% | Upper 95% | t Stat | P-value |
| Intercept | 1.348 | 0.669 | 0.033 | 2.662 | 2.015 | <0.05 |
| WS | 0.939 | 0.073 | 0.796 | 1.082 | 12.874 | <0.05 |
| BMI | 0.035 | 0.003 | −0.019 | 0.089 | 1.281 | 0.201 |
| FF to HO | Coefficients | Standard Error | Lower 95% | Upper 95% | t Stat | P-value |
| Intercept | 5.572 | 0.367 | 4.850 | 6.294 | 15.172 | <0.05 |
| WS | −0.187 | 0.040 | −0.265 | −0.108 | −4.659 | <0.05 |
| BMI | −0.039 | 0.015 | −0.068 | −0.009 | −2.565 | <0.05 |
| HO to TO | Coefficients | Standard Error | Lower 95% | Upper 95% | t Stat | P-value |
| Intercept | 0.930 | 0.207 | 0.523 | 1.337 | 4.495 | <0.05 |
| WS | 0.042 | 0.023 | −0.002 | 0.087 | 1.881 | 0.061 |
| BMI | 0.061 | 0.008 | 0.045 | 0.078 | 7.225 | <0.05 |

## 4. Discussion

The goal of this preliminary study was to identify whether ankle angular velocity or ankle torque is the better control reference parameter for implementation of stance assistance using MR brake in PICAFO. The control reference parameter must adapt to different subjects and walking situations to maximize the benefit of using PICAFO [11]. Here, different subjects were represented by BMI, while the walking situations were represented by walking speed. Therefore, a superior control reference parameter is expected to have a high correlation with the BMI and walking speed during the stance phase.

The results of the regression analysis revealed that the ankle angular velocity is the preferable control reference parameter rather than ankle torque. The ankle angular velocity has a higher correlation score with BMI and walking speed compared to ankle torque, as shown in Table 3. The overall standard error of ankle angular velocity estimation is lower than the ankle torque estimation, which strengthens the correlation score result. The result of estimation and t-test of the critical parameter coefficient also shows the superiority of ankle angular velocity as control reference parameter where all the critical parameter coefficients were statistically significant not zero as shown in Table 4. However, the presented result cannot conclude the relationship between control reference and critical parameter due to a lack of sufficient participating subjects and regression model testing, which is a limitation of this study.

In the context of critical parameters, the results revealed that the combination of BMI and walking speed produced better estimations than a stand-alone parameter. Single-handedly, the walking speed alone already has enough correlation with both control reference parameters, especially ankle angular velocity, as shown in Table 3. This result agrees with the previous work by Kikuchi et al. in which the ankle angular velocity during IC to FF was predicted using the walking speed [32,33]. However, in this preliminary research, additional parameters such as BMI have been shown to improve the overall correlation score. Also, the standard error results support the correlation analysis. The standard error reduced when a combination of walking speed and BMI is used for estimation of ankle angular velocity, as shown in Table 3.

To sum up, the ankle angular velocity is the better choice for use as a control reference parameter, which can be estimated based on walking speed and BMI as revealed by the results. The implementation of the control reference parameter using the MR brake is also not difficult, because the feedback signal can be measured directly by using a rotary encoder. Ankle velocity can also be used to classify the gait phases [36]. This means that only rotary encoder is necessary as the sensor for both classification and control function in future implementation. Further study should be conducted in the future, which mainly focused on reducing the standard error of the control reference estimation. Improvement can be made by comparing a different kind of regression model and adding the sample sizes (subject number and walking speed). After obtaining a better fit estimation, the PICAFO system can implement the control reference parameter for stance assistance. Then, in a training session with the patient, for example, the therapist can optimally configure the PICAFO system simply by inserting the patient's walking speed and BMI.

**Author Contributions:** Conceptualization, D.A. and M.A.A.R.; methodology, N.N. and M.H.M.A.; formal analysis, D.A. and J.K.; investigation, D.A. and U.; resources, M.A.A.R, U. and S.A.M.; data curation, D.A. and M.K.S.; writing—original draft preparation, D.A..; writing—review and editing, D.A., M.A.A.R., U., N.N. and M.K.S.; supervision, M.A.A.R., U., S.A.M., and J.K.; funding acquisition, M.A.A.R. and U.

**Funding:** This research was funded by the Ministry of Education Malaysia, grant number 06G16 and the APC was funded by Malaysia Japan International Institute of Technology, Universiti Teknologi Malaysia. Some of the hardware was financially supported by Universitas Sebelas Maret (UNS) through Hibah Kolaborasi Internasional 2020 as well as partial funding from USAID through the Sustainable Higher Education Research Alliances (SHERA) Program, NCSTT with Contract No. IIE00000078-ITB-1.

**Acknowledgments:** The authors would like to express their appreciation to the Ministry of Education Malaysia, Universiti Teknologi Malaysia, Universitas Sebelas Maret, National Center for Sustainable Transportation Technology, and Institut Teknologi Telkom Surabaya for their financial support in this research.

**Conflicts of Interest:** The authors declare no conflict of interest.

## References

1. Burridge, J.; Taylor, P.; Hagan, S.; Swain, I. Experience of clinical use of the Odstock dropped foot stimulator. *Artif. Organs* **1997**, *21*, 254–260. [CrossRef] [PubMed]
2. Huo, W.; Mohammed, S.; Moreno, J.C.; Amirat, Y. Lower limb wearable robots for assistance and rehabilitation: A state of the art. *IEEE Syst. J.* **2016**, *10*, 1068–1081. [CrossRef]
3. Alam, M.; Choudhury, I.A.; Mamat, A.B. Mechanism and design analysis of articulated ankle foot orthoses for drop-foot. *Sci. World J.* **2014**, *2014*. [CrossRef] [PubMed]
4. Roche, N.; Bonnyaud, C.; Geiger, M.; Bussel, B.; Bensmail, D. Relationship between hip flexion and ankle dorsiflexion during swing phase in chronic stroke patients. *Clin. Biomech.* **2015**, *30*, 219–225. [CrossRef]
5. Chisholm, A.E.; Perry, S.D.; McIlroy, W.E. Correlations between ankle-foot impairments and dropped foot gait deviations among stroke survivors. *Clin. Biomech.* **2013**, *28*, 1049–1054. [CrossRef]
6. Tanida, S.; Kikuchi, T.; Kakehashi, T.; Otsuki, K.; Ozawa, T.; Fujikawa, T.; Yasuda, T.; Furusho, J.; Morimoto, S.; Hashimoto, Y. Intelligently controllable Ankle Foot Orthosis (I-AFO) and its application for a patient of Guillain-Barre syndrome. In Proceedings of the 2009 IEEE International Conference on Rehabilitation Robotics, Kyoto, Japan, 23–26 June 2009; pp. 857–862.
7. Mahon, C.E.; Farris, D.J.; Sawicki, G.S.; Lewek, M.D. Individual limb mechanical analysis of gait following stroke. *J. Biomech.* **2015**, *48*, 984–989. [CrossRef]
8. Collins, S.H.; Bruce Wiggin, M.; Sawicki, G.S. Reducing the energy cost of human walking using an unpowered exoskeleton. *Nature* **2015**, *522*, 212–215. [CrossRef]
9. Mickelborough, J.; van der Linden, M.L.; Tallis, R.C.; Ennos, A.R. Muscle activity during gait initiation in normal elderly people. *Gait Posture* **2004**, *19*, 50–57. [CrossRef]
10. Mishra, A.K.; Srivastava, A.; Tewari, R.P.; Mathur, R. EMG analysis of lower limb muscles for developing robotic exoskeleton orthotic device. *Procedia Eng.* **2012**, *41*, 32–36. [CrossRef]
11. Adiputra, D.; Nazmi, N.; Bahiuddin, I.; Ubaidillah, U.; Imaduddin, F.; Rahman, M.A.; Mazlan, S.A.; Zamzuri, H. A review on the control of the mechanical properties of ankle foot orthosis for gait assistance. *Actuators* **2019**, *8*, 10. [CrossRef]
12. Delafontaine, A.; Gagey, O.; Colnaghi, S.; Do, M.-C.; Honeine, J.-L. Rigid ankle foot orthosis deteriorates mediolateral balance control and vertical braking during gait initiation. *Front. Hum. Neurosci.* **2017**, *11*, 214. [CrossRef] [PubMed]
13. Bregman, D.J.J.; de Groot, V.; van Diggele, P.; Meulman, H.; Houdijk, H.; Harlaar, J. Polypropylene ankle foot orthoses to overcome drop-foot gait in central neurological patients: A mechanical and functional evaluation. *Prosthet. Orthot. Int.* **2010**, *34*, 293–304. [CrossRef] [PubMed]
14. Tavernese, E.; Petrarca, M.; Rosellini, G.; Stanislao, E.D.; Pisano, A.; Rosa, G.D.; Castelli, E. Carbon Modular Orthosis (Ca.M.O.): An innovative hybrid modular ankle-foot orthosis to tune the variable rehabilitation needs in hemiplegic cerebral palsy. *Neurorehabilitation* **2017**, *40*, 447–457. [CrossRef] [PubMed]
15. Schrank, E.S.; Hitch, L.; Wallace, K.; Moore, R.; Stanhope, S.J. Assessment of a virtual functional prototyping process for the rapid manufacture of passive-dynamic ankle-foot orthoses. *J. Biomech. Eng.* **2013**, *135*, 101011. [CrossRef] [PubMed]
16. Frascarelli, F.; Masia, L.; Rosa, G.D.; Cappa, P.; Petrarca, M.; Castelli, E.; Krebs, H.I. The impact of robotic rehabilitation in children with acquired or congenital movement disorders. *Eur. J. Phys. Rehabil. Med.* **2009**, *45*, 135–141.
17. Adiputra, D.; Mazlan, S.U.; Zamzuri, H.; Rahman, M.A. Fuzzy logic control for ankle foot equipped with magnetorheological brake. *J. Teknol.* **2016**, *11*, 25–32. [CrossRef]
18. Adiputra, D.; Rahman, M.A.A.; Tjahjana, D.D.D.P.U.; Widodo, P.J.; Imaduddin, F. Controller development of a passive control ankle foot orthosis. In Proceedings of the International Conference on Robotics, Automation and Sciences, Melaka, Malaysia, 27–29 November 2017. [CrossRef]
19. Adiputra, D.; Mazlan, S.A.; Zamzuri, H.; Rahman, M.A.A. Development of controller for Passive Control Ankle Foot Orthoses (PICAFO) based on Electromyography (EMG) signal and angle. In Proceedings of the Joint International Conference on Electric Vehicular Technology and Industrial, Mechanical, Electrical, and Chemical Engineering (ICEVT & IMECE), Surakarta, Indonesia, 4–5 November 2015; pp. 200–206.
20. Nazmi, N.; Rahman, M.A.; Yamamoto, S.-I.; Ahmad, S.; Zamzuri, H.; Mazlan, S. A review of classification techniques of EMG signals during isotonic and isometric contractions. *Sensors* **2016**, *16*, 1304. [CrossRef]

21. Nazmi, N.; Rahman, M.A.A.; Yamamoto, S.I.; Ahmad, S.A. Walking gait event detection based on electromyography signals using artificial neural network. *Biomed. Signal Process. Control* **2019**, *47*, 334–343. [CrossRef]
22. Holgate, M.A.; Böhler, A.W.; Sugar, T.G. Control algorithms for ankle robots: A reflection on the state-of-the-art and presentation of two novel algorithms. In Proceedings of the 2nd Biennial IEEE/RAS-EMBS International Conference on Biomedical Robotics and Biomechatronics, Scottsdale, AZ, USA, 19–22 October 2008; pp. 97–102.
23. Boehler, A.W.; Hollander, K.W.; Sugar, T.G.; Shin, D. Design, implementation and test results of a robust control method for a powered ankle foot orthosis (AFO). In Proceedings of the IEEE International Conference on Robotics and Automation, Pasadena, CA, USA, 19–23 May 2008; pp. 2025–2030.
24. Blaya, J.A.; Herr, H. Adaptive control of a variable-impedance ankle-foot orthosis to assist drop-foot gait. *IEEE Trans. Neural Syst. Rehabil. Eng.* **2004**, *12*, 24–31. [CrossRef]
25. Chen, B.; Zhao, X.; Ma, H.; Qin, L.; Liao, W.-H. Design and characterization of a magnetorheological series elastic actuator for a lower extremity exoskeleton. *Smart Mater. Struct.* **2017**, *26*, 105008. [CrossRef]
26. Gordon, K.E.; Sawicki, G.S.; Ferris, D.P. Mechanical performance of artificial pneumatic muscles to power an ankle-foot orthosis. *J. Biomech.* **2006**, *39*, 1832–1841. [CrossRef] [PubMed]
27. Gordon, K.E.; Ferris, D.P. Learning to walk with a robotic ankle exoskeleton. *J. Biomech.* **2007**, *40*, 2636–2644. [CrossRef] [PubMed]
28. Fleischer, C.; Hommel, G. EMG-driven human model for orthosis control. In *Human Interaction with Machines Workshop*; Springer: Dordrecht, The Netherlands, 2006; pp. 69–76.
29. Emmens, A.R.; van Asseldonk, E.H.F.; van der Kooij, H. Effects of a powered ankle-foot orthosis on perturbed standing balance. *J. Neuroeng. Rehabil.* **2018**, *15*, 50. [CrossRef]
30. Kikuchi, T.; Tanida, S.; Otsuki, K.; Yasuda, T.; Furusho, J. Development of third-generation intelligently controllable ankle-foot orthosis with compact MR fluid brake. In Proceedings of the IEEE International Conference on Robotics and Automation, Anchorage, AK, USA, 3–7 May 2010; pp. 2209–2214.
31. Jiménez-Fabián, R.; Verlinden, O. Review of control algorithms for robotic ankle systems in lower-limb orthoses, prostheses, and exoskeletons. *Med Eng. Phys.* **2012**, *34*, 397–408. [CrossRef]
32. Kikuchi, T.; Tanida, S.; Yasuda, T.; Fujikawa, T. Automatic adjustment of initial drop speed of foot for intelligently controllable ankle foot orthosis. In Proceedings of the 2013 6th IEEE/SICE International Symposium on System Integration, Kobe, Japan, 15–17 December 2013; pp. 276–281.
33. Naito, H.; Akazawa, Y.; Tagaya, K.; Matsumoto, T.; Tanaka, M. An ankle-foot orthosis with a variable-resistance ankle joint using a magnetorheological-fluid rotary damper. *J. Biomech. Sci. Eng.* **2009**, *4*, 182–191. [CrossRef]
34. Guanziroli, E.; Cazzaniga, M.; Colombo, L.; Basilico, S.; Legnani, G.; Molteni, F. Assistive powered exoskeleton for complete spinal cord injury: Correlations between walking ability and exoskeleton control. *Eur. J. Phys. Rehabil. Med.* **2019**, *55*, 209–216. [CrossRef]
35. Winter, D.A. *Biomechanics and Motor Control of Human Movement*; John Wiley & Sons: Hoboken, NJ, USA, 2009. [CrossRef]
36. Grimmer, M.; Schmidt, K.; Duarte, J.E.; Neuner, L.; Koginov, G.; Riener, R. Stance and swing detection based on the angular velocity of lower limb segments during walking. *Front. Neurorobot.* **2019**, *13*, 57. [CrossRef]

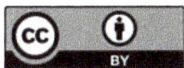

© 2019 by the authors. Licensee MDPI, Basel, Switzerland. This article is an open access article distributed under the terms and conditions of the Creative Commons Attribution (CC BY) license (http://creativecommons.org/licenses/by/4.0/).

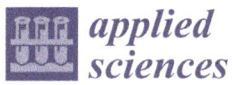 

Article

# Modeling of Motorized Orthosis Control

Iñigo Aramendia [1], Ekaitz Zulueta [2,*], Daniel Teso-Fz-Betoño [2], Aitor Saenz-Aguirre [2] and Unai Fernandez-Gamiz [1]

1. Nuclear Engineering and Fluid Mechanics Department, University of the Basque Country UPV/EHU, 01006 Vitoria-Gasteiz, Araba, Spain; inigo.aramendia@ehu.eus (I.A.); unai.fernandez@ehu.eus (U.F.-G.)
2. Automatic Control and System Engineering Department, University of the Basque Country, UPV/EHU, 01006 Vitoria-Gasteiz, Spain; daniel.teso@ehu.eus (D.T.-F.-B.); asaenz012@ikasle.ehu.eus (A.S.-A.)
* Correspondence: ekaitz.zulueta@ehu.eus; Tel.: +34-945-014-066

Received: 26 April 2019; Accepted: 13 June 2019; Published: 15 June 2019

**Abstract:** Orthotic devices are defined as externally applied devices that are used to modify the structural and functional characteristics of the neuro-muscular and skeletal systems. The aim of the current study is to improve the control and movement of a robotic arm orthosis by means of an intelligent optimization system. Firstly, the control problem settlement is defined with the muscle, brain, and arm model. Subsequently, the optimization control, which based on a differential evolution algorithm, is developed to calculate the optimum gain values. Additionally, a cost function is defined in order to control and minimize the effort that is made by the subject and to assure that the algorithm follows as close as possible the defined setpoint value. The results show that, with the optimization algorithm, the necessary development force of the muscles is close to zero and the neural excitation level of biceps and triceps signal values are getting lower with a gain increase. Furthermore, the necessary development force of the biceps muscle to overcome a load added to the orthosis control system is practically the half of the one that is necessary without the optimization algorithm.

**Keywords:** orthosis control; muscle modeling; arm; Hill muscle; swarm optimization

## 1. Introduction

The research carried out in biomechanics gives rise to continuous improvements to the health and life quality of the human being, and therefore is considered as a rising field of knowledge than can offer scientific and technological solutions in the near future, as described in the overviews of Dollar and Herr [1] and Lo and Xie [2]. People with physical disabilities have to face many barriers to participate in any life activity area. The development and study of assistive devices in order to improve the limb functionality began in the 1940s due to the polio epidemic, where the survivors presented arms that were too weak to carry out basic activities, such as feeding themselves. With years and technological advances, these types of devices have been improved to be used for other activities of daily living and to treat different types of upper extremity malfunctions [3]. They are what we know nowadays as orthotic devices or arm supports. Van der Heide et al. [4] made an extensive review and classified all of the different dynamic arm supports for people with deceased arm function. According to the ISO 9999:2016 [5], they are defined as "externally applied devices used to modify the structure and functional characteristics of the neuro-muscular and skeletal systems".

Tsagarakis et al. [6] developed an orthosis prototype for the upper arm training and rehabilitation. It provided seven DOFs that corresponded to the natural movement of the human arm from the shoulder to the wrist with the help of pneumatic-muscle actuator. Kiguchi et al. [7] introduced a robotic exoskeleton for the assistance of the upper-limb motion with a hierarchical neuro-fuzzy controller. The system was experimentally tested with three healthy human subjects, showing a reduction in the electromyography (EMG) signals when this type of exoskeleton assisted the subjects. Pratt et al. [8]

developed an exoskeleton system, RoboKnee, to assist the wearer in tasks, such as climbing stairs strengthening the knee movement. A linear series-elastic actuator powers the device and the actuator force is provided by a positive-feedback controller. Peternel et al. [9] developed an exoskeleton control method for the adaptive learning of assistive joint torque profiles in periodic tasks. Combined with adaptive oscillators, it was tested with real robot experiments in subjects wearing an elbow exoskeleton.

Cavallaro et al. [10] presented the development, optimization, and integration of real-time myoprocessors as a human machine interface (HMI) for an upper limb powered exoskeleton that was based on the Hill muscle model. Their results, offering a high correlation between joint moment prediction of the model and the measured data, proved the feasibility and robustness of myoprocessors for its integration into the exoskeleton control system. Tang et al. [11] developed an upper-limb power-assist exoskeleton and studied its behavior under four different experimental conditions. The results showed that the user can control the exoskeleton in real-time by to improve the arm performance. Recently, Williams [12] carried out a pilot study with an upper arm support in subjects who suffered a severe to moderate stroke. Most of them presented faster and more accurate results while using support at the upper limb, with a decrease in the effort to lift the arm and reduced biceps activity.

In order to advance in this field, new muscle models have been developed to make real-time simulations and to reproduce the operation of the muscles as well as possible. In this context, one of the most interesting approaches has been the development of the real-time model that was studied by Chadwick et al. [13], which describes the complex dynamics of the arm by means of the creation of a virtual arm. Using an implicit method that was based on first order functions of Rosenbrock, it allows for simulating the complex muscle and joint dynamics in real time and to make real-time experiments with the participation of real subjects, achieving faster simulations with the same precision as the slower explicit methods. Previously, Chadwick et al. [14] have been carried out approximations in which the simulation of the arm dynamics of the subject was made by means of a direct dynamics model, which described the complex dynamics of the activation and contraction of the muscles as well as the non-linear characteristics of these muscles and the coupling of the muscular skeleton. In direct dynamics, the muscles activations or neuronal excitations are specified, and mathematically described how those signals are transformed into movement. However, the simulation of direct dynamics by explicit numerical methods requires very small times of execution, which makes the processing to be slow and, in no case, closer to real time. The precision of the implicit method was checked in the work of van den Bogert et al. [15], where the same simulation was performed while using two different methods: the implicit Rosenbrock method and an explicit second-order Runge-Kutta method.

Within the most sophisticated models, designs using electromyography (EMG) signals make use of the electrical power that is generated by the remaining muscles of the harmed arm; they have both high cost and learning curve. Three different aspects must be taken into account in an EMG control system: the intuitiveness of actuating control, the accuracy of movement selection, and the response time of the control system. Tsai et al. [16] carried out a comparison of upper-limb motion pattern recognition while using multichannel EMG signals from the shoulder and elbow during dynamic and isometric muscle contractions. Suberbiola et al. [17] captured the biceps and triceps EMG signals and found more precise movement with the use of algorithms that are based on autoregressive models and artificial neural networks Recently, Desplenter and Trejos [18] have evaluated seven muscle activation models by means of an EMG-driven elbow motion model. Many differences were found between models suggesting that further evaluation and improvements of motion models is still necessary in order to increase the safety and feasibility of the wearable assistive devices.

The application of mathematical models in biological systems are very powerful tools when it is wanted to model a complex system. In our case of study, muscle dynamics depends on several factors or effects that are all working at the same time, introducing a significant complexity in muscle fiber analysis. The model that is applied in the present study is mathematically defined in [13]. This model will be used due to its simplicity to be applied in control system modeling and because it is realistic enough to correctly explain the arm's muscles dynamics.

This study has been carried out in order to improve the control and movement of a robotic arm prosthesis or orthosis. We hypothesized that the application of an optimization algorithm could contribute to decreasing the necessary development force of the biceps muscle carried out for a patient to overcome a load. These man-machine interfaces have become very important for physically disabled people to carry out specific jobs or operations and they will become even more important in the future. The purpose of this orthosis is to aid people who lost the ability to move the upper arm or who lost strength in the muscles. The arm orthosis is custom made and it can be seen in Figure 1. Two surface EMG sensors and a goniometer capture the EMG signals and transmit it to a biomedical amplifier system, which transmits the amplified signals to a data acquisition card to process the signals on a computer with MATLAB software that is installed. From the computer, i the possibility to control the arm orthosis exists, which two linear actuators power. Figure A1 of Appendix A illustrates the main Simulink diagram that is used in this study to control the orthosis.

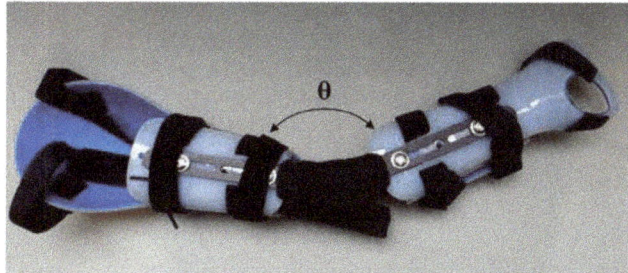

**Figure 1.** Custom made arm orthosis used in the present study, where θ represents the forearm angle.

## 2. Motorized Orthosis Control Problem Settlement

The proposed model is a Single Input Single Output (SISO) system. The muscle model input is a neural signal that expresses the command that is given by the human subject to activate the muscle, whereas the output signal of the model is the force that is generated by the muscle, as shown in Figure A2. This model has several parameters that are known by the literature (Chadwick et al. [13]), which have high sensibility in our system's response. The mechanical characteristics have also high influence in this response. In this study, we have supposed that muscles only develop a force in a single direction. This assumption is good enough for control objectives. In [19], Hill defined the three element model that was presented in Figure 2; the contractile element (CE), an elastic element (PEE) in parallel connection with the contractile element, and finally another elastic element (SEE) in series connection with the contractile element. Thelen [20] adjusted the parameters of the Hill-type muscle model to reflect the observed age-related changes in dynamic muscle contractions.

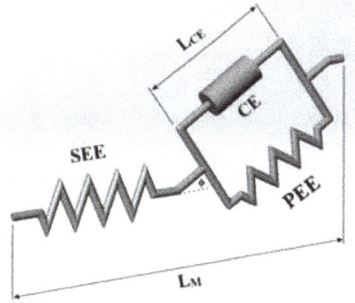

**Figure 2.** Hill muscle model.

## 2.1. Muscle-Skeletal Dynamic

This process is described by the non-linear first order differential Equation (1), as shown in the work of He et al. [21].

$$\frac{da}{dt} = \left(\frac{u}{T_{act}} + \frac{1-u}{T_{deact}}\right)(u-a) \qquad (1)$$

where the activation dynamics a is the activation level of this muscle and 'u' is the neural excitation level that is acquired by the muscle. The activation and deactivation time constants $T_{act}$ and $T_{deact}$ values were obtained from the work of Winters and Stark [22]. The total force generated by the muscle, as described by Equation (2), is calculated by the mechanical model that is proposed in Figure 2.

$$F_{total} = (F_{active} + f_{PEE}(L_{CE}))\cos\phi = f_{SEE}(L_M - L_{CE}\cos\phi) \qquad (2)$$

where $L_{CE}$ is the contractile element's length, $L_M$ is the muscle's length, and $\phi$ is the pennation angle. $F_{active}$, $f_{PEE}$, and $f_{SEE}$ correspond to the forces that are applied into CE, PEE and SEE points, respectively. The value of the pennation angle has been set to s = $L_{CE}\cos\phi$ in order to avoid singularity problems, as used in the work of Van den Vogert et al. [15].

## 2.2. Muscle Model

The contractile element active force is calculated, as shown in Equation (3):

$$F_{active} = a \cdot F_{max} \cdot f_{FL}(L_{CE}) \cdot f_{FV}(\dot{L}_{CE}) \qquad (3)$$

where a is the activation level and $F_{max}$ is the maximum isometric force. This parameter is estimated for each muscle, where several studies in human bodies give a 100 N/cm$^2$ value for transversal force stress (see Klein-Breteler et al. [23] and Holzbaur et al. [24]). The Gaussian like function of Equation (4) describes the mathematical relationship between the normalized force and the contractile element's length ($L_{CE}$).

$$f_{FL}(L_{CE}) = e^{-\left(\frac{L_{CE}-L_{CEopt}}{w \cdot L_{CEopt}}\right)^2} \qquad (4)$$

$L_{CE}$ is the contractile element's length, $L_{CEopt}$ its optimal length (values are given in the work of Klein-Breteler [23]), and the force versus length curve w parameter has been set to 0.56. The pennation angle and the optimal length values have been set to values that are given in [23].

$f_{FV}(\dot{L}_{CE})$ is the force versus speed function, as defined by Equation (5), based on the mathematical expression of McLean et al. [25]:

$$f_{FV}(V_{CE}) \begin{cases} \frac{V_{max}+V_{CE}}{V_{max}-\frac{V_{CE}}{A}} & if \ V_{CE} \leq 0 \\ \frac{g_{max} \cdot V_{CE}+c_3}{V_{CE}+c_3} & if \ V_{CE} > 0 \end{cases} \qquad (5)$$

where $V_{CE}$ is the contractile element's contraction speed, the A parameter is set to 0.25 according to Herzog [26], and the maximum activation speed, $V_{max}$, is set to 10 m/s. The parameter $g_{max}$ is assumed to be 1.5, following to [25], whereas the parameter $c_3$ is calculated from $f_{FV}(V_{CE})$ function's first derivate when $V_{CE} = 0$, as shown in Equation (6).

$$c_3 = \frac{V_{max} \cdot A(g_{max}-1)}{A+1} \qquad (6)$$

The parallel elastic element (PEE) and series elastic element (SEE), as determined by Equation (7), are modeled as passive non linear springs:

$$F(L)\begin{cases} K_1(L-L_{slack}) \text{ if } L \leq L_{slack} \\ K_1(L-L_{slack}) + K_2(L-L_{slack})^2 \text{ if } L > L_{slack} \end{cases} \quad (7)$$

$K_1$ term is set to 10 N/m. This value is low, but it is necessary to give some rigidity to the muscle models. Actually, a null value can generate singularity problems. The $K_2$ term is assumed to have a null value. In SEE, the $L_{slack}$ parameter, which is the length of the element when it is relaxed, is set by means of the results that were obtained in the cadaver studies, whereas, in PEE, the $L_{CEopt}$ value is identical with the exception of some muscle elements that support high passive forces. These values are calculated in the work of Chadwick et al. [27].

### 2.3. Brain Model

We have assumed that the human brain behavior can be modelled as a proportional controller in position. The signal is distributed in the $u_{biceps}$ and $u_{triceps}$ signals, as represented in the Equations (8) and (9):

$$u_{biceps}(t)\begin{cases} (\theta_{sp}-\theta)K_p \text{ if } (\theta_{sp}-\theta) \geq 0 \\ 0 \text{ if } (\theta_{sp}-\theta) < 0 \end{cases} \quad (8)$$

$$u_{triceps}(t)\begin{cases} -K_p(\theta_{sp}-\theta) \text{ if } (\theta_{sp}-\theta) < 0 \\ 0 \text{ if } (\theta_{sp}-\theta) \geq 0 \end{cases} \quad (9)$$

where $\theta$ is the angular position of the forearm, $\theta_{sp}$ is the instruction of the angular position of the forearm, and $K_p$ is the gain between the error of the angular position and its instruction. $u_{biceps}$ and $u_{triceps}$ are the neural excitation level of biceps and triceps, respectively. Each signal has a saturation block to remain within an interval and the $u_{triceps}$ signal has a negative gain, since the triceps muscles exerts a force opposed to the biceps muscle, as illustrated in Figure A3. That is, if the biceps muscle is extended, then the triceps muscle is relaxed.

### 2.4. Arm Model

Equation (1) has been also used, since the arm activation dynamics is similar to the muscle model. Therefore, Equations (10) and (11), along with Equation (1), describe the modeling procedure of the biceps and triceps muscles, where the $f_{SEE}$ force is calculated.

$$F_{Total} = (F_{active} + f_{PEE}(L_{CE}))\cos\phi = f_{SEE}(L_M - L_{CE}\cos\phi) \quad (10)$$

$$F(L)\begin{cases} K_1(L-L_{slack}) \text{ if } L \leq L_{slack} \\ K_1(L-L_{slack}) + K_2(L-L_{slack})^2 \text{ if } L > L_{slack} \end{cases} \quad (11)$$

From Equations (10) and (11), we are able to obtain Equation (12):

$$L_T = L_M - L_{CE}\cos\phi \quad (12)$$

where $L_T$ is the length of the SEE element. Once $L_T$ is calculated, the value of $f_{SEE}$ is obtained and then the value of $L_{CE}$. When it comes to considering the model, different options have been studied and the integration method was chosen. The $L_{CE}$ variable is calculated depending on two situations, as shown in Figure A4.

1. When the activation is not null, it is achieved with the inversion of the differential equation that relates the active force and the relation $V_{CE}$.
2. When the activation is null, the influence of the element CE disappears. The force that is achieved as a consequence of the extinction of the CE element is the one that is only caused by the elements SEE and PEE, and this is possible when the contractile element's length is equal to the slack length ($L_{CE} = L_{slack}$).

The calculation of the variable L$_{CE}$ is achieved by means of Equations (13)–(16):

$$F_{active} = a \cdot F_{max} \cdot f_{FL}(L_{CE}) \cdot f_{FV}(\dot{L}_{CE}) \tag{13}$$

$$f_{FL}(L_{CE}) = e^{-\left(\frac{L_{CE}-L_{CEopt}}{w \cdot L_{CEopt}}\right)^2} \tag{14}$$

$$f_{FV}(V_{CE}) \begin{cases} \frac{V_{max}+V_{CE}}{V_{max}-\frac{V_{CE}}{A}} & if \ V_{CE} \leq 0 \\ \frac{g_{max} \cdot V_{CE}+c_3}{V_{CE}+c_3} & if \ V_{CE} > 0 \end{cases} \tag{15}$$

$$F(L) \begin{cases} K_1(L-L_{slack}) & if \ L \leq L_{slack} \\ K_1(L-L_{slack}) + K_2(L-L_{slack})^2 & if \ L > L_{slack} \end{cases} \tag{16}$$

Once defined the muscle model, it is necessary to describe the dynamics of the arm by means of the Equation (17), as shown in Figure A5. The momentum of inertia J$_{arm}$ is obtained with the Equation (18) in order to achieve the arm dynamics.

$$J_{arm} \frac{d^2\theta}{dt^2} = R_{muscle} \cdot (F_{Biceps} - F_{Triceps}) + T_{control} + T_{load} \tag{17}$$

$$J_{arm} = I_g + m_{arm} \cdot d^2 \tag{18}$$

where I$_g$ is the forearm inertia with respect to its center of gravity, m$_{arm}$ is the mass of the arm, and $d$ is the distance between the mass center of the forearm and its center of rotation.

The forces F$_{Biceps}$ and F$_{Triceps}$ muscles are obtained through the R$_{muscle}$ parameter, creating a force momentum.

## 3. Proposed Control Scheme and Control Parameter Adjustment

As illustrated in the control block of Figure A6, the K$_{pbi}$ and K$_{ptri}$ gain values are calculated by the intelligent algorithm that is explained later in this study. The goal of this block is to provide the necessary assistant force to move the muscle. It is obtained with the K$_{pbi}$ and K$_{ptri}$ gain values of the Equation (19). K$_{control}$ is a gain value that is set to 0.1 or to 0.3, with the aim of achieving enough torque assistance. K$_{pbi}$ and K$_{ptri}$ are set in order to define the relative strength between the biceps and triceps EMG signals in order to achieve the best dynamics response (see Equation (20)).

$$T_{control} = K_{control} \cdot (K_{pbi} \cdot u_{Biceps} - K_{ptri} \cdot u_{Triceps}) \tag{19}$$

The proposed control law has two inputs: u$_{biceps}$, the neural excitation level of biceps and u$_{triceps}$, the neural excitation level of triceps. These two inputs, which are captured and estimated by surface EMG signal sensors, are calculated as the rectified and filtered values of surface EMG sensors located in biceps and triceps. The proportional gains models the weight of each signal in torque assistance. An intelligent optimization algorithm, as described below, must set these parameters.

The authors proposed this control, since it is simple enough to be executed by a real time processor and it takes into account the main variables that define the system state (the excitation levels of triceps and biceps). This control law does not take into account the real setpoint, because it is unknown, so the control measures the excitation level in order to know which the desired forearm angle is. Table 1 represents the parameters that were used in the proposed control scheme.

Table 1. Parameter values used in the proposed control scheme.

| Parameter | Value | Units |
|---|---|---|
| Human height (h) | 1.90 | m |
| Human weight (M) | 100 | kg |

Table 1. Cont.

| Parameter | Value | Units |
|---|---|---|
| Distance (d) | $0.0725 \times H$ | m |
| Turning radius ($R_g$) | $0.303 \times d$ | m |
| Arm weight ($m_{arm}$) | $0.016 \times M$ | kg |
| Moment of inertia ($I_g$) | $m_{arm} \times (R_g)^2$ | $kg \times m^2$ |
| Forearm moment of inertia ($J_{arm}$) | $J_{arm} = I_g + m_{arm} \times (d^2)$ | $kg/m^2$ |
| Arm length ($R_{arm}$) | $R_{arm} = 2 \times d/10$ | m |
| Friction coefficient | 0.1 | N·m/rad·s |

## 3.1. Control Parameter Optimization

A cost function has been described within the optimization algorithm by means of the Equation (20). The goal of this function is to minimize the effort that is made by the subject and to assure that the algorithm follows as close as possible the defined setpoint value.

$$Cost\ function = \alpha_1(\overline{|\theta_{sp} - \theta|}) + \alpha_2 \left(\frac{1}{T}\int_0^T \left[u_{biceps}(t)\right]^2\right) + \alpha_3 \left(\frac{1}{T}\int_0^T \left[u_{triceps}(t)\right]^2\right) \\ + \alpha_4\left(max(|\theta_{sp} - \theta|)\right) \quad (20)$$

where $\theta$ is the angular position of the forearm, $\theta_{sp}$ is the instruction of the angular position of the forearm, and $\alpha_j$ are the different weights of different relevant design criteria: the mean absolute error, the maximum absolute error, and the effort made by biceps and triceps (described by the square mean value of biceps and triceps excitations levels) and T is the time horizon.

## 3.2. Optimization Algorithm Description

The differential evolution (DE) is applied in the resolution of complex problems being an optimization method within the evolutionary computation. As other intelligent or swarm optimization algorithms, the DE algorithm proposes different agents set. All agents in this set are evaluated, crossed, mutated and selected. All these steps are made in order to improve the agent set.

Algorithms, the variables that are wanted to be optimized in the problem, take real values, as they were codified from a vector. The length of these vectors (n) and the quantity of variables of the problem is the same. In order to define a vector, the nomenclature $x_p^g$ has been used, where p is the indicator of the individual population (p = 1 ... NP) and g is the corresponding generational number. The vectors are also completed with the problem variable $x_{p,m}^g$, where m is the indicator of the variable of the population (m = 1 ... n).

The problem field variables reach the minimum and maximum values at $x_m^{min}$ and $x_m^{max}$, respectively. In the current case, the variables $K_{pbi}$ y $K_{ptri}$ have been limited to 50. The DE algorithm has four stages:

- Initialization
- Mutation
- Recombination
- Election

The initialization algorithm is executed each time that it takes place. However, the mutation, recombination, and election algorithms are indefinitely repeated until one of the next elements is satisfied (the generational quantity, the past time, the quality of the solution achieved). The function of each one of these stages is explained below.

### 3.2.1. Initialization

The population is randomly initialized, while taking into account the maximum and minimum values of each variable, as described in Equation (21):

$$x^1_{p,m} = x^{min}_m + rand(0,1) \cdot (x^{max}_m - x^{min}_m) \tag{21}$$

where p = 1 ... NP, m = 1 ... n and rand(0,1), (0,1) is any value of the interval.

3.2.2. Mutation

The mutations NP have as a goal the origin of the vectors. These vectors are created choosing three elements ($x_a$, $x_b$, $x_c$), and they are achieved with the Equation (22):

$$n^t_p = x_c + F \cdot (x_a - x_b) \tag{22}$$

where a, b, and c cannot be the same value and p = 1 ... NP. F is a parameter that controls the mutation rate founded in the interval (0,2).

3.2.3. Recombination

When the random vectors NP have been obtained, their recombination is also randomly carried out in comparison with the original vectors ($x_p$,$g$). In this way, the new agent proposal ($t^g_m$) is achieved by Equation (23):

$$t^g_{p,m} \begin{cases} n^g_{p,m} \; if \; rand([0,1]) < GR \\ x^g_{p,m} \; if \; any \; other \; case \end{cases} \tag{23}$$

where p = 1 ... NP, m = 1 ... n and GR is the parameter that controls the recombination rate. Subsequently, a variable-variable comparison is carried out, thus, the test vector NP can be considered as a mixture between the vectors and the original vectors.

3.2.4. Election

In the election process, the cost function is calculated by means of the element that is achieved in the recombination. From this value, it is compared with the value of the function that is wanted to be represented and it will get with the cost that provides the best value.

## 4. Results and Discussion

Table 2 summarized the three different cases that have been simulated, depending on the application of the optimization algorithm and the addition of a load, respectively.

Table 2. Test cases studied for the orthosis control system.

|  | Without Load | With Load |
|---|---|---|
| No optimization algorithm | 1. Comparison between a $K_{control}$ value of 0.1 and 0.3, respectively | 3. Comparison between a case without the optimization algorithm and with the application of the optimization algorithm |
| Optimization algorithm activated | 2. Comparison between a $K_{control}$ value of 0.1 and 0.3, respectively | |

The results that are presented in Figures 3 and 4 correspond to a case without the optimization algorithm described earlier and they were obtained with a $K_{control}$ gain value of 0.1 and 0.3, respectively. The first subplot shows the θ and $θ_{sp}$ forearm angle values and how the reference signals continue in a suitable way. The following two subplots illustrate the $u_{biceps}$ and $u_{triceps}$ signals. As previously mentioned, these muscles are antagonistic, so, when one of these muscles is activated, the other is deactivated and vice versa. Subsequently, the subplots with $F_{Biceps}$ and $F_{Triceps}$ are represented, which express the force value of each muscle when they are activated. Finally, the subplot with w represents the arm angular velocity (rad/s).

Analyzing the results, it was observed that an increase in the $K_{control}$ gain value leads to a decrease in the effort that is necessary to bear the weight of the arms. This behavior was expected, since we are assisting the arm by means of the gain, and therefore the force that is necessary to carry out the movements is reduced.

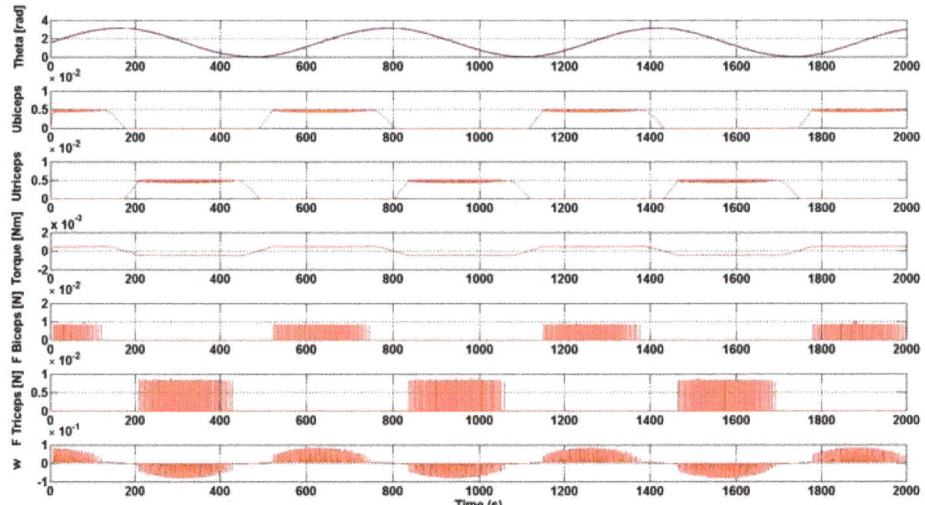

**Figure 3.** Results without the optimization algorithm and with a $K_{control}$ gain value of 0.1.

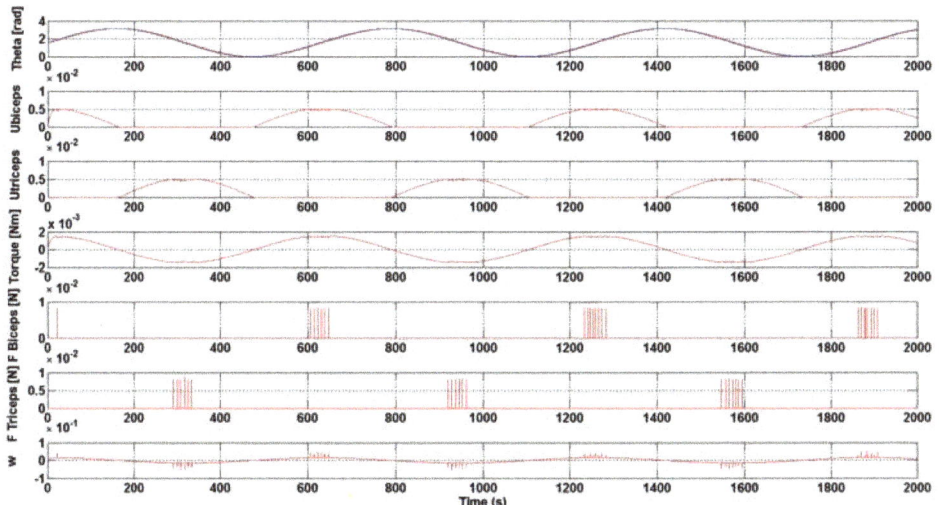

**Figure 4.** Results without the optimization algorithm and with a $K_{control}$ gain value of 0.3.

Currently, the DE algorithm has been executed to calculate the optimum gain value $K_{pbi}$ and $K_{ptri}$. In our case, 100 particles and 100 iterations have been used to carry out this calculation and the gain values have been limited between 0 and 50. The best results are achieved with the maximum $K_{control}$ gain value, according to the $F_{biceps}$ and $F_{triceps}$ values of Figures 3 and 4, that is, the force that is made by the muscle from the beginning to carry out the movements is lower. Subsequently, the previous data and the optimum gain values $K_{pbi}$ and $K_{ptri}$ are used.

Once analyzing the results that were obtained in Figures 5 and 6, it is clearly visible that the necessary development force of the muscles, $F_{Biceps}$ and $F_{Triceps}$, is very low, close to zero. It is also clear that the $u_{biceps}$ and $u_{triceps}$ signal values are getting lower with a $K_{control}$ gain increase. Taking into account the aforementioned, the optimum $K_{pbi}$ and $K_{ptri}$ gain values have great importance for the muscles to do less effort when it comes to making any movement.

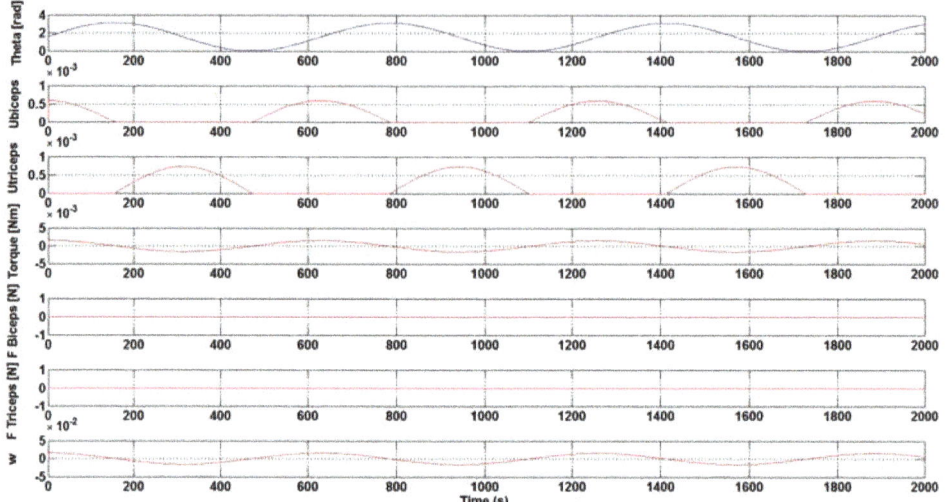

**Figure 5.** Results with the optimization algorithm and with a $K_{control}$ gain value of 0.1.

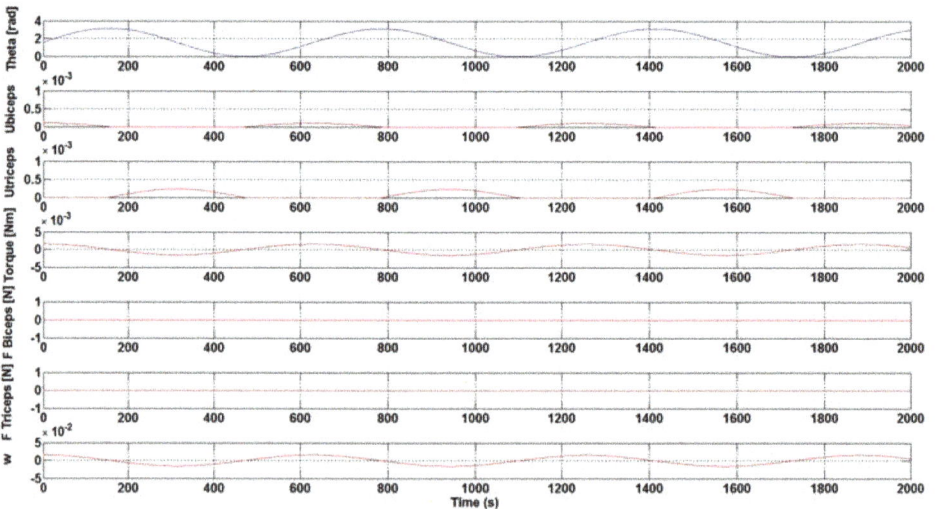

**Figure 6.** Results with the optimization algorithm and with a $K_{control}$ gain value of 0.3.

The next step has been to introduce a load to the control system of the orthosis in order to study the necessary force that is to be carried out by the biceps. As shown in Figures 7 and 8, a load of 1 N·m was introduced 50 seconds after the simulation starts. The results show the perturbation produced when the load is applied. Furthermore, the results show how, without the optimization algorithm, the required development force of the biceps muscle to overcome the load is practically double with respect to the case with the optimization algorithm. Specifically, a value of 0.1 N has been achieved for $F_{Biceps}$ without applying the optimization algorithm, as illustrated in Figure 7. However, when the optimization algorithm has been used a value of 0.05 N has been obtained, see Figure 8.

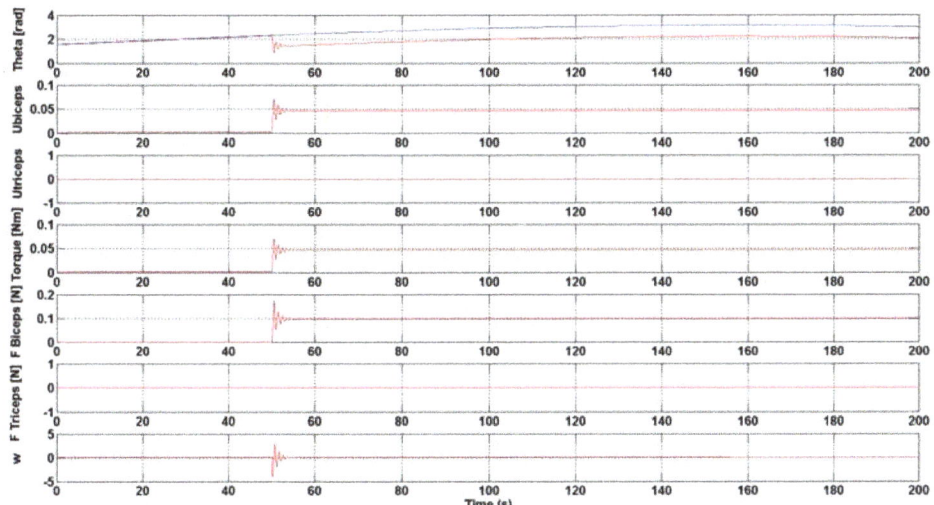

**Figure 7.** Results without the optimization algorithm and with the application of a load.

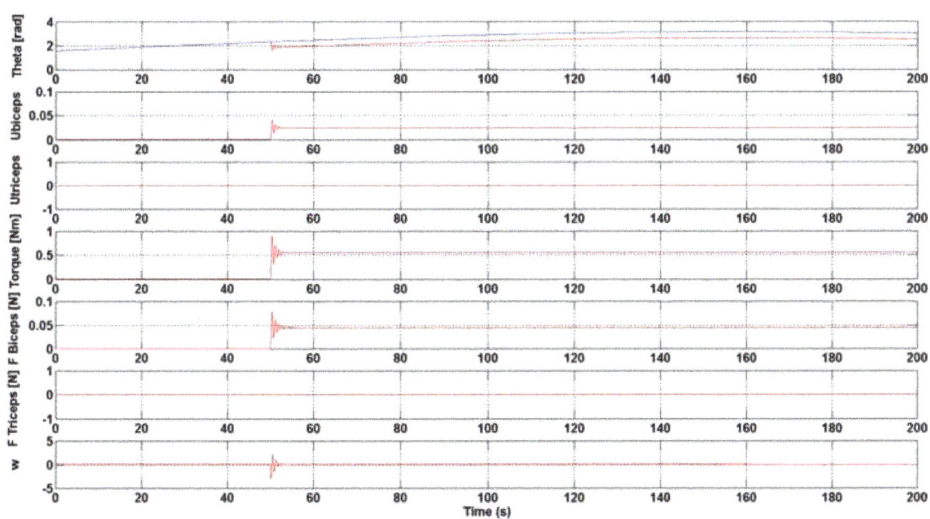

**Figure 8.** Results with the optimization algorithm and with the application of a load.

It was observed that an increase in the $K_{control}$ gain value led to a decrease in the effort that is necessary to bear the weight of the arms. With the execution of the DE algorithm to calculate the optimum gain values, $K_{pbi}$ and $K_{ptri}$, it was clearly visible that the necessary development force of the muscles is very small, being close to zero. Additionally, the $u_{biceps}$ and $u_{triceps}$ signal values were getting lower, with a gain increase highlighting the importance of the optimum gain values for the muscles in order to carry out less effort. The introduction of a load in the control system showed that the necessary development force of the biceps muscle to overcome the load is practically the double with respect to the case with the optimization algorithm without the optimization algorithm.

The major novelty of the current research is the implementation of an optimization algorithm based on differential evolution (DE) to improve the control and movement of the orthosis. This method, which is based on evolutionary principles, has been chosen due to its simplicity, small number of configuration parameters, and good performance. Sanz-Merodio et al. [28] combined the use of different gains and passive elements to reduce the energy consumption while applying a static optimization. Additionally, Belkadi et al. [29] proposed a PID adaptive controller based on modified particle swarm optimization algorithm, where the controller is initialized with the desired position and velocity instead of EMG signals, as made in this work. Experimental studies, as the one carried out with eight subjects by Song et al. [30], showed improvements in the upper limb functions with the use of a controlled robotic system with one degree-of-freedom. Recently, in the study of McCabe et al. [31], a clinical case of an upper limb orthosis can be found for use in assisting the user to perform the flexion/extension of the elbow demonstrating the feasibility of the implementation of an upper limb myoelectric orthosis. Stein et al. [32] developed a novel device, the Active Joint Brace (AJB), which combined an exoskeletal robotic brace with EMG control algorithms. They confirmed the feasibility of using an EMG-controlled powered exoskeletal orthosis for exercise training. The control and optimization algorithm that was carried out in the current research to assist the elbow movement could contribute to the improvement of devices as the one studied by Page et al. [33], which enables the bidirectional control at the elbow into flexion or extension. New wearable devices, as the one developed by Rong et al. [34], combining a neuromuscular electrical stimulation (NMES) and robot hybrid system, have also showed improvements in the coordination of agonist/antagonist pairs when performing sequencing limb movements.

In the previous study that was made by Suberbiola et al. [17], a similar EMG based orthosis control was proposed. However, this work did not explain how the control parameters can be obtained. Recently, Dao et al. [35] developed a modified computed torque controller to enhance the tracking performance of a robotic orthosis of the lower limb. Their control laws proposed have similar concepts, but with different objectives and approaches. In the current study, we follow the movements of the human being, whereas, in [35], they try to teach or show the correct forces and torques that must be applied to follow the desired trajectory.

## 5. Conclusions

Computational methods are tools quite useful and powerful for making a test of the muscle unit. These procedures are more comfortable and less expensive in comparison with the experimental method. In the present study, a numerical model of a muscle, arm, and orthosis has been developed and different cases have been tested.

The optimum gain values that were obtained with the DE optimization algorithm, $K_{pbi}$ and $K_{ptri}$, showed necessary development forces close to zero, which highlighted the importance of these values for the muscles to carry out less effort. Improvements were also observed with the introduction of a load of 0.1 N and the application of the DE optimization algorithm, where practically half of the development biceps force was necessary to overcome the load.

An important contribution of the present study has been the implementation of a numerical model of a muscle, arm, and orthosis. In this case, a singularity was created when the activation took a value of zero. In fact, the muscle was deactivated and the arm stayed without force when the activation was null. However, the singularity has been avoided, because the force of the serial element does not take immediately the zero value. Thus, even though the activation was zero, the muscle force does not immediately drop to zero. Additionally, an intelligent optimization system has been developed in order to calculate the value of two important non-linear parameters, $K_{pbi}$ and $K_{ptri}$, in the orthosis control law.

**Author Contributions:** I.A., E.Z. and U.F.-G. performed the new control algorithm and carried out the Formal Analysis. D.T.-F.-B. and A.S.-A. supervised the methodology and contributed to the preparation and creation of the manuscript.

**Funding:** The authors are grateful to the Government of the Basque Country and the University of the Basque Country UPV/EHU through the SAIOTEK (S-PE11UN112) and EHU12/26 research programs, respectively.

The Regional Development Agency of the Basque Country (SPRI) is gratefully acknowledged for economic support through the research project KK-2018/00109, ELKARTEK.

**Acknowledgments:** This research was partially funded by Fundation VITAL Fundazioa.

**Conflicts of Interest:** The authors declare no conflict of interest.

## Appendix A

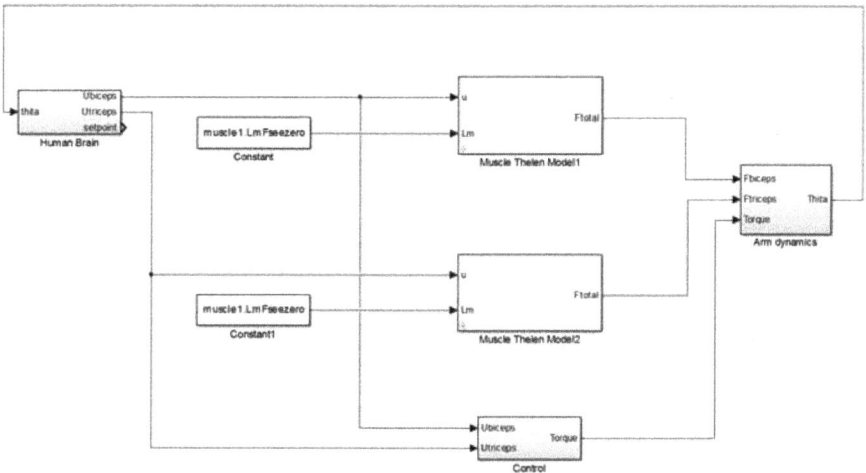

**Figure A1.** General Simulink diagram used in the orthosis control.

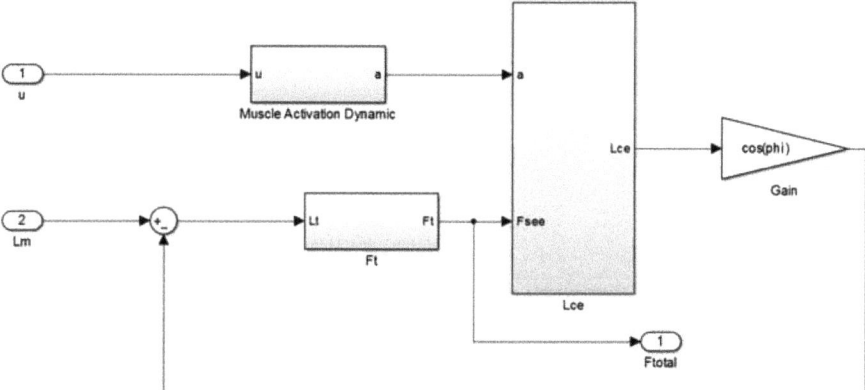

**Figure A2.** Implementation of Thelen Model.

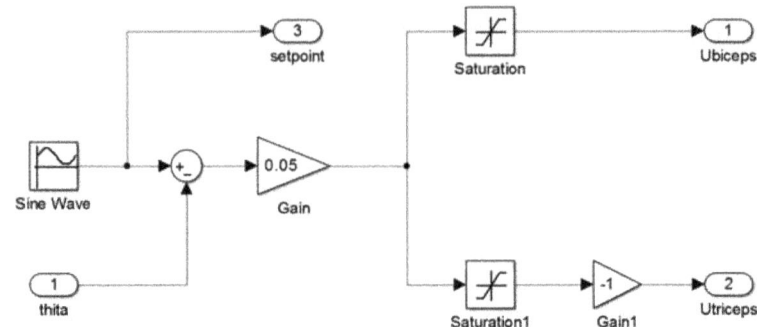

**Figure A3.** Human Brain's behavior model.

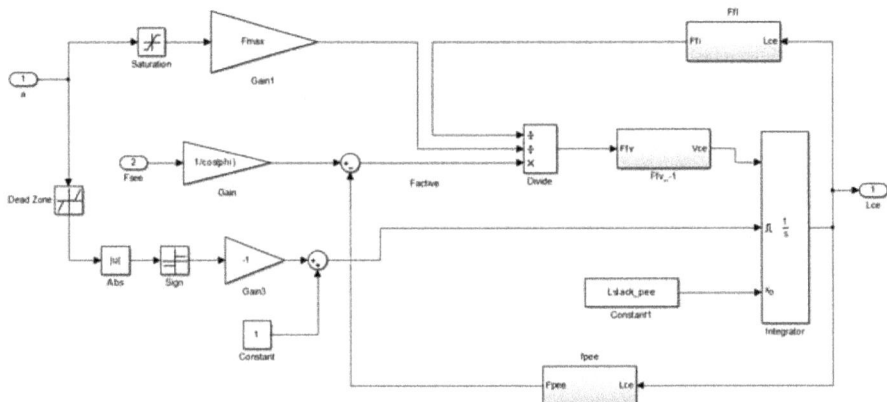

**Figure A4.** Block diagram representing the contractile element's length (Lce).

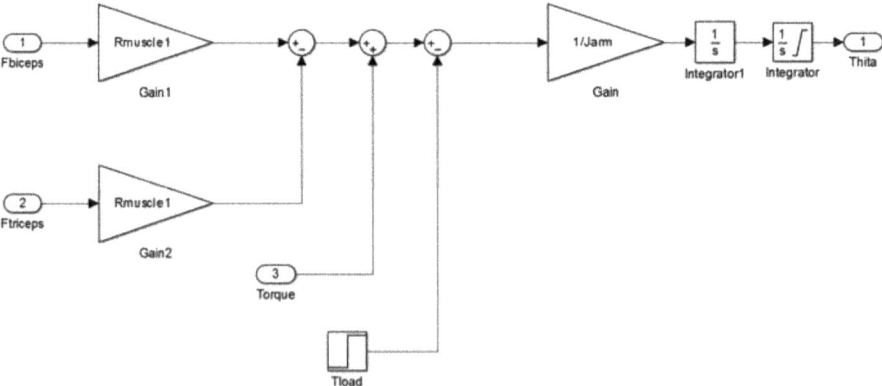

**Figure A5.** Arm dynamics model.

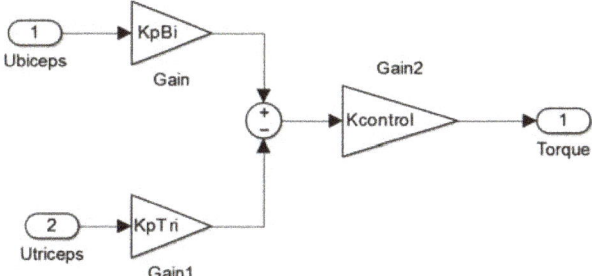

**Figure A6.** Control law proposal. The optimum $K_{pbi}$ and $K_{ptri}$ values are calculated through the optimization algorithm.

## References

1. Dollar, A.M.; Herr, H. Lower extremity exoskeletons and active orthoses: Challenges and state-of-the-art. *IEEE Trans. Robot.* **2008**, *24*, 144–158. [CrossRef]
2. Lo, H.S.; Xie, S.Q. Exoskeleton robots for upper-limb rehabilitation: State of the art and future prospects. *Med. Eng. Phys.* **2012**, *34*, 261–268. [CrossRef] [PubMed]
3. Kiguchi, K.; Hayashi, Y. An EMG-Based Control for an Upper-Limb Power-Assist Exoskeleton Robot. *IEEE Trans. Syst. Man Cybern. Part B Cybern.* **2012**, *42*, 1064–1071. [CrossRef] [PubMed]
4. Van der Heide, L.A.; van Ninhuijs, B.; Bergsma, A.; Gelderblom, G.J.; van der Pijl, D.J.; de Witte, L.P. An overview and categorization of dynamic arm supports for people with decreased arm function. *Prosthet. Orthot. Int.* **2014**, *38*, 287–302. [CrossRef] [PubMed]
5. ISO. *9999 Assistive Products for Persons with Disability—Classification and Terminology*; ISO: Geneva, Switzerland, 2011.
6. Tsagarakis, N.; Caldwell, D. Development and control of a 'soft-actuated' exoskeleton for use in physiotherapy and training. *Auton. Robot.* **2003**, *15*, 21–33. [CrossRef]
7. Kiguchi, K.; Tanaka, T.; Fukuda, T. Neuro-fuzzy control of a robotic exoskeleton with EMG signals. *IEEE Trans. Fuzzy Syst.* **2004**, *12*, 481–490. [CrossRef]
8. Pratt, J.; Krupp, B.; Morse, C.; Collins, S. The RoboKnee: An exoskeleton for enhancing strength and endurance during walking. In Proceedings of the 2004 IEEE International Conference on Robotics and Automation, New Orleans, LA, USA, 26 April–1 May 2004; pp. 2430–2435. [CrossRef]
9. Peternel, L.; Noda, T.; Petric, T.; Ude, A.; Morimoto, J.; Babic, J. Adaptive Control of Exoskeleton Robots for Periodic Assistive Behaviours Based on EMG Feedback Minimisation. *PLoS ONE* **2016**, *11*, e0148942. [CrossRef]
10. Cavallaro, E.E.; Rosen, J.; Perry, J.C.; Burns, S. Real-time myoprocessors for a neural controlled powered exoskeleton arm. *IEEE Trans. Biomed. Eng.* **2006**, *53*, 2387–2396. [CrossRef]
11. Tang, Z.; Zhang, K.; Sun, S.; Gao, Z.; Zhang, L.; Yang, Z. An Upper-Limb Power-Assist Exoskeleton Using Proportional Myoelectric Control. *Sensors* **2014**, *14*, 6677–6694. [CrossRef]
12. Williams, M.R. A pilot study into reaching performance after severe to moderate stroke using upper arm support. *PLoS ONE* **2018**, *13*, e0200787. [CrossRef]
13. Chadwick, E.K.; Blana, D.; Kirsch, R.F.; van den Bogert, A.J. Real-Time Simulation of Three-Dimensional Shoulder Girdle and Arm Dynamics. *IEEE Trans. Biomed. Eng.* **2014**, *61*, 1947–1956. [CrossRef] [PubMed]
14. Chadwick, E.K.; Blana, D.; Simeral, J.D.; Lambrecht, J.; Kim, S.P.; Cornwell, A.S.; Taylor, D.M.; Hochberg, L.R.; Donoghue, J.P.; Kirsch, R.F. Continuous neuronal ensemble control of simulated arm reaching by a human with tetraplegia. *J. Neural Eng.* **2011**, *8*, 034003. [CrossRef]
15. Van den Bogert, A.J.; Blana, D.; Heinrich, D. Implicit methods for efficient musculoskeletal simulation and optimal control. *Procedia IUTAM* **2011**, *2*, 297–316. [CrossRef]
16. Tsai, A.; Hsieh, T.; Luh, J.; Lin, T. A comparison of upper-limb motion pattern recognition using EMG signals during dynamic and isometric muscle contractions. *Biomed. Signal Process. Control* **2014**, *11*, 17–26. [CrossRef]

17. Suberbiola, A.; Zulueta, E.; Manuel Lopez-Guede, J.; Etxeberria-Agiriano, I.; Grana, M. Arm Orthosis/Prosthesis Movement Control Based on Surface EMG Signal Extraction. *Int. J. Neural Syst.* **2015**, *25*, 1550009. [CrossRef] [PubMed]
18. Desplenter, T.; Trejos, A.L. Evaluating Muscle Activation Models for Elbow Motion Estimation. *Sensors* **2018**, *18*, 1004. [CrossRef] [PubMed]
19. Hill, A. The heat of shortening and the dynamic constants of muscle. *Proc. R. Soc. Ser. B Biol. Sci.* **1938**, *126*, 136–195. [CrossRef]
20. Thelen, D. Adjustment of muscle mechanics model parameters to simulate dynamic contractions in older adults. *J. Biomech. Eng. Trans. ASME* **2003**, *125*, 70–77. [CrossRef]
21. He, J.; Levine, W.; Loeb, G. Feedback Gains for Correcting Small Perturbations to Standing Posture. *IEEE Trans. Autom. Control* **1991**, *36*, 322–332. [CrossRef]
22. Winters, J.; Stark, L. Analysis of Fundamental Human Movement Patterns through the Use of In-Depth Antagonistic Muscle Models. *IEEE Trans. Biomed. Eng.* **1985**, *32*, 826–839. [CrossRef]
23. Breteler, M.; Spoor, C.; Van der Helm, F. Measuring muscle and joint geometry parameters of a shoulder for modeling purposes. *J. Biomech.* **1999**, *32*, 1191–1197. [CrossRef]
24. Holzbaur, K.; Murray, W.; Delp, S. A model of the upper extremity for simulating musculoskeletal surgery and analyzing neuromuscular control. *Ann. Biomed. Eng.* **2005**, *33*, 829–840. [CrossRef] [PubMed]
25. McLean, S.; Su, A.; van den Bogert, A. Development, and validation of a 3-D model to predict knee joint loading-during, dynamic movement. *J. Biomech. Eng. Trans ASME* **2003**, *125*, 864–874. [CrossRef] [PubMed]
26. Herzog, W. Muscle. In *Biomechanics of the Musculoskeletal System*, 2nd ed.; Nigg, M., Herzog, W., Eds.; Wiley: New York, NY, USA, 1999; pp. 148–188.
27. Chadwick, E.K.; Blana, D.; van den Bogert, A.J.; Kirsch, R.F. A Real-Time, 3-D Musculoskeletal Model for Dynamic Simulation of Arm Movements. *IEEE Trans. Biomed. Eng.* **2009**, *56*, 941–948. [CrossRef]
28. Sanz-Merodio, D.; Cestari, M.; Carlos Arevalo, J.; Garcia, E. Control Motion Approach of a Lower Limb Orthosis to Reduce Energy Consumption Regular Paper. *Int. J. Adv. Robot. Syst.* **2012**, *9*, 232. [CrossRef]
29. Belkadi, A.; Oulhadj, H.; Touati, Y.; Khan, S.A.; Daachi, B. On the robust PID adaptive controller for exoskeletons: A particle swarm optimization based approach. *Appl. Soft Comput.* **2017**, *60*, 87–100. [CrossRef]
30. Song, R.; Tong, K.; Hu, X.; Li, L. Assistive control system using continuous myoelectric signal in robot-aided arm training for patients after stroke. *IEEE Trans. Neural Syst. Rehabil. Eng.* **2008**, *16*, 371–379. [CrossRef]
31. Mccabe, J.P.; Henniger, D.; Perkins, J.; Skelly, M.; Tatsuoka, C.; Pundik, S. Feasibility and clinical experience of implementing a myoelectric upper limb orthosis in the rehabilitation of chronic stroke patients: A clinical case series report. *PLoS ONE* **2019**, *14*, e0215311. [CrossRef] [PubMed]
32. Stein, J.; Narendran, K.; McBean, J.; Krebs, K.; Hughes, R. Electromyography-controlled exoskeletal upper-limb-powered orthosis for exercise training after stroke. *Am. J. Phys. Med. Rehabil.* **2007**, *86*, 255–261. [CrossRef]
33. Page, S.J.; Hill, V.; White, S. Portable upper extremity robotics is as efficacious as upper extremity rehabilitative therapy: A randomized controlled pilot trial. *Clin. Rehabil.* **2013**, *27*, 494–503. [CrossRef] [PubMed]
34. Rong, W.; Li, W.; Pang, M.; Hu, J.; Wei, X.; Yang, B.; Wai, H.; Zheng, X.; Hu, X. A Neuromuscular Electrical Stimulation (NMES) and robot hybrid system for multi-joint coordinated upper limb rehabilitation after stroke. *J. NeuroEng. Rehabil.* **2017**, *14*, 34. [CrossRef] [PubMed]
35. Dao, Q.; Yamamoto, S. Assist-as-Needed Control of a Robotic Orthosis Actuated by Pneumatic Artificial Muscle for Gait Rehabilitation. *Appl. Sci.* **2018**, *8*, 499. [CrossRef]

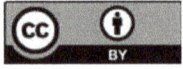

© 2019 by the authors. Licensee MDPI, Basel, Switzerland. This article is an open access article distributed under the terms and conditions of the Creative Commons Attribution (CC BY) license (http://creativecommons.org/licenses/by/4.0/).

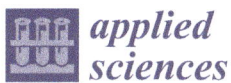 

Article

# Discrete-Time Fractional Order Integral Sliding Mode Control of an Antagonistic Actuator Driven by Pneumatic Artificial Muscles

Quy-Thinh Dao [1,2,*], Manh-Linh Nguyen [2] and Shin-ichiroh Yamamoto [3]

1. Graduate School of Engineering and Science, Shibaura Institute of Technology, Saitama 337-8570, Japan
2. Department of Industrial Automation, Hanoi University of Science and Technology, Ha Noi 11615, Vietnam; linh.nguyenmanh@hust.edu.vn
3. Department of Bioscience and Engineering, Shibaura Institute of Technology, Saitama 337-8570, Japan; yamashin@se.shibaura-it.ac.jp
* Correspondence: nb16505@shibaura-it.ac.jp or thinh.daoquy@hust.edu.vn; Tel.: +81-80-9307-9301

Received: 22 May 2019; Accepted: 18 June 2019; Published: 19 June 2019

**Abstract:** Recently, pneumatic artificial muscles (PAMs), a lightweight and high-compliant actuator, have been increasingly used in assistive rehabilitation robots. PAM-based applications must overcome two inherent drawbacks. The first is the nonlinearity due to the compressibility of the air, and the second is the hysteresis due to its geometric construction. Because of these drawbacks, it is difficult to construct not only an accurate mathematical model but also a high-performance control scheme. In this paper, the discrete-time fractional order integral sliding mode control approach is investigated to deal with the drawbacks of PAMs. First, a discrete-time second order plus dead time mathematical model is chosen to approximate the characteristics of PAMs in the antagonistic configuration. Then, the fractional order integral sliding mode control approach is employed together with a disturbance observer to improve the trajectory tracking performance. The effectiveness of the proposed control method is verified in multi-scenario experiments using a physical actuator.

**Keywords:** pneumatic artificial muscle; sliding mode control; fractional calculus; antagonistic actuator

## 1. Introduction

In recent years, high-compliant and low-cost pneumatic artificial muscles (PAMs) have been widely implemented in rehabilitation systems [1–4]. PAMs are shortened in the longitudinal direction and enlarged in the radial direction when being inflated, and they will turn back to their initial form when being completely deflated. PAMs act similar to the human muscle, e.g., the longer muscles produce bigger force and vice versa. Furthermore, these pneumatic muscles are also inherently compliant, which makes them suitable for applying in human-robotic systems. In comparison with the motorized actuators, PAMs are lightweight and have a high power-to-weight ratio. In addition to the aforementioned advantages, the PAM-based applications also have inherent drawbacks, such as very high nonlinearity and uncertainty, and slow response in force generation. These drawbacks make it difficult to model and control PAMs.

Using a nonlinear mathematical model to describe the nonlinear characteristic of the PAMs is the most common choice of researchers. In 2003, D. B. Reynolds et al. introduced a three-elements model of PAM, which consists of a contractile (force-generating) element, spring element, and damping element in parallel [5]. Using this type of model, K. Xing et al. developed the sliding mode control (SMC) based on a nonlinear disturbance observer to improve the tracking performance of a single PAM-mass system [6]. A boundary layer augmented SMC and its modified versions have also been developed for both antagonistic configuration of PAMs and robot orthosis actuated by PAMs [4,7–12].

However, the procedure to identify this model's parameters remains complicated with at least two separate experiments: one experiment for determining spring ($K$) and contractile ($F$) coefficients and another experiment for estimating damping ($B$) coefficient. Each experiment must be carried out in three steps [6]. Besides, the parameters of the damping ($B$) coefficient must be obtained by measuring the load's acceleration, which is very sensitive to external noise. For this reason, it is difficult to obtain the model's parameters with high accuracy.

To deal with hysteresis of PAMs, many hysteresis models have been proposed recently, e.g., Maxwell-slip model [13], Prandtl–Ishlinskii model [14], and Preisach model [15]. In these reports, the dynamic characteristic of PAMs was described by an equivalent pressure/length hysteresis model. The obtained models were used in the feedforward term of the cascade position control scheme for hysteresis compensation. The inner loop of the controllers was designed to regulate the inside pressure of the muscles. The outer loops were designed to deal with the nonlinearity of the PAMs characteristic. Both of the loops use PID-based control strategy. Consequently, some authors continued to develop the modified hysteresis model for both single PAM-mass system and PAMs in antagonistic configuration [16,17]. However, they mainly focused on modelling of PAMs. Only the trajectory-tracking experiments with low frequency, e.g., up to 0.2 Hz, were conducted in literature. Furthermore, enhanced PID control methods, which were most widely used in these studies, could not deal with hysteresis of PAMs.

Another common way to identify the model of PAM-based actuator is the grey-box experiment method [18–21]. In 2015, to deal with uncertain nonlinearity of PAMs, Dang Xuan Ba et al. introduced a grey-box experimental model, which consisted of uncertain, unknown, and nonlinear terms. Based on the built-in model, the authors employed a sliding mode control strategy [18] and an integrated intelligent nonlinear control approach [19] for the tracking purpose. The control performance was significantly improved, and the system could track the 10° amplitude sinusoidal signal with 1.5 Hz frequency. The grey-box method was also reported by Robinson et al. in 2016 [20] and by L. Cveticanin et al. in 2018 [21]. The relationships angle/torque and force/pressure were thoroughly investigated in the wide range of pressure. However, only the mathematical model was considered and verified in [20]. The low rate of desired trajectories was tracked in [21].

The mechanism-based model [22,23] is another method in which the behaviour of PAMs was described based on their physical properties: length, diameter, and volume of PAMs, etc. However, as most of nonlinear models mentioned above, these types of models also require a complex procedure to derive the model parameters.

To obtain the model of PAMs in a more simple way with a good enough accuracy, the linear mathematical model has recently been applied to approximate the characteristic of PAMs [24–28]. In these studies, the uncertain nonlinearity of PAM was considered as the system disturbance and solved by extended state observer (ESO) together with an active disturbance rejection controller (ADRC). The control performance is considerably improved with 0.5 Hz of sinusoidal reference signal frequency.

In this research, a discrete-time fractional order integral sliding mode control (DFISMC) is employed to improve tracking performance of an antagonistic actuator driven by PAMs. First, a linear discrete-time second order plus dead time (SOPDT) model is chosen to describe the nonlinear dynamic behaviour of the antagonistic actuator. In this approximation, a nonlinear term in characteristics of PAM is considered as a disturbance. Then, the DFISMC is designed based on the fractional order integral (FOI) calculus and a disturbance observer (DSO) for the trajectory tracking purpose. Finally, the effectiveness of the proposed control technique is confirmed through multi-scenario experiments. The proposed method shows many advantages in both mathematical model and control technique. The linear discrete-time SOPDT can approximate the behaviour of antagonistic actuator at a good accuracy. Besides, the identification procedure is also simplified. By employing the FOI function together with a DSO, the DFISMC controller is able to reduce the "chattering" problem in sliding mode control systems. In addition, the proposed is designed in a discrete-time domain, therefore, it can be easily implemented by any digital control system.

## 2. System Description

*2.1. Experiment Platform*

A typical configuration of antagonistic configuration of PAMs is shown in Figure 1a, and the proposed experiment platform is demonstrated in Figure 1b. The experimental system consisted of two PAMs which had 1.0 inches of diameter and 22 inches of length. The PAMs were fabricated at our local institute. The pressure inside each PAMs was regulated by two proportional electric control valves series ITV 2030-212S-X26 from SMC company. One potentiometer CP-20H from Midori Precision (Japan) was used to measure the actuator's angle. All the control systems were implemented by using computer-based controller NI cDAQ-9178 from National Instrument (USA). The real-time controller collected the data from the potentiometer via analogue input module and sends the control signal to the electric control valve via analogue output modules. The developed control algorithm was implemented and compiled by LabView software before downloading it to the hardware controller.

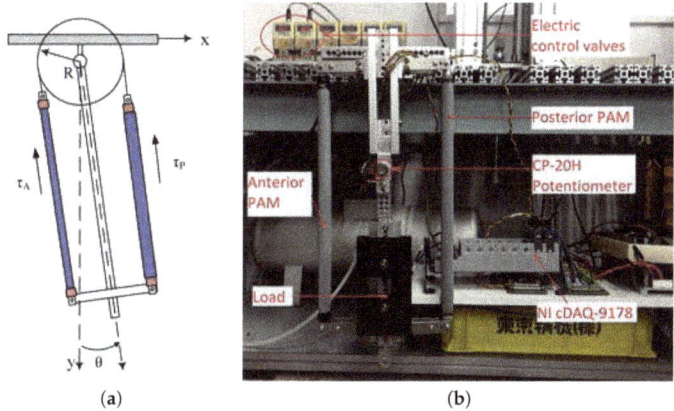

**Figure 1.** (a) Typical antagonistic configuration of two pneumatic artificial muscles (PAMs) and (b) experiment platform of an antagonistic actuator powered by PAMs.

*2.2. System Modeling*

Based on the geometry of the typical antagonistic configuration, which is illustrated in Figure 1a, the length of each PAMs can be obtained from the measured joint angle, as in the following equations:

$$y_A = y_{AN} + R\theta \tag{1a}$$

$$y_P = y_{PN} - R\theta, \tag{1b}$$

where $y_{AN}$ and $y_{PN}$ are the nominal length of the anterior and posterior PAMs when the joint angle $\theta = 0$, and $R$ is the rotation radius of the actuator. Because two similar PAMs are used in the system, we can consider that $y_{AN} = y_{PN} = y_N$. Following that, the relationship between contraction of PAMs and the measured angle can be expressed as

$$\varepsilon_A = \frac{y_0 - y_A}{y_0} \times 100\% = \frac{y_0 - (y_N + R\theta)}{y_0} \times 100\% \tag{2a}$$

$$\varepsilon_P = \frac{y_0 - y_P}{y_0} \times 100\% = \frac{y_0 - (y_N - R\theta)}{y_0} \times 100\% \tag{2b}$$

where $y_0$ is the length of PAMs in the complete deflation state. In (2), $y_0$ and $y_N$ are fixed by the deflation and nominal lengths of PAMs. Therefore, the contraction of PAMs can be expressed as the function of the measured joint angle $\theta$. As a result, the dynamic behaviour of an antagonistic muscle can be described by a single input single output (SISO) system, in which the input is the difference pressure of two PAMs ($\Delta P$), and the output is the measured angle $\theta$. The input pressure inside the anterior and posterior PAMs can be expressed as

$$P_P = P_0 + \Delta P \tag{3a}$$
$$P_A = P_0 - \Delta P, \tag{3b}$$

where $P_0$ is the nominal pressure which determines the initial position of antagonistic actuator. The nominal pressure can be chosen so that the joint has the desired compliance for a specific application. It was fixed, so $\Delta P$ was chosen as a control variable of trajectory-tracking controller. All the system parameters $P_0$, $y_0$, and $y_N$ are provided as in Table 1. In this research, the following discrete-time SISO system was chosen to describe the model of antagonistic actuator:

$$y_{k+1} = -\sum_{i=1}^{n} a_i y_{k-i+1} + \sum_{j=1}^{m} b_j u_{k-j-d+1} + p_k, \tag{4}$$

where $u_k$ represents the control pressure $\Delta P$, $y_k$ is the joint angle, $d$ is a positive integer representing the dead time of the system (as a number of the sampling time), $p_k$ is the unknown disturbance of the system, $a_i$ and $b_j$ are the model parameters with $b_1 \neq 0$, $n$ and $m$ are integers which satisfy $n \leq m$. The model parameters of the system are obtained by the identification experiment. To verify the mathematical model of PAM, the following experiment procedure was carried out.

Step 1: The initial position of the actuator was set at $0°$ by supplying nominal pressure $P_0$ to each PAMs of the actuator.

Step 2: The actuator angle can be changed by sending different types of control signal to the electrical control valves. Three types of control signals were used in this experiment:

- Step response: the control signal was a step wave with the final values 0.2, 0.4, 0.5, and 0.8 MPa.
- Sinusoidal signal: The control signal is the 0.2 MPa amplitude sinusoidal signal, where frequency varies from 0.2 to 1.0 Hz.
- A sine wave signal with time-varying amplitude and frequency, as in the following equation:

$$u(t) = A\sin(2\pi f t) + 0.8A\sin(2\pi 0.2 f t) + 0.5A\sin(2\pi 1.5 f t) + 0.2A\sin(2\pi 3 f t), \tag{5}$$

where $A = 0.05$ MPa and $f = 0.5$ Hz are the basis amplitude and frequency of the control signal, respectively.

All the data, including control signals and measured angles of actuator, were recorded with sampling time $T_s = 5$ ms for further analysis.

Step 3: The discrete-time SOPDT, in which $m = n = 2$, was chosen as the mathematical model of the actuator with good accuracy. The precise values of the model's parameters are estimated by using the MATLAB software and provided in Table 2.

Table 1. Initial parameters of pneumatic artificial muscles (PAMs).

| Parameters | $y_0$ [in] | $y_N$ [in] | $P_0$ [MPa] |
|---|---|---|---|
| Values | 22 | 15 | 0.2 |

**Table 2.** Identified parameters of the antagonistic actuator.

| Model Parameters | $a_1$ | $a_2$ | $b_1$ | $b_2$ | $d$ |
|---|---|---|---|---|---|
| Value (Mean ± SD) | −1.9139 ± 0.0182 | 0.9164 ± 0.0180 | 0.0472 ± 0.0064 | 0.0460 ± 0.0061 | 22 ± 3 |

Figure 2 shows identification results: (a) the control inputs are step of 0.4 MPa, (b) 0.5 Hz sine wave signal, and (c) time-varying amplitude and frequency sinusoidal signal. The discrete-time SOPDT mathematical model depicts a good approximation of nonlinear behaviour of the antagonistic actuator. The maximum error of the estimated angle (dash red line) from the measured one (blue line) was less than 5.0°, and the root mean square error did not exceed 2.5°. The mean values and standard deviations (SD) of the model parameters obtained by different types of control signals are provided in Table 2. As seen in Table 2, the standard deviations of the model parameters were much smaller than their mean values. Therefore, we can conclude that the model parameters obtained by different methods have similar values. As a result, we can use any aforementioned method for the identification purpose. The model parameters, which were identified by time-varying amplitude and frequency, are chosen to design the controller in Section 3 of this paper.

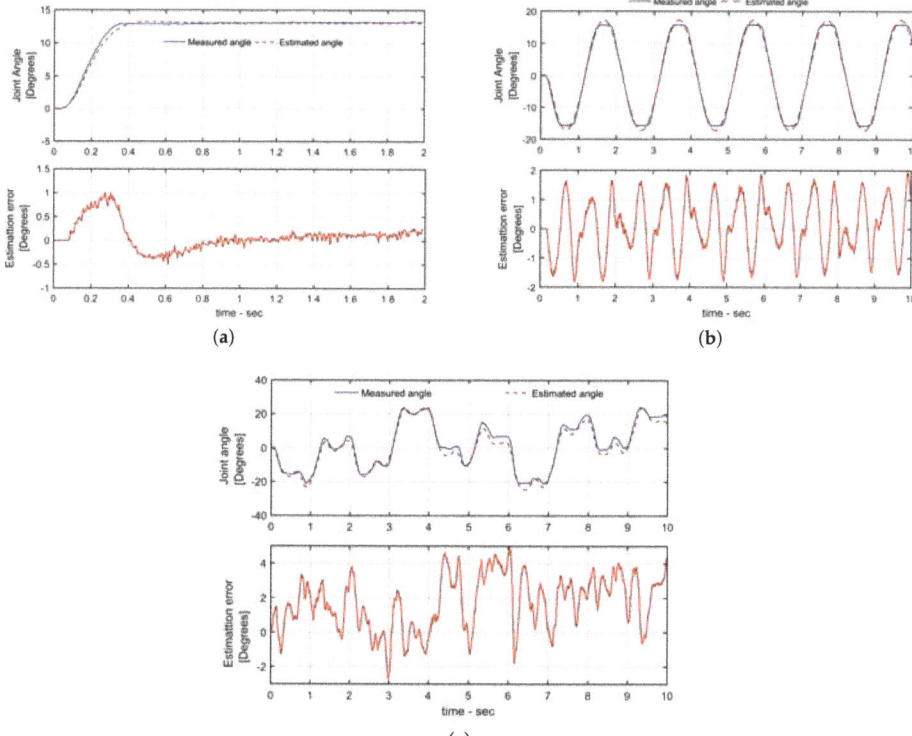

**Figure 2.** Identification results of the antagonistic actuator: (**a**) the step input of 0.4 MPa, (**b**) the 0.5 Hz sinusoidal signal, and (**c**) the time-varying amplitude and frequency control input. Upper sub-figures show measured (blue line) and estimated (dash red line) show value of the actuator angle. Lower sub-figures show the estimation error of the mathematical model.

## 3. Control Design

Recently, SMC has been employed for designing the controller for PAMs or systems powered by PAMs [4,6–11]. SMC is able to provide highly accurate tracking performance with a bounded error; however, "chattering" problem is a big challenge that SMC must overcome. SMC is a suitable control approach for PAM-based systems to deal with their uncertain, nonlinear and time varying characteristics. In this research, we addressed a DFISMC to improve the tracking performance of the antagonistic actuator powered by PAMs. The fractional order integral is implemented together with disturbance observer to deal with the "chattering" problem. Figure 3 illustrates the block diagram of the proposed control system.

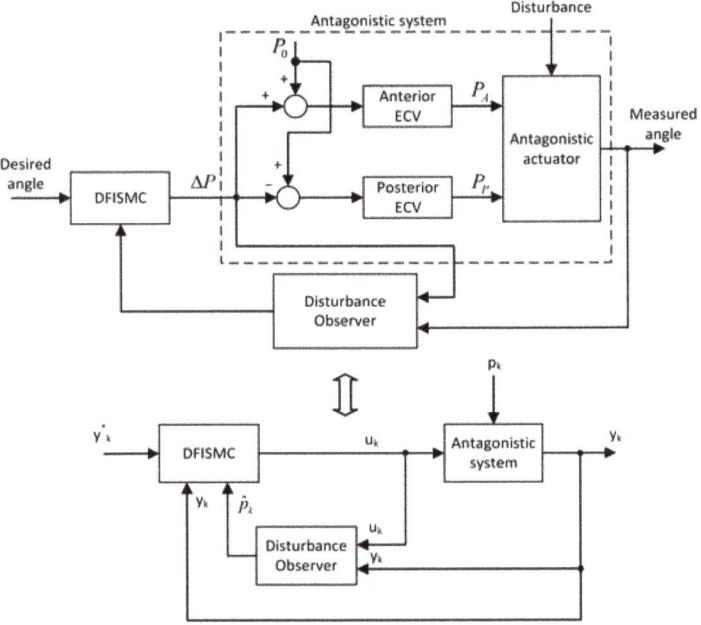

**Figure 3.** Block diagram of the discrete-time fractional integral sliding mode control.

We consider the following fractional integral sliding surface:

$$S_k = e_k + {}^\alpha \Xi_{e,k} \tag{6}$$

where $e_k = y_k^* - y_k$ is the tracking error with the desired trajectory $y_k^*$, and ${}^\alpha \Xi_{e,k}$ is the integral of the tracking error with fractional order $\alpha$ and integral gain $K_I$. ${}^\alpha \Xi_{e,k}$ can be calculated as follows:

$${}^\alpha \Xi_{e,k} = {}^\alpha \Xi_{e,k-1} + K_I \left( \sum_{j=2}^{N} \Omega_j \tilde{e}_{k-N+j} + \Omega_1 e_{k-N+1} \right) \tag{7}$$

and ${}^\alpha \Xi_{e,0} = \omega_N e_0$ at the initial state. Please refer to Appendix A for details about fractional integral approximation. We also obtain

$${}^\alpha \Xi_{e,k+1} = {}^\alpha \Xi_{e,k} + K_I \left( \sum_{j=2}^{N} \Omega_j \tilde{e}_{k-N+j+1} + \Omega_1 \tilde{e}_{k-N+2} \right) \tag{8}$$

From (6)–(8), we can obtain

$$S_{k+1} = e_{k+1} + S_k - e_k + K_I \left( \sum_{j=2}^{N} \Omega_j \tilde{e}_{k-N+j+1} + \Omega_1 \tilde{e}_{k-N+2} \right) \quad (9)$$

Therefore,

$$S_{k+1} - S_k = (1 + K_I \Omega_N) e_{k+1} - (1 + K_I \tilde{\Omega}_N) e_k - K_I \sum_{j=2}^{N-1} \tilde{\Omega}_j e_{k-N+j} \quad (10)$$

where $e_k + 1$ is one-step-ahead tracking error, which can be computed from the SISO model of the actuator in (4) as

$$e_{k+1} = y^*_{k+1} + \sum_{i=1}^{n} a_i y_{k-i+1} - \sum_{j=1}^{m} b_j u_{k-d-j+1} - p_k, \quad (11)$$

where $y^*_{k+1}$ is one step ahead of the desired trajectory, which is considered to be known when apply the model to a specific application. In (4), disturbance $p_k$ is unknown and needs to be estimated. In this study, one-step delayed technique was used to estimate $p_k$. This technique is based on the following assumptions:

**Assumption 1.** *Sampling time $T_s$ was sufficiently small and system disturbance $p_k$ is bounded, so the difference between two consecutive time samples is also bounded, i.e.,*

$$p_k - p_{k-1} = O(T_s) \quad (12)$$
$$p_k - 2p_{k-1} + p_{k-2} = O(T_s^2), \quad (13)$$

where $O(T_s)$ is the thickness boundary layer. It means there always exist constants $A$ and $B$, $\forall k > 0$, such that

$$|p_k - p_{k-1}| \leq A T_s \quad (14)$$
$$|p_k - 2p_{k-1} + p_{k-2}| \leq B T_s^2. \quad (15)$$

The aforementioned assumption was based on the Taylor expansion described in Appendix B. Estimation $\hat{p}_k$ of disturbance $p_k$ can be computed based on (4) as

$$\hat{p}_k = 2p_{k-1} - p_{k-2}, \quad (16)$$

where

$$p_{k-1} = y_k + \sum_{i=1}^{n} a_i y_{k-i} - \sum_{j=1}^{m} b_j u_{k-j}. \quad (17)$$

Hence, the error of estimation $\tilde{p}_k$ is

$$\tilde{p}_k = p_k - \hat{p}_k$$
$$= p_k - 2p_{k-1} + p_{k-2} = O(T_s^2). \quad (18)$$

Finally, the one-step-ahead tracking error (11) can be expressed by

$$e_{k+1} = y_{d,k+1} + \sum_{i=1}^{n} a_i y_{k-i+1} - \sum_{j=1}^{m} b_j u_{k-j+1} - \hat{p}_k - \tilde{p}_k. \quad (19)$$

When substituting $e_{k+1}$ in (11) and $p_k = \hat{p}_k + \tilde{p}_k$ into (10), we can obtain

$$S_{k+1} - S_k = -(1 + K_I \tilde{\Omega}_N)e_k - K_I \sum_{j=2}^{N-1} \tilde{\Omega}_j e_{k-N+j}$$

$$+ (1 + K_I \Omega_N) \left( y_{k+1}^* + \sum_{i=1}^{n} a_i y_{k-i+1} - \sum_{j=1}^{m} b_j u_{k-j-d+1} - \hat{p}_k - \tilde{p}_k \right) \quad (20)$$

Disturbance estimation error $\tilde{p}_k$ is unknown in practice; however, it is very small and bounded by assumption 1. Control signal $u_k$ can be obtained by solving the reaching law $S_{k+1} = 0$ with the absence of $\tilde{p}_k$ as follows:

$$u_k = b_1^{-1} \left( y_{k+1}^* + \sum_{i=1}^{n} a_i y_{k-i+1} - \sum_{j=1}^{m} b_j u_{k-j-d+1} - \hat{p}_k \right) - \frac{(1 + K_I \tilde{\Omega}_N)e_k - K_I \sum_{j=2}^{N-1} \tilde{\Omega}_j e_{k-N+j}}{b_1 (1 + K_I \Omega_N)}. \quad (21)$$

Adjusting integral gain $K_I$ and fractional order integral $\alpha$ may improve performance of the control system.

## 4. Experimental Evaluation

### 4.1. Experimental Procedure

To verify the effectiveness of the proposed control method, multiple-scenario experiment with different desired trajectories was carried out. In the first scenario of the trajectory-tracking experiment, sinusoidal signals with amplitude 20° and 0.2, 0.5, 0.8, and 1 Hz frequency were given as desired trajectories. To evaluate the applicability of the proposed control method for a rehabilitation robot, a human-like pattern signal was employed as a desired trajectory in the second scenario of the experiment. The modified knee gait data profile in textbook [29], where the maximum flexion angle is set at 28°, was used to verify the control performance. In both experimental scenarios, the system was tested under two load conditions: no load and load m = 2.5 kg.

In all experimental scenarios, the sampling time of the discrete-time control system was $T_s$ = 5 ms. All the data were recorded for ten cycles from the start time of the experiment. The data were processed by MATLAB software version R2016b. The proposed controller is also compared with the conventional discrete-time sliding mode control (DSMC) method in terms of tracking performance. The parameters of both controllers after being well-tuned are provided in Table 3.

Table 3. Parameters of the discrete-time fractional order integral sliding mode control (DFISMC) and conventional DSMC controller.

| Parameters | FDISMC | | DSMC | |
|---|---|---|---|---|
| | $\alpha$ | $K_I$ | $\lambda$ | $K_{sw}$ |
| Values | 0.8 | 0.01 | 0.1 | $1.5 \times 10^{-3}$ |

### 4.2. Experiment Result

To quantitatively evaluate the tracking performance, the maximum tracking error (MTE) and root mean square tracking error (RMSTE) are computed. The RMSTE is calculated as follows:

$$RMSTE = \sqrt{\frac{1}{N} \sum_{k=0}^{N} e_k^2}, \quad (22)$$

where $N$ is the total number of data samples, and $e_k$ is the tracking error under $k^{th}$ sample.

Figure 4 depicts the experimental results when the actuator tracks the sine wave signals without load. The sinusoidal signal had an amplitude of 20° and frequency from 0.2 Hz to 1 Hz. In the second scenario, a knee gait pattern was given as a desired trajectory. The proposed controller was evaluated with two different gait cycle (GC) times: 2.5 s and 4 s. The experimental results of this scenario are shown in Figure 5. In both Figures 4 and 5, the upper sub-figure of each image includes the desired trajectory (back line), measured angle controlled by DFISMC (dash-blue line), and measured angle controller by conventional DSMC (dash-dot red line). The lower part of each figure shows the tracking errors of both proposed controller and DSMC controller. In comparison with the traditional DSMC, the DFISMC was able to provide a better performance in both transient and steady states. As demonstrated in Figure 6, in all scenarios of the experiment, both MTE and RMSTE of the proposed control approach are smaller than the ones of the conventional DSMC control method. For example, when tracking the 1.0 Hz frequency sinusoidal signal, the RMSTEs of the DFISMC and DSMC controllers are 1.63° and 1.43°, respectively. It means that DFISMC is able to provide a better performance than the conventional DSMC controller. In particular, as seen in the error graphs in Figures 4 and 5, the finite amplitude oscillation of the tracking error in DFISMC is much smaller than in DSMC. It can be concluded that the inherent "chattering" phenomenon of SMC control is reduced with DFISMC. The numerical values of the experimental results in all scenarios are given in Table 4.

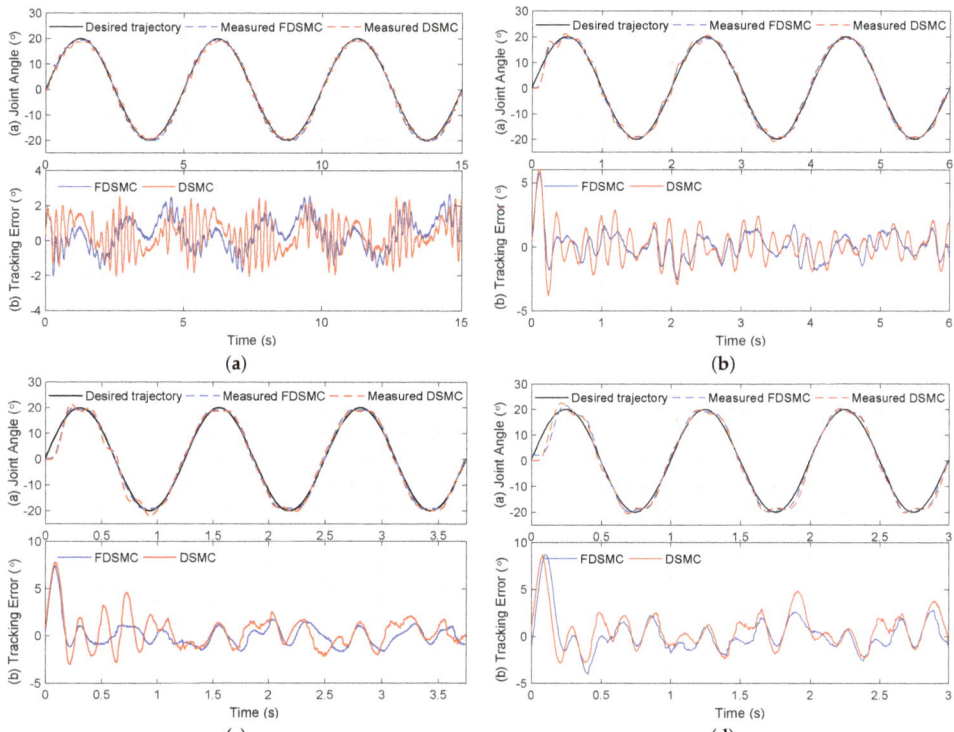

**Figure 4.** Experiment results without a load for tracking a sinusoidal trajectory: (**a**) 0.2 Hz, (**b**) 0.5 Hz, (**c**) 0.8 Hz, and (**d**) 1.0 Hz of signal frequency.

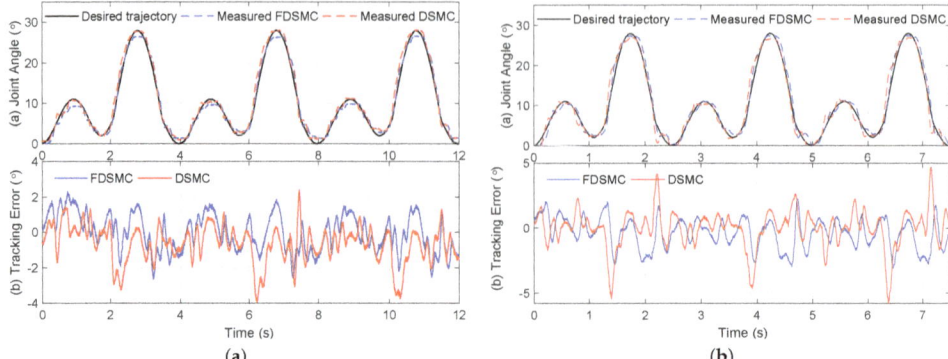

**Figure 5.** Experiment results of the proposed controller and conventional DSMC controller when tracking the human-gait pattern signal: (**a**) 4 s and (**b**) 2.5 s of gait cycle time. The experiment was carried out without a load.

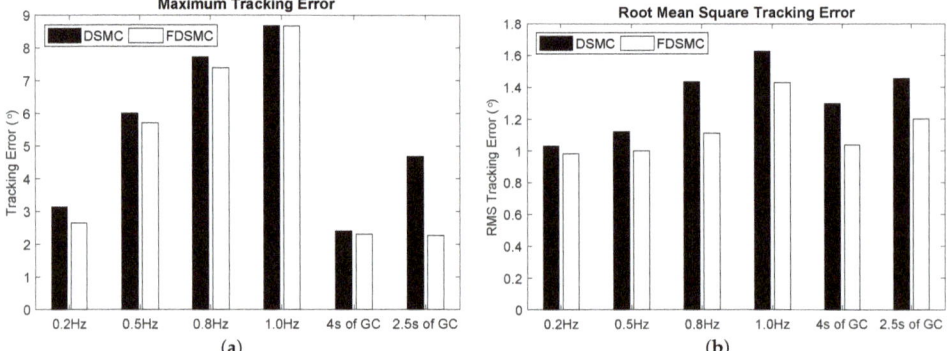

**Figure 6.** Maximum tracking error (MTE) and root mean square tracking error (RMSTE) of the proposed controller and conventional DSMC controller with 0.2 Hz, 0.5 Hz, 0.8 Hz, and 1.0 Hz of the desired signal frequency in case of no load.

**Table 4.** Maximum tracking error (MTE) and root mean square tracking error (RMSTE) of the proposed control method and conventional DSMC control method in case of no load.

| Signal Frequency | MTE (°) | | RMSTE (°) | |
|---|---|---|---|---|
| | DSMC | DFISMC | DSMC | DFISMC |
| 0.2 Hz | 3.14 | 2.65 | 1.03 | 0.98 |
| 0.5 Hz | 6.01 | 5.71 | 1.12 | 1.00 |
| 0.8 Hz | 7.73 | 7.39 | 1.43 | 1.11 |
| 1.0 Hz | 8.68 | 8.67 | 1.63 | 1.43 |
| 4 s of GC | 2.40 | 2.31 | 1.30 | 1.04 |
| 2.5 s of GC | 4.69 | 2.26 | 1.45 | 1.20 |

Figures 7 and 8 show the control performances of the system when tracking the sinusoidal signals and human-gait pattern with a load of 2.5 kg, respectively. When the antagonistic actuator carries a load m = 2.5 kg, the difference between the DFISMC and DSMC is not significant in terms of MTE. However, the RMSTE of the DFISMC controller are smaller than the ones of the DSMC controller, as shown in Figure 9. For example, when tracking the 2.5 s human-gait trajectory, the RMSTEs of the DFISMC and DSMC controllers are 1.22° and 1.68°, respectively. Furthermore, the same conclusion about the *"chattering"* phenomenon is drawn out in this experiment scenario. All numerical values of MTE and RMSTE in this experimental scenario are also shown in Table 5.

From experimental results with multiple scenarios, we can conclude that the DFISMC controller obtains a better tracking performance than the conventional DSMC controller which used the "sign" function of tracking errors. In addition, the implemented disturbance observer and fractional order integral term are able to deal with the finite-amplitude oscillation of sliding mode implementations. As a result, the "chattering" phenomenon is reduced.

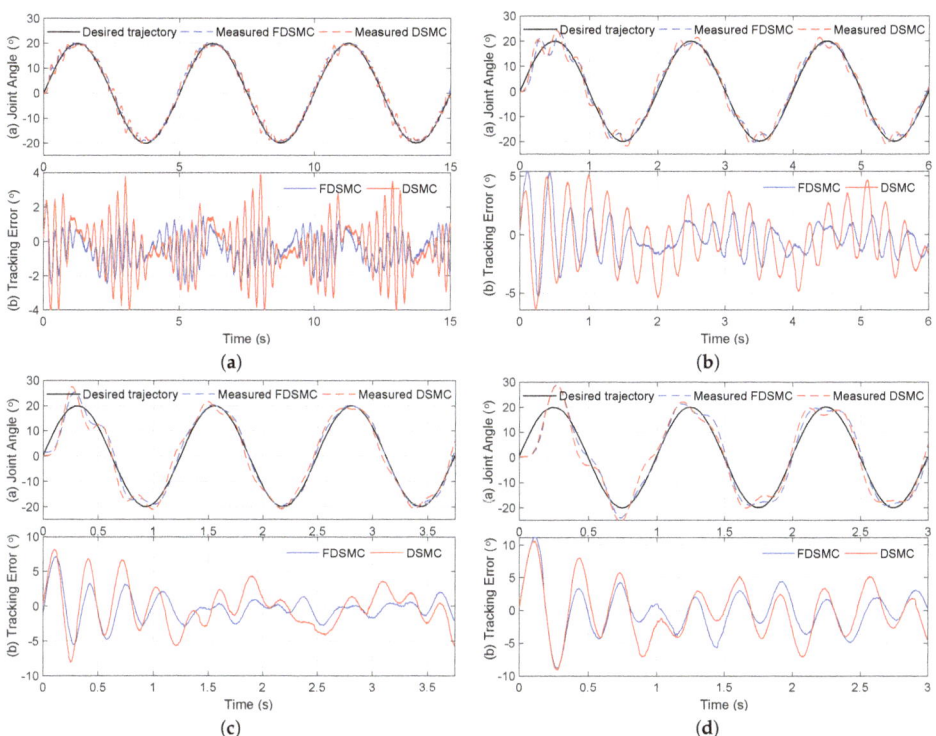

**Figure 7.** Experiment results with 2.5 kg of load for tracking a sinusoidal trajectory: (**a**) 0.2 Hz, (**b**) 0.5 Hz, (**c**) 0.8 Hz, and (**d**) 1.0 Hz of the desired signal frequency.

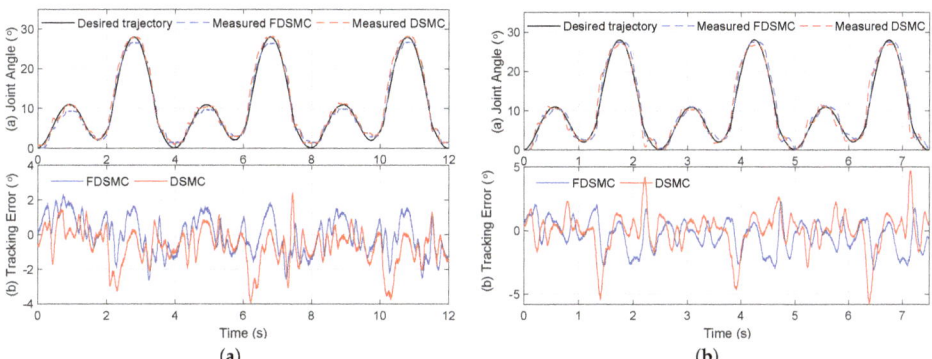

**Figure 8.** Experiment results for the proposed controller and conventional DSMC controller when tracking the human-gait pattern signal with a load m = 2.5 kg: (**a**) 4 s and (**b**) 2.5 s of gait cycle time.

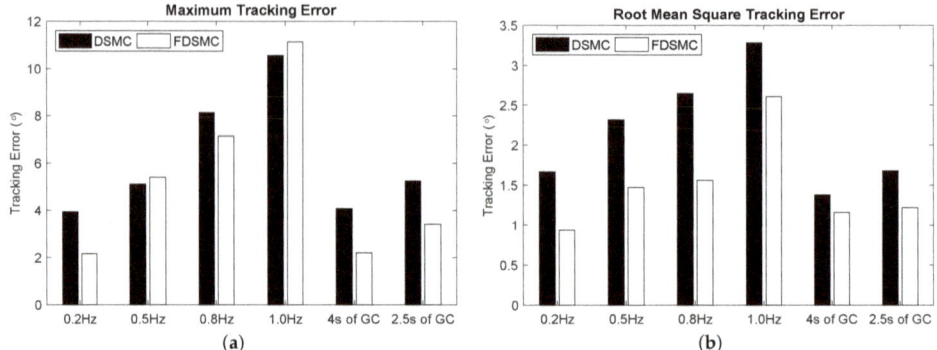

**Figure 9.** MTE and RMSTE of the proposed controller and conventional DSMC controller with 0.2 Hz, 0.5 Hz, 0.8 Hz, and 1.0 Hz of the desired signal frequency and load m = 2.5 kg.

**Table 5.** MTE and RMSTE of the proposed control method and conventional DSMC control method with load m = 2.5 kg.

| Signal Frequency | MTE (°) | | RMSTE (°) | |
| --- | --- | --- | --- | --- |
| | DSMC | DFISMC | DSMC | DFISMC |
| 0.2 Hz | 3.94 | 2.16 | 1.67 | 0.93 |
| 0.5 Hz | 5.11 | 5.39 | 2.31 | 1.47 |
| 0.8 Hz | 8.13 | 7.13 | 2.64 | 1.56 |
| 1.0 Hz | 10.56 | 11.13 | 3.28 | 2.61 |
| 4 s of GC | 4.09 | 2.20 | 1.38 | 1.16 |
| 2.5 s of GC | 5.23 | 3.41 | 1.68 | 1.22 |

## 5. Discussion and Conclusions

This paper proposed an advanced SMC control strategy for PAMs in antagonistic configuration. First, the discrete-time SOPDT is chosen to describe the dynamic behaviour of the antagonistic actuator. The chosen model demonstrated a good approximation of nonlinear characteristics of the actuator: the root mean square errors between estimated and measured values are less than 2.5°. Based on the built-in model, an DFISMC controller, which employed a fractional order integral of tracking error together with a disturbance observer, was proposed for the tracking purpose. The implemented approximation of FOI and DO was able to reduce the *"chattering"* phenomenon, which often occurs in SMC implementations. The reduction of the *"chattering"* phenomenon is very important for applications of the PAMs in rehabilitation robot field. Finally, multi-scenario experiments were carried out to compare the tracking performances between the DFISMC and the conventional DSMC.

In comparison with the three-elements model [5], hysteresis model [13–15], and mechanism-based model [22,23], the identification procedure of the proposed method is simplified. Besides, this procedure does not need to measure the load's acceleration, which is very sensitive to noise. Experiments show that, in comparison with DSMC, the DFISMC was able to significantly enhance the tracking performance of 20° amplitude sinusoidal signals with frequency up to 1.0 Hz. In particular, when the actuator drove a load of m = 2.5 kg, the RMSTEs of DFISMC were about two times less than those of conventional DSMC in most of the desired trajectory frequencies. For example, with a frequency of 0.2 Hz, the RMSTEs are 0.93° and 1.67° for DFISMC and DSMC, respectively. The proposed controller achieves a performance comparable to the experimental results with similar configuration and desired trajectory in [23,24]. In [23], when tracking a 0.4 Hz frequency and 5° sinusoidal signal, the residual error amplitude is 0.5 ° equivalent to 10%. When tracking a 0.5 Hz frequency and 20° amplitude sinusoidal signal, the RMSTE of the DFISMC is 1.47 °, equivalent to

7.35% of amplitude. This result was better than the one in [24], in which a sinusoidal signal with 40° amplitude and frequency 0.25 Hz is used as a desired trajectory. The experiments also show that the proposed controller can track a human-gait pattern with the MTE of less than 6°. This result is in accordance with the commercial gait training system LOKOMAT [30], in which the MTE is 15°. It is shown that the built-in model and proposed controller can be applied in robot gait training system. Furthermore, the proposed DFISMC is designed in discrete-time domain, so that it is convenient for implementing in any digital industrial controller, e.g., the NI instrument in this research.

In summary, this paper presents the control of an antagonistic actuator powered by PAMs. The dynamic behaviour of the antagonistic actuator is described by a discrete-time SOPDT model, which requires a simpler identification procedure. The DFISMC controller based on a DSO and the approximated FOI is used to improve the tracking performance. The implementation of DSO and FOI also helps the system reduce the "chattering" phenomenon. The experimental results illustrate the applicability of the proposed model and controller to a robotic gait training system with a human-gait pattern trackable ability. Future work will involve the impedance control of the antagonistic actuator to increase applicability of PAMs in the field of rehabilitation. The impedance of the actuator can be regulated by manipulating the nominal pressure $P_0$ of two PAMs. To integrate the impedance controller into the system, the relationship between the actuator compliance and nominal pressure $P_0$ would be considered and modelled in future work.

**Author Contributions:** Q.-T.D. conceived the methodology and designed the experiment; he also performed the experiment. Q.-T.D. and M.-L.N. analyzed data and wrote the paper. S.-i.Y. led the research efforts and preparation of this paper.

**Conflicts of Interest:** The authors declare no conflict of interest.

## Abbreviations

The following abbreviations are used in this manuscript:

| | |
|---|---|
| PAM | Pneumatic artificial muscle |
| PID | Proportional integral derivative |
| SOPDT | Second order plus dead time |
| SISO | Single input single output |
| SMC | Sliding mode control |
| DSMC | Discrete-time sliding mode control |
| DFISMC | Discrete-time fractional order integral sliding mode control |
| MTE | Maximum tracking error |
| RMSTE | Root mean square tracking error |
| ESO | Extended state observer |
| ADRC | Active disturbance rejection controller |
| DSO | Disturbance observe |
| SD | Standard deviation |
| FOI | Fractional order integral |
| GC | Gait cycle |

## Appendix A. Fractional Integral Approximation

Fractional-order calculus is a generalization of the integration and differentiation from integer to non-integer order. This appendix introduces only definitions which are widely used in the area of control systems. First, gamma function $\Gamma(z)$, which is the extension of the factorial for non-integer number $z$, is introduced as

$$\Gamma(z) = \int_0^\infty e^{-t} t^{z-1} dt \tag{A1}$$

The most important property of the gamma function is

$$z\Gamma(z) = \Gamma(z+1) \tag{A2}$$

Then, the definition of integral of order $\alpha \in \mathbb{R}$ is presented. In continuous-time domain, the most often used one is the *Riemann-Liouville* definition:

$$^{\alpha}\Xi e(t) = \frac{1}{\Gamma(\alpha)} \int_0^t (t-\tau)^{(\alpha-1)} e(\tau) d\tau \tag{A3}$$

At this time, the FOI is not supported in any programming language. For this reason, its numerical approximation is required to implement the FOI in any real-time control system. In a digital control system with sampling time $T_s$, interval $(0, t)$ can be approximated by $k = \frac{t}{T_s}$ sub-intervals. Therefore,

$$^{\alpha}\Xi e(t) = \frac{1}{\Gamma(\alpha)} \sum_{j=1}^{k} \int_{jT_s}^{(j+1)T_s} (t-\tau)^{(\alpha-1)} e(\tau) d\tau \tag{A4}$$

Consider that $T_s$ is small enough, so that $e$ is constant in each sub-interval. Therefore,

$$^{\alpha}\Xi e(t) \approx ^{\alpha}\Xi_{e,k} = \frac{1}{\Gamma(\alpha)} \sum_{j=1}^{k} \int_{jT_s}^{(j+1)T_s} (t-\tau)^{(\alpha-1)} e(\tau) d\tau \tag{A5}$$

Following that,

$$^{\alpha}\Xi_{e,k} = \sum_{j=1}^{k} [(k-j+1)^{\alpha} - (k-j)^{\alpha}] \frac{T_s^{\alpha}}{\alpha \Gamma(\alpha)} e_{j+1} \tag{A6}$$

From (A2) and (A6), we have

$$^{\alpha}\Xi_{e,k} = \sum_{j=1}^{k} w_j e_j \tag{A7}$$

with the weighting factor $w_j$ as follows:

$$w_j = [(k-j+1)^{\alpha} - (k-j)^{\alpha}] \frac{T_s^{\alpha}}{\alpha \Gamma(\alpha)}. \tag{A8}$$

Because of the infinite data in (A7), the approximation of FIO cannot be directly implemented in any digital system. In this research, the recursive approximation of FIO in [31] is employed. Denote $\Xi_{e,k-1}$ as FIO of the tracking error in the last step, and it can be computed as

$$^{\alpha}\Xi_{e,k-1} = \sum_{j=2}^{k} w_j e_{j-1} \tag{A9}$$

From (A7) and (A9), we have

$$^{\alpha}\Xi_{e,k} = ^{\alpha}\Xi_{e,k-1} + \sum_{j=2}^{k} w_j \tilde{e}_{j-1} + w_1 e_1 \tag{A10}$$

where $\tilde{e}_j = e_j - e_{j-1}$. We apply the short memory principle to (A10) and we can consider two cases:
(a). If $k < N$, where $N = \left[\frac{L}{T_s}\right]$ is the number of considered data samples, then

$$^{\alpha}\Xi_{e,k} = ^{\alpha}\Xi_{e,k-1} + \sum_{j=N-k+2}^{N} \Omega_j \tilde{e}_{N-k+j} + \Omega_{N-k+1} e_1 \tag{A11}$$

(b). If $k \geq N$,
$$^\alpha \Xi_{e,k} = ^\alpha \Xi_{e,k-1} + \sum_{j=2}^{N} \Omega_j \tilde{e}_{k-N+j} + \Omega_1 e_{k-N+1} \quad (A12)$$

where
$$\Omega_j = [(N-j+1)^\alpha - (N-j)^\alpha] \frac{T_s^\alpha}{\Gamma(\alpha+1)} \quad (A13)$$

The FIO is approximated by Equations (A11) and (A12), which can be easily implemented in any digital control system.

## Appendix B. Proof of Assumption 1

Assumption 1 is based on the Taylor expansion and can be explained as follows. For a very small constant $T_s$, we have

$$p(t-T_s) = p(t) - \frac{dp(t)}{dt} T_s + \sum_{i=2}^{\infty} (-1)^i \frac{d^{(i)} p(t)}{dt^i} \frac{T_s^i}{i!} \quad (A14)$$

Then, it can be derived from (A14) that

$$p(t) - p(t-Ts) = \frac{dp(t)}{dt} T_s - \sum_{i=2}^{\infty} (-1)^i \frac{d^{(i)} p(t)}{dt^i} \frac{T_s^i}{i!}$$
$$\approx \frac{dp(t)}{dt} T_s + O(T_s^2) \quad (A15)$$

Assume that signal $p(t)$ is smooth, and its differential is bounded. Then there exists a constant $A$ such that

$$|p(t) - p(t-T_s)| \leq A T_s + O(T_s^2) \quad (A16)$$

which means
$$P(t) - p(t-T_s) = O(T_s) \quad (A17)$$

and (12) holds.

Now, ignore the small term $O(T_s^2)$ and differentiate both sides of (A15). This gives us

$$\frac{dp(t)}{dt} - \frac{dp(t-T_s)}{dt} \approx \frac{d^2 p(t)}{dt^2} T_s \quad (A18)$$

By using (A15) on the left side of (A18),

$$p(t) - 2p(t-T_s) + p(t-2T_s) \approx \frac{d^2 p(t)}{dt^2} T_s^2 \quad (A19)$$

Again, assume that the second order differential of $p(t)$ is bounded by a constant $B$, then it leads to

$$|p(t) - 2p(t-T_s) + p(t-2T_s)| \leq B T_s^2 \quad (A20)$$

which means that (15) holds.

**References**

1. Banala, S.K.; Kim, S.H.; Agrawal, S.K.; Scholz, J.P. Robot Assisted Gait Training with Active Leg Exoskeleton (ALEX). *IEEE Trans. Neural Syst. Rehabil. Eng.* **2009**, *17*, 2–8. [CrossRef]
2. Beyl, P.; Knaepen, K.; Duerinck, S.; Van Damme, M.; Vanderborght, B.; Meeusen, R.; Lefeber, D. Safe and Compliant Guidance by a Powered Knee Exoskeleton for Robot-Assisted Rehabilitation of Gait. *Adv. Robot.* **2011**, *25*, 513–535. [CrossRef]
3. Dao, Q.-T.; Yamamoto, S.-I. Assist-as-Needed Control of a Robotic Orthosis Actuated by Pneumatic Artificial Muscle for Gait Rehabilitation. *Appl. Sci.* **2018**, *8*, 499. [CrossRef]
4. Hussain, S.; Xie, S.Q.; Jamwal, P.K. Control of a robotic orthosis for gait rehabilitation. *Robot. Auton. Syst.* **2013**, *61*, 911–919. [CrossRef]
5. Reynolds, D.B.; Repperger, D.W.; Phillips, C.A.; Bandry, G. Dynamic characteristics of pneumatic muscle. *Ann. Biomed. Eng.* **2003**, *31*, 310–317. [CrossRef]
6. Xing, K.; Huang, J.; Wang, Y.; Wu, J.; Xu, Q.; He, J. Tracking control of pneumatic artificial muscle actuators based on sliding mode and non-linear disturbance observer. *IET Control Theory Appl.* **2010**, *4*, 2058–2070. [CrossRef]
7. Lilly, J.H.; Quesada, P.M. A two-input sliding-mode controller for a planar arm actuated by four pneumatic muscle groups. *IEEE Trans. Neural Syst. Rehabil. Eng.* **2004**, *12*, 349–359. [CrossRef]
8. Lilly, J.H.; Yang, L. Sliding mode tracking for pneumatic muscle actuators in opposing pair configuration. *IEEE Trans. Control Syst. Technol.* **2005**, *13*, 550–558. [CrossRef]
9. Choi, T.Y.; Lee, J.J. Control of Manipulator Using Pneumatic Muscles for Enhanced Safety. *IEEE Trans. Ind. Electron.* **2010**, *57*, 2815–2825. [CrossRef]
10. Choi, T.Y.; Choi, B.S.; Seo, K.H. Position and Compliance Control of a Pneumatic Muscle Actuated Manipulator for Enhanced Safety. *IEEE Trans. Control Syst. Technol.* **2011**, *19*, 832–842. [CrossRef]
11. Hussain, S.; Xie, S.Q.; Jamwal, P.K. Adaptive Impedance Control of a Robotic Orthosis for Gait Rehabilitation. *IEEE Trans. Cybern.* **2013**, *43*, 1025–1034. [CrossRef]
12. Merola, A.; Colacino, D.; Cosentino, C.; Amato, F. Model-based tracking control design, implementation of embedded digital controller and testing of a biomechatronic device for robotic rehabilitation. *Mechatronics* **2018**, *52*, 70–77. [CrossRef]
13. Minh, T.V.; Tjahjowidodo, T.; Ramon, H.; Brussel, H.V. Cascade position control of a single pneumatic artificial muscle-mass system with hysteresis compensation. *Mechatronics* **2010**, *20*, 402–414. [CrossRef]
14. Xie, S.; Mei, J.; Liu, H.; Wang, Y. Hysteresis modeling and trajectory tracking control of the pneumatic muscle actuator using modified Prandtl—Ishlinskii model. *Mech. Mach. Theory* **2018**, *120*, 213–224. [CrossRef]
15. Kosaki, T.; Minesaki, A.; Sano, M. Adaptive Hysteresis Compensation with a Dynamic Hysteresis Model for Control of a Pneumatic Muscle Actuator. *J. Environ. Eng.* **2012**, *7*, 53–65. [CrossRef]
16. Vo-Minh, T.; Tjahjowidodo, T.; Ramon, H.; Brussel, H.V. A new approach to modeling hysteresis in a pneumatic artificial muscle using the Maxwell-slip model. *IEEE/ASME Trans. Mechatron.* **2011**, *16*, 177–186. [CrossRef]
17. Minh, T.V.; Kamers, B.; Ramon, H.; Brussel, H.V. Modeling and control of a pneumatic artificial muscle manipulator joint- part i: Modeling of a pneumatic artificial muscle manipulator joint with accounting for creep effect. *Mechatronics* **2012**, *22*, 923–933. [CrossRef]
18. Ba, D.X.; Ahn, K.K. Indirect sliding mode control based on gray-box identification method for pneumatic artificial muscle. *Mechatronics* **2015**, *32*, 1–11. [CrossRef]
19. Ba, D.X.; Dinh, T.Q.; Ahn, K.K. An integrated intelligent nonlinear control method for a pneumatic artificial muscle. *IEEE/ASME Trans. Mechatron.* **2016**, *21*, 1835–1845. [CrossRef]
20. Robinson, R.M.; Kothera, C.S.; Sanner, R.M.; Wereley, N.M. Nonlinear Control of Robotic Manipulators Driven by Pneumatic Artificial Muscles. *IEEE/ASME Trans. Mechatron.* **2016**, *21*, 55–68. [CrossRef]
21. Cveticanin, L.; Zukovic, M.; Biro, I.; Sarosi, J. Mathematical investigation of the stability condition and steady state position of a pneumatic artificial muscle—Mass system. *Mech. Mach. Theory* **2018**, *125*, 196–206. [CrossRef]
22. Yang, H.; Yu, Y.; Zhang, J. Angle tracking of a pneumatic muscle actuator mechanism under varying load conditions. *Control Eng. Pract.* **2017**, *61*, 1–10. [CrossRef]

23. Zhao, L.; Li, Q.; Liu, B.; Cheng, H. Trajectory Tracking Control of a One Degree of Freedom Manipulator Based on a Switched Sliding Mode Controller with a Novel Extended State Observer Framework. *IEEE Trans. Syst. Man Cybern. Syst.* **2019**, *49*, 1110–1118. [CrossRef]
24. Andrikopoulos, G.; Nikolakopoulos, G.; Manesis, S. Advanced Nonlinear PID-Based Antagonistic Control for Pneumatic Muscle Actuators. *IEEE Trans. Ind. Electron.* **2014**, *61*, 6926–6937. [CrossRef]
25. Yuan, Y.; Yu, Y.; Guo, L. Nonlinear Active Disturbance Rejection Control for the Pneumatic Muscle Actuators With Discrete-Time Measurements. *IEEE Trans. Ind. Electron.* **2019**, *66*, 2044–2053. [CrossRef]
26. Zhao, L.; Liu, X.; Wang, T. Trajectory tracking control for double-joint manipulator systems driven by pneumatic artificial muscles based on a nonlinear extended state observer. *Mech. Syst. Signal Process.* **2019**, *122*, 307–320. [CrossRef]
27. Zhao, L.; Cheng, H.; Xia, Y.; Liu, B. Angle Tracking Adaptive Backstepping Control for a Mechanism of Pneumatic Muscle Actuators via an AESO. *IEEE Trans. Ind. Electron.* **2019**, *66*, 4566–4576. [CrossRef]
28. Yuan, Y.; Yu, Y.; Wang, Z.; Guo, L. A Sampled-Data Approach to Nonlinear ESO-Based Active Disturbance Rejection Control for Pneumatic Muscle Actuator Systems with Actuator Saturations. *IEEE Trans. Ind. Electron.* **2019**, *66*, 4608–4617. [CrossRef]
29. Winter, D.A. *Biomechanics and Motor Control of Human Movement*, 3rd ed.; University of Waterloo Press: Waterloo, ON, Canada, 1990.
30. Riener, R.; Lunenburger, L.; Jezernik, S.; Anderschitz, M.; Colombo, G.; Dietz, V. Patient-cooperative strategies for robot-aided treadmill training: First experimental results. *IEEE Trans. Neural Syst. Rehabil. Eng.* **2005**, *13*, 380–394. [CrossRef]
31. Nguyen, M.L.; Chen, X. Discrete-Time Fractional Order Integral Sliding Mode Control for Piezoelectric Actuators with Improved Performance Based on Fuzzy Tuning. In Proceedings of the 2018 13th World Congress on Intelligent Control and Automation (WCICA), Changsha, China, 4–8 July 2018; pp. 554–559. [CrossRef]

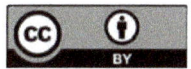

© 2019 by the authors. Licensee MDPI, Basel, Switzerland. This article is an open access article distributed under the terms and conditions of the Creative Commons Attribution (CC BY) license (http://creativecommons.org/licenses/by/4.0/).

MDPI  
St. Alban-Anlage 66  
4052 Basel  
Switzerland  
Tel. +41 61 683 77 34  
Fax +41 61 302 89 18  
www.mdpi.com

*Applied Sciences* Editorial Office  
E-mail: applsci@mdpi.com  
www.mdpi.com/journal/applsci

www.ingramcontent.com/pod-product-compliance
Lightning Source LLC
LaVergne TN
LVHW071935080526
838202LV00064B/6611